I0044660

Recent Progress in Arthritis Treatment

Recent Progress in Arthritis Treatment

Edited by Grenn Jones

hayle
medical

New York

Hayle Medical,
750 Third Avenue, 9th Floor,
New York, NY 10017, USA

Visit us on the World Wide Web at:
www.haylemedical.com

© Hayle Medical, 2019

This book contains information obtained from authentic and highly regarded sources. Copyright for all individual chapters remain with the respective authors as indicated. All chapters are published with permission under the Creative Commons Attribution License or equivalent. A wide variety of references are listed. Permission and sources are indicated; for detailed attributions, please refer to the permissions page and list of contributors. Reasonable efforts have been made to publish reliable data and information, but the authors, editors and publisher cannot assume any responsibility for the validity of all materials or the consequences of their use.

ISBN: 978-1-63241-716-9

Trademark Notice: Registered trademark of products or corporate names are used only for explanation and identification without intent to infringe.

Cataloging-in-Publication Data

Recent progress in arthritis treatment / edited by Grenn Jones.
    p. cm.
Includes bibliographical references and index.
ISBN 978-1-63241-716-9
1. Arthritis--Treatment. 2. Arthritis. 3. Joints--Diseases. I. Jones, Grenn.
RC933 .R43 2019
616.722--dc23

Contents

Preface

I am honored to present to you this unique book which encompasses the most up-to-date data in the field. I was extremely pleased to get this opportunity of editing the work of experts from across the globe. I have also written papers in this field and researched the various aspects revolving around the progress of the discipline. I have tried to unify my knowledge along with that of stalwarts from every corner of the world, to produce a text which not only benefits the readers but also facilitates the growth of the field.

Arthritis refers to the disorders which affect the joints. Some common symptoms include joint pain, redness, stiffness, swelling and reduced motion of affected joints. Osteoarthritis and rheumatoid arthritis are two of the most common types of arthritis. Usually arthritis is a common disorder in old age. Blood tests and X-rays are two primary ways to assess joint problems associated with arthritis. Treatment methods of arthritis generally involve alternate application of heat and ice on the affected area, weight loss, joint resting, joint replacement and pulsed electromagnetic field therapy. This book contains some path-breaking studies in the treatment of arthritis. It aims to shed light on some of the unexplored aspects of arthritis and the recent researches in this field. For all readers who are interested in arthritis, the case studies included in this book will serve as an excellent guide to develop a comprehensive understanding.

Finally, I would like to thank all the contributing authors for their valuable time and contributions. This book would not have been possible without their efforts. I would also like to thank my friends and family for their constant support.

Editor

Cortical bone loss is an early feature of nonradiographic axial spondyloarthritis

Anna Neumann[1†], Judith Haschka[1,2†], Arnd Kleyer[1], Louis Schuster[1], Matthias Englbrecht[1], Andreas Berlin[1], Camille P. Figueiredo[1,3], David Simon[1], Christian Muschitz[2], Roland Kocijan[2], Heinrich Resch[2], Jürgen Rech[1] and Georg Schett[1*]

Abstract

Background: In the present study, we investigated bone geometry, microstructure, and volumetric bone mineral density (vBMD) in a cohort of patients with nonradiographic axial spondyloarthritis (nr-axSpA) in order to define the early bone changes occurring in axial spondyloarthritis (axSpA) and to define potential factors for deterioration of bone microstructure.

Methods: Patients with axSpA ($n = 107$) and healthy control subjects ($n = 50$) of similar age and sex were assessed for geometric, volumetric, and microstructural parameters of bone using high-resolution peripheral quantitative computed tomography (HR-pQCT) at the radius. Additionally, demographic and disease-specific characteristics of patients with axSpA were recorded.

Results: Patients with nr-axSpA and control subjects were comparable in age, sex, and body mass index. Geometric and microstructural analysis by HR-pQCT revealed a significantly reduced cortical area ($p = 0.022$) and cortical thickness ($p = 0.006$) in patients with nr-axSpA compared with control subjects. Total and cortical vBMD were significantly reduced in patients with nr-axSpA ($p = 0.042$ and $p = 0.007$, respectively), whereas there was no difference in trabecular vBMD. Patients with a short disease duration (< 2 years; $n = 46$) also showed significant reduction of cortical thickness and cortical area compared with control subjects. Patients with disease duration > 2 years ($n = 55$) additionally developed a decrease of cortical and total vBMD. Multiple regression models identified male sex to be associated with lower cortical vBMD and female sex to be associated with lower trabecular vBMD.

Conclusions: Bone microstructure in patients with nr-axSpA is characterized primarily by deterioration of cortical bone. Cortical bone loss starts early and is evident within the first 2 years of the disease.

Keywords: Spondyloarthritis, Bone loss, Computed tomography

Background

Spondyloarthritis (SpA) comprises a group of diseases with shared genetic and pathophysiologic backgrounds affecting the axial and peripheral skeleton. Axial disease comprises nonradiographic axial SpA (nr-axSpA) and ankylosing spondylitis (AS). Axial inflammation leads to local bone formation with progressive ankylosis of sacroiliac joints as well as syndesmophyte formation. Nonetheless, systemic bone loss and increased vertebral and nonvertebral fracture risk have been described in AS [1].

Authors of a recent review of the literature on bone mass in AS reported a prevalence of osteoporosis varying from 3% to 47% according to different measurement techniques and patient selection criteria, whereas osteopenia has been reported in up to 88% of patients [2]. These variations may be based on the fact that bone analysis in nr-axSpA and AS is challenging, particularly in the axial skeleton, where it is confounded by local new bone formation. Especially in patients with syndesmophytes, dual-energy X-ray absorptiometry (DXA) is unreliable because it sums up new bone formation with bone loss owing to its two-dimensional nature [3, 4].

* Correspondence: georg.schett@uk-erlangen.de
†Anna Neumann and Judith Haschka contributed equally to this work.
[1]Department of Internal Medicine 3, Friedrich Alexander University Erlangen-Nurnberg and Universitätsklinikum Erlangen, Ulmenweg 18, 91054 Erlangen, Germany
Full list of author information is available at the end of the article

However, bone loss has also been found at the hip of patients with AS [5–8]. Furthermore, quantitative computed tomography (QCT), which separately measures trabecular and cortical volumetric bone density, has supported the occurrence of bone loss in AS, showing reduced trabecular volumetric bone mineral density (vBMD) in the lumbar spine in severe AS with syndesmophyte formation [9].

Systemic inflammation is at least partly responsible for systemic bone loss in patients owing to proinflammatory cytokines leading to a direct activation of osteoclastogenesis [10]. In prior studies, patients with AS showed significant bone loss as measured by DXA at the lumbar spine compared with patients with mechanical back pain [11]. Further, in the DESIR (DEvenir des Spondyloarthrites Indifférenciées Récentes) cohort, 71.4% of patients with inflammatory back pain fulfilled Assessment of Spondyloarthritis international Society (ASAS) classification criteria for axial spondyloarthritis (axSpA), and in multiple logistic regression analyses, bone marrow edema seen on magnetic resonance imaging scans, markers of inflammation such as C-reactive protein (CRP) and erythrocyte sedimentation rate (ESR), and male sex were associated with lower bone mineral density (BMD) at any site [12]. Inhibition of tumor necrosis factor (TNF)-α has been reported to show a beneficial effect on BMD and bone turnover markers of patients with AS, thereby supporting the role of systemic inflammation on bone metabolism [13–15]. In accordance with this, vertebral fractures in patients with AS are associated with the longer disease duration independent of age [16].

Bone strength depends not only on BMD but also on bone geometry and microarchitectural aspects of cancellous and cortical bone [17, 18]. High-resolution quantitative computed tomography (HR-pQCT) permits a noninvasive, three-dimensional assessment of bone geometry, volumetric BMD, and microarchitecture, which resembles a virtual bone biopsy of peripheral bone [19, 20]. HR-pQCT data have been shown to correlate with BMD results obtained by DXA and with incident fracture risk in the radius, hip, and spine in postmenopausal women [21, 22].

The aim of the present study was to investigate bone microstructure, geometry, and vBMD using HR-pQCT in a large cohort of patients with nr-axSpA in early stages of disease and to search for potential risk factors for deterioration of bone microstructure. In this context, it is important to mention that patients with AS with long-standing disease are characterized by reduction of total and cortical vBMD and cortical thickness, as well as increased cortical porosity [23, 24]. Data on early disease, however, which may reflect the initial changes of bone in nr-axSpA, are missing to date.

Methods

Patients and control subjects

A total of 107 Caucasian patients with a diagnosis of nr-axSpA were recruited at the Department of Internal Medicine 3 of the University of Erlangen-Nuremberg, Germany. All patients fulfilled the ASAS classification criteria. Patients with AS were not included in this study because we were specifically seeking to study a population with early bone changes. Recruitment of healthy control subjects has been described elsewhere, and these individuals were matched by age and sex [25]. Briefly, exclusion criteria for being a healthy control subject were (1) presence or history of chronic joint pain/swelling, (2) presence of systemic diseases, (3) documented osteopenia/osteoporosis, (4) present or past use of bisphosphonates or prednisolone, and (5) positivity for anticitrullinated protein antibodies (ACPA) or rheumatoid factor. This study was approved by the local ethics committee and the national radiation safety agency (Bundesamt fur Strahlenschutz). Informed consent was obtained from each patient, and the study was performed in accordance with the Declaration of Helsinki.

Demographic and disease-specific characteristics

Demographic characteristics, disease duration, features of SpA (psoriasis, inflammatory bowel disease [IBD], uveitis), human leukocyte antigen (HLA)-B27 status, ESR, and serum CRP levels were recorded in all patients. Current disease activity was determined by Ankylosing Spondylitis Disease Activity Score (ASDAS-CRP; inactive disease ASDAS-CRP < 1.3, 1.3–2.0 moderate disease activity, 2.1–3.5 high disease activity, > 3.5 very high disease activity). Spinal mobility was assessed by Bath Ankylosing Spondylitis Metrology Index (BASMI). For the assessment of present enthesitis, the Maastricht Ankylosing Spondylitis Enthesitis Score was used. Peripheral arthritis was assessed by 78 tender and 76 swollen joint counts. The Spondylitis Disease Activity Index (BASDAI) was assessed as a secondary disease activity measure, and the Bath Ankylosing Spondylitis Functional Index (BASFI) was used for patient-reported outcomes.

The use of conventional disease-modifying antirheumatic drugs (methotrexate, sulfasalazine, azathioprine, leflunomide, chloroquine, gold) and biologic agents (TNF inhibitors [TNFi]) was recorded. Further, the current or previous use of systemic glucocorticoid (GC) treatment exceeding continuous treatment with 5 mg of prednisolone-equivalent daily for more than 3 months was assessed. Treatment with nonsteroidal anti-inflammatory drugs was also recorded (on demand, daily). History of nontraumatic fractures, diagnosis of osteoporosis, and previous or ongoing antiresorptive treatment or supplementation of 25(OH)vitamin D_3 and calcium was taken.

High-resolution peripheral quantitative computed tomography

HR-pQCT imaging was performed in all patients and 50 healthy age- and sex-matched control subjects using the XtremeCT scanner (SCANCO Medical, Brüttisellen, Switzerland). The scan region was selected according to the manufacturer's standard in vivo protocol of the ultradistal radius of the dominant hand. For measurement, the patient's hand was immobilized using a carbon fiber shell to reduce movement. Standardization of measurements was ensured by daily cross-calibrations with a standardized control phantom (QRM, Moehrendorf, Germany). The ROI was determined with an anteroposterior scout view and was fixed 9.5 mm proximal from the reference line. The effective dose for each scan was < 3 μSv. The reference line was set manually. The scan ROI was examined in 110 parallel slices (82-μm voxel size) with a total measurement time of 2.8 minutes. All measurements and evaluations were performed using the manufacturer's standard software. Motion grading (1–5) of each scan was performed using SCANCO Medical standard operating procedure scale, and scans graded > 3 were excluded from analysis.

vBMD, bone microstructure, and geometry were measured with HR-pQCT. Three-dimensional vBMD of the total radius (total BMD in mg of hydroxyapatite [HA]/cm^3), the cortical shell (Ct. BMD, mg HA/cm^3), and the trabecular compartment (Tb.BMD, mg HA/cm^3) were extracted. Additional, distinctive results of trabecular BMD adjacent to bone cortex (mg HA/cm^3) and central medullary trabecular BMD (mg HA/cm^3) were expressed. Results of bone microstructure included bone volume fraction (BV/TV, %), trabecular number (mm^{-1}), trabecular thickness (μm), trabecular separation (Tb.Sp, μm), inhomogeneity of the trabecular network (μm), cortical thickness (Ct.Th, μm), and cortical porosity (Ct.Po, %). Furthermore, bone geometry was represented by total, cortical, and trabecular bone area (mm^2). All these parameters were calculated by using automated software. Reliability of the automated contouring method of the Xtreme CT scanner software has recently been shown [26].

Statistical analysis

Data were collected, organized, and analyzed using IBM SPSS Statistics software (IBM, Armonk, NY, USA). If not stated otherwise, categorical variables are presented as number and percent, and continuous variables are provided as median (IQR). Inferential comparisons comprised chi-square tests for categorical variables (indicated as number and percent in the tables) to check for observed deviations from expected frequencies, as well as the Kruskal-Wallis and Mann-Whitney U tests to compare data derived from interval scales. To investigate potential relationships of total, cortical, and trabecular

vBMD with disease-related or demographic parameters, multiple linear regression models were computed with an enter procedure including all predictors at a single step. The first model incorporated sex, age, BMI, and smoking status. The second model included sex, age, BMI, remission status, disease duration, treatment with TNFi, prior GC treatment, HLA-B27 status, and peripheral arthritis. A p value less than 0.05 was considered significant.

Results

Characteristics of patients with nr-axSpA and healthy control subjects

A total of 107 patients with nr-axSpA and 50 healthy control subjects were recruited for this bone analysis. Six patients with nr-axSpA could not be further analyzed, owing to unacceptable motion artefacts, leaving 101 patients with nr-axSpA to be analyzed. Demographic and disease-specific characteristics are shown in Table 1. Patients with nr-axSpA and control subjects were comparable in age (median [IQR], 45.0 [15.0] vs. 44.76 [26.0] years, $p = 0.917$), sex (females, 41.6% vs. 40%, $p = 0.852$), and BMI (median [IQR], 26.3 [6.5] vs. 23.8 [5.2], $p = 0.118$). Of the patients, 37.6% were former or current smokers, with no significant difference compared with healthy control subjects.

Of patients with nr-axSpA, 75% showed HLA-B27 positivity, and 12.9% of the patients had psoriasis, 7.9% had anterior uveitis, and 6.9% had IBD in their medical history. Systemic inflammation markers were only minimally elevated, with CRP at 6.2 (4.0) mg/L and ESR at 12.7 (10.5) mm. Median disease duration was 6.5 (9.0) years. Disease activity as assessed by ASDAS-CRP was 2.1 (1.4). Only 14.9% of patients were in ASDAS-CRP remission, despite 58.4% of patients being on TNFi treatment with a median (IQR) duration of 2.0 (4.0) years of treatment. Details on the characteristics of patients with nr-axSpA receiving a TNFi and those without a TNFi are summarized in Additional file 1. Clinical assessment by BASMI showed mild impairment of spinal mobility with a median (IQR) score of 1.1 (2) units, whereas patient-reported outcomes revealed a BASDAI of 3.5 (3.6) units and a BASFI of 2.9 (3.8).

Serum 25(OH)vitamin D$_3$ level (median (IQR)) was 32.4 (16.3) ng/ml. Fractures after inadequate trauma were reported in seven patients (6.9%), five patients had prior or current antiresorptive treatment, 7.9% had supplementation with calcium, and 25.7% had supplementation with 25(OH)vitamin D$_3$.

Bone geometry and vBMD in patients with nr-axSpA

Bone geometry showed a significant difference in the cortical area between patients with nr-axSpA and control subjects ($p = 0.022$), whereas there was no difference in the total bone area ($p = 0.700$) or the trabecular area ($p = 0.374$) (Table 2). Cortical vBMD suggested a

Table 1 Demographic and disease-specific characteristics of patients with nonradiographic axial spondyloarthritis and healthy control subjects

	Nr-axSpA (n = 101)	Control subjects (n = 50)	p Value
Demographic characteristics			
Female sex, n (%)	42 (41.6)	20 (40)	0.852
Age, yr	45.0 (15.0)	44.76 (26.0)	0.917
Height, m	1.74 (0.1)	1.74 (0.1)	0.997
Weight, kg	81.1 (21.5)	76.0 (18.5)	0.054
Body mass index, kg/m^2	26.3 (6.5)	23.8 (5.2)	0.118
Current or previous smoking, n (%)	38 (37.6)	11 (24.4)	0.119
Disease-specific characteristics			
HLA-B27 positivity, n (%)	75 (75.0)	–	–
Duration of disease, yr	6.5 (9.0)	–	–
Disease remission, n (%)	15 (14.9)	–	–
ASDAS-CRP, units	2.1 (1.4)	–	–
BASDAI, units	3.5 (3.6)	–	–
C-reactive protein, mg/L	6.2 (4.0)	–	–
ESR, mm	12.7 (10.5)	–	–
BASFI, units	2.9 (3.8)	–	–
BASMI, units	1.1 (2)	–	–
Peripheral arthritis, n (%)	35 (34.7)	–	–
Dactylitis, n (%)	2 (2.0)	–	–
Enthesitis, n (%)	17 (16.8)	–	–
MASES, units	1.1 (1)	–	–
Psoriasis, n (%)	13 (12.9)	–	–
Uveitis, n (%)	8 (7.9)	–	–
Inflammatory bowel disease, n (%)	7 (6.9)	–	–
Low trauma fracture, n (%)	7 (6.9)	–	–
25(OH)vitamin D$_3$, ng/ml	32.4 (16.3)	–	–
Treatment modalities			
Current biologic therapy[a], n (%)	59 (58.4)	–	–
Duration of biologic therapy, yr	2.0 (4.0)		
Current DMARD therapy[b], n (%)	28 (27.7)	–	–
NSAID, n (%)	68 (67.3)	–	–
NSAID daily, n (%)	22 (21.8)	–	–
NSAID on demand, n (%)	46 (45.5)	–	–
Prednisolone ≥ 5 mg > 3 months[c], n (%)	32 (31.7)	–	–
Calcium substitution, n (%)	8 (7.9)	–	–
25(OH)vitamin D$_3$ substitution, n (%)	26 (25.7)	–	–
Antiresorptive treatment, n (%)	5 (5.0)	–	–

Abbreviations: axSpA Axial spondyloarthritis, ESR Erythrocyte sedimentation rate, 25(OH)vitamin D$_3$ 25-Hydroxyvitamin D$_3$, ASDAS-CRP Ankylosing Spondylitis Disease Activity Score, defined as inactive < 1.3, moderate < 2.1, high < 3.5, very high > 3.5 disease activity, disease remission defined as ASDAS-CRP < 1.3, BASDAI Bath Ankylosing Spondylitis Disease Activity Index, BASFI Bath Ankylosing Spondylitis Functional Index, BASMI Bath Ankylosing Spondylitis Metrology Index, MASES Maastrich Ankylosing Spondylitis Enthesitis Score, DMARD Disease-modifying antirheumatic drug, NSAID Nonsteroidal anti-inflammatory drug
Results are median (IQR) or absolute value and percent
[a]Tumor necrosis factor inhibitors
[b]Methotrexate, sulfasalazine, azathioprine, leflunomide, mesalazine
[c]History of treatment with ≥ 5 mg prednisolone for ≥ 3 months

Table 2 Bone microstructure in patients with nonradiographic axial spondyloarthritis assessed by high-resolution peripheral quantitative computed tomography

	axSpA (n = 101)	Control subjects (n = 50)	p Value
Bone geometry			
Total bone area, mm²	334 (108)	326 (116)	0.700
Ct. area, mm²	60 (20)	65 (23)	**0.022**
Tb. area, mm²	265 (78)	254 (83)	0.374
Volumetric bone mineral density			
Total BMD, HA/cm³	313 (70)	334 (61)	**0.042**
Ct. BMD, HA/cm³	823 (66)	846 (78)	**0.007**
Tb. BMD, HA/cm³	174 (44)	183 (68)	0.376
Tb. meta BMD, HA/cm³	234 (43)	243 (61)	0.310
Tb. inn BMD, HA/cm³	133 (47)	141 (72)	0.491
Bone microstructure			
BV/TV, %	14.5 (3.7)	15.2 (5.7)	0.383
Tb. N, mm⁻¹	2.08 (0.31)	2.11 (0.42)	0.799
Tb. Th, μm	70 (15)	72 (17)	0.486
Tb. Sp, μm	417 (83)	410 (104)	0.602
Inhomogeneity, μm	172 (44)	169 (47)	0.828
Ct. Th, μm	767 (190)	840 (160)	**0.006**
Ct. Po, %	2.4 (1.66)	2.2 (1.57)	0.685

Abbreviations: axSpA Axial spondyloarthritis, Ct. Cortical, Tb. Trabecular, Tb. meta BMD Peripheral trabecular density adjacent to cortex, Tb. inn BMD Central medullary trabecular density, BV/TV Trabecular bone volume, Th Thickness, Sp Separation, Po Porosity
Bone geometry, microstructure, and volumetric bone mineral density (BMD) determined by high-resolution peripheral quantitative computed tomography at the ultradistal radius. Results are median (interquartile range)
Bold indicates significant differences (p < 0.05)

reduction in patients with axSpA (compared with control subjects; $p = 0.007$), whereas trabecular BMD showed no difference ($p = 0.376$). Also, no difference between nr-axSpA and control subjects was found for the central medullary and peripheral trabecular density adjacent to cortex ($p = 0.310$ and $p = 0.941$, respectively). Overall total vBMD was different in patients with axSpA, showing lower values than in control subjects ($p = 0.042$), which was based on the differences in cortical BMD.

Bone microstructure in patients with nr-axSpA
Assessment of parameters of bone microstructure showed results very consistent with bone geometry and vBMD with reduced cortical thickness ($p = 0.006$). Trabecular bone structure showed no reduction in trabecular bone volume ($p = 0.383$), number ($p = 0.799$), thickness ($p = 0.486$), or increased inhomogeneity ($p = 0.828$) or trabecular separation ($p = 0.602$). Further cortical analysis showed no increases in cortical porosity ($p = 0.685$) or in

pore volume and pore diameter ($p = 0.919$ and $p = 0.827$, respectively). (Figs. 1 and 2a).

Bone microarchitecture and vBMD with respect to disease duration in patients with nr-axSpA
The overall disease duration was 6.5 (9) years, with men having longer disease duration than women (5.0 [10] vs. 2.0 [4], $p = 0.021$). To assess the impact of disease duration on bone microstructure and vBMD, patients were divided into two groups. Forty-six patients had a disease duration of less than 2 years. Comparison between the two groups and healthy control subjects revealed a significant difference in cortical vBMD ($p = 0.012$), cortical thickness ($p = 0.015$), and cortical pore diameter ($p = 0.007$). No difference in trabecular bone density and microstructure was observed (Table 3). Further intergroup comparisons showed that cortical vBMD is decreased in patients with long-standing disease compared with control subjects ($p = 0.004$), whereas there was only a trend in early SpA ($p = 0.096$). Cortical thickness, however, is already decreased in early nr-axSpA ($p = 0.050$), but the decrease is more prominent in patients with long-standing disease than in control subjects ($p = 0.007$).

Bone microarchitecture and vBMD with respect to glucocorticoid treatment in patients with nr-axSpA
Patients were divided into two groups according to their prior exposure to GC treatment (> 5 mg of prednisolone equivalent over ≥ 3 months) in their medical history. Patients treated with GC showed a reduced trabecular vBMD compared with GC-naïve patients ($p = 0.044$), whereas there was no difference in total or cortical vBMD. Further, especially vBMD of the centrally located trabecular network ($p = 0.014$) showed a reduction, whereas there was no difference of trabecular bone adjacent to cortex ($p = 0.209$). Bone microstructure showed deterioration of the trabecular network with reduced trabecular bone volume (BV/TV; $p = 0.045$) as well as increased inhomogeneity index ($p = 0.007$) and Tb.Sp ($p = 0.037$) in patients treated with prednisolone. Cortical thickness showed no significant difference ($p = 0.959$). (Fig. 2b).

Factors associated with cortical bone changes in nr-axSpA
The first multiple logistic regression model for demographic variables included sex, age, BMI, and smoking status. Male sex was associated with lower cortical vBMD ($p = 0.001$), whereas female sex was associated with lower trabecular vBMD ($p < 0.001$). The model for total vBMD revealed no demographic predictor (Table 4). In a second model, sex, age, BMI, remission status, disease duration, treatment with TNFi, prior GC treatment, HLA-B27 status, and peripheral arthritis were included. In these models, male sex again was associated with lower cortical vBMD ($p = 0.004$), whereas female sex was

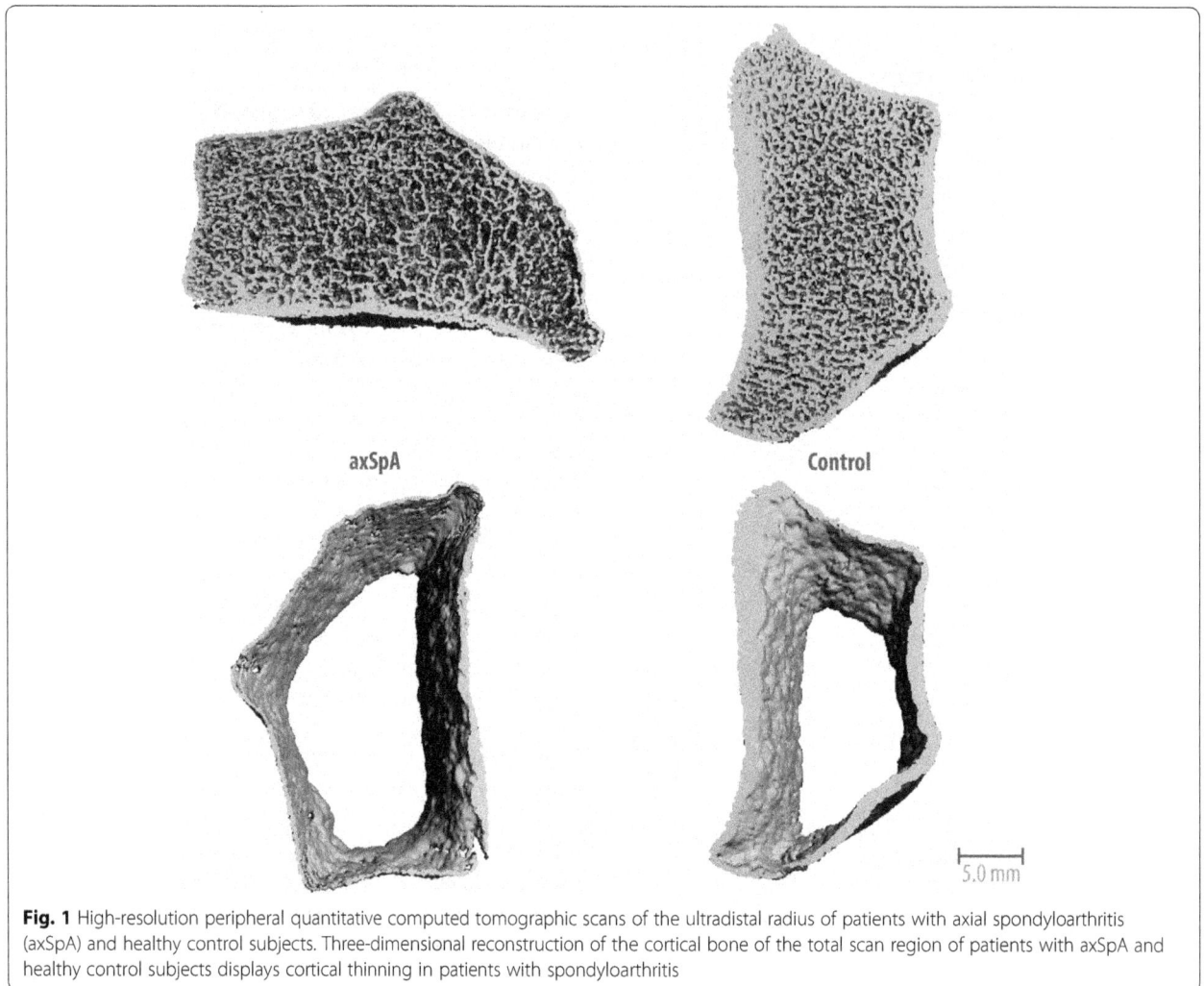

Fig. 1 High-resolution peripheral quantitative computed tomographic scans of the ultradistal radius of patients with axial spondyloarthritis (axSpA) and healthy control subjects. Three-dimensional reconstruction of the cortical bone of the total scan region of patients with axSpA and healthy control subjects displays cortical thinning in patients with spondyloarthritis

associated with lower trabecular vBMD ($p = 0.001$). The model for total vBMD identified no predictors. Prior GC treatment was associated with lower trabecular vBMD ($p = 0.041$). Interestingly, disease duration was positively associated with trabecular vBMD ($p = 0.010$). All further parameters, including age, BMI, remission status, treatment with TNFi, HLA-B27 status, and peripheral arthritis, did not show significant results.

Discussion

Bone loss is a well-known phenomenon in axSpA, especially in long-standing disease. In the present study, we performed a detailed analysis of bone microstructure in a large cohort of patients with axSpA, with disease duration of less than 2 years in nearly 50% of patients. Our analysis shows that patients with nr-axSpA are characterized by a virtually exclusive cortical but not trabecular bone pathology, which is remarkable. Cortical bone changes characterized by changed geometry, BMD, and

microstructure were found early in the disease course of axSpA.

To date, different structural and compartmental changes in bone have been identified using HR-pQCT in systemic inflammatory diseases. Whereas in rheumatoid arthritis a significant deterioration of cortical and trabecular bone has been described, especially in ACPA-positive patients, patients with psoriatic arthritis show predominantly changes of trabecular bone [27, 28]. In contrast, in patients with IBD, primarily a loss of cortical bone has been found [29]. The described changes of cortical bone in nr-axSpA reflect bone structural changes found in patients with IBD.

Our study shows that cortical bone loss as evidenced by cortical thinning happens early in axSpA and can already be found within the first 2 years of disease. In accordance with this, a previous HR-pQCT study of male patients with established AS showed a reduction of cortical vBMD and increased cortical porosity [24]. In this study, however, patients had long-standing disease, with

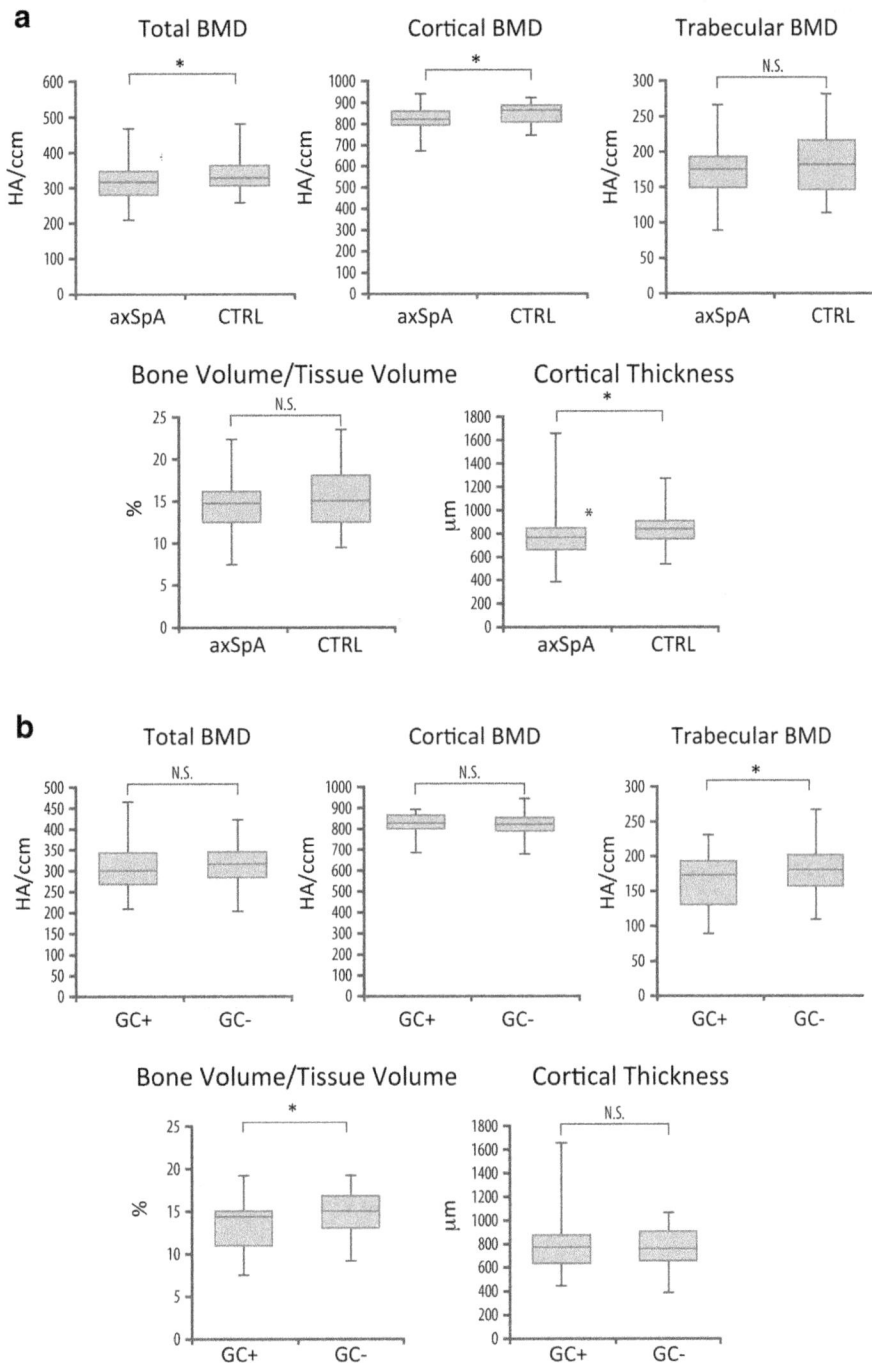

Fig. 2 Differences in bone microarchitecture in patients with nonradiographic axial spondyloarthritis (nr-axSpA). **a** Changes of total, cortical, and trabecular bone mineral density (BMD) and bone microarchitecture reflected by total bone volume (BV/TV) and cortical thickness (Ct.Th) between patients with axial spondyloarthritis (SpA) and healthy control subjects. **b** Changes of total, cortical, and trabecular BMD and bone microarchitecture reflected by BV/TV and Ct.Th between patients with nr-axSpA with or without a history of treatment with > 5 mg prednisolone equivalent for more than 3 months. *GC* Glucocorticoids, *N.S.* Not significant, *HA* Hydroxyapatite. *$p < 0.05$

a median duration of symptoms longer than 20 years. Cortical thinning and low cross-sectional area in the peripheral skeleton in patients with AS were strongly associated with the presence of vertebral fractures [24]. These findings are in accordance with the previously described association of cortical thinning and loss of cortical BMD at the radius and the tibia with the occurrence of vertebral fractures in men in the general population [30]. The median disease duration in our study was much shorter (6.5 years) than in the aforementioned

Table 3 Bone microstructure in patients with nonradiographic axial spondyloarthritis with short and longer disease duration and in healthy control subjects

	axSpA < 2 yr (n = 46)	axSpA > 2 yr (n = 55)	Control subjects (n = 50)	axSpA < 2 yr vs. axSpA > 2 years vs. control subjects	axSpA < 2 yr vs. control subjects	axSpA < 2 yr vs. axSpA > 2 yr	axSpA > 2 yr vs. control subjects
Bone geometry							
Total bone area, mm^2	317 (114)	349 (94)	326 (116)	0.060	0.322	**0.023**	0.136
Ct. area, mm^2	59 (18)	61 (22)	65 (23)	0.068	**0.032**	0.703	0.066
Tb. area, mm^2	250 (95)	277 (88)	254 (83)	0.068	0.628	**0.041**	0.062
Volumetric bone mineral density							
Total BMD, HA/cm^3	317 (49)	309 (75)	334 (61)	0.096	0.170	0.423	**0.036**
Ct. BMD, HA/cm^3	833 (62)	814 (65)	846 (78)	**0.012**	0.096	0.167	**0.004**
Tb. BMD, HA/cm^3	173 (44)	175 (47)	183 (68)	0.571	0.289	0.564	0.610
Tb. meta BMD, HA/cm^3	233 (38)	234 (51)	243 (61)	0.561	0.294	0.728	0.465
Tb. inn BMD, HA/cm^3	132 (47)	135 (52)	141 (72)	0.618	0.359	0.464	0.753
Bone microstructure							
BV/TV, %	14.4 (3.7)	14.6 (3.9)	15.2 (5.7)	0.575	0.288	0.564	0.628
Tb. N, mm^{-1}	2.12 (0.30)	2.05 (0.41)	2.11 (0.42)	0.534	0.739	0.263	0.480
Tb. Th, μm	68 (15)	71 (15)	72 (17)	0.244	0.171	0.120	0.946
Tb. Sp, μm	410 (66)	423 (107)	410 (104)	0.677	0.956	0.480	0.424
Inhomogeneity, μm	165 (41)	178 (48)	169 (47)	0.351	0.575	0.149	0.399
Ct. Th, μm	775 (160)	759 (235)	840 (160)	**0.015**	**0.050**	0.245	**0.007**
Ct. Po, %	2.0 (1.46)	2.8 (1.72)	2.2 (1.57)	0.064	0.373	**0.020**	0.157

Abbreviations: BMD Bone mineral density, *SpA* Spondyloarthritis, *Ct.* Cortical, *Tb.* Trabecular, *Tb. meta* Bone mineral density peripheral trabecular density adjacent to cortex, *Tb. inn* Bone mineral density central medullary trabecular density, *BV/TV* Trabecular bone volume, *Th* Thickness, *Sp* Separation, *Po* Porosity
Bone geometry, microstructure, and volumetric BMD by high-resolution peripheral quantitative computed tomography at the ultradistal radius. Results are median (IQR)
Bold indicates significant differences ($p < 0.05$)

study. Nonetheless, about half of the patients with nr-axSpA did not have early disease (< 2 years) anymore and were treated with TNFi. The fact that some patients had a disease duration longer than 2 years may also explain the observation that 7% of the patients with axSPA already had a history of low traumatic fracture. Overall, however, our data show systemic deterioration of cortical bone microstructure even at an early stage of disease in patients with nr-axSpA.

Data are so far limited regarding the factors that influence bone microarchitecture in patients with nr-axSpA and patients with AS. Multiple logistic regression identified male sex to be associated with lower cortical vBMD.

Interestingly, loss of cortical vBMD was independent of standard disease-related features such as age, BMI, remission status, anti-TNF treatment, HLA-B27 status, and peripheral arthritis. In contrast to cortical vBMD, trabecular vBMD was lower in women than in men. These findings are in accordance with previous population-based studies showing higher trabecular vBMD in men, whereas cortical vBMD is higher in women [31]. Disease duration was associated positively with higher trabecular vBMD in the present study, which can be explained by longer disease duration in men than in women. These results confirm previous findings of Haroon et al., who investigated sex

Table 4 Predictors of reduced total, cortical, and trabecular bone mineral density in patients with nonradiographic axial spondyloarthritis

	Total BMD			Ct. BMD			Trab. BMD		
	β	T	p	β	T	p	β	T	p
Model 1									
Age	0.006	0.068	0.946	−0.038	−0.449	0.654	−0.073	−0.952	0.342
Sex (male vs. female)	−0.143	−1.730	0.086	0.285	3.523	**0.001**	−0.466	−6.324	**< 0.001**
BMI	0.079	0.915	0.362	−0.004	−0.042	0.966	0.083	1.080	0.282
Smoking (yes/no)	0.118	1.415	0.159	−0.041	−0.505	0.615	0.103	1.378	0.171
Intercept	–	11.570	**< 0.001**	–	29.784	**< 0.001**	–	12.765	**< 0.001**
R^2 adjusted	–	0.016	–	–	0.059	–	–	0.219	–
Model 2									
Age	−0.109	−0.913	0.364	−0.094	−0.858	0.393	−0.151	−1.498	0.138
Sex	−0.095	−0.847	0.399	0.300	2.937	**0.004**	−0.420	−4.448	**< 0.001**
BMI	0.115	1.036	0.303	0.017	0.164	0.870	0.159	1.689	0.095
Remission	−0.017	−0.150	0.881	0.015	0.147	0.883	0.048	0.512	0.610
Disease duration	0.157	1.241	0.218	−0.169	−1.460	0.148	0.280	2.625	**0.010**
Anti-TNF	−0.094	−0.776	0.440	−0.131	−1.176	0.243	−0.160	−1.557	0.123
GC (yes/no)	−0.132	−1.131	0.261	0.109	1.023	0.309	−0.205	−2.078	**0.041**
HLA-B27 positivity	−0.027	−0.254	0.800	0.002	0.020	0.984	0.027	0.304	0.762
Peripheral arthritis	0.011	0.095	0.924	−0.041	−0.404	0.687	−0.093	−0.987	0.327
Intercept	–	8.522	**< 0.001**	–	23.225	**< 0.001**	–	9.761	**< 0.001**
R^2 adjusted	–	−0.038	–	–	0.130	–	–	0.258	–

Abbreviations: BMD Bone mineral density, *Ct. BMD* Cortical bone mineral density, *Trab. BMD* Trabecular bone mineral density, *axSpA* axial spondyloarthritis, *BMI* Body mass index, *Anti-TNF* Current treatment with anti-tumor necrosis factor α inhibitor, *GC* History of glucocorticoid treatment with ≥ 5 mg prednisolone equivalent daily for > 3 mo
Remission status according to Ankylosing Spondylitis Disease Activity Score (ASDAS-CRP, inactive disease ASDAS-CRP < 1.3)
Bold indicates significant differences ($p < 0.05$)

differences among patients with AS and showed decreased cortical vBMD in men, whereas trabecular vBMD was worse in women [23].

Although nr-axSpA specifically affects cortical bone, an evaluation of those patients treated with GCs > 5 mg daily for > 3 months in the past showed specific loss of trabecular bone associated with reduction of trabecular vBMD, lower total bone volume, and higher trabecular separation and inhomogeneity. Sutter et al. investigated postmenopausal women treated with oral GCs for > 3 months and age-/race-matched control subjects using HR-pQCT and DXA. In their study, despite no difference in areal BMD, GC-treated women showed an impairment of cortical and trabecular vBMD and bone microarchitecture [32]. Moreover, later stages of the disease, particularly in patients with severe AS with syndesmophyte formation, also trabecular vBMD appears to decrease, which is reflected by a study from Devogelaer and colleagues [9].

The strength of the present study is a detailed assessment of bone macro- and microarchitecture using HR-pQCT in patients with axSpA. To date, this is the largest nr-axSpA cohort with detailed bone analysis by HR-pQCT. A further strength and novelty of this work is

the assessment of patients with short disease duration. A limitation is, of course, that HR-pQCT cannot analyze the spine but is confined to peripheral sites. However, several studies have previously shown that structural changes in the peripheral bones reflect bone changes as well as fracture risk in the axial skeleton [22, 23].

The reason why nr-axSpA virtually exclusively affects cortical bone is not entirely clear. It can be speculated that such changes reflect increased cortical bone remodeling. For instance, it has long been known that the remodeling of cortical bone is highly dependent on strain [33], and later concepts even suggested that cortical bone remodeling may even be entirely dependent on microcracks [34]. Hence, altered bone responses to mechanical forces in nr-axSpA may be triggers for increased cortical bone remodeling and bone loss. In accordance with this, prostaglandin E_2, a prototype inflammatory mediator released upon injury and having a central role in nr-axSpA, has been shown to enhance cortical bone remodeling [35]. The disbalance in cortical bone in patients with nr-axSpA, however, may stem from cytokines such as interleukin-17, which effectively suppress bone formation but at the same time increase bone resorption [36, 37].

Conclusions

In this study, we show that axSpA specifically leads to an early and virtually exclusive loss of cortical bone, thereby contrasting with many other inflammatory diseases but resembling features of bone loss observed in patients with IBD. In contrast, trabecular bone does not appear to be directly influenced by axSpA.

Abbreviations

ACPA: Anticitrullinated protein antibodies; AS: Ankylosing spondylitis; ASAS: Assessment of Spondyloarthritis international Society; ASDAS: Ankylosing Spondylitis Disease Activity Score; BASDAI: Bath Ankylosing Spondylitis Disease Activity Index; BASMI: Bath Ankylosing Spondylitis Metrology Index; BMD: Bone mineral density; BMI: Body mass index; BV/TV: Bone volume per tissue volume; CRP: C-reactive protein; Ct: Cortical bone; Ct.Po: Cortical porosity; Ct.Th: Cortical thickness; DMARD: Disease-modifying antirheumatic drug; DXA: Dual-energy x-ray absorptiometry; ESR: Erythrocyte sedimentation rate; GC: Glucocorticoid; HA: Hydroxyapatite; HLA-B27: Human leukocyte antigen B27; HR-pQCT: High-resolution quantitative computed tomography; IBD: Inflammatory bowel disease; MASES: Maastricht Ankylosing Spondylitis Enthesitis Score; SpA: Spondyloarthritis; Tb: Trabecular bone; Tb.Sp: Trabecular separation; TNF: Tumor necrosis factor α; TNFi: Inhibition of tumor necrosis factor α; vBMD: Volumetric bone mineral density

Acknowledgements

This study was supported by the Bundesministerium fuer Bildung und Forschung (BMBF project METARTHROS), the Deutsche Forschungsgemeinschaft (CRC1181), the Marie Curie project Osteoimmune and the Innovative Medicines Initiative-funded project Be The Cure (BTCure). CPF was supported by Cienciassem Fronteiras from Conselho Nacional de Desenvolvimento Cientifico e Tecnologico (CNPq), Brazil.

Funding

This study was supported by the Deutsche Forschungsgemeinschaft (CRC1181), the Bundesministerium für Bildung und Forschung (BMBF; project METARTHROS) and the Innovative Medicine Initiative-funded project Rheuma Tolerance for Cure (RTCure).

Authors' contributions

AN, JH, and AK collected and analyzed the data. LS performed the scan evaluation and motion grading. JH and ME performed the statistical analysis. AB provided data of healthy control subjects. AN, JH, AK, ME, CPF, DS, CM, RK, HR, JR, and GS interpreted the data and revised the manuscript. AN, JH, and GS wrote the manuscript. The present work was performed in fulfillment of the requirements for obtaining the 'Dr. med.' degree by AN. All authors read and approved the final manuscript.

Competing interests

The authors declare that they have no competing interests.

Author details

[1]Department of Internal Medicine 3, Friedrich Alexander University Erlangen-Nurnberg and Universitätsklinikum Erlangen, Ulmenweg 18, 91054 Erlangen, Germany. [2]St. Vincent Hospital, VINFORCE Study Group, Medical University of Vienna, Vienna, Austria. [3]Division of Rheumatology, Faculdade de Medicina da Universidade de São Paulo, São Paulo, Brazil.

References

1. Donnelly S, Doyle DV, Denton A, Rolfe I, McCloskey EV, Spector TD. Bone mineral density and vertebral compression fracture rates in ankylosing spondylitis. Ann Rheum Dis. 1994;53:117–21.
2. Kilic E, Ozgocmen S. Bone mass in axial spondyloarthritis: a literature review. World J Orthop. 2015;6:298–310.
3. Klingberg E, Lorentzon M, Mellstrom D, Geijer M, Gothlin J, Hilme E, et al. Osteoporosis in ankylosing spondylitis - prevalence, risk factors and methods of assessment. Arthritis Res Ther. 2012;14:R108.
4. Lange U, Kluge A, Strunk J, Teichmann J, Bachmann G. Ankylosing spondylitis and bone mineral density—what is the ideal tool for measurement? Rheumatol Int. 2005;26:115–20.
5. Speden DJ, Calin AI, Ring FJ, Bhalla AK. Bone mineral density, calcaneal ultrasound, and bone turnover markers in women with ankylosing spondylitis. J Rheumatol. 2002;29:516–21.
6. Karberg K, Zochling J, Sieper J, Felsenberg D, Braun J. Bone loss is detected more frequently in patients with ankylosing spondylitis with syndesmophytes. J Rheumatol. 2005;32:1290–8.
7. Meirelles ES, Borelli A, Camargo OP. Influence of disease activity and chronicity on ankylosing spondylitis bone mass loss. Clin Rheumatol. 1999; 18:364–8.
8. Singh A, Bronson W, Walker SE, Allen SH. Relative value of femoral and lumbar bone mineral density assessments in patients with ankylosing spondylitis. South Med J. 1995;88:939–43.
9. Devogelaer JP, Maldague B, Malghem J, Nagant de Deuxchaisnes C. Appendicular and vertebral bone mass in ankylosing spondylitis: a comparison of plain radiographs with single- and dual-photon absorptiometry and with quantitative computed tomography. Arthritis Rheum. 1992;35:1062–7.
10. Schett G, David JP. The multiple faces of autoimmune-mediated bone loss. Nat Rev Endocrinol. 2010;6:698–706.
11. Akgol G, Kamanli A, Ozgocmen S. Evidence for inflammation-induced bone loss in non-radiographic axial spondyloarthritis. Rheumatology (Oxford). 2014;53:497–501.
12. Briot K, Durnez A, Paternotte S, Miceli-Richard C, Dougados M, Roux C. Bone oedema on MRI is highly associated with low bone mineral density in patients with early inflammatory back pain: results from the DESIR cohort. Ann Rheum Dis. 2013;72:1914–9.
13. Allali F, Breban M, Porcher R, Maillefert JF, Dougados M, Roux C. Increase in bone mineral density of patients with spondyloarthropathy treated with anti-tumour necrosis factor α. Ann Rheum Dis. 2003;62:347–9.
14. Arends S, Spoorenberg A, Houtman PM, Leijsma MK, Bos R, Kallenberg CG, et al. The effect of three years of TNFα blocking therapy on markers of bone turnover and their predictive value for treatment discontinuation in patients with ankylosing spondylitis: a prospective longitudinal observational cohort study. Arthritis Res Ther. 2012;14:R98.
15. Kang KY, Ju JH, Park SH, Kim HY. The paradoxical effects of TNF inhibitors on bone mineral density and radiographic progression in patients with ankylosing spondylitis. Rheumatology (Oxford). 2013;52:718–26.
16. Klingberg E, Geijer M, Gothlin J, Mellstrom D, Lorentzon M, Hilme E, Hedberg M, Carlsten H, Forsblad-D'Elia H. Vertebral fractures in ankylosing spondylitis are associated with lower bone mineral density in both central and peripheral skeleton. J Rheumatol. 2012;39:1987–95.
17. Seeman E, Delmas PD. Bone quality—the material and structural basis of bone strength and fragility. N Engl J Med. 2006;354:2250–61.
18. Stein EM, Kepley A, Walker M, Nickolas TL, Nishiyama K, Zhou B, et al. Skeletal structure in postmenopausal women with osteopenia and fractures is characterized by abnormal trabecular plates and cortical thinning. J Bone Miner Res. 2014;29:1101–9.
19. Boutroy S, Bouxsein ML, Munoz F, Delmas PD. In vivo assessment of trabecular bone microarchitecture by high-resolution peripheral quantitative computed tomography. J Clin Endocrinol Metab. 2005;90:6508–15.
20. Cheung AM, Adachi JD, Hanley DA, Kendler DL, Davison KS, Josse R, et al. High-resolution peripheral quantitative computed tomography for the assessment of bone strength and structure: a review by the Canadian Bone Strength Working Group. Curr Osteoporos Rep. 2013;11:136–46.
21. Amstrup AK, Jakobsen NF, Moser E, Sikjaer T, Mosekilde L, Rejnmark L. Association between bone indices assessed by DXA, HR-pQCT and QCT scans in post-menopausal women. J Bone Miner Metab. 2016;34:638–45.
22. Engelke K, Libanati C, Fuerst T, Zysset P, Genant HK. Advanced CT based in vivo methods for the assessment of bone density, structure, and strength. Curr Osteoporos Rep. 2013;11:246–55.
23. Haroon N, Szabo E, Raboud JM, McDonald-Blumer H, Fung L, Josse RG, et al. Alterations of bone mineral density, bone microarchitecture and strength in patients with ankylosing spondylitis: a cross-sectional study using high-resolution peripheral quantitative computerized tomography and finite element analysis. Arthritis Res Ther. 2015;17:377.

24. Klingberg E, Lorentzon M, Gothlin J, Mellstrom D, Geijer M, Ohlsson C, et al. Bone microarchitecture in ankylosing spondylitis and the association with bone mineral density, fractures, and syndesmophytes. Arthritis Res Ther. 2013;15:R179.

25. Simon D, Kleyer A, Stemmler F, Simon C, Berlin A, et al. Age- and sex-dependent changes of intra-articular cortical and trabecular bone structure and the effects of rheumatoid arthritis. J Bone Miner Res. 2017;32:722–30.

26. de Waard EAC, Sarodnik C, Pennings A, de Jong JJA, Savelberg HHCM, van Geel TA, et al. The reliability of HR-pQCT derived cortical bone structural parameters when using uncorrected instead of corrected automatically generated endocortical contours in a cross-sectional study: the Maastricht study. Calcif Tissue Int. 2018; https://doi.org/10.1007/s00223-018-0416-2.

27. Kocijan R, Finzel S, Englbrecht M, Engelke K, Rech J, Schett G. Differences in bone structure between rheumatoid arthritis and psoriatic arthritis patients relative to autoantibody positivity. Ann Rheum Dis. 2014;73:2022–8.

28. Kocijan R, Englbrecht M, Haschka J, Simon D, Kleyer A, Finzel S, et al. Quantitative and qualitative changes of bone in psoriasis and psoriatic arthritis patients. J Bone Miner Res. 2015;30:1775–83.

29. Haschka J, Hirschmann S, Kleyer A, Englbrecht M, Faustini F, Simon D, et al. High-resolution quantitative computed tomography demonstrates structural defects in cortical and trabecular bone in IBD patients. J Crohns Colitis. 2016;10:532–40.

30. Szulc P, Boutroy S, Vilayphiou N, Chaitou A, Delmas PD, Chapurlat R. Cross-sectional analysis of the association between fragility fractures and bone microarchitecture in older men: the STRAMBO study. J Bone Miner Res. 2011;26:1358–67.

31. Khosla S, Riggs BL, Atkinson EJ, Oberg AL, McDaniel LJ, Holets M, et al. Effects of sex and age on bone microstructure at the ultradistal radius: a population-based noninvasive in vivo assessment. J Bone Miner Res. 2006; 21:124–31.

32. Sutter S, Nishiyama KK, Kepley A, Zhou B, Wang J, McMahon DJ, et al. Abnormalities in cortical bone, trabecular plates, and stiffness in postmenopausal women treated with glucocorticoids. J Clin Endocrinol Metab. 2014;99:4231–40.

33. Carter DR. Mechanical loading histories and cortical bone remodeling. Calcif Tissue Int. 1984;36:S19–24.

34. Martin RB. Is all cortical bone remodeling initiated by microdamage? Bone. 2002;30:8–13.

35. Jee WS, Mori S, Li XJ, Chan S. Prostaglandin E_2 enhances cortical bone mass and activates intracortical bone remodeling in intact and ovariectomized female rats. Bone. 1990;11:253–66.

36. Uluckan O, Jimenez M, Karbach S, Jeschke A, Graña O, Keller J, et al. Chronic skin inflammation leads to bone loss by IL-17-mediated inhibition of Wnt signaling in osteoblasts. Sci Transl Med. 2016;8:330ra337.

37. Kotake S, Udagawa N, Takahashi N, Matsuzaki K, Itoh K, Ishiyama S, et al. IL-17 in synovial fluids from patients with rheumatoid arthritis is a potent stimulator of osteoclastogenesis. J Clin Invest. 1999;103:1345–52.

2

The frequency of ANCA-associated vasculitis in a national database of hospitalized patients

Jiannan Li[1], Zhao Cui[1], Jian-yan Long[2], Wei Huang[3], Jin-wei Wang[1], Haibo Wang[2,4], Luxia Zhang[1,5], Min Chen[1] and Ming-hui Zhao[1,6]*

Abstract

Background: Anti-neutrophil cytoplasmic autoantibody (ANCA)-associated vasculitis (AAV) is a group of life-threatening autoimmune diseases. The epidemiological data on AAV in China are limited. The aim of the present study is to investigate the frequency, geographical distribution, and ethnic distribution of AAV in hospitalized patients in China, and its association with environmental pollution.

Methods: We investigated the hospitalized patients in a national inpatient database covering 54.1% tertiary hospitals in China from 2010 to 2015. Diagnosis of AAV was extracted according to the definition of International Classification of Diseases (ICD)-10 codes and free text. Variables from the front page of inpatient records were collected and analyzed, including frequency, geographic distribution, demographic characteristics and seasonal variations of AAV. The association between various environmental pollutants and frequency of AAV was further analyzed.

Results: Among 43.7 million inpatients included in the study period, 0.25‰ (10,943) were diagnosed as having AAV. The frequency of AAV was relatively stable during the study period (from 0.34‰ in 2010 to 0.27‰ in 2015). The proportion of AAV increased with latitude (0.44‰ in Northern China and 0.27‰ in Southern China in 2015). Hospitalizations were mostly observed in winter (30.2%). The Dong population, an ethnic minority of the Chinese population, had the highest frequency of patients with AAV (0.67‰). We also found a positive association between the exposure to carbon monoxide and the frequency of AAV ($R^2 = 0.172$, $p = 0.025$). In Yunnan province, the frequency of AAV increased 1.37-fold after the Zhaotong earthquake, which took place in 2014.

Conclusions: Our present investigation of hospitalized patients provided epidemiological information on AAV in China for the first time. A spatial and ethnic clustering trend and an association between pollution and the frequency of AAV were observed.

Keywords: ANCA, Vasculitis, Frequency, Hospitalized population

* Correspondence: mhzhao@bjmu.edu.cn
[1]Renal Division, Department of Medicine, Peking University First Hospital, Peking University Institute of Nephrology, Key Laboratory of Renal Disease, Ministry of Health of China, Key Laboratory of CKD Prevention and Treatment, Ministry of Education of China, Beijing, China
[6]Peking-Tsinghua Center for Life Sciences, Beijing, People's Republic of China
Full list of author information is available at the end of the article

Background

Anti-neutrophil cytoplasmic autoantibody (ANCA) associated vasculitis (AAV) is a group of life-threatening autoimmune diseases affecting mainly small-to-medium vessels [1], with a poor prognosis if left untreated [2–8]. According to the 2012 classification of the Chapel Hill Consensus Conference (CHCC) [9], the phenotypes include four clinical syndromes, namely, granulomatosis with polyangiitis (GPA, formerly known as Wegener's granulomatosis), microscopic polyangiitis (MPA), eosinophilic granulomatosis with polyangiitis (EGPA, formerly known as Churg-Strauss syndrome), and single-organ AAV (for example, renal-limited AAV). The serological marker for AAV is ANCA [10].

The epidemiological characteristics of AAV have been investigated worldwide. The annual incidence and prevalence of AAV varies according to latitude in both the southern and northern hemispheres [11]. Several environmental factors are associated with the development of AAV. Exposure to silicons and subsequent modification of myeloperoxidase (MPO) by air pollution is suspected to be a risk factor for AAV [12–14]. Earthquake might also be a source of silicons, which might subsequently result in the incremental incidence of AAV with more rapid deteriotion of renal function [15, 16]. However, this phenomenon was not supported by a similar study in New Zealand [17]. Infections might contribute to the onset of AAV, especially *Staphylococcus aureus* infections [18–20]. Moreover, certain genetic backgrounds might lead to greater susceptiblity to AAV [21], especially in specific races [22]. However, although AAV was first reported in 1993 in China [23, 24], only limited single-center surveys of AAV have been carried out [25, 26] and nationwide epidemiological investigations are not yet available. The purpose of the present study was to investigate the proportion and characteristics of AAV patients and their clinical phenotypes in hospitalized patients in China.

Methods
Study population
The study population included 43,677,829 inpatients from 878 tertiary hospitals from 1 Jan 2010 to 31 Dec 2015, covering 54.1% of tertiary hospitals in 31 provinces nationwide.

The database we used is the Hospital Quality Monitoring System (HQMS), which is a registration database of the standardized electronic inpatient discharge records of tertiary hospitals in China. Under the administration of the Bureau of Medical Administration and Medical Service Supervision, National Health and Family Planning Commission of the People's Republic of China, tertiary hospitals in China have mandatorily and automatically submitted electronic discharge records daily to HQMS, since 1 Jan 2013. Data from 1 Jan 2010 to 31 Dec 2012 were collected retrospectively. Demographic characteristics, clinical diagnoses, procedures, pathological diagnoses, and expenditures were extracted from the front page of the hospital medical record.

Physicians were responsible for filing the data on the front page, and the diagnosis were coded by certified professional medical coders at every hospital according to the International Classification of Diseases-10 (ICD-10) coding system. Data quality was controlled automatically at the time of data submission to ensure completeness, consistency, and accuracy.

For patients with multiple admissions, only the first admission was included for analysis. We identified 288,804 patients for analysis from 1 Jan 2013 to 31 Dec 2015, and 11,102 patients from 1 Jan 2010 to 31 Dec 2012. Identification numbers and telephone numbers were combined to define the place of patient residence. Urban/rural residency was identified by the type of health insurance (basic medical insurance or free medical insurance for urban residency, and new rural cooperative medical care for rural residency). The ethics committee of Peking University First Hospital approved the study.

Definition of AAV
The ICD-10 coding of discharged diagnoses and free text were used to identify patients with AAV compromising granulomatosis with polyangiitis (GPA), microscopic polyangitis (MPA), eosinophilic granulomatosis with polyangiitis (EGPA) and kidney-limited vasculitis (relevant ICD-10 coding in Appendix 1). The definition of AAV had to exclude large vessel vasculitis (e.g., Takayasu arteritis, giant cell arteritis), medium vessel vasculitis (e.g., polyarteritis nodosa, Kawasaki disease), and immune complex small vessel vasculitis (SVV) (e.g., rheumatoid vasculitis, sarcoid vasculitis, and others) (relevant ICD-10 coding in Appendix 2), from which, 6844 patients were excluded. Nephrotic syndrome, rapidly progressive glomerulonephritis, nephritis syndrome, and related complications are also listed in Appendix 2.

Demographic data and other covariates
Information on age, gender, ethnicity, occupation, residence, health insurance, type of admission, and intensive care unit (ICU) stay were collected from the front page of the medical records. Outcome data on expenditure, length of stay, and in-hospital mortality were also extracted. The survival status of each patient was

verified based on discharge status, and combined with information from autopsy reporting.

Geographic latitude

The latitude and longitude of each province and each capital city in China were acquired from the National Bureau of Statistics (http://www.stats.gov.cn/). The range of latitude of Northeastern China is 38.7° N to 53.6° N, of Northern China it is 34.9° N to 53.4° N, of Northwestern China it is 31.7° N to 48.2° N, of Central China it is 24.6° N to 36.4° N, of Eastern China it is 23.5° N to 38.4° N, of Southern China it is 18.2° N to 26. 4° N, and of Southwestern China it is 20° N to 34.3° N.

Pollution exposure assessment

The National Bureau of Statistics of China has published the average concentrations of air pollutants in each city, including main pollutant emission in waste gas, which contained particulate matter (PM) of 2.5 ($\mu g/m^3$) (PM 2.5) in 2015, PM of 10 ($\mu g/m^3$) (PM 10) since 2010, carbon monoxide (CO) ($\mu g/m^3$), inhalable particulate (10,000 tons), nitrogen dioxide (NO_2) (10,000 tons), sulfur oxide (SO_2) (10,000 tons) since 2002; main pollutant emission in waste water, which contains the total volume of waste water discharged (10,000 tons), ammonia nitrogen (10,000 tons), total nitrogen (10,000 tons), total phosphorus (10,000 tons), petroleum (ton), volatile phenol (ton), plumbum (kg), mercury (kg); and general industrial solid waste per year since 2002, which contains household garbage and industrial solid wastes, with various kinds of pollutants, including nitrogenous wastes, organic pollutants, such as polycyclic aromatic hydrocarbons, which mainly affects soil and water. Data on polycyclic aromatic hydrocarbon pollution in soil has been provided by Ma et al. [27] Data on seasonal PM 2.5 and PM 10 in 2014–2015 has been provided by Zhang et al. [28] Data on annual average temperature, humidity, and precipitation were acquired from the National Meteorological Center (http://data.cma.cn). Detailed data on pollutants are listed in Additional files 1, 2, and 3.

Statistical analyses

The proportion and absolute number of patients with AAV were identified and further analyzed. Patients with AAV were stratified by age, gender, geographic regions, and rural/urban residency. General demographic characteristics, costs, length of stay and in-hospital mortality were compared among patients with GPA, MPA, and EGPA. Continuous data were analyzed as mean ± standard deviation, or as median (inter-quartile range) for highly skewed variables. Categorical variables were analyzed as proportions with 95% confidence interval (CI).

The association between the frequency of AAV in the hospitalized population and exposure to ambient environmental pollution were analyzed using Pearson correlation models and generalized linear regression models. Data on air pollutants were adjusted for annual average temperature, humidity, and precipitation. The proportions of patients with AAV were adjusted for average age and gender. The analysis of populations of patients with AAV was based on individual patients instead of admissions, since the number of patients was more relevant to the prevalence of AAV. All analyses were performed using SAS software, version 9.1 (SAS Institute Inc., Cary, NC, USA).

Results
Demographic characteristics of patients with AAV in 2015
The frequency of AAV was relatively stable in the study period (from 0.34‰ in 2010 to 0.27‰ in 2015). There were 4440 patients (0.27‰ of all inpatients) identified as having AAV in 2015 and these were included for further analysis. The demographic characteristics of patients with AAV in 2015 are shown in Table 1. Patients with AAV were most commonly admitted by the nephrology division ($n = 1971$ (44.4%)), followed by the respiratory division ($n = 584$ (13.2%)), and the rheumatology division ($n = 509$ (11.5%)). Most admissions were in winter (30.2%) (Fig. 1). The age of patients with AAV at diagnosis was 60.0 ± 15.6 years, and the majority were older than 50 years (Fig. 2).

There was a greater frequency of hospitalized patients with AAV in Northern China (0.44‰ of all inpatients in Northern China vs. 0.27‰ in Southern China) (Fig. 3). We analyzed the association between the frequency of AAV and the latitude of major cities in China; however, no significant association was found.

The ethnic distribution of AAV in the study period
Dong, Zhuang, and Li ethnic people had the highest frequency of AAV, with a frequency of 0.67‰, 0.61‰, and 0.42‰, respectively (Fig. 4). The Dong and Zhuang populations are mostly distributed in Southern China. However, there was no significant correlation between the proportion of ethnic groups in each province and the frequency of AAV.

The distribution of AAV according to pollution
The pathogenesis of AAV is reported to be associated with silicon pollution [15]. We further investigated the association between various pollutants and the frequency of AAV. We analyzed the association

Table 1 Demographic information on patients with AAV in 2015 in China

	AAV	GPA	MPA	EGPA
Number	4440	385	396	223
Age (years)	60.0 ± 15.6	50.7 ± 15.6	62.3 ± 17.2	50.3 ± 15.6
Age group, %				
0–17	1.3	1.6	3.5	3.1
18–30	5.0	11.4	2.8	9.4
31–40	4.8	10.4	2.8	11.2
41–50	11.8	23.9	7.4	20.2
51–60	20.6	24.4	17.4	27.8
61–70	29.9	17.1	34.8	21.5
> 80	26.6	11.2	31.3	6.6
Male, %	46.4(45.0,47.9)	49.9(44.9,54.9)	48.5(43.6,53.4)	52.5(45.9,59.0)
Occupation, %				
Professional or semi-professional	9.1 (8.2,10.0)	14.7 (10.9,18.4)	8.5 (5.6,11.4)	16.1 (11.1,21.1)
Worker	2.9 (2.4,3.4)	2.9 (1.1,4.6)	2.5 (0.9,4.2)	3.9 (1.3,6.6)
Farmer	25.7 (24.3,27.0)	22.4 (18.0,26.8)	25.4 (20.9,30.0)	22.0 (16.3,27.6)
Retired	20.4 (19.1,21.6)	12.9 (9.4,16.5)	24.3 (19.8,28.8)	15.6 (10.6,20.6)
Unemployed	7.2 (6.4,8.0)	6.9 (4.2,9.6)	7.9 (5.1,10.7)	4.4 (1.6,7.2)
Others	34.7 (33.3,36.2)	40.2 (35.1,45.4)	31.4 (26.5,36.2)	38.0 (31.4,44.7)
Medical insurance				
Basic Medical Insurance	44.4 (43.0,45.9)	38.2 (33.3,43.0)	44.4 (39.6,49.3)	45.7 (39.2,52.3)
New Rural Co-operative Medical Care	24.1 (22.9,25.4)	24.7 (20.4,29.0)	21.7 (17.7,25.8)	25.1 (19.4,30.8)
Other insurance	16.0 (14.9,17.1)	16.1 (12.4,19.8)	21.5 (17.4,25.5)	17.9 (12.9,23.0)
No insurance	15.4 (14.4,16.5)	21.0 (17.0,25.1)	12.4 (9.1,15.6)	11.2 (7.1,15.4)
Admission place				
Emergency	12.6 (11.6,13.6)	15.0 (11.3,18.7)	11.5 (8.2,14.7)	16.4 (11.5,21.4)
Routine	79.9 (78.7,81.1)	76.7 (72.3,81.0)	83.1 (79.2,86.9)	77 (71.3,82.6)
Other	7.5 (6.7,8.3)	8.3 (5.5,11.2)	5.5 (3.1,7.8)	6.6 (3.2,9.9)
ICU stay, %	2.2 (1.7,2.6)	0.3 (0,0.8)	3.5 (1.7,5.4)	0.4 (0,1.3)
Costs (10,000 RMB), median (Q1–Q3)	13 (7–23)	10 (6–19)	14 (8–24)	11 (7–18)
Length of stay (days), median (Q1–Q3)	12 (8–19)	12 (7–18)	13 (8–21)	12 (8–16)
In-hospital mortality, %	1.8 (1.4,2.2)	1.3 (0.2,2.4)	2.8 (1.2,4.4)	0.4 (0,1.3)

Abbreviations: AAV anti-neutrophil cytoplasmic autoantibody associated vasculitis, *GPA* granulomatosis with polyangiitis, *MPA* microscopic polyangiitis, *EGPA* eosinophilic granulomatosis with polyangiitis, *ICU* intensive care unit, *RMB* Renminbi, which is Chinese currency.

between particular molecules and AAV using data from 946 stations covering 190 cities within 2014–2015, published by the National Air Quality Monitoring Network [28] in China, and analyzed aerosol optical depth (AOD) data from 1998 to 2014 provided by the National Aeronautics and Space Administration (NASA). Data on air sulfur dioxide, carbon dioxide, and dust were obtained from the National Bureau of Statistics. We found positive correlation between exposure to carbon monoxide and the frequency of AAV (R^2 = 0.172, P = 0.025). However, there was no significant correlation between the frequency of AAV and air pollutents (PM 2.5, PM 10, other inhalable particulates, NO_2, SO_2) or water pollution.

The increasing frequency of AAV after the severe earthquake

On 3 Aug 2014, a major earthquake hit Yunnan province and threatened more than 1 million lives. The frequency of AAV in Yunnan province increased 1.37-fold after the earthquake, from 0.19‰ in 2013 to 0.26‰ in 2014 (Fig. 5).

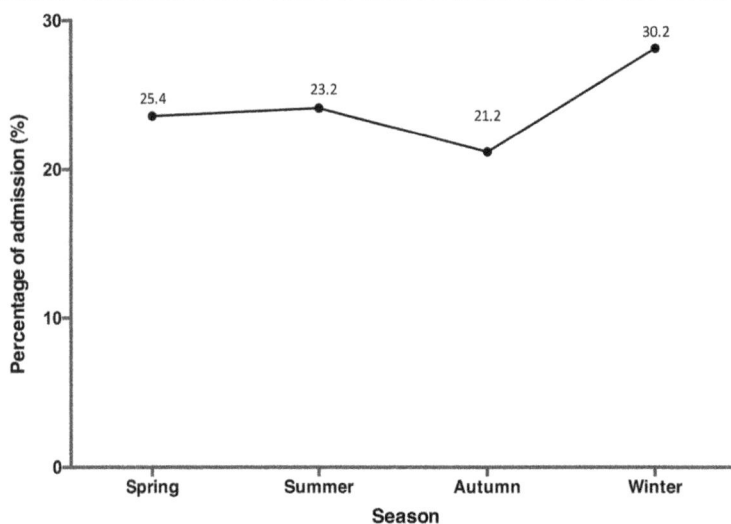

Fig. 1 The distribution of anti-neutrophil cytoplasmic autoantibody associated vasculitis (AAV) in different seasons in 2015. The highest frequency of admissions for AAV were in winter (30.2%)

Discussion

Using a large national inpatient database covering 43,677,829 patients from 2010 to 2015, we described the epidemiological characteristics of AAV in China for the first time. We observed a changing frequency of AAV according to latitude and seasonal variations. In addition, the Dong ethnic minority had the highest proportion of patients with AAV. We also noticed that exposure to carbon monoxide (CO) might increase the frequency of AAV.

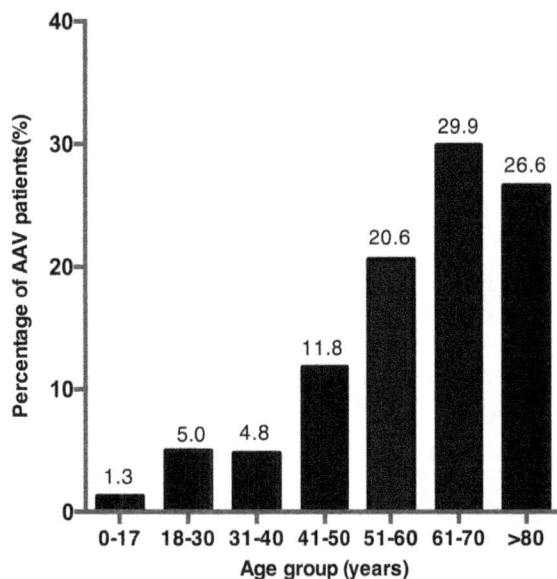

Fig. 2 The age distribution of anti-neutrophil cytoplasmic autoantibody associated vasculitis (AAV) in 2015. Most patients with AAV were older than 50 years, with a peak age at 61–70 years (29.9%)

Incidence studies performed in Japan and European countries suggest that there are geographic variations in AAV [11, 29] in the northern hemisphere, while studies in Austrilia and New Zealand showed a similar trend [30, 31] (Additional file 1: Table S1). The reason is explained as genetic variation and the ultraviolet radiation gradient according to latitude [32, 33]. In the present study, the inpatients in Northern China (34.9° N to 53.4° N) had the highest proportion of patients with AAV (0.42‰), while in Central China (24.63° N to 36.37° N), Southwestern China (23.5° N to 38.4° N) and Southern China (18.2° N to 26. 4° N) the proportions were lower (0.23‰, 0.25‰, 0.28‰, respectively), which is consistent with previous reports. However, most physicians in China do not make a precise diagnosis of each subtype of AAV, i.e., GPA, MPA, or EGPA on the first page of the inpatients' documents, probably due to the similar treatment strategy for each pathological type of AAV; thus GPA, MPA, and EGPA were not analyzed further. In addition, our data were from a hospital-based database, which can not be used to compare our data with the incidence or prevalence of AAV in other countries. However, we could still find that the disease spectrum is different between China and Japan, since the incidence of GPA in Japan is much lower than that of MPA (2.1 (0.6, 3.5) vs. 18.2 (14.3, 22.0)/million in adults, and 2.7 (– 0.8, 6.3)/million vs. 50.7 (38.3, 63.0)/million in seniors) [34], while in China it is almost the same as for MPA.

The Chinese Dong population had the highest proportion of patients with AAV in China, with incidence twofold higher than the national average. They are mainly distributed in Southwestern China and Southern China, which might also contribute to the

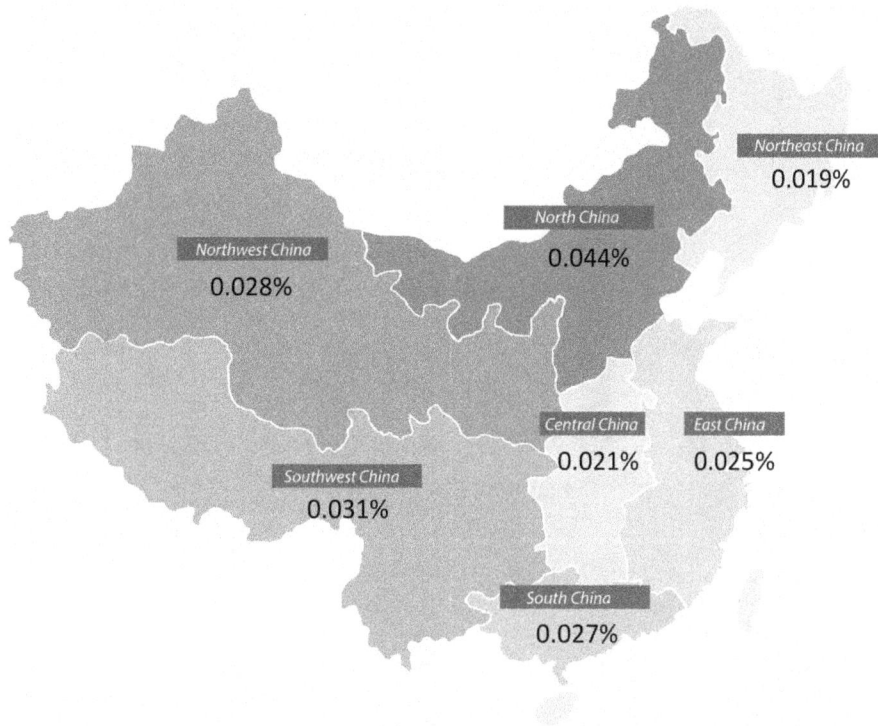

Fig. 3 The distribution of anti-neutrophil cytoplasmic autoantibody associated vasculitis (AAV) according to Chinese geographical regions in 2015. The frequency of AAV in all inpatients in seven geographical regions, with the highest in North China (0.44‰)

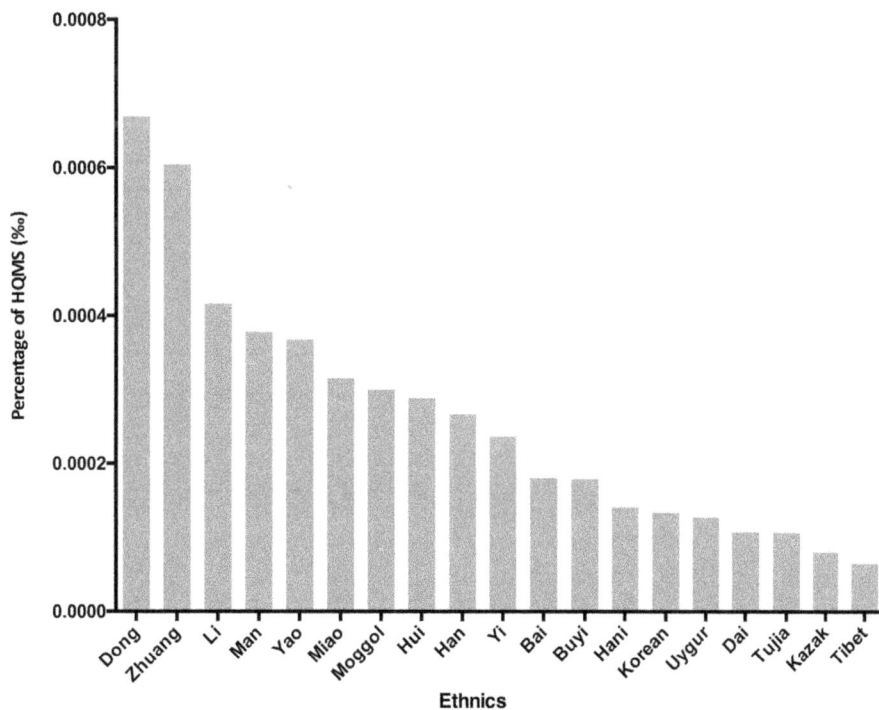

Fig. 4 Ethnic distribution of anti-neutrophil cytoplasmic autoantibody associated vasculitis (AAV) in the Chinese population. The Dong, Zhuang and Li ethnic minorities had the highest frequencies of AAV, with a frequency of 0.67‰, 0.61‰ and 0.42‰, respectively. HQMS, Hospital Quality Monitoring System

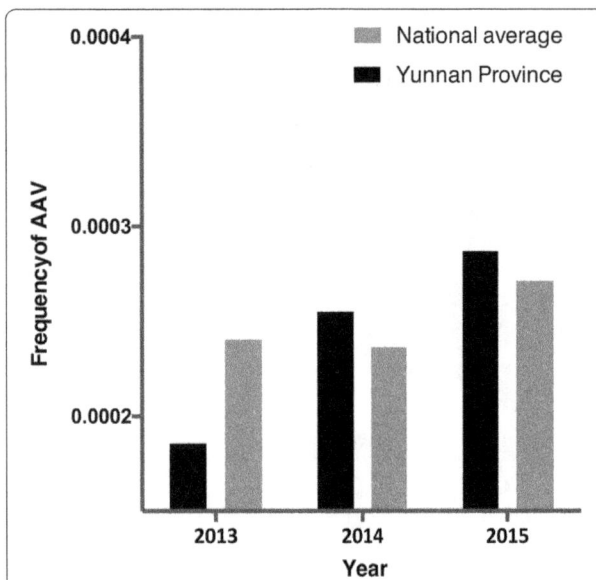

Fig. 5 The proportion of anti-neutrophil cytoplasmic autoantibody associated vasculitis (AAV) in Yunnan province and the national average value since 2013. The frequency of AAV in Yunnan province has increased annually since 2013

relatively high proportion of patients with AAV compared to the provinces in the same latitude, such as Eastern China. Genome-wide association studies (GWAS) have shownd that HLA-DP (rs3117242) variants contribute to the pathogenesis of MPO-ANCA associated vasculitis, while PRTN3 (rs 62,132,295) variants might contribute to PR3-ANCA associated vasculitis [21, 34–37]. Phylogenic studies have revealed that the Chinese Dong population is a distinct population from the Han population, along with the Li and Yao populations, which also had a relatively high frequency of AAV [38]. The Dong population has been shown to have a low prevalence of type II diabetes mellitus (T2D), and seven loci were identified by GWAS to be associated with T2D in the Dong population [39]. Further genetic studies might be able to reveal the genetic variants related to AAV in this race, which might provide a promising opportunity to further explore the pathogenesis of AAV.

Earthquake and the subsequent releasing of silicon has been reported to be associated with the onset of AAV, and to exacerbate disease severity in Kobe, Japan [15, 40]. However, data from New Zealand showed an opposite result [17]. On 3 Aug 2014, there were major earthquakes in Yunnan Province in China, of which the biggest reached 6.5 on the Richter scale. According to the air pollution data published by the National Bureau of Statistics from 2010 to 2015, although there was no significant increase in PM 10, the proportion of AAV had increased 1.37-fold by 2014 in Yunnan province. This phenomenon in our present study supports the hypothesis that release of environment pollutants after earthquake might contribute to the pathogenesis of AAV. However, since our only analysis only included data from 2 years after the earthquake, we might need more follow-up data to finalize our conclusion.

In our study, we found exposure to carbon monoxide (CO) increased the frequency of AAV (R^2 = 0.172, P = 0.025), which seems to be contradictory to the anti-inflammatory effect of CO [41]. It has been proved in animal models that CO might inhibit the activation of T cells in systematic lupus erythematosus (SLE) [42], and alleviate the inflammatory effect of peripheral mononuclear cell-derived MPO in vessels [43, 44]. However, CO could bind hemoglobin and might subsequently prevent oxygen transportation and thus result in oxygen deficiency or hypoxia in cells, which might injure the endothelium. This might suggest harmful effects of CO in vessel inflammation, which still needs in-depth exploration.

This study has several limitations. First, the data in the present study covered only 54.1% of tertiary hospitalized populations in China. Second, the diagnosis of AAV, especially GPA, MPA, and EGPA, in hospitalized patients was based on ICD-10 coding and free text from single hospitalizations with relatively low sensitivity and no laboratory data on patterns and antigenicity in patients with ANCA. Third, 77.4% of patients with AAV had not been classified according to the 2012 CHCC classification, and each subtype was not further analyzed.

Conclusions

In conclusion, in the present study, we provided the first epidemiological data on AAV in hospitalized patients in China, which showed evident seasonal variation, geographic and ethnic clustering, and association with pollution.

Appendix 1

Table 2 The International Classification of Diseases-10 coding of AAV

Disease	ICD-10 coding
AAV	M31.802
MPA	M31.701[#] M31.700[†], M31.702 + G63.5[*†]
GPA	M31.301, K13.407[#] M31.300[†], M31.301, M31.302 + J99.1[*†], M31.303 + N08.5[*†]
EGPA	M30.101

[#]Applicable for ICD-10 (Beijing Version 4.0) only
[†]Applicable for ICD-10 (National Standard Version1.0) only
Abbreviations: ICD-10 International Classification of Diseases-10, AAV anti-neutrophil cytoplasmic autoantibodies associated vasculitis, GPA granulomatosis with polyangiitis, MPA microscopic polyangiitis, EGPA eosinophilic granulomatosis with polyangiitis

Appendix 2

Table 3 The International Classification of Diseases-10 coding of exclusion criteria of AAV and complications

Disease	ICD-10 coding
TAK	M31.401
GCA	M31.501[#], M31.601[#] M31.500[†], M31.600[†]
PAN	M30.002[#] M30.000[†], M30.001 + G73.7[*†], M30.002 + G63.5[*†], M30.003 + G63.5[*†], M30.800[†]
KD	M30.301[#] M30.300[†]
RA	M05.391[#], M05.392[#], M06.811[#], M06.821[#], M06.831[#], M06.841[#], M06.851[#], M06.861[#], M06.871[#], M06.872[#], M06.991[#], M08.091[#] M05.101 + J99.0[*†], M05.102 + J99.0[*†], M05.300+[†], M05.301 + G63.6[*†], M05.302 + I52.8[*†], M05.303 + G73.7[*†], M05.304 + I52.8[*†], M05.305 + I32.8[*†], M05.306 + I41.8[*†], M05.307 + I39.8[*†], M05.308[†], M05.800[†], M05.900, M06.000[†], M06.800[†], M06.900[†], M06.901[†], M06.902[†], M06.903[†], M06.904[†], M06.905[†], M06.906[†], M06.907[†], M06.909[†], M08.800[†], M08.001[†], M08.002[†]
SLE	F06.921[#], M32.001[#], M32.101 + G05.8[*#], M32.102 + I32.8[*#], M32.104 + J99.1[*#], M32.105 + N08.5[*#], M32.107 + J99.1[*#], M32.108 + G63.5[*#], M32.109 + G99.2[*#], M32.110 + G63.5[*#], M32.111 + K67.8[*#], M32.112 + N08.5[*#], M32.113 + N16.4[*#], M32.901[#] M32.000[†], M32.100+[†], M32.101 + N08.5[*†], M32.102 + N16.4[*†], M32.103 + J99.1[*†], M32.104 + I43.8[*†], M32.105 + I32.8[*†], M32.106 + G63.5[*†], M32.107 + G99.2[*†], M32.108 + K77.8[*†], M32.110 + G73.7[*], M32.111 + D77[*], M32.112 + K93.8[*], M32.113 + H36.8[*], M32.114 + G94.8[*†], M32.115[†], M32.800[†], M32.900[†], M32.901[†]
Sarcoidosis	D86.001[#], D86.301[#], D86.102[#], D86.201[#], D86.301[#], D86.802 + G53.2[*#], D86.803 + H22.1[*#], D86.804 + M63.3[*#], D86.805 + I41.8[*#], D86.806 + M14.8[*#], D86.901[#], K13.408[#] D86.000[†], D86.100[†], D86.200[†], D86.300[†], D86.800[†], D86.801[†], D86.802[†], D86.900[†], D86.901[†]
IBD	K50.002, K50.003[#], K50.004[#], K50.005[#], K50.006[#], K50.101, K50.102, K50.103, K50.104, K50.803[#], K50.901[#], K50.902 + M07.4[*#], K51.001[#], K51.002, K51.201[#], K51.301, K51.901, K51.902, K51.903 + M07.5[*#] K50.000[†], K50.001[†], K50.100[†], K50.800[†], K50.801[†], K50.900[†], K50.901[†], K50.902 + M07.4[*†], K51.000[†], K51.001[†], K51.003[†], K51.004[†], K51.005[†], K51.200[†], K51.201[†], K51.202[†], K51.203[†], K51.300[†], K51.302[†], K51.303[†], K51.400[†], K51.401[†], K51.800[†], K51.900[†], K51.903[†], K51.904 + M07.5[*†]
LVV	I77.601[#]; I77.602[#]; I77.603[#]; I77.604[#] M31.400[†]; M31.401[†]
HBV	54.808[#], B18.102[#], B18.103[#], B18.104[#], B18.105[#], B18.106[#], Z22.501[#], Z22.502[#], B16.001[#], B16.002[#], B16.101[#], B16.103[#], B16.104[#], B16.105[#], B16.201[#], B16.202#, B16.901[#], B16.902[#], B16.903[#], B16.905[#], B18.004[#], B18.005[#], B18.006[#], B18.101[#], B18.102[#], B18.103[#], B18.104[#], B18.105[#], B18.106[#] Z22.502[†], Z22.503[†], Z22.504[†], B16.000[†], B16.001[†], B16.100[†], B16.101[†], B16.200[†], B16.201[†], B16.202[†], B16.203[†], B16.204[†], B16.205[†], B16.206[†], B16.900[†], B16.901[†], B16.902[†], B16.903[†], B16.904[†], B16.905[†], B17.000[†], B18.103 + N08.0[*†], B18.104[†], B18.105[†], B18.106[†], B18.107[†], K74.602[†]
HCV	O98.402[#], Z22.591[#], B17.101[#], B17.102[#], B17.103[#], B17.104[#], B17.105[#], B18.201[#], B18.202[#], B18.203[#], B18.205[#], B18.207[#], B18.208[#] Z22.501[†], B18.205 + N08.0[*†], K74.603[†], B17.100[†], B17.101[†], B17.102[†], B17.103[†], B18.200[†], B18.201[†], B18.202[†], B18.203[†], B18.204[†]
Syphillis	A51, A52
Carcinoma	C00-D49
RPGN	N01.701[#], N01.803[#], N01.901[#], N01.902[#], N01.903[#] N01.700[†], N01.800[†], N01.900[†]
Acute nephritis syndrome	N00.901[#], N00.902[#], N00.903[#], N00.801[#], N17.002[#], N17.102[#], N17.201[#], N17.901[#], N17.902[#], N17.903[#], N17.904[#] N00.000[†], N00.100[†], N00.200[†], N00.300[†], N00.400[†], N00.500[†], N00.600[†], N00.700[†], N00.800[†], N00.900[†], N00.902[†]
NS	N04

[#]Applicable for ICD-10 (Beijing Version 4.0) only
[†]Applicable for ICD-10 (National Standard Version1.0) only
Abbreviations: ICD-10 International Classification of Diseases-10, TAK Takayasu arteritis, GCA giant cell arteritis, PAN polyarteritis nodosa, KD Kawasaki disease, LVV large vessel vasculitis, IBD inflammatory bowel disease, SLE systemic lupus erythematosus, RA rheumatoid arthritis, NS nephrotic syndrome, RPGN rapidly progressive glomerulonephritis

Abbreviations

AAV: Anti-neutrophil cytoplasmic autoantibody associated vasculitis; ANCA: Anti-neutrophil cytoplasmic autoantibody; AOD: Aerosol optical depth; CHCC: Chapel Hill Consensus Conference; CI: Confidence interval; CO: Carbon monoxide; EGPA: Eosinophilic granulomatosis with polyangiitis; GPA: Granulomatosis with polyangiitis; GWAS: Genome-wide association study; HLA: Human leukocyte antigen; HQMS: Hospital Quality Monitoring System; ICD: International Classification of Diseases; ICU: Intensive care unit; MPA: Microscopic polyangiitis; MPO: Myeloperoxidase; NASA: National Aeronautics and Space Administration; NO2: Nitrogen dioxide; PM: Particulate matter; SLE: Systemic lupus erythematosus; SO2: Sulfur oxide

Funding

This work is supported by grants of Natural Science Foundation of China to the Innovation Research Group (81621092), the Outstanding Young Scholar (81622009), and other programs (81330020, 81370801). The authors thank the Bureau of Medical Administration and Medical Service Supervision, National Health and Family Planning Commission of the People's Republic of China for the support of this study.

Authors' contributions

JNL and ZC defined the search strategy and analysis; JNL wrote the manuscript; JYL performed data analysis. WH and JWW helped modify the data analysis. HBW, LXZ, MC, and MHZ designed and directed the study, and revised the manuscript. All authors have read and approved the final manuscript.

Consent for publication

Not applicable.

Competing interests

The authors declare that they have no competing interests.

Author details

[1]Renal Division, Department of Medicine, Peking University First Hospital, Peking University Institute of Nephrology, Key Laboratory of Renal Disease, Ministry of Health of China, Key Laboratory of CKD Prevention and Treatment, Ministry of Education of China, Beijing, China. [2]Clinical Trial Unit, First Affiliated Hospital of Sun Yat-Sen University, Guangzhou, China. [3]Department of Occupational and Enviromental Health, Peking University School of Public Health, Beijing, China. [4]China Standard Medical Information Research Center, Shenzhen, Guangdong, China. [5]Peking University, Center for Data Science in Health and Medicine, Beijing, China. [6]Peking-Tsinghua Center for Life Sciences, Beijing, People's Republic of China.

References

1. Furuta S, Jayne DRW. Antineutrophil cytoplasm antibody-associated vasculitis: recent developments. Kidney Int. 2013;84:244–9.
2. Goupil R, Brachemi S, Nadeau-Fredette A-C, Déziel C, Troyanov Y, Lavergne V, Troyanov S. Lymphopenia and treatment-related infectious complications in ANCA-associated vasculitis. Clin J Am Soc Nephrol. 2013;8:416–23.
3. Koldingsnes W, Jacobsen EA, Sildnes T, Hjalmarsen A, Nossent HC. Pulmonary function and high-resolution CT findings five years after disease onset in patients with Wegener's granulomatosis. Scand J Rheumatol. 2005; 34:220–8.
4. Cartin-Ceba R, Diaz-Caballero L, Alqadi MO, Tryfon S, Fervenza FC, Ytterberg SR, Specks U. Diffuse alveolar hemorrhage secondary to ANCA-associated vasculitis: predictors of respiratory failure and clinical outcomes. Arthritis Rheumatol 2016;68(6):1467–76.
5. Bligny D, Mahr A, Toumelin PL, Mouthon L, Guillevin L. Predicting mortality in systemic Wegener's granulomatosis: a survival analysis based on 93 patients. Arthritis Rheum. 2004;51:83–91.
6. Li PKT, Ho KKL, Szeto CC, Yu L, Lai FM-M. Prognostic indicators of IgA nephropathy in the Chinese–clinical and pathological perspectives. Nephrol Dial Transplant. 2002;17:64–9.
7. Wong L, Harper L, Little MA. Getting the balance right: adverse events of therapy in anti-neutrophil cytoplasm antibody vasculitis. Nephrol Dial Transplant. 2015;30(Suppl 1);i164–70.
8. Falk RJ, Hogan S, Carey TS, Jennette JC. Clinical course of anti-neutrophil cytoplasmic autoantibody-associated glomerulonephritis and systemic vasculitis. The Glomerular Disease Collaborative Network. Ann Intern Med. 1990;113:656–63.
9. Jennette JC, Falk RJ, Bacon PA, Basu N, Cid MC, Ferrario F, Flores-Suarez LF, Gross WL, Guillevin L, Hagen EC, Hoffman GS, Jayne DR, Kallenberg CGM, Lamprecht P, Langford CA, Luqmani RA, Mahr AD, Matteson EL, Merkel PA, Ozen S, Pusey CD, Rasmussen N, Rees AJ, Scott DGI, Specks U, Stone JH, Takahashi K, Watts RA. 2012 revised International Chapel Hill Consensus Conference Nomenclature of Vasculitides; 2013. p. 1–11.
10. Falk RJ, Jennette JC. Anti-neutrophil cytoplasmic autoantibodies with specificity for myeloperoxidase in patients with systemic vasculitis and idiopathic necrotizing and crescentic glomerulonephritis. N Engl J Med. 1988;318:1651–7.
11. Kobayashi S, Fujimoto S. Epidemiology of vasculitides: differences between Japan, Europe and North America. Clin Exp Nephrol. 2013;17:611–4.
12. Gómez-Puerta JA, Gedmintas L, Costenbader KH. The association between silica exposure and development of ANCA-associated vasculitis: systematic review and meta-analysis. Autoimmun Rev. 2013;12:1129 35.
13. Pelclová D, Bartůnková J, Fenclová Z, Lebedová J, Hladíková M, Benáková H. Asbestos exposure and antineutrophil cytoplasmic antibody (ANCA) positivity. Arch Environ Health. 2003;58:662–8.
14. Wichmann I, Sanchez-Roman J, Morales J, Castillo MJ, Ocaña C, Nuñez-Roldan A. Antimyeloperoxidase antibodies in individuals with occupational exposure to silica. Ann Rheum Dis. 1996;55:205–7.
15. Yashiro M, Muso E, Itoh-Ihara T, Oyama A, Hashimoto K, Kawamura T, Ono T, Sasayama S. Significantly high regional morbidity of MPO-ANCA-related angitis and/or nephritis with respiratory tract involvement after the 1995 great earthquake in Kobe (Japan). Am J Kidney Dis. 2000;35:889–95.
16. Gatenby PA. Anti-neutrophil cytoplasmic antibody-associated systemic vasculitis: nature or nurture? Intern Med J. 2012;42:351–9.
17. Farquhar HJ, McGettigan B, Chapman PT, O'Donnell JL, Frampton C, Stamp LK. Incidence of anti-neutrophil cytoplasmic antibody-associated vasculitis before and after the February 2011 Christchurch earthquake. Intern Med J. 2017;47:57–61.
18. Stegeman CA, Tervaert JW, Sluiter WJ, Manson WL, de Jong PE, Kallenberg CG. Association of chronic nasal carriage of Staphylococcus aureus and higher relapse rates in Wegener granulomatosis. Ann Intern Med. 1994;120:12–7.
19. Popa ER, Stegeman CA, Kallenberg CGM, Tervaert JWC. Staphylococcus aureus and Wegener's granulomatosis. Arthritis Res. 2002;4:77–9.
20. Hamidou MA, Audrain M, Ninin E, Robillard N, Muller J-Y, Bonneville M. Staphylococcus aureus, T-cell repertoire, and Wegener's granulomatosis. Joint Bone Spine. 2001;68:373–7.
21. Lyons PA, Rayner TF, Trivedi S, Holle JU, Watts RA, Jayne DRW, Baslund B, Brenchley P, Bruchfeld A, Chaudhry AN, Cohen Tervaert JW, Deloukas P, Feighery C, Gross WL, Guillevin L, Gunnarsson I, Harper L, Hrušková Z, Little MA, Martorana D, Neumann T, Ohlsson S, Padmanabhan S, Pusey CD, Salama AD, Sanders J-SF, Savage CO, Segelmark M, Stegeman CA, Tesař V, Vaglio A, Wieczorek S, Wilde B, Zwerina J, Rees AJ, Clayton DG, Smith KGC. Genetically distinct subsets within ANCA-associated vasculitis. N Engl J Med. 2012;367:214–23.
22. Sreih AG, Mandhadi R, Aldaghlawi F, Khan A, Irshad V, Finn K, Block JA. ANCA-associated vasculitis in Hispanic Americans: an unrecognized severity. Clin Rheumatol. 2014;34:943–8.
23. Bjørneklett R, Vikse BE, Svarstad E, Aasarød K, Bostad L, Langmark F, Iversen BM. Long-term risk of cancer in membranous nephropathy patients. Am J Kidney Dis. 2007;50:396–403.
24. Ponticelli C, Passerini P, Salvadori M, Manno C, Viola BF, Pasquali S, Mandolfo S, Messa P. A randomized pilot trial comparing methylprednisolone plus a cytotoxic agent versus synthetic adrenocorticotropic hormone in idiopathic membranous nephropathy. Am J Kidney Dis. 2006;47:233–40.
25. Chen M, Yu F, Zhang Y, Zou W-Z, Zhao M-H, Wang H-Y. Characteristics of Chinese patients with Wegener's granulomatosis with anti-myeloperoxidase autoantibodies. Kidney Int. 2005;68:2225–9.
26. Chen M, Yu F, Wang S-X, Zou W-Z, Zhang Y, Zhao M-H, Wang H-Y. Renal histology in Chinese patients with anti-myeloperoxidase autoantibody-positive Wegener's granulomatosis. Nephrol Dial Transplant. 2007;22:139–45.
27. Ma WL, Liu LY, Tian CG, Qi H, Jia HL, Song WW, Li YF. Polycyclic aromatic hydrocarbons in Chinese surface soil: occurrence and distribution. Environ Sci Pollut Res Int. 2015;22:4190–200.
28. Zhang Y-L, Cao F. Fine particulate matter (PM 2.5) in China at a city level. Sci Rep. 2015;5:14884.
29. Watts RA, Gonzalez-Gay MA, Lane SE, Garcia-Porrua C, Bentham G, Scott DG. Geoepidemiology of systemic vasculitis: comparison of the incidence in two regions of Europe. Ann Rheum Dis. 2001;60:170–2.
30. Ormerod AS, Cook MC. Epidemiology of primary systemic vasculitis in the Australian Capital Territory and South-Eastern New South Wales. Intern Med J. 2008;38:816–23.
31. O'Donnell JL, Stevanovic VR, Frampton C, Stamp LK, Chapman PT. Wegener's granulomatosis in New Zealand: evidence for a latitude-dependent incidence gradient. Intern Med J. 2007;37:242–6.
32. Gatenby PA. Anti-neutrophil cytoplasmic antibody-associated systemic vasculitis: nature or nurture? Intern Med J. 2012;42:1066–7.
33. Gatenby PA, Lucas RM, Engelsen O, Ponsonby A-L, Clements M. Antineutrophil cytoplasmic antibody-associated vasculitides: could geographic patterns be explained by ambient ultraviolet radiation? Arthritis Rheum. 2009;61:1417–24.

34. Fujimoto S, Watts RA, Kobayashi S, Suzuki K, Jayne DR, Scott DG, Hashimoto H, Nunoi H. Comparison of the epidemiology of anti-neutrophil cytoplasmic antibody-associated vasculitis between Japan and the UK. Rheumatology. 2011;50(10):1916–20.

35. Tsuchiya N, Kobayashi S, Kawasaki A, Kyogoku C, Arimura Y, Yoshida M, Tokunaga K, Hashimoto H. Genetic background of Japanese patients with antineutrophil cytoplasmic antibody-associated vasculitis: association of HLA-DRB1*0901 with microscopic polyangiitis. J Rheumatol. 2003;30:1534–40.

36. Tsuchiya N, Kobayashi S, Hashimoto H, Ozaki S, Tokunaga K. Association of HLA-DRB1*0901-DQB1*0303 haplotype with microscopic polyangiitis in Japanese. Genes Immun. 2006;7:81–4.

37. Nakamaru Y, Maguchi S, Takizawa M, Fukuda S, Inuyama Y. The association between human leukocyte antigens (HLA) and cytoplasmic-antineutrophil cytoplasmic antibody (cANCA)-positive Wegener's granulomatosis in a Japanese population. Rhinology. 1996;34:163–5.

38. Chu JY, Huang W, Kuang SQ, Wang JM, Xu JJ, Chu ZT, Yang ZQ, Lin KQ, Li P, Wu M, Geng ZC, Tan CC, Du RF, Jin L. Genetic relationship of populations in China. Proc Natl Acad Sci USA. 1998;95(20):11763–8.

39. Liu L, Chen L, Li Z, Li L, Qu J, Xue J. Association between gene polymorphisms of seven newly identified loci and type 2 diabetes and the correlate quantitative traits in Chinese dong populations. Iran J Public Health. 2014;43:1345–55.

40. Yashiro M, Muso E, Itoh T, Oyama A, Ono T, Sasayama S. Significantly high incidence and high morbidity of acute renal failure with respiratory tract involvement of p-ANCA-related angitis revealed in Kobe city and the environs after the Kobe earthquake in 1995. Clin Nephrol. 1999;51:190–1.

41. Nagao S, Taguchi K, Sakai H, Yamasaki K, Watanabe H, Otagiri M, Maruyama T. Carbon monoxide-bound hemoglobin vesicles ameliorate multiorgan injuries induced by severe acute pancreatitis in mice by their anti-inflammatory and antioxidant properties. Int J Nanomedicine. 2016;11:5611–20.

42. Mackern-Oberti JP, Obreque J, Méndez GP, Llanos C, Kalergis AM. Carbon monoxide inhibits T cell activation in target organs during systemic lupus erythematosus. Clin Exp Immunol. 2015;182:1–13.

43. Patterson EK, Fraser DD, Capretta A, Potter RF, Cepinskas G. Carbon monoxide-releasing molecule 3 inhibits myeloperoxidase (MPO) and protects against MPO-induced vascular endothelial cell activation/dysfunction. Free Radic Biol Med. 2014;70:167–73.

44. Wang X, Qin W, Song M, Zhang Y, Sun B. Exogenous carbon monoxide inhibits neutrophil infiltration in LPS-induced sepsis by interfering with FPR1 via p38 MAPK but not GRK2. Oncotarget. 2016;7:34250–65.

3

Interferon-λ3/4 genetic variants and interferon-λ3 serum levels are biomarkers of lupus nephritis and disease activity

Ji-Yih Chen[1*], Chin-Man Wang[2], Tai-Di Chen[3], Yeong-Jian Jan Wu[1], Jing-Chi Lin[1], Ling Ying Lu[4*] and Jianming Wu[5*]

Abstract

Background: Type III interferons (IFNs) or IFN-λs are the newly discovered cytokines that primarily target the cells of epithelial and myeloid lineages, which are major components of kidneys. The current study aimed to investigate whether IFN-λs are involved in the pathogenesis of systemic lupus erythematosus (SLE) and lupus nephritis.

Methods: TaqMan allele discrimination assays were used to determine *IFNL3/4* SNP genotypes of 1620 healthy controls and 1013 SLE patients (two independent cohorts consisting of 831 and 182 subjects, respectively) from Taiwan. The distributions of *IFNL3/4* SNP genotypes and allele frequencies were compared between SLE patients and healthy controls and among SLE patients stratified by clinical phenotypes. ELISA was used to determine the serum IFN-λ3 concentrations of SLE patients.

Results: All major *IFN3/4* SNP alleles were significantly associated with the risk for lupus nephritis (rs8099917T, $P_{FDR} = 0.0021$, OR 1.75, 95% CI 1.24–2.47; rs12979860C, $P_{FDR} = 0.0034$, OR 1.65, 95% CI 1.18–2.30; rs4803217C, $P_{FDR} = 0.0021$, OR 1.76, 95% CI 1.25–2.48; and ss469415590TT, $P_{FDR} = 0.0021$, OR 1.73, 95% CI 1.23–2.42) among SLE patients. Similarly, the major *IFNL3/4* SNP haplotype rs8099917T-ss469415590TT-rs12979860C-rs4803217C (or T-TT-C-C) was a significant risk factor for lupus nephritis ($P = 0.0015$, OR 1.68, 95% CI 1.22–2.32). Additionally, all minor *IFN3/4* SNP alleles were significantly associated with SLE susceptibility in nephritis-negative SLE patients as compared to normal healthy controls (rs8099917G, $P_{FDR} = 0.00177$, OR 1.68, 95% CI 1.24–2.28; rs12979860T, $P_{FDR} = 0.00299$, OR 1.58, 95% CI 1.18–2.32; rs4803217A, $P_{FDR} = 0.00176$, OR 1.65, 95% CI 1.22–2.23; and ss469415590ΔG, $P_{FDR} = 0.00176$, OR 1.70, 95% CI 1.26–2.29). Furthermore, the elevated serum levels of IFN-λ3 were significantly correlated with the complement depression and the high SLE disease activities in SLE patients.

Conclusions: *IFN-λ3/4* genetic variants play a unique role in the development of lupus nephritis and SLE.

Keywords: Interferon λ, Lupus nephritis, Systemic lupus erythematosus

* Correspondence: jychen31@adm.cgmh.org.tw; lylu@vghks.gov.tw; jmwu@umn.edu
[1]Department of Medicine, Division of Allergy, Immunology and Rheumatology, Chang Gung Memorial Hospital, Chang Gung University College of Medicine, No. 5, Fu-Shin St. Kwei-Shan, Tao-Yuan, Taiwan
[4]Department of Medicine, Division of Allergy Immunology and Rheumatology, Kaohsiung Veterans General Hospital, No. 386, Dazhong 1st Rd, Zuoying District, Kaohsiung City 81362, Taiwan
[5]Department of Veterinary and Biomedical Sciences, Department of Medicine, University of Minnesota, 235B Animal Science/Vet. Med. Bldg, 1988 Fitch Avenue, St. Paul, MN 55108, USA
Full list of author information is available at the end of the article

Background

Systemic lupus erythematosus (SLE) is a prototypic auto-immune disease resulting from abnormal immune responses of immune cells including dendritic cells (DCs), macrophages, monocytes, neutrophils, and lymphocytes [1, 2]. In addition, nonimmune cells such as endothelial, epithelial, and renal tubular cells contribute to the development of SLE [3]. Genetic studies have identified multiple genes involved in the pathogenesis of SLE. However, the functional roles of various risk genes in the development of SLE remain incompletely understood.

Type III interferons (IFNs) or IFN-λs (IFNLs) are newly discovered cytokines that mediate diverse immune functions [4]. Located at chromosome 19q13, the IFN-λ gene family consists of four newly identified members: IL-29 (IFN-λ1 or IFNL1), IL-28A (IFN-λ2 or IFNL2), IL-28B (IFN-λ3 or IFNL3), and IFN-λ4 (IFNL4). IFN-λs are mainly produced by monocytes, macrophages, DCs, and bronchial epithelial cells in response to viral infections [4]. IFN-λs bind to a distinct receptor complex (IL-28RA/IL-10Rβ) that is primarily expressed by cells of epithelial origin (respiratory, intestinal, and reproductive tract epithelial cells, hepatocytes, and keratinocytes) and myeloid linage [4]. IFN-λs exert highly circumscribed antiviral effects through intracellular activation of anti-viral host factors in the infected cells, similar to the type I IFNs [5]. Accumulating evidence suggests that IFN-λs have a unique role in regulating innate and adaptive immune responses targeting microbial infections of epithelial cells expressing cognate receptor complexes [4, 6].

Type I IFNs (IFN-α, IFN-β, IFN-ε, and IFN-ω) initiate signal transduction cascades leading to expression of IFN-stimulated genes (ISGs) that control virus replication [7]. The expression of type I IFNs and type I IFN-inducible genes is significantly increased in patients with SLE, pointing to a role of type I IFNs in SLE pathogenesis [7–10]. High levels of circulating type I IFNs and type I IFN-induced cell activation are heritable traits in families with SLE, suggesting that the alleles responsible for a strong type I IFN activation pathway are risk factors for the development of SLE [11–13]. While IFN-λs mediate antiviral functions similar to the type I IFNs [4], the role of IFN-λs in the development of SLE remains unknown as the IFNL locus was not revealed by genome-wide association studies (GWAS) [14, 15]. In particular, the IFN-λ3 SNPs (rs8099917, rs12979860, and rs4803217) in strong linkage disequilibrium with the IFN-λ4 SNP rs368234815 (TT/ΔG) have been suggested to influence IFN-λ3 mRNA stability, IFN-λ3/4 expression, ISG levels, and the response to IFN-α treatment [16]. The present study was aimed to investigate whether the IFN-λ3/4 genes are associated with SLE susceptibility and disease phenotypes in Taiwanese.

Methods

Study participants and disease activity assessment

SLE patients were recruited at the Rheumatology Clinics of Chang Gung Memorial Hospital. All SLE patients fulfilled the 1982 and 1997 American College of Rheumatology (ACR) criteria for the classification of SLE [17]. Lupus activity was assessed according to the SLE Disease Activity Index (SLEDAI) [18], which defines SLEDAI > 4 as high SLE disease activity. Ethnically matched healthy controls were recruited following a questionnaire survey to ensure that the control subjects were free of any autoimmune diseases. The human study was approved by the ethics committees of Chang Gung Memorial Hospital. All subjects provided written consent to participate in human studies according to the Declaration of Helsinki.

Genomic DNA extraction

Genomic DNA was extracted from anticoagulated peripheral blood using the Gentra Puregene DNA isolation kit.

SNP genotype assays

Validated made-for-order TaqMan SNP assays (Applied Biosystems, Foster City, CA, USA) were used for genotype analyses of the SNPs at the *IFNL3/4* locus. The TaqMan allele discrimination assays were carried out on an ABI ViiA 7 Real-time PCR System (Applied Biosystems) using probes labeled with fluorescent dyes (FAM and VIC) and nonfluorescent quencher according to the vendor's instructions.

Serum complement assay

Serum concentrations of complement C4 and C3 were determined by nephelometry. Complement depression was defined as the detection of both lower serum C4 (concentration < 100 mg/L) and C3 (concentration < 700 mg/L).

Serum IFNL3 assay

An IFNL3 ELISA kit (catalog no. CSB-E13296h; CUSABIO, College Park, MD, USA) was used to measure serum IFNL levels of SLE patients according to the manufacturer's instructions.

Immunohistochemistry to detect IL-28B and IL-28 receptor in kidney tissue

The presence of IL-28B and expression of IL-28 receptor in kidney tissue were examined using kidney biopsies of lupus patients. Slides with the kidney biopsy sections were blocked with goat serum before being incubated with primary anti-IFNL3 antibodies (catalog no. A12908; ABclonal) and anti-IL-28 receptor alpha antibodies (catalog no. ab224395; Abcam) for 30 min at room temperature. The slides were washed three times with PBS before the addition of HRP-conjugated goat anti-mouse secondary antibodies. After extensive washing,

DAB substrate was added to the slides for the detection of IFNL3 and IL-28 receptor.

Statistical analysis

The Hardy–Weinberg equilibrium (HWE) was examined for all SNPs using chi-square tests. Three chi-square tests (the genotype test, the allele test, and the Cochran–Armitage trend test) were carried out with the SAS/Genetics software package release 8.2 (SAS Institute, Cary, NC, USA) to determine associations between individual SNPs and SLE susceptibility. To investigate the association between SNPs and SLE clinical manifestations, we stratified the clinical phenotypes according to SLE diagnosis criteria and assigned those SLE patients positive for a phenotype as "+" cases and assigned those negative as "–" cases. The allele and genotype distributions of SNPs between "+" cases and "–" cases were compared. The additive, dominant, and recessive models were used to analyze associations between SNP genotypes and phenotypes. To investigate the independent association between SLE clinical characteristics and SNP alleles/genotypes, multivariate logistic regressions were performed. The additive, dominant, and recessive allele effects for each SNP were modeled as the response variables and two categories of cases ("+" cases, "–" cases) were used as the independent variables pertaining to each clinical phenotype. In addition, logistic regressions adjusted for age and sex were used to calculate P values, odds ratios (ORs), and 95% confidence intervals (CIs) of risk alleles or genotypes. To account for multiple testing, Benjamini and Hochberg's linear step-up method was carried out using the SAS MULTTEST procedure [19]. The false discovery rate (FDR)-adjusted P values are defined in a step-up fashion, with less conservative multipliers and control. A corrected P value (P_{FDR}) less than 0.05 was considered statistically significant.

Linkage disequilibrium patterns of the IFNL3/4 locus SNPs (Additional file 1: Figure S1) were analyzed by Haploview 4.2 (Broad Institute, Cambridge, MA, USA; http://www.broad.mit.edu/mpg/haploview). Haplotype information was inferred and frequencies were estimated using the HAPLOTYPE procedure of SAS 9.2 (SAS Institute). Haplotype frequency differences were then assessed between SLE cases and controls and between cases positive for and cases negative for a specific phenotype among SLE patients. To evaluate the independent association of each haplotype category, the permutation ($N = 10,000$) P values were calculated using the EM algorithm conditioned on the other haplotypes. Logistic regressions adjusted for sex and age were used to investigate the association between haplotype and SLE susceptibility and between cases positive for nephritis and cases negative for nephritis. Unpaired t tests were used to analyze the serum IFNL3 levels among SLE

patients using GraphPad Prism 6.0 (GraphPad, La Jolla, CA, USA). $P < 0.05$ was considered significant.

Results
Characteristics of SLE patients

SLE patients (71 males and 760 females) and healthy controls (701 males and 919 females) were used in the genetic analyses of four SNPs (rs8099917, rs12979860, rs3682134815, and rs4803217) at the IFNL3/4 locus (Additional file 1: Figure S1). The age onset of 831 SLE cases ranged from 8 to 77 years with an average age of 30.77 years (SD = 11.73) (Table 1). SLE cases consisted of 8.54% (71/831) males with an average age of 31.72 years (SD = 12.36) and 91.46% (760/831) females with an average age of 30.68 years (SD = 11.68). The ages of 1620 healthy controls ranged from 18 to 64 years and the average age of healthy controls was 41.22 years (SD = 10.47). The healthy controls consisted of 43.27% (701/1620) males with an average age of 40.26 years (SD = 9.26) and 56.73% (919/1620) females with an average age of 40.23 years (SD = 12.02). The clinical characteristics of the 831 SLE patients are presented in Table 1. Among the SLE patients, 55.48% (461/831) were positive for lupus nephritis (Table 1) according to the 1997 ACR diagnostic criteria either persistent proteinuria of greater than 0.5 g/d (or 3+ proteins on dipstick) or cellular casts of any type. For confirmation, another cohort of 182 SLE (100 with nephritis and 82 without nephritis) patients was used for lupus nephritis findings.

Association of IFNL3/4 SNPs with SLE susceptibility in patients negative for nephritis

Among four IFNL4 SNPs, the distributions of three SNP genotypes were consistent with the Hardy–Weinberg equilibrium in both SLE patients and healthy controls. Only the IFNL4 SNP ss469415590TT>ΔG (or rs3682134815) genotype distribution deviated from Hardy–Weinberg equilibrium, which is likely caused by the positive selection of the ss469415590TT allele favorable for humans fighting against viral infections [20–24]. We examined the single-locus association of four candidate SNPs in 831 SLE patients and 1620 healthy controls. As shown in Table 2, all four minor IFNL3/4 SNP alleles (rs8099917G, rs12979860T, rs4803217A, and ss469415590ΔG) tended to associate with SLE susceptibility in the Cochran–Armitage trend test (rs8099917G, $P_{FDR} = 0.009$; rs12979860T, $P_{FDR} = 0.0225$; rs4803217A, $P_{FDR} = 0.009$; ss469415590ΔG, $P_{FDR} = 0.0398$). Nevertheless, the association between IFNL3/4 SNPs and SLE susceptibility was not significant after adjustment for sex and age ($P_{FDR} > 0.10$). Subsequently, we analyzed the association between IFNL3/4 SNPs and SLE susceptibility after stratifying SLE patients based on positivity of lupus nephritis. As shown in Table 2, all minor IFNL3/4 SNP

Table 1 Clinical characteristics of 831 Taiwanese SLE patients

	Count/available (%)	Male (N = 71)	Female (N = 760)
SLE case	831/831 (100.00%)	71/831 (8.54%)	760/831 (91.46%)
Age (years), mean ± standard deviation	30.77 ± 11.73	31.72 ± 12.36	30.68 ± 11.68
Oral ulcer	218/831 (26.23%)	14/71 (19.72%)	204/760 (26.84%)
Arthritis	522/831 (62.82%)	39/71 (54.93%)	483/760 (63.55%)
Malar rash	459/831 (55.23%)	39/71 (54.93%)	420/760 (55.26%)
Discoid rash	160/831 (19.25%)	18/71 (25.35%)	142/760 (18.68%)
Photosensitivity	187/831 (22.5%)	14/71 (19.72%)	173/760 (22.76%)
Pleural effusion	158/831 (19.01%)	12/71 (16.9%)	146/760 (19.21%)
Pericardial effusion	100/831 (12.03%)	13/71 (18.31%)	87/760 (11.45%)
Ascites	43/831 (5.17%)	3/71 (4.23%)	40/760 (5.26%)
Total counts for nephritis status	831 (100%)	71 (100%)	760 (100%)
Nephritis negative	370/831 (44.52%)	25/71 (35.21%)	345/760 (45.39%)
Nephritis positive	461/831 (55.48%)	46/71 (64.79%)	415/760 (54.61%)
Neuropsychiatric manifestations	133/831 (16%)	10/71 (14.08%)	123/760 (16.18%)
Leukopenia (WBC count < 3500/µl)	466/831 (56.08%)	41/71 (57.75%)	425/760 (55.92%)
Anemia (hemoglobin < 9 g/dl)	252/831 (30.32%)	11/71 (15.49%)	241/760 (31.71%)
Thrombocytopenia (platelet count < 10^5/µl)	215/831 (25.87%)	23/71 (32.39%)	192/760 (25.26%)
Anti-dsDNA	618/813 (76.01%)	54/70 (77.14%)	564/743 (75.91%)
Complement depressed	632/818 (77.26%)	54/69 (78.26%)	578/749 (77.17%)
Anti-RNP	292/677 (43.13%)	24/62 (38.71%)	268/615 (43.58%)
Anti-Sm	256/678 (37.76%)	28/63 (44.44%)	228/615 (37.07%)
Anti-SSA	362/560 (64.64%)	30/48 (62.5%)	332/512 (64.84%)
Anti-SSB	149/560 (26.61%)	8/48 (16.67%)	141/512 (27.54%)
Anticardiolipin IgG	184/655 (28.09%)	12/50 (24%)	172/605 (28.43%)
Anticardiolipin IgM	55/600 (9.17%)	4/48 (8.33%)	51/552 (9.24%)

Data presented as count/available (%)
SLE systemic lupus erythematosus, *WBC* white blood cell

alleles were significantly associated with SLE susceptibility in patients negative for nephritis compared to healthy controls adjusted for sex and age (rs8099917G, P_{FDR} = 0.00177, OR 1.68, 95% CI 1.24–2.28; rs12979860T, P_{FDR} = 0.00299, OR 1.58, 95% CI 1.18–2.32; rs4803217A, P_{FDR} = 0.00176, OR 1.65, 95% CI 1.22–2.23; and ss469415590ΔG, P_{FDR} = 0.00176, OR 1.70, 95% CI 1.26–2.29). In contrast, *IFN3/4* SNPs were not associated with SLE susceptibility in nephritis-positive patients (P_{FDR} > 0.9). Our data suggest that IFN-λ genetic variants may be a risk factor for the development of SLE in the subset of lupus nephritis-negative patients.

Association of *IFNL3/4* SNPs with lupus nephritis
As a common phenotype, lupus nephritis represents a severe form of SLE. We subsequently analyzed whether *IFNL3/4* SNPs were associated with lupus nephritis among SLE patients. Table 3 shows that all major alleles of four *IFNL3/4* SNPs were significantly associated with the risk for nephritis (logistic regression analyses adjusted

for sex and age: rs8099917T, P_{FDR} = 0.0021, OR 1.75, 95% CI 1.24–2.47; rs12979860C, P_{FDR} = 0.0034, OR 1.65, 95% CI 1.18–2.30; rs4803217C, P_{FDR} = 0.0021, OR 1.76, 95% CI 1.25–2.48; and ss469415590TT, P_{FDR} = 0.0021, OR 1.73, 95% CI 1.23–2.42). Our data show that the homozygosity of major alleles of four *IFNL3/4* SNPs is a major risk for lupus nephritis in SLE patients (Table 3). However, *IFNL3/4* SNPs were not significant associated with other manifestations such as arthritis, malar rash, leukopenia, positivity of anti-dsDNA/anti-RNP autoantibodies, and depressed complement levels among SLE patients (data not shown).

Association of *IFNL3/4* SNP haplotypes with lupus nephritis
IFNL3/4 SNPs are in strong linkage disequilibrium (Additional file 1: Figure S2). Subsequently, we used haplotype analysis to determine whether *IFNL3/4* SNP haplotypes (rs8099917, ss469415590, rs12979860, and rs4803217) are associated with the risk for nephritis

Table 2 Association of *IFNL3/4* SNPs with SLE susceptibility

SNP	Risk allele frequency	Genotype frequency			P_{Trend}[a]	P_{FDR}	Unadjusted[b]			Adjusted for sex and age[b]		
							P	P_{FDR}	OR (95% CI)	P	P_{FDR}	OR (95% CI)
rs809991T > G	G	GG	GT	TT								
SLE	129 (7.76%)	3 (0.36%)	123 (14.8%)	705 (84.84%)	0.0035	0.009	0.0033	0.0084	1.42 (1.12–1.79)	0.1144	0.1144	1.26 (0.95–1.67)
Nephritis negative	75 (10.14%)	2 (0.54%)	71 (19.19%)	297 (80.27%)	0	0	8.57E–06	2.14E–05	1.90 (1.43–2.52)	0.00077	0.00177	1.68 (1.24–2.28)
Nephritis positive	54 (5.86%)	1 (0.22%)	52 (11.28%)	408 (88.50%)	0.7508	0.9401	0.74389	0.90622	1.05 (0.77–1.44)	0.91081	0.99622	1.02 (0.72–1.44)
Control	181 (5.57%)	8 (0.49%)	165 (10.16%)	1451 (89.35%)								
rs12979860C > T	T	CC	CT	TT								
SLE	133 (8%)	702 (84.48%)	125 (15.04%)	4 (0.48%)	0.0135	0.0225	0.0121	0.0202	1.34 (1.07–1.67)	0.0968	0.1144	1.26 (0.96–1.66)
Nephritis negative	76 (10.27%)	297 (80.27%)	70 (18.92%)	3 (0.81%)	0.0004	0.0005	7.19E–05	8.99E–05	1.75 (1.33–2.30)	0.00239	0.00299	1.58 (1.18–2.12)
Nephritis positive	57 (6.18%)	405 (87.85%)	55 (11.93%)	1 (0.22%)	0.9401	0.9401	0.89714	0.90622	1.02 (0.76–1.38)	0.87007	0.99622	1.03 (0.74–1.43)
Control	197 (6.07%)	1437 (88.49%)	177 (10.90%)	10 (0.62%)								
rs4803217C > A	A	AA	AC	CC								
SLE	131 (7.88%)	3 (0.36%)	125 (15.04%)	703 (84.6%)	0.0036	0.009	0.0029	0.0084	1.43 (1.13–1.8)	0.0386	0.1137	1.35 (1.02–1.8)
Nephritis negative	76 (10.27%)	2 (0.54%)	72 (19.46%)	296 (80.00%)	0	0	2.37E–05	3.96E–05	1.82 (1.38–2.41)	0.00106	0.00176	1.65 (1.22–2.23)
Nephritis positive	55 (5.97%)	1 (0.22%)	53 (11.50%)	407 (88.29%)	0.9368	0.9401	0.90622	0.90622	1.02 (0.75–1.38)	0.99622	0.99622	1.00 (0.71–1.40)
Control	190 (5.86%)	9 (0.56%)	172 (10.61%)	1440 (88.83%)								
ss469415590TT>ΔG[b]	ΔG	ΔG/ΔG	ΔG/TT	TT/TT								
SLE	142 (8.6%)	10 (1.21%)	122 (14.77%)	694 (84.02%)			0.0293	0.0367	1.26 (1.02–1.55)	0.0571	0.1137	1.28 (0.99–1.65)
Nephritis negative	76 (10.35%)	3 (0.82%)	70 (19.07%)	294 (80.11%)	0	0	7.87E–06	2.14E–05	1.89 (1.43–2.50)	0.00058	0.00176	1.70 (1.26–2.29)
Nephritis positive	54 (5.88%)	1 (0.22%)	52 (11.33%)	406 (88.45%)	0.875	0.9401	0.83482	0.90622	1.03 (0.76–1.41)	0.98182	0.99622	1.00 (0.71–1.40)
Control	185 (5.70%)	8 (0.49%)	169 (10.41%)	1446 (89.09%)								

Data presented as *n* (%)

SLE systemic lupus erythematosus, *SNP* single-nucleotide polymorphism, *OR* odds ratio, *CI* confidence interval

[a]Trend test *P* values generated from 10,000 permutations

[b]Additive model used to test mode of inheritance

Table 3 Association of *IFNL3/4* SNPs with lupus nephritis among SLE patients

SNP	Risk allele frequency	Genotype frequency			P_{Trend}[a]	P_{FDR}	Test for mode of inheritance unadjusted				Test for mode of inheritance adjusted for sex and age			
								P	P_{FDR}	OR (95% CI)		P	P_{FDR}	OR (95% CI)
rs8099917 T > G	T	GG	GT	TT			Additive				Additive			
Nephritis+	1058 (94.30%)	1 (0.18%)	62 (11.05%)	498 (88.77%)	0.001	0.0016		0.0018	0.0024	1.73 (1.23–2.45)		0.0016	0.0021	1.75 (1.24–2.47)
Cohort 1	868 (94.14%)	1 (0.22%)	52 (11.28%)	408 (88.5%)			TT + GT vs GG	0.45681	0.657	2.49 (0.23–27.60)	TT vs GT + GG	0.4705	0.684	2.42 (0.22–26.82)
Cohort 2	190 (95.00%)	0 (0.00%)	10 (10.00%)	90 (90.00%)										
Nephritis−	818 (90.69%)	2 (0.44%)	80 (17.74%)	369 (81.82%)			TT vs GT + GG	0.0019	0.0025	1.76 (1.23–2.50)	TT + GT vs GG	0.0016	0.0022	1.77 (1.24–2.53)
Cohort 1	665 (89.86%)	2 (0.54%)	71 (19.19%)	297 (80.27%)										
Cohort 2	153 (94.44%)	0 (0.00%)	9 (11.11%)	72 (88.89%)										
rs12979860 T > C	C	CC	CT	TT			Additive				Additive			
Nephritis+	1053 (93.85%)	494 (88.06%)	65 (11.59%)	2 (0.36%)	0.0042	0.0042		0.0036	0.0036	1.64 (1.18–2.29)		0.0034	0.0034	1.65 (1.18–2.30)
Cohort 1	865 (93.82%)	405 (87.85%)	55 (11.93%)	1 (0.22%)			CC + CT vs TT	0.4949	0.4949	1.87 (0.31–11.22)	CC vs CT + TT	0.5153	0.5153	1.81 (0.30–10.91)
Cohort 2	188 (94.00%)	89 (89.00%)	10 (10.00%)	1 (1.00%)										
Nephritis−	817 (90.38%)	368 (81.42%)	81 (17.92%)	3 (0.66%)			CC vs CT + TT	0.0034	0.0136	1.68(1.19–2.38)	CC + CT vs TT	0.0031	0.0123	1.69 (1.19–2.40)
Cohort 1	664 (89.73%)	297 (80.27%)	70 (18.92%)	3 (0.81%)										
Cohort 2	153 (93.29%)	71 (86.59%)	11 (13.41%)	0 (0.00%)										
rs4803217 C > A	C	AA	AC	CC			Additive				Additive			
Nephritis+	1055 (94.20%)	2 (0.36%)	61 (10.89%)	497 (88.75%)	0.0012	0.0016		0.0012	0.0024	1.76(1.25–2.47)		0.0011	0.0021	1.76 (1.25–2.48)
Cohort 1	867 (94.03%)	1 (0.22%)	53 (11.5%)	407 (88.29%)			CC + AC vs AA	0.8300	0.83	1.24 (0.17–8.84)	CC vs AC + AA	0.8531	0.8531	1.20 (0.17–8.58)
Cohort 2	188 (94.95%)	1 (1.01%)	8 (8.08%)	90 (90.91%)										
Nephritis−	817 (90.38%)	2 (0.44%)	83 (18.36%)	367 (81.19%)			CC vs AC + AA	0.0008	0.0025	1.83 (1.28–2.60)	CC + AC vs AA	0.0007	0.0022	1.84 (1.29–2.61)
Cohort 1	664 (89.73%)	2 (0.54%)	72 (19.46%)	296 (80%)										
Cohort 2	153 (93.29%)	0 (0.00%)	11 (13.41%)	71 (86.59%)										
ss469415590 TT > ΔG[b]	TT	ΔG/ΔG	ΔG/TT	TT/TT			Additive				Additive			
Nephritis+	1052 (94.10%)	2 (0.36%)	62 (11.09%)	495 (88.55%)	0.0011	0.0016		0.0015	0.0024	1.72 (1.23–2.42)		0.0015	0.0021	1.73(1.23–2.42)
Cohort 1	858 (93.46%)	4 (0.87%)	52 (11.33%)	403 (87.8%)			BB + AB vs AA	0.4927	0.657	1.87 (0.31–11.26)	2TT vs GTT + GG	0.513	0.684	1.82 (0.30–10.94)
Cohort 2	188 (94.00%)	1 (1.00%)	10 (10.00%)	89 (89.00%)										
Nephritis−	811 (90.31%)	3 (0.67%)	81 (18.04%)	365 (81.29%)			BB vs AB + AA	0.0013	0.0025	1.78 (1.25–2.53)	2TT + GTT vs GG	0.0012	0.0022	1.79 (1.26–2.54)
Cohort 1	652 (88.83%)	6 (1.63%)	70 (19.07%)	291 (79.29%)										
Cohort 2	153 (93.29%)	0 (0.00%)	11 (13.41%)	71 (86.59%)										

Data presented as *n* (%)

SLE systemic lupus erythematosus, *SNP* single-nucleotide polymorphism, *OR* odds ratio, *CI* confidence interval

[a] Trend test *P* values generated from 10,000 permutations

[b] Genotypes of ΔG/ΔG, ΔG/TT, and TT/TT are also named GG, GTT, and 2TT, respectively

Table 4 Association of *IFN3/4* locus SNP haplotypes (rs8099917-ss469415590-rs12979860-rs4803217) with lupus nephritis among SLE patients

Haplotype	Estimated frequency (%)			Permutation	Logistic regression		Logistic regression adjusted for sex and age	
	Nephritis⁺	Nephritis⁻	SLE cases	P*	P	OR (95% CI)	P	OR (95% CI)
	(N = 461)	(N = 370)	(N = 831)					
T-TT-C-C	91.74	86.99	89.62	0.0024	0.0018	1.66 (1.21–2.28)	0.0015	1.68 (1.22–2.32)
G-ΔG-T-A	4.44	8.23	6.13	0.0019	0.0016	0.52 (0.34–0.78)	0.0011	0.5 (0.33–0.76)
Others	3.83	4.78	4.25		0.3472	0.79 (0.49–1.28)	0.3690	0.8 (0.49–1.3)

Data presented as *n* (%)
*The *p*-values for the estimated haplotype were generated from 10,000 permutations using the EM algorithm
SLE systemic lupus erythematosus, *SNP* single-nucleotide polymorphism, *OR* odds ratio, *CI* confidence interval

among SLE patients. As shown in Table 4, the most common haplotype (T-TTC-C) was significantly associated with the risk for lupus nephritis (logistic regression adjusted for sex and age: $P = 0.0015$, OR 1.68, 95% CI 1.22–2.32) while the minor haplotype (G-ΔG-T-A) was associated with the low risk for lupus nephritis (adjusted $P = 0.0011$, OR 0.50, 95% CI 0.33–0.76). A combination of two cohorts of SLE patients revealed similar significant findings (Additional file 1: Table S1). However, *IFNL3/4* SNP haplotypes were not associated with other manifestations including oral ulcer, arthritis, malar rash, discoid rash, photosensitivity, pleural effusion, pericardial effusion, ascites, neuropsychiatric manifestations, leukopenia, anemia, thrombocytopenia, anti-dsDNA, complement depressed, anti-RNP, anti-Sm, anti-SSA, anti-SSB, anticardiolipin IgG, and anticardiolipin IgM) when compared among SLE patients (data not shown). Our data suggest that IFN-λs have a unique role in the development of lupus nephritis.

IFNL-λ3 (IFNL3) levels correlated with SLE disease activity and complement depression

We subsequently performed correlation analyses of serum IFNL3 levels with traditional clinical and laboratory parameters. As shown in Fig. 1, we found that the serum IFNL3 levels were significantly increased in SLE patients with high SLE disease activity index (SLEDAI > 4, $N = 19$; IFNL3 concentration 9.190 ± 1.351 pg/ml) as compared to the patients with low disease activity (SLEDAI ≤ 4, $N = 51$; IFNL3 concentration 3.413 ± 0.3171 pg/ml) ($P < 0.0001$). In addition, SLE patients with both depressed C3 and C4 had significantly higher serum IFNL3 ($N = 14$) than those without complement C3 plus C4 depression ($N = 56$) (IFNL3 concentration 8.288 ± 1.696 pg/ml vs 4.154 ± 0.4514 pg/ml; $P = 0.0013$). We confirmed that IFNL3 levels were significantly associated with SLEDAI in an independent cohort (Additional file 1: Figure S3A). However, IFNL3 levels were not significantly different (unpaired *t* test $t = 1.650$, $P = 0.103$) between nephritis-positive patients and nephritis-negative patients (Additional file 1: Figure S3B). Our data suggest that serum IFNL3 could be used as a disease activity biomarker for SLE.

Detection of IL-28B and IL-28 receptors in kidney tissue of SLE patients
Since *IFNL3/4* SNP haplotypes were associated with lupus nephritis, we carried out immunohistochemistry analyses to examine the presence of IFNL and its receptor in kidney tissues of three SLE patients with nephritis. IFNL3 were detected on parietal cells (red arrow), podocytes (yellow arrows), and tubular cells (blue arrows)

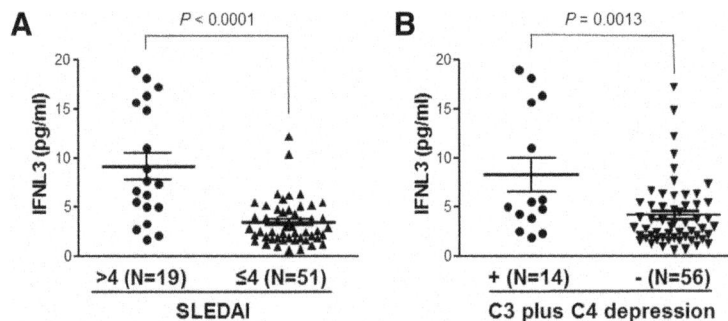

Fig. 1 Association of serum IFNL3 levels with SLEDAI and complement depression. **a** IFNL3 levels significantly (unpaired *t* test $t = 5.974$, $P < 0.0001$) increased in high SLEDAI SLE patients (SLEDAI > 4, $N = 19$; IFNL3 concentration 9.190 ± 1.351 pg/ml) compared to low SLEDAI SLE patients (SLEDAI ≤ 4, $N = 51$; IFNL3 concentration 3.413 ± 0.3171 pg/ml). **b** IFNL3 levels also significantly (unpaired *t* test $t = 3.362$, $P = 0.0013$) higher in SLE patients ($N = 14$) with complement C3 plus C4 depression (IFNL3 concentration 8.288 ± 1.696 pg/ml) than in those ($N = 56$) without complement C3 plus C4 depression (IFNL3 concentration 4.154 ± 0.4514 pg/ml). IFNL3 interferon-λ3, SLEDAI Systemic Lupus Erythematosus Disease Activity Index

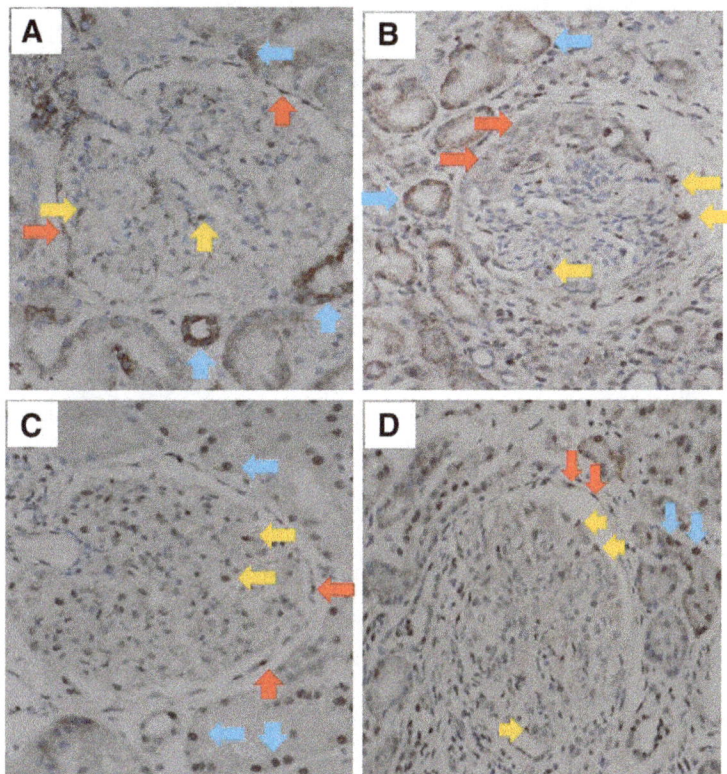

Fig. 2 Detection of IL-28B (IFNL3) and IL-28 receptor alpha (IL-28RA) in kidney tissue of lupus patients with nephritis. IFNL3 detected on parietal cells (red arrow), podocytes (yellow arrows), and tubular cells (blue arrows) of kidney from lupus patient with minimal change disease (**a**) and lupus patient with class IV proliferative nephritis (**b**). IL-28RA expressed in parietal cells (red arrow), podocytes (yellow arrows), and tubular cells (blue arrows) of kidney from patient with minimal change disease (**c**) and lupus patient with class IV proliferative nephritis (**d**)

(Fig. 2a, b), which expressed IL-28 receptor alpha (IL-28RA) (Fig. 2c, d). Our data support the concept that kidney tissue is a target of IFNLs.

Discussion

IFN-λs (IFNLs) play critical roles in innate and adaptive immune responses [4]. Recent genetic studies revealed that IFN-λ genes contribute to the spontaneous resolution of HCV and that IFN-λ genetic variants are reliable biomarkers for treatment outcomes of HCV infections [5]. SLE is a heterogeneous disease with varied clinical phenotypes. In the current study, we demonstrated that *IFNL3/4* genetic variants were significantly associated with SLE susceptibility in lupus nephritis-negative patients. Specifically, minor alleles of all *IFNL3/4* SNPs are risk factors for SLE development in patients without nephritis. In contrast, the major alleles of *IFNL3/4* SNPs are a significant risk factor for the development of nephritis among SLE patients. Our study is the first to reveal that IFN-λ genes play a unique role in the development of SLE and lupus nephritis, indicating that IFN-λ genetic variants could be potential biomarkers for SLE susceptibility and lupus nephritis.

Type I IFNs contribute to the breakdown of immune tolerance by enhancing the differentiation of immature myeloid dendritic cells (mDCs) into mature DCs that drive the expansion and differentiation of autoreactive T cells and B cells. Type I IFN-matured DCs also activate cytotoxic CD8$^+$ T cells that kill susceptible target cells. Type I IFNs are key cytokines in the pathogenesis of SLE [25]. Mouse models confirmed that type I IFNs accelerate disease progression through the increase of autoantibody production and the development of nephritis [26, 27]. IFN-λs (IFN-λ1, IFN-λ2, IFN-λ3, and IFN-λ4) are structurally related to the IL-10 family that transduces cellular signals through a heterodimeric IFN-λ receptor complex composed of a unique IL28RA/IFN-λR1 (IFN-λ-specific ligand binding chain) and a shared IL-10Rβ chain (a subunit of the receptors for IL-10, IL-22, and IL-26) [6, 28, 29]. The binding of IFN-λs to the IFN-λ-receptor complex activates the Janus kinase–signal transducer and activator of transcription (Jak–STAT) pathway, leading to the expressions of IFN-regulated genes (ISGs) that inhibit viral replication [4, 28, 30, 31].

IFN-λ-stimulated DCs express high levels of MHC class I and MHC class II but low levels of costimulatory molecules. IFN-λ-exposed DCs specifically induce IL-2-dependent proliferation of CD4$^+$CD25$^+$Foxp3$^+$ suppressive T cells that inhibit the T-cell proliferation driven by mature DCs. Therefore, IFN-λs favor the generation of tolerogenic DCs that thwart type I IFN functions [32]. Interestingly, as an important target of IFN-λs, neutrophils also express high levels of IL28RA/IFN-λR1. IFN-λs inhibit neutrophil recruitment and activation, preventing the amplification of inflammation. Furthermore, IFN-λs could completely halt and reverse the development of collagen-induced arthritis [33]. As a key regulator to inhibit B-cell immune responses, IFN-λ3 treatment dramatically reduced antigen-stimulated B-cell proliferation and IgG production through suppressing Th2 cytokine production [34]. Taken together, IFN-λs appear to inhibit chronic inflammation through the actions of DCs, suppressive T cells, neutrophils, and B cells [33].

IFNL3/4 locus SNPs are strongly associated with clearance of HCV [35–42]. *IFNL3* 3′-untranslated region (UTR) SNP rs4803217 significantly influences AU-rich element-mediated *IFNL3* mRNA decay. *IFNL3* mRNA containing the minor rs4803217A allele is much less stable than that with the major rs4803217C allele. Therefore, the major rs4803217C allele is a high IFN-λ3 producer while the minor rs4803217A allele is a low IFN-λ3 producer [43]. It is reasonable to assume that the most common *IFNL3/4* SNP haplotype rs8099917T/ss469415590/rs12979860C/rs4803217C containing the rs4803217C allele is a high producer of IFN-λ3, which is assumed to suppress the development of autoimmune inflammation [33]. We found that the most common *IFNL3/4* SNP haplotype containing the rs4803217C allele was significantly associated with the low risk for SLE in nephritis-negative patients, confirming that a high producer of IFN-λ3 may have a protective role against SLE.

Notably, the newly identified *IFNL4* SNP ss469415590 TT>ΔG alters the *IFNL4* reading frame and the rs368234815ΔG allele results in the open reading frame *IFNL4* mRNA. Nevertheless, IFN-λ4 peptide produced from the *IFNL4* ss469415590ΔG allele is a dysfunctional cytokine [22], which may explain the defective HCV clearance in Africans, Europeans, and Asians with the *IFNL4* ss469415590ΔG allele [20, 22–24, 44, 45]. On the other hand, the major ss469415590TT allele with a disrupted *IFNL4* open reading frame is associated with the increased expression of IFN-λ3 [21, 23, 24]. Our study revealed that the minor rs3682134815ΔG allele carrier is also a risk for SLE susceptibility in the subset of SLE patients negative for lupus nephritis, indicating that the expression of dysfunctional IFN-λ4 in combination with the low IFN-λ3 production has a role in the pathogenesis of SLE. IFN-λ3 levels have been linked to SLE disease activity, complement, and autoantibody (anti-Ro/SSA) status [46]. In the current study, we found

that high levels of IFN-λ3 were significantly associated with high SLEDAI and complement depression. The increased production of IFN-λ3 in SLE patients with a high SLEDAI may reflect an intrinsic mechanism to suppress chronic inflammation. IFN-λ3 levels may be a useful biomarker for SLE disease activity.

Paradoxically, our study revealed that the most common *IFNL3/4* SNP haplotype rs8099917T/rs12979860C/rs4803217C (high IFN-λ3 producer) was significantly associated with the risk for lupus nephritis, while the minor haplotype rs8099917G/rs12979860T/rs4803217A (low IFN-λ3 producer) had a protective role against lupus nephritis. We speculate several possible explanations. First, IFN-λs possess the highest cytotoxic potential as they induce more robust cell death than type I IFNs and type II IFNs [47]. Kidney cells express the IFN-λ3 receptor and could be very susceptible to IFN-λ-induced apoptosis, leading to necrotic inflammation and kidney injury. Indeed, we have detected both IFN-λ3 (IFNL3) and IL-28 receptor alpha in kidney tissue, suggesting a pathogenic mechanism of IFN-λ3 in the development of SLE nephritis. Second, the high levels of proinflammatory cytokines such as type I IFNs and IL-6 in SLE patients may reverse the anti-inflammatory action of IFN-λs, which subsequently exacerbates kidney injury under the circumstances of inflammation. Indeed, in patients with chronic hepatitis C (CHC), while the favorable genotypes responsible for high levels of IFN-λ production increase viral clearance, patients with the high IFN-λ-producer genotypes were twice as likely to develop adverse clinical outcomes [48, 49]. Finally, the *IFNL3/4* risk SNP haplotype may be in linkage disequilibrium with unidentified causative SNPs and/or may interact with other genes to cause lupus nephritis. Nevertheless, the *IFNL3/4* locus at chromosome 19q13 has never been identified to contain risk gene(s) for SLE susceptibility by GWAS [14, 15]. The absence of association of *IFNL3/4* SNPs with SLE in previous studies could be explained by our observation that the *IFNL3/4* SNPs are a risk factor for SLE susceptibility in the subset of lupus nephritis-negative patients. Further mechanistic studies are needed to pinpoint the precise role of IFN-λs in the development of lupus nephritis.

Nevertheless, the current study has several limitations. First, the cross-sectional serum IFNL3 levels were determined in a modest number of SLE patients. Studies with large clinical samples and longitudinal data are required to establish the association between serum IFNL3 levels and SLE disease activity. Second, since IFNL3 production could be affected by disease activity, a large number of SLE patients in quiescent disease status need to be used to determine the effect of *IFNL3/4* SNPs on IFNL3 production. Finally, extensive in-vivo and in-vitro studies are required to delineate the mechanistic roles of IFNLs in SLE development and lupus nephritis.

Conclusions

IFNL3/4 SNPs are significantly associated with SLE susceptibility and lupus nephritis in Taiwanese. High levels of IFN-λs may have a protective role against the development of SLE in the initial stage, but the increased and persistent production of IFN-λs may predispose SLE patients to the development of lupus nephritis. Our data point to a distinctive role of IFN-λs in the development of autoimmune diseases and phenotypes. IFN-λs may be a potential therapeutic target in treating lupus nephritis.

Abbreviations

CHC: Chronic hepatitis C; HWE: Hardy–Weinberg equilibrium; IFN: Interferon; ISG: IFN-regulated gene; JAK: Janus kinase; mDC: Myeloid dendritic cell; SLE: Systemic lupus erythematosus; SLEDAI: Systemic Lupus Erythematosus Disease Activity Index; SNP: Single-nucleotide polymorphism; STAT: Signal transducer and activator of transcription; UTR: Untranslated region

Acknowledgements

The authors greatly appreciate Shin Chu Blood Donor Center for sample collection.

Funding

This study was supported by funding from the Chang Gung Memorial Hospital (CMRPG3B1823 and CMRPG3E05313) and the Ministry of Science and Technology (103-2314-B-182-067-MY3). JWu's work was supported by a NIH grant (AI125729).

Authors' contributions

JYC and JW performed the study design, manuscript preparation, and coordination. YJJW and JCL participated in sample acquisition and data interpretation. TDC performed the kidney biopsy preparation and reading. LYL collected the SLE samples and performed data interpretation of the second cohort. CMW conceived of the study, participated in its design, and helped draft the manuscript. All authors reviewed, read, and approved the final manuscript.

Consent for publication

Not applicable.

Competing interests

The authors declare that they have no competing interests.

Author details

[1]Department of Medicine, Division of Allergy, Immunology and Rheumatology, Chang Gung Memorial Hospital, Chang Gung University College of Medicine, No. 5, Fu-Shin St. Kwei-Shan, Tao-Yuan, Taiwan. [2]Department of Rehabilitation, Chang Gung Memorial Hospital, Chang Gung University College of Medicine, No. 5, Fu-Shin St. Kwei-Shan, Tao-Yuan, Taiwan. [3]Department of Anatomic Pathology, Chang Gung Memorial Hospital, Chang Gung University College of Medicine, Tao-Yuan, Taiwan. [4]Department of Medicine, Division of Allergy Immunology and Rheumatology, Kaohsiung Veterans General Hospital, No. 386, Dazhong 1st Rd, Zuoying District, Kaohsiung City 81362, Taiwan. [5]Department of Veterinary and Biomedical Sciences, Department of Medicine, University of Minnesota, 235B Animal Science/Vet. Med. Bldg, 1988 Fitch Avenue, St. Paul, MN 55108, USA.

References

1. Tsokos GC. Systemic lupus erythematosus. N Engl J Med. 2011;365(22):2110–21.
2. Azevedo PC, Murphy G, Isenberg DA. Pathology of systemic lupus erythematosus: the challenges ahead. Methods Mol Biol. 2014;1134:1–16.
3. Kow NY, Mak A. Costimulatory pathways: physiology and potential therapeutic manipulation in systemic lupus erythematosus. Clin Dev Immunol. 2013;2013:245928.
4. Galani IE, Koltsida O, Andreakos E. Type III interferons (IFNs): emerging master regulators of immunity. Adv Exp Med Biol. 2015;850:1–15.
5. Kelly C, Klenerman P, Barnes E. Interferon lambdas: the next cytokine storm. Gut. 2011;60(9):1284–93.
6. Zdanov A. Structural analysis of cytokines comprising the IL-10 family. Cytokine Growth Factor Rev. 2010;21(5):325–30.
7. Sozzani S, Bosisio D, Scarsi M, Tincani A. Type I interferons in systemic autoimmunity. Autoimmunity. 2010;43(3):196–203.
8. Ronnblom L, Alm GV, Eloranta ML. The type I interferon system in the development of lupus. Semin Immunol. 2011;23(2):113–21.
9. Ronnblom L, Eloranta ML. The interferon signature in autoimmune diseases. Curr Opin Rheumatol. 2013;25(2):248–53.
10. Obermoser G, Pascual V. The interferon-alpha signature of systemic lupus erythematosus. Lupus. 2010;19(9):1012–9.
11. Bennett L, Palucka AK, Arce E, Cantrell V, Borvak J, Banchereau J, Pascual V. Interferon and granulopoiesis signatures in systemic lupus erythematosus blood. J Exp Med. 2003;197(6):711–23.
12. Bronson PG, Chaivorapol C, Ortmann W, Behrens TW, Graham RR. The genetics of type I interferon in systemic lupus erythematosus. Curr Opin Immunol. 2012;24(5):530–7.
13. Sandling JK, Garnier S, Sigurdsson S, Wang C, Nordmark G, Gunnarsson I, Svenungsson E, Padyukov L, Sturfelt G, Jonsen A, et al. A candidate gene study of the type I interferon pathway implicates IKBKE and IL8 as risk loci for SLE. Eur J Hum Genet. 2011;19(4):479–84.
14. Morris DL, Sheng Y, Zhang Y, Wang YF, Zhu Z, Tombleson P, Chen L, Cunninghame Graham DS, Bentham J, Roberts AL, et al. Genome-wide association meta-analysis in Chinese and European individuals identifies ten new loci associated with systemic lupus erythematosus. Nat Genet. 2016;48(8):940–6.
15. Teruel M, Alarcon-Riquelme ME. The genetic basis of systemic lupus erythematosus: what are the risk factors and what have we learned. J Autoimmun. 2016;74:161–75.
16. Boisvert M, Shoukry NH. Type III interferons in hepatitis C virus infection. Front Immunol. 2016;7:628.
17. Hochberg MC. Updating the American College of Rheumatology revised criteria for the classification of systemic lupus erythematosus. Arthritis Rheum. 1997;40(9):1725.
18. Bombardier C, Gladman DD, Urowitz MB, Caron D, Chang CH. Derivation of the SLEDAI. A disease activity index for lupus patients. The committee on prognosis studies in SLE. Arthritis Rheum. 1992;35(6):630–40.
19. Benjamini Y, Hochberg Y. Controlling the false discovery rate: a practical and powerful approach to multiple testing. J R Stat Soc Ser B Methodol. 1995;57:289–300.
20. Aka PV, Kuniholm MH, Pfeiffer RM, Wang AS, Tang W, Chen S, Astemborski J, Plankey M, Villacres MC, Peters MG, et al. Association of the IFNL4-DeltaG allele with impaired spontaneous clearance of hepatitis C virus. J Infect Dis. 2014;209(3):350–4.
21. Bibert S, Roger T, Calandra T, Bochud M, Cerny A, Semmo N, Duong FH, Gerlach T, Malinverni R, Moradpour D, et al. IL28B expression depends on a novel TT/−G polymorphism which improves HCV clearance prediction. J Exp Med. 2013;210(6):1109–16.
22. Hamming OJ, Terczynska-Dyla E, Vieyres G, Dijkman R, Jorgensen SE, Akhtar H, Siupka P, Pietschmann T, Thiel V, Hartmann R. Interferon lambda 4 signals via the IFNlambda receptor to regulate antiviral activity against HCV and coronaviruses. EMBO J. 2013;32(23):3055–65.
23. Prokunina-Olsson L, Muchmore B, Tang W, Pfeiffer RM, Park H, Dickensheets H, Hergott D, Porter-Gill P, Mumy A, Kohaar I, et al. A variant upstream of IFNL3 (IL28B) creating a new interferon gene IFNL4 is associated with impaired clearance of hepatitis C virus. Nat Genet. 2013;45(2):164–71.
24. Key FM, Peter B, Dennis MY, Huerta-Sanchez E, Tang W, Prokunina-Olsson L, Nielsen R, Andres AM. Selection on a variant associated with improved viral clearance drives local, adaptive pseudogenization of interferon lambda 4 (IFNL4). PLoS Genet. 2014;10(10):e1004681.
25. Banchereau J, Pascual V. Type I interferon in systemic lupus erythematosus and other autoimmune diseases. Immunity. 2006;25(3):383–92.
26. Liu Z, Bethunaickan R, Huang W, Lodhi U, Solano I, Madaio MP, Davidson A. Interferon-alpha accelerates murine systemic lupus erythematosus in a T cell-dependent manner. Arthritis Rheum. 2011;63(1):219–29.

27. Liu Z, Bethunaickan R, Huang W, Ramanujam M, Madaio MP, Davidson A. IFN-alpha confers resistance of systemic lupus erythematosus nephritis to therapy in NZB/W F1 mice. J Immunol. 2011;187(3):1506–13.

28. Gad HH, Hamming OJ, Hartmann R. The structure of human interferon lambda and what it has taught us. J Interf Cytokine Res. 2010;30(8):565–71.

29. Commins S, Steinke JW, Borish L. The extended IL-10 superfamily: IL-10, IL-19, IL-20, IL-22, IL-24, IL-26, and IL-28, and IL-29. J Allergy Clin Immunol. 2008; 121(5):1108–11.

30. Gad HH, Dellgren C, Hamming OJ, Vends S, Paludan SR, Hartmann R. Interferon-lambda is functionally an interferon but structurally related to the interleukin-10 family. J Biol Chem. 2009;284(31):20869–75.

31. Zheng YW, Li H, Yu JP, Zhao H, Wang SE, Ren XB. Interferon-lambdas: special immunomodulatory agents and potential therapeutic targets. J Innate Immun. 2013;5(3):209–18.

32. Mennechet FJ, Uze G. Interferon-lambda-treated dendritic cells specifically induce proliferation of FOXP3-expressing suppressor T cells. Blood. 2006;107(11):4417–23.

33. Blazek K, Eames HL, Weiss M, Byrne AJ, Perocheau D, Pease JE, Doyle S, McCann F, Williams RO, Udalova IA. IFN-lambda resolves inflammation via suppression of neutrophil infiltration and IL-1beta production. J Exp Med. 2015;212(6):845–53.

34. Egli A, Santer DM, O'Shea D, Barakat K, Syedbasha M, Vollmer M, Baluch A, Bhat R, Groenendyk J, Joyce MA, et al. IL-28B is a key regulator of B- and T-cell vaccine responses against influenza. PLoS Pathog. 2014;10(12):e1004556.

35. Ge D, Fellay J, Thompson AJ, Simon JS, Shianna KV, Urban TJ, Heinzen EL, Qiu P, Bertelsen AH, Muir AJ, et al. Genetic variation in IL28B predicts hepatitis C treatment-induced viral clearance. Nature. 2009;461(7262):399–401.

36. Rauch A, Kutalik Z, Descombes P, Cai T, Di Iulio J, Mueller T, Bochud M, Battegay M, Bernasconi E, Borovicka J, et al. Genetic variation in IL28B is associated with chronic hepatitis C and treatment failure: a genome-wide association study. Gastroenterology. 2010;138(4):1338–45. 1345.e1–7

37. Suppiah V, Moldovan M, Ahlenstiel G, Berg T, Weltman M, Abate ML, Bassendine M, Spengler U, Dore GJ, Powell E, et al. IL28B is associated with response to chronic hepatitis C interferon-alpha and ribavirin therapy. Nat Genet. 2009;41(10):1100–4.

38. Tanaka Y, Nishida N, Sugiyama M, Kurosaki M, Matsuura K, Sakamoto N, Nakagawa M, Korenaga M, Hino K, Hige S, et al. Genome-wide association of IL28B with response to pegylated interferon-alpha and ribavirin therapy for chronic hepatitis C. Nat Genet. 2009;41(10):1105–9.

39. Thomas DL, Thio CL, Martin MP, Qi Y, Ge D, O'Huigin C, Kidd J, Kidd K, Khakoo SI, Alexander G, et al. Genetic variation in IL28B and spontaneous clearance of hepatitis C virus. Nature. 2009;461(7265):798–801.

40. Duggal P, Thio CL, Wojcik GL, Goedert JJ, Mangia A, Latanich R, Kim AY, Lauer GM, Chung RT, Peters MG, et al. Genome-wide association study of spontaneous resolution of hepatitis C virus infection: data from multiple cohorts. Ann Intern Med. 2013;158(4):235–45.

41. Bota S, Sporea I, Sirli R, Neghina AM, Popescu A, Strain M. Role of interleukin-28B polymorphism as a predictor of sustained virological response in patients with chronic hepatitis C treated with triple therapy: a systematic review and meta-analysis. Clin Drug Investig. 2013;33(5):325–31.

42. Shakado S, Sakisaka S, Okanoue T, Chayama K, Izumi N, Toyoda J, Tanaka E, Ido A, Takehara T, Yoshioka K, et al. Interleukin 28B polymorphism predicts interferon plus ribavirin treatment outcome in patients with hepatitis C virus-related liver cirrhosis: a multicenter retrospective study in Japan. Hepatol Res. 2014;44:983–92.

43. McFarland AP, Horner SM, Jarret A, Joslyn RC, Bindewald E, Shapiro BA, Delker DA, Hagedorn CH, Carrington M, Gale M Jr, et al. The favorable IFNL3 genotype escapes mRNA decay mediated by AU-rich elements and hepatitis C virus-induced microRNAs. Nat Immunol. 2014;15(1):72–9.

44. Fujino H, Imamura M, Nagaoki Y, Kawakami Y, Abe H, Hayes CN, Kan H, Fukuhara T, Kobayashi T, Masaki K, et al. Predictive value of the IFNL4 polymorphism on outcome of telaprevir, peginterferon, and ribavirin therapy for older patients with genotype 1b chronic hepatitis C. J Gastroenterol. 2014;49(12):1548–56.

45. Lu YF, Goldstein DB, Urban TJ, Bradrick SS. Interferon-lambda4 is a cell-autonomous type III interferon associated with pre-treatment hepatitis C virus burden. Virology. 2015;476:334–40.

46. Amezcua-Guerra LM, Marquez-Velasco R, Chavez-Rueda AK, Castillo-Martinez D, Masso F, Paez A, Colin-Fuentes J, Bojalil R. Type III interferons in systemic lupus erythematosus: association between interferon lambda3, disease activity, and anti-Ro/SSA antibodies. J Clin Rheumatol. 2017;23(7):368–75.

47. Li W, Lewis-Antes A, Huang J, Balan M, Kotenko SV. Regulation of apoptosis by type III interferons. Cell Prolif. 2008;41(6):960–79.

48. Noureddin M, Wright EC, Alter HJ, Clark S, Thomas E, Chen R, Zhao X, Conry-Cantilena C, Kleiner DE, Liang TJ, et al. Association of IL28B genotype with fibrosis progression and clinical outcomes in patients with chronic hepatitis C: a longitudinal analysis. Hepatology. 2013;58(5):1548–57.

49. Petta S, Grimaudo S, Camma C, Cabibi D, Di Marco V, Licata G, Pipitone RM, Craxi A. IL28B and PNPLA3 polymorphisms affect histological liver damage in patients with non-alcoholic fatty liver disease. J Hepatol. 2012;56(6):1356–62.

4

The role of RORα in salivary gland lesions in patients with primary Sjögren's syndrome

Xiuhong Weng[1], Yi Liu[2], Shun Cui[3*] and Bo Cheng[1*]

Abstract

Background: The orphan nuclear receptors retinoic acid-related receptor α and γt (RORα and RORγt) are critical in the development of T helper 17 (Th17) cells, and ROR-specific synthetic ligands have proven efficacy in several mouse models of autoimmunity. However, the pathological significance of RORα in primary Sjögren's syndrome (pSS) remains to be elucidated. The present study was designed to clarify the significance of RORα in the pathogenesis of pSS.

Methods: RORα expression in the labial salivary gland (LSG) was determined by immunohistochemical analysis using a quantitative scoring system in 34 patients with pSS. The correlation between RORα expression in LSGs and the focus score (FS) was determined, and Th17 and IL-17 receptor A (1L-17RA) levels in LSGs were determined. To investigate the effect of RORs and the therapeutic potential of targeting RORs in pSS, we administered SR1001, a selective RORα/γt inverse agonist, to non-obese diabetic (NOD) mice.

Results: The expression of RORα was significantly increased in LSGs of patients with pSS and intensified with disease stage/FS, showing a similar increasing trend with IL-17A and IL-17RA. SR1001 significantly improved salivary gland secretory function and relieved sialadenitis in treated mice.

Conclusion: Our data reveal the importance of RORα in controlling pathologic lymphocytic infiltration of the salivary glands and suggest that RORα may be a druggable target in treating pSS.

Keywords: Primary Sjögren's syndrome, RORα, Focus score, Th17 cells, Inverse agonist

Background

Primary Sjögren's syndrome (pSS) is a chronic, systemic autoimmune disease characterized by lymphocyte infiltration into exocrine glands, such as salivary and lacrimal glands. The main clinical manifestations include xerostomia, xerophthalmia and several systemic manifestations. In addition, the probability of developing lymphoma is significantly higher (up to 44-fold higher) in patients with pSS than in the normal population [1, 2].

Focal lymphocytic sialadenitis is the characteristic histopathological feature of pSS. Minor salivary glands are more likely to have a focus score (FS), which is an index of inflammation, of at least 1 when evaluated by an expert histopathologist [3]. In addition, high concentrations of anti-Ro/La antibodies (SSA/SSB), anti-nuclear antibody (ANA), rheumatoid factor (RF) and immunoglobulin G (IgG) are detected in the plasma of patients with a FS greater than or equal to 1 [4] . Thus, it has been suggested that the FS may be associated with disease activity. The diagnosis of pSS is based on clinical manifestations and laboratory examination [5]. Immunological studies must include a determination of autoantibodies to the SSA and SSB antigens. Minor salivary gland (MSG) biopsy is highly specific for the diagnosis of SS and is indicated principally in patients who are negative for anti-SSA/SSB antibodies.

The pathogenesis of pSS is not yet clear. Immunohistochemical studies have shown that T helper 17 (Th17) cells are among the infiltrating lymphocytes in the labial

* Correspondence: cuishun7171@foxmail.com; chengbo_01@hotmail.com
Xiuhong Weng and Yi Liu are co-first authors.
Xiuhong Weng and Yi Liu contributed equally to this work.
[3]Department of Rheumatology, Union Hospital, Tongji Medical College, Huazhong University of Science and Technology, 1277 Jiefang Ave, Jianghan District, Wuhan 430022, Hubei Province, China
[1]Department of Stomatology, Zhongnan Hospital of Wuhan University, 169 Donghu Road, Wuhan 430071, Hubei Province, China
Full list of author information is available at the end of the article

salivary glands (LSGs) and lacrimal glands [6–9] . High levels of interleukin-17 (IL-17) and Th17-related cytokines have recently been identified in the salivary glands and plasma of patients with pSS and in mouse models of pSS [6, 8, 9]. Blocking IL-17 can significantly improve salivary gland function and reduce gland inflammation in pSS animal models [10]. Retinoic acid-related orphan receptors (RORs) are transcription factors that participate in the differentiation of inflammatory Th17 cells and cytokine production [11–15]. RORα cooperates with RORγt and nuclear factor κB inhibitor ζ (IκBζ) to enhance IL-17 expression by binding directly to the regulatory region of the IL-17A gene [13, 16]. Although several studies have indicated that Th17-related cytokines may be involved in the development of pSS, there is little information on the pathological importance of RORα in pSS. To address this issue, we used the inverse agonist SR1001, which has been found to obstruct Th17 differentiation by specifically inhibiting RORα [11]. This study aimed to investigate the role of RORα in salivary gland inflammation and function in pSS and to explore its role in the progression of pSS, with the goals of providing a theoretical basis and scientific evidence for key targets in the pathogenesis of pSS and improving the clinical diagnosis, staging, and treatment of pSS.

Methods
LSG histology
LSG biopsy specimens were obtained with informed consent from 34 individuals undergoing diagnostic evaluation for sicca symptoms indicative of pSS and diagnosed by American-European Sjögren's syndrome (SS) consensus criteria. The control group consisted of 12 gender-matched individuals with subjective complaints of dry mouth or eyes but who did not fulfill the criteria for pSS and had no histopathological evidence of pSS. None of the patients had evidence of lymphoma, sarcoidosis, essential mixed cryoglobulinemia, or HIV or hepatitis B or C virus infection at the time of the study. In addition, patients' medical records were evaluated for clinical and serological parameters, including SSA and SSB antibodies, high erythrocyte sedimentation rate (ESR), and C3/C4 hypocomplementemia.

The inflammatory lesions were graded histologically (histological FS) using the following method proposed by Greenspan: FS 1, a single focus composed of ~ 50 mononuclear cells per 4 mm^2 tissue. Salivary gland histopathology and rank were evaluated by researchers who were blinded to diagnosis, and at least one tissue section from each salivary gland was examined. Biopsy specimens were fixed, embedded, sectioned (4 μm/section), deparaffinized, rehydrated in alcohol, and stained with H&E.

Immunofluorescence of human samples
Paraffin sections were placed on silane-coated slides, dewaxed, rehydrated, and heated in citric acid (pH 6.0) buffer for 7 min for antigen retrieval. The sections were incubated with ice-cold blocking solution (PBS containing 5% (vol/vol) donkey serum and 1% (wt/vol) BSA) for 1 h and the primary antibody (RORα, 1:200; Abcam, UK) diluted 1/10 in blocking solution overnight at 4 °C, followed by three washes with Tris-buffered-saline Tween (TBST), and finally incubated with 488 Donkey-Anti-Rabbit IgG (H + L) (1: 400, Jackson Immunoresearch) for 1 h. Nucleus was stained with diamidino-phenyl-indole (DAPI) (Guge, Wuhan). Staining of CD4 (1:100, Biolegend) and IL-17 (1:100, Peprotech) was as herein before. Confocal images were acquired with the same pinhole diameter for each channel.

Immunohistochemical analysis of human samples
Paraffin sections were placed on silane-coated slides, dewaxed, rehydrated and heated in citric acid (pH 6.0) buffer for antigen retrieval. Endogenous peroxidase activity was blocked with 3% H_2O_2 for 15 min. Then, sections were incubated with blocking serum (ZSGB-BIO, Beijing) for 1 h and then with IL-17RA (1:100, Sangon Biotech, Shanghai) primary antibody overnight at 4 °C. After 20-min incubation with biotinylated secondary antibody (ZSGB-BIO, Beijing), staining was developed for 20 min with an Avidin: Biotinylated Enzyme Complex (ZSGB-BIO, Beijing), followed by 3,3-diaminobenzidine (DAB) staining (ZSGB-BIO, Beijing) and counterstaining with Meyer's hematoxylin for 1 min. Slides were washed in TBST 3 × 5 minutes after each step. Staining of RORγt (1:50, Abcam) was done as herein before.

Mice
Female NOD/LtJ mice, 4 weeks old (4W) and 8 weeks old (8W) were obtained from Huafukang (Beijing) and were maintained in specific pathogen-free conditions at the Animal Experiment Center of Huazhong University of Science and Technology. NOD mice were injected intraperitoneally (i.p.) twice a day with vehicle or SR1001, which was dissolved in a 50% dimethyl sulphoxide (DMSO) and 50% normal saline (dose 2.5 mg/ml, equal to 25 mg/kg and 1 μl/g body weight). Mice were divided into four groups: 4W mice treated i.p. with SR1001 or vehicle; and 8W mice treated i.p. with SR1001 or vehicle. Each group received SR1001 or vehicle i.p. for 4 weeks. Salivary gland function (measurement of saliva flow rate) and blood glucose (Roche, Swizterland) were evaluated before and after the drug intervention. Body weight was measured every day to monitor any effects of SR1001on growth and development. After 4 weeks, mice were sacrificed, and the isolated salivary glands were H&E stained to observe salivary gland structure. The treatment effect of

SR1001 on salivary gland function was measured by saliva volume secreted in 15 min. Mesenteric lymph nodes (MLNs) and cervical lymph nodes (CLNs) were removed, and the ratio of CD4+/IL-17A+ cells was measured by flow cytometry. All experiments were performed according to the Guide for the Care and Use of Laboratory Animals at Tongji Medical College.

Measurement of stimulated saliva flow
Each NOD mouse was first anesthetized with an i.p. injection of pentobarbital (25 mg/kg/body weight, Sigma-Aldrich, USA) and a subsequent i.p. injection of pilocarpine (1.0 mg/kg/body weight, Leqi, Wuhan). At 1 min after injection of the secretagogue, saliva was collected from the oral cavity using a 200-µl micropipette for 15 min at room temperature. The volume (µl) of each saliva sample was measured and expressed relative to body weight (grams). Baseline saliva flow rates were measured 3 days before the drug injection, and final saliva flow rates in each group were measured the end of the drug injection.

Flow cytometry
Tissue was cut into small pieces for flow cytometric analysis of MLNs and CLNs cells. T cells were cultured for Th17 differentiation as previously described [17]. Staining for CD4 (1:100, BioLegend) expression was performed for 20 min using a mixture of antibodies. Intracellular staining for IL-17A (1:100, BioLegend) was performed after fixation and permeabilization according to the protocol supplied by the manufacturer (BD Biosciences). Samples were analyzed with a FACS Calibur Flow Cytometer (BD Biosciences), and data were analyzed with FlowJo software (Tree Star, Ashland, OR, USA).

Western blot
Minor saliva gland proteins were isolated, and western blotting was performed as follows. Proteins were extracted in the radio-immunoprecipitation (RIPA)-cocktail buffer and centrifuged. The supernatant was collected as the RIPA soluble fraction, and the pellet was washed with RIPA buffer, centrifuged and boiled with Laemmli buffer. The concentration of extracted proteins was measured using a BCA protein assay kit (Byotime, Shanghai). The following primary antibodies were used: rabbit anti-RORα (1:800, ab60134, Abcam), rabbit anti-IL-17RA (1:1000, Sangon Biotech, Shanghai), anti-RORγt (1:500, Invitrogen 14–6988-80), and mouse anti-GAPDH (1:5000, Santa Cruz Biotechnology, USA). Protein samples were separated on a 4–12% SDS-PAGE gel and electro-transferred onto a polyvinylidene fluoride (PVDF) membrane for 2 h. Membranes were blocked in blocking solution (TBST containing 5% (wt/vol) milk serum and 1% (wt/vol) BSA) for 1 h at room temperature and then incubated with primary antibodies overnight at 4 °C. Next, membranes were washed in TBST and then incubated with secondary HRP-conjugated anti-mouse (1:5000, Aspen, Wuhan) or anti-rabbit (1:5000, Aspen, Wuhan) antibodies for 1 h at room temperature. The signal was detected with enhanced chemiluminescence (ECL) Western Blotting Substrate (Thermo Scientific Pierce, P180196).

RNA extraction and real-time quantification PCR
Total RNA was obtained from frozen human labial gland specimens from patients with and without pSS using Trizol reagent according to the protocol supplied by the manufacturer (TaKaRa, Japan). Complementary DNA (Cdna) was synthesized from RNA using PrimeScript RT reagent Kit with gDNA Eraser (TaKaRa, Japan). Real-time PCR for H-RORγt and RORα were performed on StepOne Real-Time (Life Technologies) using the SYBR® Premix Ex Taq kit (TaKaRa, Japan), and H-GAPDH as normalization control. We used the $2^{-\Delta\Delta CT}$ method for data analysis. Each sample was tested in triplicate, and tests were replicated twice. The primer sets for RT-PCR can be found in Table 1.

Statistical analysis
Data were analyzed by the two-tailed Student's t test using Graphpad Prism. Data are presented as the mean or mean ± SEM. P values are denoted as follows: $^*P < 0.05$, $^{**}P < 0.01$, $^{***}P < 0.001$.

Results
Patients
RORα expression in LSGs was determined in 46 patients with sicca syndrome who were referred to our department. Thirty-four patients met the American-European Consensus Group criteria for pSS. The remaining 12 patients were classified as having non-SS sicca syndrome. The characteristics of these patients are shown in Table 2). The mean (± SEM) age of the patients with pSS and those with non-pSS was 34.32 ± 2.225 years and 27.25 ± 7.186 years, respectively. All patients were female.

Increased RORα expression in LSGs of patients with pSS
Typical histologic characteristics of LSGs from patients with pSS were acinus atrophy and local

Table 1 Primer sets for RT-PCR

Primer		Primer sequence	Product length (bp)
H-GAPDH	Forward	5′ - CATCATCCCTGCCTCTACTGG-3′	259
	reverse	5′ - GTGGGTGTCGCTGTTGAAGTC-3′	
H-RORγt	Forward	5′ - TGGAAGTGGTGCTGGTTAGG-3′	203
	reverse	5′ - GAGAACAAGGGCTGTGTAGAGG-3′	
H-RORα	Forward	5′ - CCGTAGGGATGTCTCGAGATG-3′	211
	reverse	5′ -TCAATGTAGTTACTGAGGTCGTCG-3′	

Table 2 Characteristics of patients with and without pSS

Variable	pSS (n = 34)	NC (n = 12)
Age, mean (SEM)	34.32 (2.225)	27.25 (7.186)
Sex (female/male)	34/0	12/0
Focus score ≥ 1, n (%)	29 (85.3)	0 (0)
Anti-Ro/SSA, n (%)	30 (88.24)	0 (0)
Anti-La/SSB, n (%)	19 (55.88)	0 (0)
Both Anti-Ro/SSA and Anti-La/SSB, n (%)	19 (55.88)	0 (0)
ANA, n (%)	32 (94.12)	0 (0)
ESR↑, n (%)	17 (50)	0 (0)
IgG > 15.9, n (%)	24 (70.59)	0 (0)
RF > 15.9KU/l, n (%)	15 (44.12)	0 (0)

pSS primary Sjögren's syndrome, *NC* normal controls, *Anti-Ro/SSA/SSB* anti-Sjögren's-syndrome-related antigen antibody A/B, *ANA* anti-nuclear antibodies, *ESR* erythrocyte sedimentation rate, *RF* rheumatoid factor

lymphocytic sialadenitis (Fig. 1a). We detected the expression of RORα in LSGs by different methods, and all indicated that RORα expression was significantly up-regulated in the LSGs of patients with pSS (Fig. 1b–d). RORα-expressing cells were observed in the LSGs of nearly all patients with sicca syndrome, even in those without obvious local lymphocytic sialadenitis (FS = 0) (Fig. 2b).

RORa expression increased with increasing FS

RORα expression was monitored in the LSGs of pSS patients with different FS and this indicated that RORα expression increased with increasing FS (Fig. 2c), which might suggest its participation in the pathogenesis of pSS. LSGs from all pSS patients with obvious focal lymphocytic accumulation (FS ≥ 1) had a high number of RORα-positive cells localized predominantly around the ducts (Fig. 2b, c). For RORα protein expression in LSG biopsy specimens intensified with disease stage/FS, there might be indicative of a correlation between RORα up-regulation and pathological manifestations in LSGs of pSS, but it remained unclear whether this deposition correlated with known markers of pSS, such as anti-Ro (SSA) and anti-La (SSB) antibodies, high erythrocyte sedimentation rate (ESR), or C3/C4.

The ratio of CD4+/IL-17A+ cells in the salivary gland was higher in patients with pSS than in control individuals

RORα-positive Th17 cells were detected in LSGs from patients with pSS (Fig. 3), indicating that RORα regulates Th17 cell differentiation and is involved in the pathogenesis of pSS. IL-17 was secreted in large amounts by inflammatory cells from patients with pSS, which can facilitate pro-inflammatory responses and tissue destruction. An elevated number of IL-17-producing cells in patients with pSS was correlated with increased glandular

inflammation, as indicated by an increased FS in the LSGs. A large number of IL-17-producing cells was observed in the vicinity of LSG lymphocytic infiltrates and in the interstitium.

IL-17RA expression was significantly higher in salivary gland tissues from patients with pSS than in that from control individuals

Immunohistochemical staining revealed substantial expression of IL-17RA in the LSGs from pSS patients (Fig. 4b), not only seen in infiltrated lymphocytes but also in acinus and ductal epithelial cells. Furthermore, high expression of IL-17RA was detected by western blot (Fig. 4a). In addition, IL-17RA expression also tended to increase with increasing disease stage/FS as did RORα. The number of IL-17+ cells may be inflated, because the widespread distribution of IL-17RA may confound quantification. It is not possible to dissociate cells that produce IL-17 from those that bind/respond to it, and multiple cell types may be responsible for secreting IL-17. Because of the difficulty in accurately quantifying IL-17RA-expressing populations by immunohistochemical analysis, we assessed IL-17RA by western blot of proteins extracted from whole LSGs from patients with pSS and control individuals (Fig. 4a). We observed higher IL-17RA expression in the LSGs of patients with pSS (n = 34) compared with control individuals (n = 12).

Synthetic RORa inverse agonist improved salivary gland function and alleviated lymphocytic infiltration of salivary glands

To verify the secretory function of salivary glands, saliva was collected from NOD mice. Significantly more saliva was collected from SR1001-treated NOD mice than from littermate vehicle controls in both the 4W and 8W groups (Fig. 5a), but the difference between the 8W groups was more significant (Fig. 5a). Then, NOD mice were sacrificed for histological analysis to determine the effect of SR1001 on sialadenitis development. More infiltrating mononuclear cells were detected in the SMGs of vehicle-treated NOD mice. SR1001 treatment significantly reduced lymphocytic infiltration of SMGs compared with littermate vehicle controls in both the 4W and 8W groups (Fig. 5b). This result might suggest that pharmacological inhibition of RORα effectively alleviated salivary gland destruction and improved salivary gland function.

Moreover, flow cytometry analysis of CD4+ T cells in MLNs and CLNs from different-aged NOD mice that received different treatments after stimulation with phorbol-12-myristate-13-acetate (PMA) and ionomycin for 6 h was performed to determine the effect of SR1001 on Th17 cell differentiation (Fig. 6). It indicated that SR1001, a synthetic RORα inverse agonist,

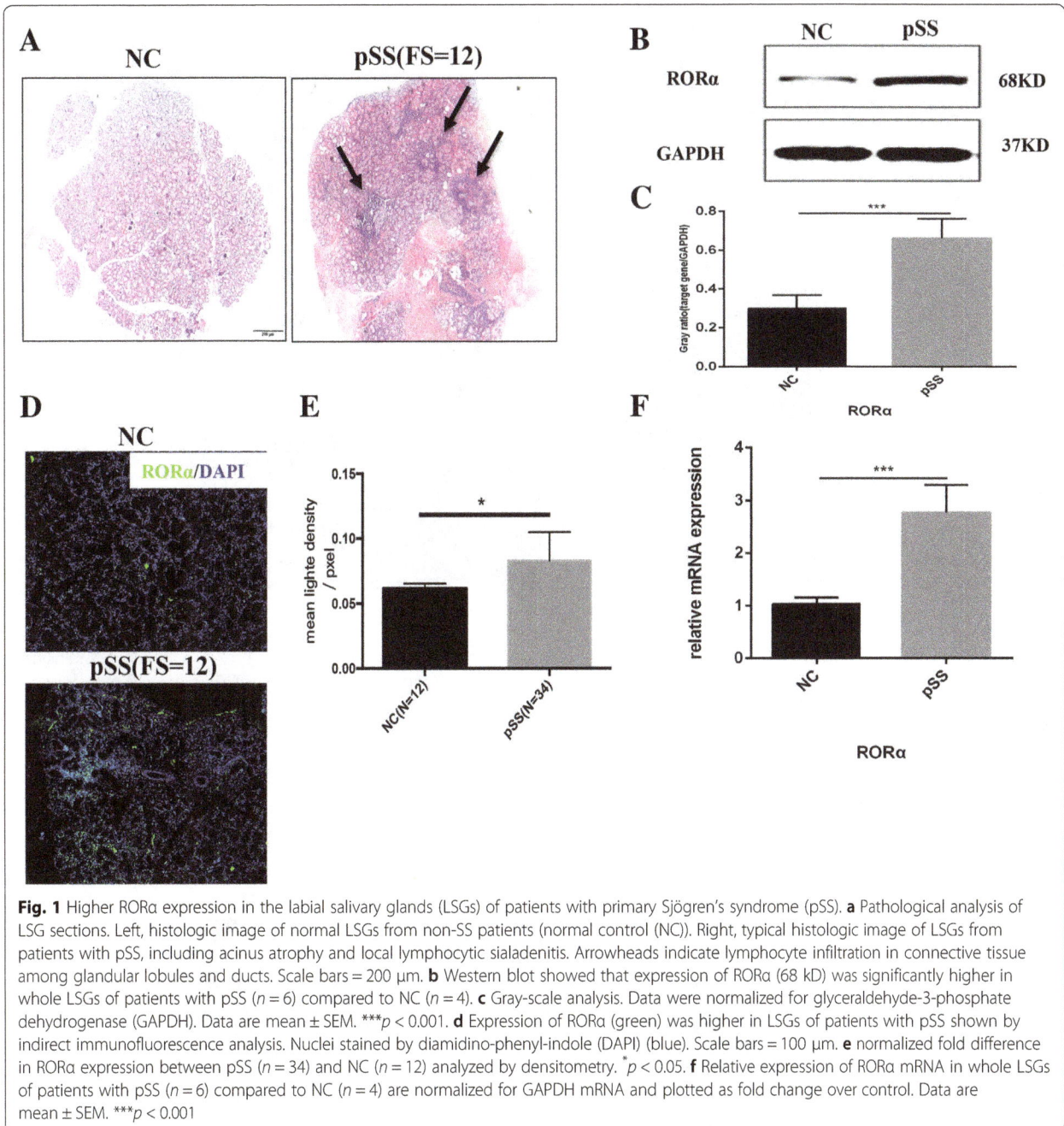

Fig. 1 Higher RORα expression in the labial salivary glands (LSGs) of patients with primary Sjögren's syndrome (pSS). **a** Pathological analysis of LSG sections. Left, histologic image of normal LSGs from non-SS patients (normal control (NC)). Right, typical histologic image of LSGs from patients with pSS, including acinus atrophy and local lymphocytic sialadenitis. Arrowheads indicate lymphocyte infiltration in connective tissue among glandular lobules and ducts. Scale bars = 200 μm. **b** Western blot showed that expression of RORα (68 kD) was significantly higher in whole LSGs of patients with pSS (n = 6) compared to NC (n = 4). **c** Gray-scale analysis. Data were normalized for glyceraldehyde-3-phosphate dehydrogenase (GAPDH). Data are mean ± SEM. ***$p < 0.001$. **d** Expression of RORα (green) was higher in LSGs of patients with pSS shown by indirect immunofluorescence analysis. Nuclei stained by diamidino-phenyl-indole (DAPI) (blue). Scale bars = 100 μm. **e** normalized fold difference in RORα expression between pSS (n = 34) and NC (n = 12) analyzed by densitometry. *$p < 0.05$. **f** Relative expression of RORα mRNA in whole LSGs of patients with pSS (n = 6) compared to NC (n = 4) are normalized for GAPDH mRNA and plotted as fold change over control. Data are mean ± SEM. ***$p < 0.001$

decreased Th17 differentiation of CD4+ T cells in MLNs and CLNs after 4-week treatment (Fig. 6). We also detected that SR1001 has the ability to regulate blood glucose in NOD mice, especially in mice at 8 weeks of age (Additional file 1B). Meanwhile, systemic treatment of SR1001 had no effect on body weight gain in NOD mice (Additional file 1A).

Discussion

Dry mouth, dry eyes and rampant caries due to a reduction in exocrine secretions are the main clinical manifestations of pSS, which cause patients considerable inconvenience and pain [18, 19]. As reported in previous studies, most patients with pSS are female [20, 21]. Lymphocytic infiltration of salivary glands and impaired saliva secretion are the main features of pSS. A variety of autoantibodies, such as high ESR, RF, and Ig, can be detected in the serum of patients with pSS. Although there have been great improvements in our knowledge and understanding of pSS, diagnosis, treatment and disease monitoring are still challenging in the clinic.

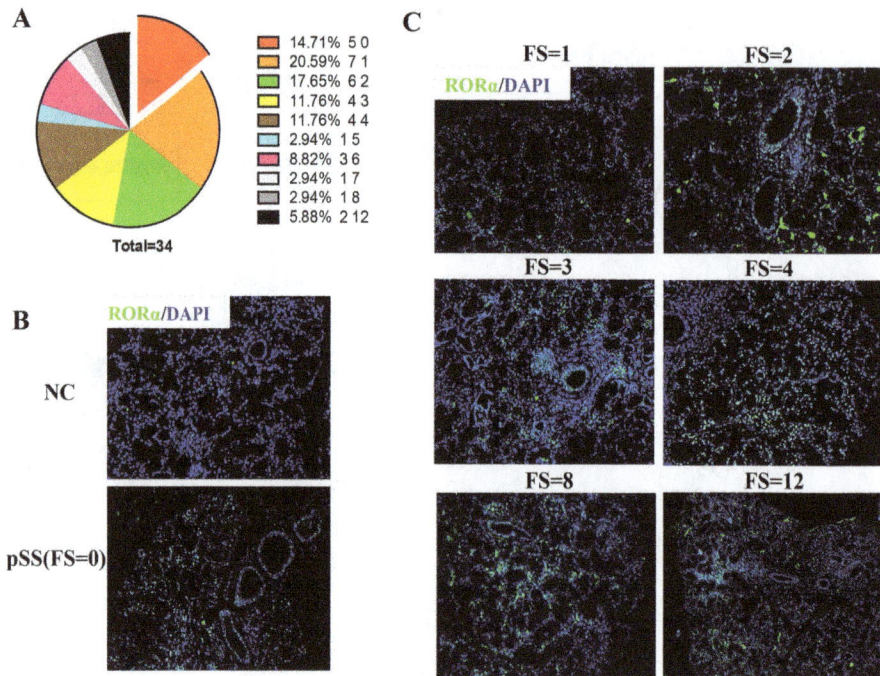

Fig. 2 RORα expression in the labial salivary glands (LSGs) of patients with primary Sjögren's syndrome (pSS) increased with increasing focus score (FS). **a** Focal index of all patients with pSS (*n* = 34) and the statistical analysis: 85.3% (*n* = 29) of pSS in our study had obvious local lymphocytic sialadenitis (FS > =1). **b** Expression of RORα expression (green) in LSG sections from patients with pSS with a FS of 0 (*n* = 5, lower panel) was still higher than in patients without pSS (normal control (NC) (*n* = 10, upper panel) assessed by indirect immunofluorescence. **c** RORα expression in patients with pSS with a different FS (*n* = 29) assessed by indirect immunofluorescence analysis suggested that the RORα expression in the LSGs in pSS increased with increasing FS. Diamidino-phenyl-indole (DAPI) staining for nuclei (blue). Scale bars = 100 μm

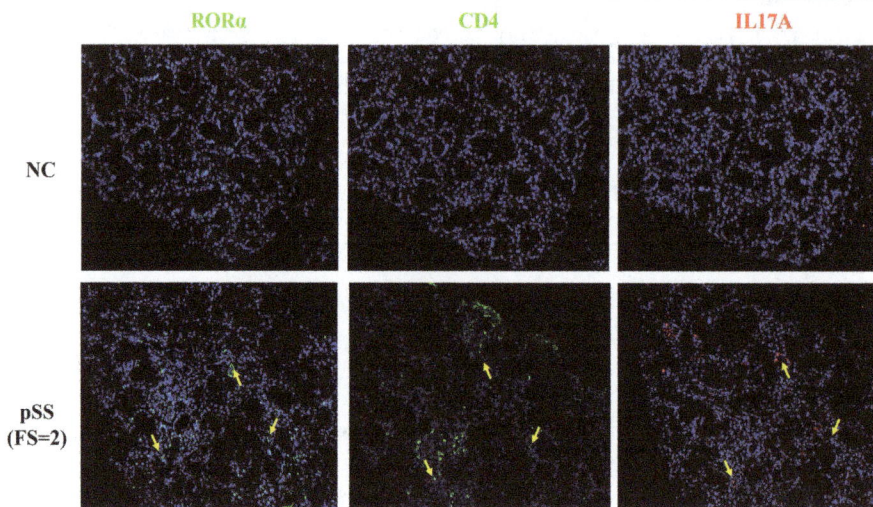

Fig. 3 Co-expression of RORα with CD4 and IL-17A in the labial salivary glands (LSGs). Indirect immunofluorescence analysis was used to assess RORα (green), CD4 (green) and IL-17A (red) expression and diamidino-phenyl-indole (DAPI) staining for nuclei (blue) in the LSG. Results are representative of 30 patients with primary Sjögren's syndrome (pSS) (lower lane) and 10 normal control individuals (NC) (upper lane). The micrographs in the lower panel showed RORα-positive T helper 17 (Th17) cells in the LSGs of patients with pSS (focus score (FS) = 2), whereas the upper panel only shows some RORα-positive cells in the LSGs of NC. It indicated RORα-positive Th17 cells in the periductal tissue of LSGs of patients with pSS. Serial sections of the LSG from the same patient, and yellow arrows (lower lane) in the same direction indicated the same cell in three serial sections. Scale bars = 100 μm

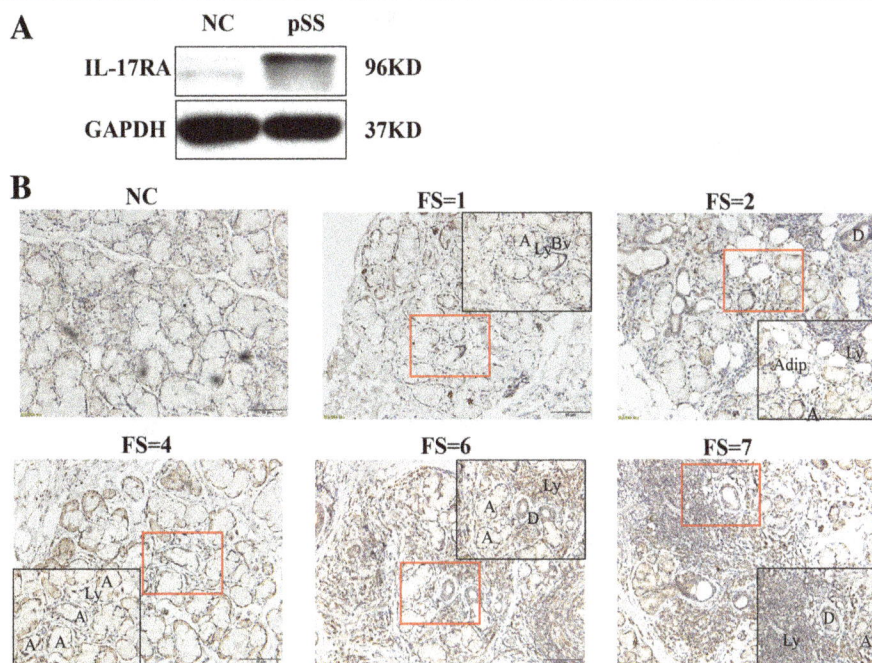

Fig. 4 Higher expression of IL-17RA in the labial salivary glands (LSGs) of patients with primary Sjögren's syndrome (pSS). **a** Protein expression level of IL-17R (96 kD) in LSGs. Expression of IL-17R in tissue with pSS ($n = 6$) was higher compared with normal control (NC) ($n = 4$). **b** Immunohistochemical analysis of local IL-17R in patients with pSS ($n = 34$) and NC ($n = 10$) LSGs. IL-17R-positive cells are significantly more numerous in the LSGs of patients with pSS compared with NC, along with an upward trend as the focus score (FS) increased. Scale bars = 50 μm; insets, ×2 magnification. Abbreviations: A, acinus; Adip, adipocytes; Bv, blood vessel; D, ductus; Ly, lymphocyte infiltration

pSS is known as an autoimmune disease caused by a group of different mechanisms, and immune disorder is important in pSS occurrence and development. Due to the complexity and integrity of the immune system, functional cells involved in immune responses may all be involved in the pathogenesis of pSS, in which the study of T/B cells predominates. The role of Th17 cells in autoimmune diseases has been widely recognized [14, 22]. In fact, lymphocytic infiltration into the exocrine glands of patients with pSS does not contain a single species but includes Th1, Th2, Th17, T regulatory (Treg), and B cells [23–25]. Treg cells are the most important immune-suppressing cells, and it is believed that the imbalance between Th17 cells and Treg cells is crucial in the progression of pSS [26, 27]. Th17 cells comprise a pro-inflammatory cell subset that can promote inflammatory reactions and secrete various pro-inflammatory factors [26]. Both patients with pSS and mouse models harbor Th17 cells and IL-17 in the salivary glands and in serum [28–30]. Furthermore, serum IL-17 levels are closely related to the degree of salivary gland damage [9].

Th17 cells and IL-17 do not directly lead to an inflammatory reaction. The pro-inflammatory effect is mainly due to pro-inflammatory cytokines, such as IL-6 and granulocyte-macrophage colony stimulating factor (GM-CSF), produced in response to IL-17 binding to IL-17RA, which occurs in the salivary glands and causes tissue damage [31, 32]. However, it has been proved that IL-17 was not essential for the development of sialadenitis by examination of IL-17-deficient mice [13]. The levels of IL-17A and IL-17RA can be regulated by each other [33, 34]; IL-17RA could be rapidly down-regulated by IL-17A binding [35], and IL-17RA has some ability to clear local IL-17A, which may reduce inflammation [36]. In the present study, we found Th17 cells and IL-17RA were significantly increased in the LSGs of patients with pSS, and the expression of IL-17RA tended to increase with increasing FS. In addition, we found lymphocytes and part of the glandular and ductal epithelial cells were IL-17RA positive. It may indicate that local increased IL-17 binding to IL-17RA promotes immune effects that cause salivary gland destruction, suggesting that IL-17RA is associated with the progression of pSS.

RORα is one member of the ROR family, which is widely expressed in a variety of tissues and participates in various biological processes, such as immune response, cerebellar development, and biological rhythms [11, 37, 38]. RORs regulate the transcription of downstream target genes in a ligand-independent manner by binding to ROR response elements with co-stimulatory transcription factors [39, 40]. RORγt and RORα are important in the differentiation and maturation of Th17

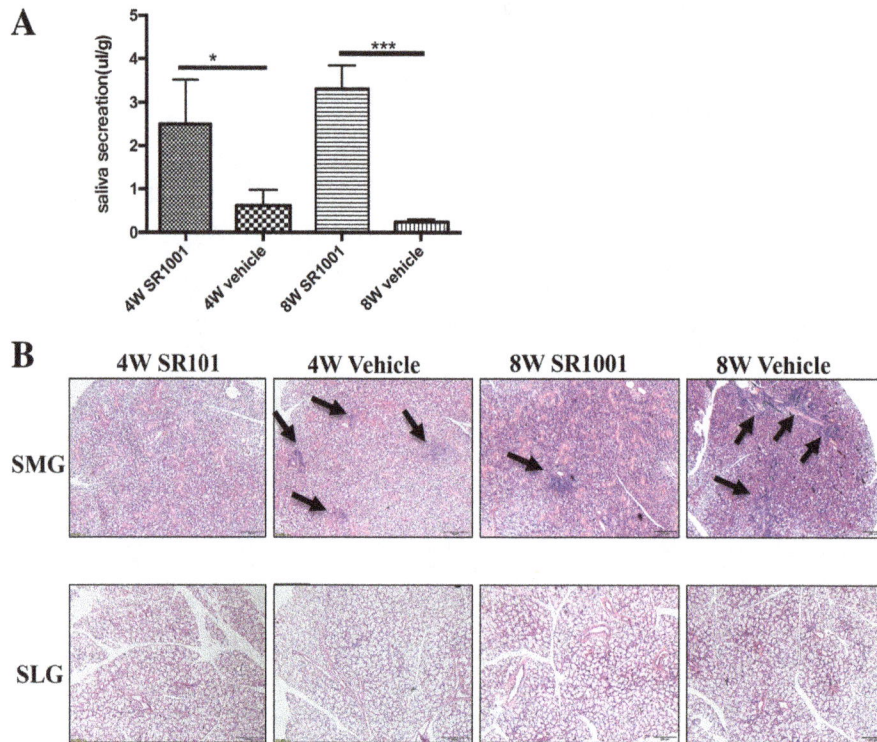

Fig. 5 SR1001 improved salivary gland function and alleviated lymphocytic infiltration of salivary glands in non-obese diabetic (NOD) mice. **a** SR1001-treated NOD mice exhibited normal salivary secretion, while significantly decreased saliva flow rate was observed in the both vehicle-treated 4-week-old (4W) and 8-week-old (8W) groups ($n = 5$ for each group); data represent means ± SEM (μl/g): $^*p < 0.05$, $^{***}p < 0.001$. **b** Histological evaluation of glandular destruction in NOD mice was performed on tissue sections of submandibular glands (SMGs) (upper lane) and sublingual glands (SLGs) (lower lane) by H&E staining ($n = 5$ for each group). Arrowheads indicate inflammatory infiltrate foci. The upper micrographs showed fewer lymphocyte infiltration foci in SMGs of 4W SR1001-treated NOD mice at both 4 and 8 weeks of age compared to vehicle groups, and older NOD mice (8W) had mild inflammatory infiltration. The lower panel indicates no obvious sialadenitis in SLGs of NOD mice ($n = 5$ for each group). Scale bars = 100 μm

cells [11, 14, 18]. In this study, we found that RORα expression was significantly higher in the LSGs of patients with pSS than in non-SS LSGs, and it showed a trend of increasing as FS increased. These data suggested that RORα expression is associated with the progression of pSS. These results may be attributed to the effects of RORα on Th17 cells, i.e., increased IL-17 synthesis and secretion, because RORα-positive Th17 cells were detected in the salivary glands of patients with pSS in our study. Approximately 25% of patients diagnosed as having pSS had no obvious evidence of sialadenitis in LSG biopsies, which is consistent with the results of previous studies [3]. Nevertheless, the LSGs in patients with pSS without obvious FS still had extensive, high RORα expression in the interstitial tissue and epithelial cells compared with LSGs in normal controls. RORα detection may distinguish patients with and without pSS among patients with suspected pSS. However, it is necessary to define the criterion for quantifying RORα. Moreover, it is unknown whether there is a relationship between RORα and disease severity, as there is for the proportion of Th17 cells and IL-17 levels in peripheral blood lymphocytes

from patients with pSS, and whether these diagnostic criteria are true in the salivary glands. If these criteria are also established in serum, it will be possible to diagnose pSS without performing an invasive lip biopsy. Since the sample size was small, the conclusion must be confirmed by further clinical case reports and experimental studies.

RORs can bind to certain small molecule ligands, such as cholesterol and oxysterols, to exert biological effects [41–43]. Recently, some synthetic ROR-specific inverse agonists have been reported and shown to be effective in controlling autoimmune diseases associated with Th17 cells in animal experiments [11, 44–48]. SR1001 is a highly selective and specific RORα/γt inverse agonist that specifically binds to RORα/γt and inhibits the differentiation of Th17 cells [44]. In our study, we investigated the effect of SR1001 in the treatment of pSS and found that SR1001 could significantly improve salivary gland function and alleviate lymphocyte infiltration into the submandibular glands; however, this effect was not obvious in the sublingual glands, since the submandibular glands in NOD mice are most likely to exhibit spontaneous sialadenitis [49]. Flow cytometry analysis showed

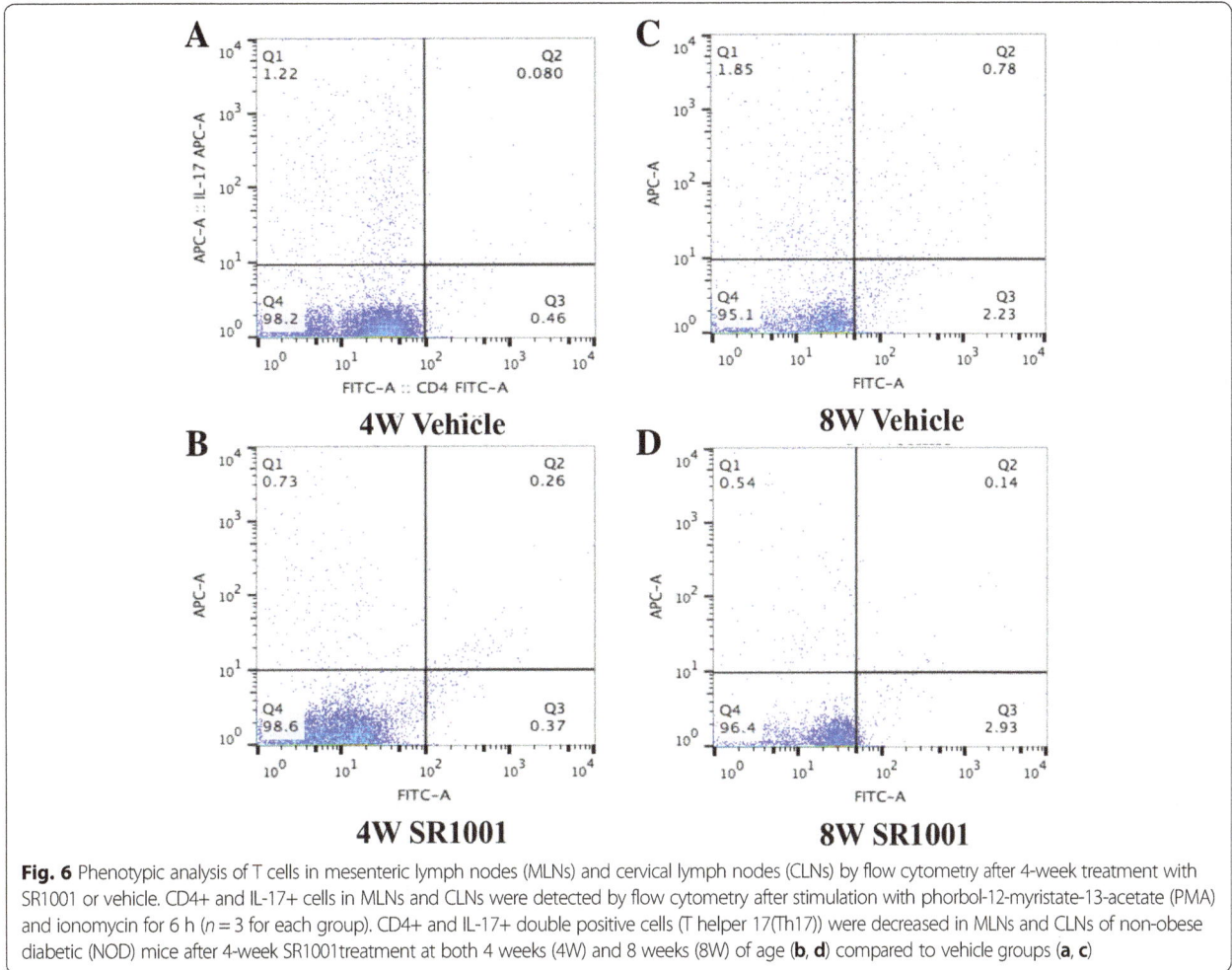

Fig. 6 Phenotypic analysis of T cells in mesenteric lymph nodes (MLNs) and cervical lymph nodes (CLNs) by flow cytometry after 4-week treatment with SR1001 or vehicle. CD4+ and IL-17+ cells in MLNs and CLNs were detected by flow cytometry after stimulation with phorbol-12-myristate-13-acetate (PMA) and ionomycin for 6 h (n = 3 for each group). CD4+ and IL-17+ double positive cells (T helper 17(Th17)) were decreased in MLNs and CLNs of non-obese diabetic (NOD) mice after 4-week SR1001treatment at both 4 weeks (4W) and 8 weeks (8W) of age (**b**, **d**) compared to vehicle groups (**a**, **c**)

that SR1001 could inhibit the differentiation of Th17 cells without affecting overall mouse development. In addition, SR1001 significantly controlled the progression of type I diabetes mellitus and had no obvious side effects on mouse development (Additional file 1). Older NOD mice had a greater improvement in salivary gland function after SR1001 treatment, so we speculated that it is possible that RORα has a different effect at different stages of pSS. At the early stage of pSS, RORα does not have a major effect because it has lower expression or activity, while at the progressive stage, it is prominent because of higher expression or activity. Although we showed that SR1001 can alleviate inflammation and improve salivary gland function, with better results in older NOD mice, additional studies are necessary to confirm this result.

Since SR1001 not only inhibits RORα, but also inhibits RORγt [44, 48], it was uncertain whether these effects stemmed from the inhibition of RORα and/or RORγt. We also detected the expression of RORγt to determine which is dominant in the process of inflammation of the LSGs. The results showed that the expression of RORγt in

the LSGs in patients with pSS was markedly higher than that in patients without pSS (Additional file 2A, B). RORγt-positive cells were seen in infiltrated lymphocytic cells and also in some acinar cells and ductal cells on immunohistochemical staining (Additional file 2C). However, we realized that the expression of RORγt displayed no obvious increasing tendency with progressive disease stage/FS, and RORγt overexpression was even more evident in scattered lymphocytes from the LSGs of patients with pSS, who had a lower histological score for inflammatory lesions. This was different from what we found about RORα in the present study. Based on this finding, we speculated that acinar cells or salivary gland duct cells themselves could have RORγt overexpression in pSS. It has been reported that RORγt overexpression induced severed spontaneous sialadenitis-like SS via RORγt overexpressed CD4+ cells and reduced Treg [13]. We hypothesized that this expression of RORγt by acinar cells or salivary gland duct cells may not be important in the differentiation of Th17 cells in patients with pSS. In addition, we did not find other data on representing relation between RORγt and pSS progression as what we found on RORα. Though several autoantigens have been identified in pSS, none of them are only pSS-specific. Data from our study might provide support to the notion that RORα may be an index sign of accessory diagnosis and classification for pSS. Nevertheless, RORα affects a wide range of biological processes, such as biological rhythms, so further studies are needed to validate potential underlying mechanisms of how RORα is involved in the progression of salivary gland inflammation in patients with pSS.

Conclusion

In summary, this is the first study of different RORα expression between patients with pSS and normal controls through the effect on Th17 cells. In patients with pSS, RORα expression increased with increasing FS, and there was positive correlation between these two factors. Specific inhibition of RORα inhibited the differentiation of Th17 cells, relieved salivary gland inflammation and improved salivary gland function. Our study may offer a new prospect for the diagnosis, classification, and treatment of pSS.

Abbreviations

ANA: Anti-nuclear antibody; BSA: Bovine serum albumin; C3: Component 3; C4: Component 4; CLNs: Cervical lymph nodes; DAPI: Diamidino-phenyl-indole; DMSO: Dimethyl Sulphoxide; ECL: Enhanced chemiluminescence; ESR: Erythrocyte sedimentation rate; FS: Focus score; GAPDH: Glyceraldehyde-3-phosphate dehydrogenase; GM-CSF: Granulocyte-macrophage colony stimulating factor; H&E: Hematoxylin and eosin; IgG: Immunoglobulin G; IL-17: Interleukin 17; IL-17RA: Interlerkin-17 receptor A; IκBζ: Nuclear factor κB inhibitor ζ; LSG: Labial salivary gland; MLNs: Mesenteric lymph nodes; MSG: Minor salivary gland; NC: Normal control; NOD: Non-obese diabetic; PBS: Phosphate-buffered saline; PCR: Polymerase chain reaction; PMA: Phorbol-12-myristate-13-acetate; pSS: Primary Sjögren's syndrome; RF: Rheumatoid factor; RIPA: Radio-immunoprecipitation assay; RORα: Orphan nuclear receptors retinoic acid-related receptor α; RORγt: Orphan nuclear receptors retinoic acid-related receptor γt; SLG: Sublingual gland; SMG: Submandibular gland; SS: Sjögren's syndrome; SSA: Anti-Sjögren's-syndrome-related antigen antibody A; SSB: Anti-Sjögren's-syndrome-related antigen antibody B; TBST: Tris-buffered-saline Tween; Th17: T helper 17; Treg: Regulatory T

Acknowledgements
We would like to thank Cong-yi Wang, Shu Zhang, and Sunchang Zhou for technical assistance, You Song for valuable discussion on the pSS study and the department of pathology of Union hospital, Wuhan for the histologic analysis of LSG sections.

Funding
The present work was supported by grants from National Natural Science Foundation of China (number 81370405).

Authors' contributions
All authors were involved in drafting the article or revising it critically for important intellectual content, and all authors approved the final version to be published. XHW carried out sample handling and collection of information, the isolation of protein and RNA, western blot, immunofluorescence, immunohistochemical analysis, animal research design and the SR1001 intervention, and the flow cytometry. YL coordinated the sample collection, isolation of protein and RNA, western-blot and real-time PCR. BC conceived and designed the study, performed data analysis, drafted the manuscript, and finalized the manuscript. SC participated in the study design, data analysis, and manuscript revision.

Consent for publication
All authors have read and approved the manuscript for publication.

Competing interests
The authors declare that they have no competing interests.

Author details
[1]Department of Stomatology, Zhongnan Hospital of Wuhan University, 169 Donghu Road, Wuhan 430071, Hubei Province, China. [2]Department of Stomatology, Union Hospital, Tongji Medical College, Huazhong University of Science and Technology, 1277 Jiefang Ave, Jianhan District, Wuhan 430022, Hubei Province, China. [3]Department of Rheumatology, Union Hospital, Tongji Medical College, Huazhong University of Science and Technology, 1277 Jiefang Ave, Jianghan District, Wuhan 430022, Hubei Province, China.

References
1. Zintzaras E, Voulgarelis M, Moutsopoulos HM. The risk of lymphoma development in autoimmune diseases: a meta-analysis. Arch Intern Med. 2005;165(20):2337–44.
2. Kassan SS, Thomas TL, Moutsopoulos HM, Hoover R, Kimberly RP, Budman DR, Costa J, Decker JL, Chused TM. Increased risk of lymphoma in sicca syndrome. Ann Intern Med. 1978;89(6):888–92.
3. Yazisiz V, Avci AB, Erbasan F, Kiris E, Terzioglu E. Diagnostic performance of minor salivary gland biopsy, serological and clinical data in Sjogren's syndrome: a retrospective analysis. Rheumatol Int. 2009;29(4):403–9.
4. Teppo H, Revonta M. A follow-up study of minimally invasive lip biopsy in the diagnosis of Sjogren's syndrome. Clin Rheumatol. 2007;26(7):1099–103.
5. Vitali C. Classification criteria for Sjogren's syndrome: a revised version of the European criteria proposed by the American-European consensus group. Ann Rheum Dis. 2002;61(6):554–8.
6. Moriyama M, Hayashida JN, Toyoshima T, Ohyama Y, Shinozaki S, Tanaka A, Maehara T, Nakamura S. Cytokine/chemokine profiles contribute to understanding the pathogenesis and diagnosis of primary Sjogren's syndrome. Clin Exp Immunol. 2012;169(1):17–26.
7. Lin X, Rui K, Deng J, Tian J, Wang X, Wang S, Ko KH, Jiao Z, Chan VS, Lau CS, et al. Th17 cells play a critical role in the development of experimental Sjogren's syndrome. Ann Rheum Dis. 2015;74(6):1302–10.
8. Ciccia F, Guggino G, Rizzo A, Ferrante A, Raimondo S, Giardina A, Dieli F, Campisi G, Alessandro R, Triolo G. Potential involvement of IL-22 and IL-22-producing cells in the inflamed salivary glands of patients with Sjogren's syndrome. Ann Rheum Dis. 2012;71(2):295–301.
9. Nguyen CQ, Hu MH, Li Y, Stewart C, Peck AB. Salivary gland tissue expression of interleukin-23 and interleukin-17 in Sjogren's syndrome: findings in humans and mice. Arthritis Rheum. 2008;58(3):734–43.
10. Wu C, Wang Z, Zourelias L, Thakker H, Passineau MJ. IL-17 sequestration via salivary gland gene therapy in a mouse model of Sjogren's syndrome suppresses disease-associated expression of the putative autoantigen Klk1b22. Arthritis Res Ther. 2015;17:198.
11. Kojetin DJ, Burris TP. REV-ERB and ROR nuclear receptors as drug targets. Nat Rev Drug Discov. 2014;13(3):197–216.
12. Ruan Q, Kameswaran V, Zhang Y, Zheng S, Sun J, Wang J, DeVirgiliis J, Liou HC, Beg AA, Chen YH. The Th17 immune response is controlled by the Rel-RORgamma-RORgamma T transcriptional axis. J Exp Med. 2011;208(11):2321–33.
13. Iizuka M, Tsuboi H, Matsuo N, Asashima H, Hirota T, Kondo Y, Iwakura Y, Takahashi S, Matsumoto I, Sumida T. A crucial role of RORgammat in the development of spontaneous Sialadenitis-like Sjogren's syndrome. J Immunol. 2015;194(1):56 67.
14. Yang XO, Pappu BP, Nurieva R, Akimzhanov A, Kang HS, Chung Y, Ma L, Shah B, Panopoulos AD, Schluns KS, et al. T helper 17 lineage differentiation is programmed by orphan nuclear receptors ROR alpha and ROR gamma. Immunity. 2008;28(1):29–39.
15. Ivanov II, McKenzie BS, Zhou L, Tadokoro CE, Lepelley A, Lafaille JJ, Cua DJ, Littman DR. The orphan nuclear receptor RORgammat directs the differentiation program of proinflammatory IL-17+ T helper cells. Cell. 2006;126(6):1121–33.
16. Okamoto K, Iwai Y, Oh-Hora M, Yamamoto M, Morio T, Aoki K, Ohya K, Jetten AM, Akira S, Muta T, et al. IkappaBzeta regulates T (H)17 development by cooperating with ROR nuclear receptors. Nature. 2010;464(7293):1381–5.

17. Yang M, Deng J, Liu Y, Ko KH, Wang X, Jiao Z, Wang S, Hua Z, Sun L, Srivastava G, et al. IL-10-producing regulatory B10 cells ameliorate collagen-induced arthritis via suppressing Th17 cell generation. Am J Pathol. 2012; 180(6):2375–85.

18. Hermann GA, Vivino FB, Goin JE. Scintigraphic features of chronic sialadenitis and Sjogren's syndrome: a comparison. Nucl Med Commun. 1999;20(12):1123–32.

19. Nikolov NP, Illei GG. Pathogenesis of Sjogren's syndrome. Curr Opin Rheumatol. 2009;21(5):465–70.

20. Alamanos Y, Tsifetaki N, Voulgari PV, Venetsanopoulou AI, Siozos C, Drosos AA. Epidemiology of primary Sjogren's syndrome in north-West Greece, 1982-2003. Rheumatology (Oxford). 2006;45(2):187–91.

21. Bournia VK, Vlachoyiannopoulos PG. Subgroups of Sjogren syndrome patients according to serological profiles. J Autoimmun. 2012;39(1–2):15–26.

22. Xu J, Racke MK, Drew PD. Peroxisome proliferator-activated receptor-alpha agonist fenofibrate regulates IL-12 family cytokine expression in the CNS: relevance to multiple sclerosis. J Neurochem. 2007;103(5):1801–10.

23. Bikker A, Moret FM, Kruize AA, Bijlsma JW, Lafeber FP, van Roon JA. IL-7 drives Th1 and Th17 cytokine production in patients with primary SS despite an increase in CD4 T cells lacking the IL-7Ralpha. Rheumatology (Oxford). 2012;51(6):996–1005.

24. Abdulahad WH, Kroese FG, Vissink A, Bootsma H. Immune regulation and B-cell depletion therapy in patients with primary Sjogren's syndrome. J Autoimmun. 2012;39(1–2):103–11.

25. Cornec D, Devauchelle-Pensec V, Tobon GJ, Pers JO, Jousse-Joulin S, Saraux A. B cells in Sjogren's syndrome: from pathophysiology to diagnosis and treatment. J Autoimmun. 2012;39(3):161–7.

26. Littman DR, Rudensky AY. Th17 and regulatory T cells in mediating and restraining inflammation. Cell. 2010;140(6):845–58.

27. Abdulahad WH, Boots AM, Kallenberg CG. FoxP3+ CD4+ T cells in systemic autoimmune diseases: the delicate balance between true regulatory T cells and effector Th-17 cells. Rheumatology (Oxford). 2011; 50(4):646–56.

28. Xuan J, Shen L, Malyavantham K, Pankewycz O, Ambrus JL Jr, Suresh L. Temporal histological changes in lacrimal and major salivary glands in mouse models of Sjogren's syndrome. BMC Oral Health. 2013;13:51.

29. Katsifis GE, Rekka S, Moutsopoulos NM, Pillemer S, Wahl SM. Systemic and local interleukin-17 and linked cytokines associated with Sjogren's syndrome immunopathogenesis. Am J Pathol. 2009;175(3):1167–77.

30. Mieliauskaite D, Dumalakiene I, Rugiene R, Mackiewicz Z. Expression of IL-17, IL-23 and their receptors in minor salivary glands of patients with primary Sjogren's syndrome. Clin Dev Immunol. 2012;2012:187258.

31. Chung Y, Chang SH, Martinez GJ, Yang XO, Nurieva R, Kang HS, Ma L, Watowich SS, Jetten AM, Tian Q, et al. Critical regulation of early Th17 cell differentiation by interleukin-1 signaling. Immunity. 2009;30(4):576–87.

32. Sherlock JP, Joyce-Shaikh B, Turner SP, Chao CC, Sathe M, Grein J, Gorman DM, Bowman EP, McClanahan TK, Yearley JH, et al. IL-23 induces spondyloarthropathy by acting on ROR-gammat+ CD3+CD4-CD8- entheseal resident T cells. Nat Med. 2012;18(7):1069–76.

33. Shen F, Hu Z, Goswami J, Gaffen SL. Identification of common transcriptional regulatory elements in interleukin-17 target genes. J Biol Chem. 2006;281(34):24138–48.

34. Maitra A, Shen F, Hanel W, Mossman K, Tocker J, Swart D, Gaffen SL. Distinct functional motifs within the IL-17 receptor regulate signal transduction and target gene expression. Proc Natl Acad Sci U S A. 2007;104(18):7506–11.

35. Gaffen SL. Structure and signalling in the IL-17 receptor family. Nat Rev Immunol. 2009;9(8):556–67.

36. Lindemann MJ, Hu Z, Benczik M, Liu KD, Gaffen SL. Differential regulation of the IL-17 receptor by gammac cytokines: inhibitory signaling by the phosphatidylinositol 3-kinase pathway. J Biol Chem. 2008;283(20):14100–8.

37. Hamilton BA, Frankel WN, Kerrebrock AW, Hawkins TL, FitzHugh W, Kusumi K, Russell LB, Mueller KL, van Berkel V, Birren BW, et al. Disruption of the nuclear hormone receptor RORalpha in staggerer mice. Nature. 1996; 379(6567):736–9.

38. Steinmayr M, Andre E, Conquet F, Rondi-Reig L, Delhaye-Bouchaud N, Auclair N, Daniel H, Crepel F, Mariani J, Sotelo C, et al. Staggerer phenotype in retinoid-related orphan receptor alpha-deficient mice. Proc Natl Acad Sci U S A. 1998;95(7):3960–5.

39. Jetten AM, Kurebayashi S, Ueda E. The ROR nuclear orphan receptor subfamily: critical regulators of multiple biological processes. Prog Nucleic Acid Res Mol Biol. 2001;69:205–47.

40. Lechtken A, Zundorf I, Dingermann T, Firla B, Steinhilber D. Overexpression, refolding, and purification of polyhistidine-tagged human retinoic acid related orphan receptor RORalpha4. Protein Expr Purif. 2006; 49(1):114–20.

41. Kallen J, Schlaeppi JM, Bitsch F, Delhon I, Fournier B. Crystal structure of the human RORalpha ligand binding domain in complex with cholesterol sulfate at 2.2 a. J Biol Chem. 2004;279(14):14033–8.

42. Wang Y, Kumar N, Crumbley C, Griffin PR, Burris TP. A second class of nuclear receptors for oxysterols: regulation of RORalpha and RORgamma activity by 24S-hydroxycholesterol (cerebrosterol). Biochim Biophys Acta. 2010;1801(8):917–23.

43. Wang Y, Kumar N, Solt LA, Richardson TI, Helvering LM, Crumbley C, Garcia-Ordonez RD, Stayrook KR, Zhang X, Novick S, et al. Modulation of retinoic acid receptor-related orphan receptor alpha and gamma activity by 7-oxygenated sterol ligands. J Biol Chem. 2010;285(7):5013–25.

44. Solt LA, Kumar N, Nuhant P, Wang Y, Lauer JL, Liu J, Istrate MA, Kamenecka TM, Roush WR, Vidovic D, et al. Suppression of TH17 differentiation and autoimmunity by a synthetic ROR ligand. Nature. 2011;472(7344):491–4.

45. Kumar N, Kojetin DJ, Solt LA, Kumar KG, Nuhant P, Duckett DR, Cameron MD, Butler AA, Roush WR, Griffin PR, et al. Identification of SR3335 (ML-176): a synthetic RORalpha selective inverse agonist. ACS Chem Biol. 2011;6(3): 218–22.

46. Wang Y, Kumar N, Nuhant P, Cameron MD, Istrate MA, Roush WR, Griffin PR, Burris TP. Identification of SR1078, a synthetic agonist for the orphan nuclear receptors RORalpha and RORgamma. ACS Chem Biol. 2010;5(11): 1029–34.

47. Kumar N, Solt LA, Conkright JJ, Wang Y, Istrate MA, Busby SA, Garcia-Ordonez RD, Burris TP, Griffin PR. The benzenesulfoamide T0901317 [N-(2,2,2-trifluoroethyl)-N-[4-[2,2,2-trifluoro-1-hydroxy-1-(trifluoromethyl) ethyl]phenyl]-benzenesulfonamide] is a novel retinoic acid receptor-related orphan receptor-alpha/gamma inverse agonist. Mol Pharmacol. 2010;77(2): 228–36.

48. Solt LA, Banerjee S, Campbell S, Kamenecka TM, Burris TP. ROR inverse agonist suppresses insulitis and prevents hyperglycemia in a mouse model of type 1 diabetes. Endocrinology. 2015;156(3):869–81.

49. Lavoie TN, Lee BH, Nguyen CQ. Current concepts: mouse models of Sjogren's syndrome. J Biomed Biotechnol. 2011;2011:549107.

5

Monosodium urate crystals reduce osteocyte viability and indirectly promote a shift in osteocyte function towards a proinflammatory and proresorptive state

Ashika Chhana[1], Bregina Pool[1], Karen E. Callon[1], Mei Lin Tay[1], David Musson[1], Dorit Naot[1], Geraldine McCarthy[2], Susan McGlashan[3], Jillian Cornish[1] and Nicola Dalbeth[1,4*]

Abstract

Background: Bone erosion is a frequent complication of gout and is strongly associated with tophi, which are lesions comprising inflammatory cells surrounding collections of monosodium urate (MSU) crystals. Osteocytes are important cellular mediators of bone remodeling. The aim of this study was to investigate the direct effects of MSU crystals and indirect effects of MSU crystal-induced inflammation on osteocytes.

Methods: For direct assays, MSU crystals were added to MLO-Y4 osteocyte cell line cultures or primary mouse osteocyte cultures. For indirect assays, the RAW264.7 macrophage cell line was cultured with or without MSU crystals, and conditioned medium from these cultures was added to MLO-Y4 cells. MLO-Y4 cell viability was assessed using alamarBlue® and LIVE/DEAD® assays, and MLO-Y4 cell gene expression and protein expression were assessed by real-time polymerase chain reaction (PCR) and enzyme-linked immunosorbent assay (ELISA), respectively. Histological analysis was used to examine the relationship between MSU crystals, inflammatory cells, and osteocytes in human joints affected by tophaceous gout.

Results: In direct assays, MSU crystals reduced MLO-Y4 cell and primary mouse osteocyte viability but did not alter MLO-Y4 cell gene expression. In contrast, conditioned medium from MSU crystal-stimulated RAW264.7 macrophages did not affect MLO-Y4 cell viability but significantly increased MLO-Y4 cell expression of osteocyte-related factors including E11, connexin 43, and RANKL, and inflammatory mediators such as interleukin (IL)-6, IL-11, tumor necrosis factor (TNF)-α and cyclooxygenase-2 (COX-2). Inhibition of COX-2 in MLO-Y4 cells significantly reduced the indirect effects of MSU crystals. In histological analysis, CD68[+] macrophages and MSU crystals were identified in close proximity to osteocytes within bone. COX-2 expression was also observed in tophaceous joint samples.

Conclusions: MSU crystals directly inhibit osteocyte viability and, through interactions with macrophages, indirectly promote a shift in osteocyte function that favors bone resorption and inflammation. These interactions may contribute to disordered bone remodeling in gout.

Keywords: Gout, Osteocyte, Inflammation, Urate, Bone erosion

* Correspondence: n.dalbeth@auckland.ac.nz
[1]Department of Medicine, Bone & Joint Research Group, University of Auckland, Auckland, New Zealand
[4]Department of Medicine, Faculty of Medical and Health Sciences, University of Auckland, 85 Park Rd, Grafton, Auckland, New Zealand
Full list of author information is available at the end of the article

Background

Bone erosion is a common complication of tophaceous gout [1]. Tophi are ordered structures containing inflammatory cells and tissue surrounding collections of monosodium urate (MSU) crystals [2]. Both MSU crystals and the soft tissue components of the tophus are strongly and independently associated with bone erosion in gout [3].

Joints affected by tophaceous gout show evidence of disordered bone remodeling, with increased osteoclast-mediated bone resorption [4, 5] and impaired osteoblast-mediated bone formation [6]. Osteocytes are the most abundant cell type found within bone and are important regulators of bone remodeling, controlling both bone resorption and bone formation [7, 8]. Embedded within the mineralized matrix, osteocytes communicate with each other and other cells on the bone surface through dendrites. Osteocytes are also a source of soluble factors that can target local and distant tissues [9]. We have previously reported that osteocyte-derived soluble factors mediate the relationship between tophus and erosion in gout [10], suggesting that osteocytes may contribute to the development of bone erosion in gout. The aim of this study was to investigate the direct effects of MSU crystals and indirect effects of MSU crystal-induced inflammation on osteocyte viability and function.

Methods

Ethical approvals

Human sample collection was approved by the Northern Regional Ethics Committee and all participants provided written informed consent. Protocols involving animals were approved by the University of Auckland Animal Ethics Committee. Use of human cadaveric tissue was in accordance with the New Zealand Human Tissue Act 2008.

Cell culture

MLO-Y4 cells (a kind gift from Professor Lynda Bonewald, Indiana University) were cultured in α-minimum essential medium (MEM) containing L-glutamine and nucleosides (Gibco, Life Technologies, Thermo Fisher Scientific, Waltham, USA) and supplemented with 2.5% heat-inactivated fetal bovine serum (FBS; Gibco) and 2.5% heat-inactivated newborn calf serum (Hyclone, GE Healthcare Life Sciences, Logan, USA). The MLO-Y4 cell line is widely used for in-vitro studies of osteocytes; these cells have similar properties to primary osteocytes with high expression of osteocalcin and connexin 43. MLO-Y4 cells also have dendritic processes and can communicate via gap junctions, similar to primary osteocytes [11, 12].

Primary mouse osteocytes were isolated from the long bones of 6-week-old C57BL/6 male mice using a modified method of Stern et al. [13]. The long bones (femur,

tibia, and humerus) were harvested, the epiphyses removed, and bone marrow flushed out with α-MEM. Bones were then cut into small pieces and sequentially digested nine times using 300 U/mL collagenase (Sigma-Aldrich, St. Louis, USA; digests 1–3, 5, 7, and 9; 25 min per digest) and 5 mM EDTA (Sigma-Aldrich; digests 4, 6, and 8; 40 min per digest) at 37 °C. Bone chips were washed with Hank's balanced salt solution (Gibco) between digests. Osteocyte-like cells were grown out from the digested bone chips onto collagen-coated surfaces with the same medium that was used for MLO-Y4 cells.

For all experiments, MLO-Y4 cells or primary mouse osteocytes were seeded in three-dimensional (3D) collagen gels in 24-well plates (1×10^4 cells/50 μL gel; 1 gel/well) as previously described [14]. Briefly, rat collagen type I (Corning Inc., Corning, USA) was neutralized with 1 M NaOH and diluted to a final concentration of 3 mg/mL. Cells were seeded in 50 μL collagen gels and allowed to set at 37 °C for 1 h prior to the addition of 1 mL culture medium. Cells were cultured in the collagen gels for 4 days (MLO-Y4 cells) or 24 h (primary mouse osteocytes) before the media were replaced and experiments commenced.

The RAW264.7 macrophage cell line (ATCC, Manassas, USA) was maintained in Iscove's modified Dulbecco's medium supplemented with 1 mM L-glutamine (both from Sigma-Aldrich) and 10% FBS.

MSU crystal synthesis

Endotoxin-free MSU crystals were prepared by recrystallization from uric acid as previously described [15].

Preparation of conditioned medium from RAW264.7 macrophages

RAW264.7 cells were seeded in 24-well plates at 1×10^6 cells/well. The following day, the medium was changed to α-MEM containing L-glutamine and nucleosides, supplemented with 2.5% heat-inactivated FBS and 2.5% heat-inactivated newborn calf serum, and 0.5 mg/mL MSU crystals were added for 24 h. Conditioned medium was then harvested and filtered using a 0.2-μm filter to remove any residual MSU crystals. The absence of MSU crystals was confirmed by polarizing light microscopy. Control conditioned medium from RAW264.7 macrophages alone (no added MSU crystals) was also prepared at the same time. There were up to 18 wells in each treatment group.

alamarBlue® assay for cell viability

For direct assays, various concentrations of MSU crystals were added to MLO-Y4 cells or primary mouse osteocytes for 24 h. Cells were then washed to remove MSU crystals and alamarBlue® reagent (Life Technologies) was added (5% final concentration in a well) for 6 h at 37 °C. At the same time, 1 U/mL uricase (Sigma-Aldrich) was added to remove residual MSU crystals to prevent interference with the assay [6]. Cell viability was assessed both 24 and 48 h after the addition of MSU crystals by measuring fluorescence (excitation 540 nm; emission 630 nm) using a Synergy 2 multidetection microplate reader (BioTek Instruments Inc., Winooski, VT). In separate experiments, calcium pyrophosphate dihydrate (CPPD) crystals (Integrated Sciences, Sydney, Australia), basic calcium phosphate (BCP) crystals (synthesized as described previously [16]) and aluminum particulates (Sigma-Aldrich) were also added to MLO-Y4 cells for viability assays.

For indirect assays, 5%, 20%, or 40% control conditioned medium or MSU crystal-stimulated conditioned medium (from the RAW264.7 macrophage assays) was added to MLO-Y4 cells for 24 h. Cells were then washed, and viability assessed using alamarBlue® as above. There were up to six wells in each treatment group for all experiments.

LIVE/DEAD® assay for cell viability
MSU crystals (0.1 or 0.3 mg/mL) were added to MLO-Y4 cells for 24 h. Cells were washed, and crystals completely removed. Cells were then stained with calcein-AM (live cells) and ethidium homodimer-1 (dead cells) using the LIVE/DEAD® Viability/Cytotoxicity Kit (Life Technologies), either 24 or 48 h after the addition of MSU crystals. Fluorescence microscopy was used to take 10 paired images of stained cells (live and dead) within three separate layers of the collagen gel (top, middle, and bottom). ImageJ software (https://imagej.nih.gov/ij/) was used to count the number of living or dead cells in each gel layer and the percentage of dead cells was calculated.

Gene and protein expression assays
For direct assays, 0.1 mg/mL MSU crystals were added to MLO-Y4 cells for 0, 1, 6, and 24 h. For indirect assays, 40% RAW264.7 conditioned medium (control or MSU crystal-stimulated) was added to MLO-Y4 cells for 0, 1, 6, and 24 h. MLO-Y4 cells were harvested for gene expression analysis, and MLO-Y4 cell supernatants and RAW264.7 macrophage conditioned medium preparations were harvested for secreted protein analysis. For each experiment, there were 6–12 wells in each treatment group.

Quantitative real-time polymerase chain reaction (PCR)
Purification of total cellular RNA, synthesis of cDNA, and real-time PCR was performed as previously described [14]. 18S rRNA endogenous control was used to correct for variations in cell numbers between samples.

The $\Delta\Delta Ct$ method was used to calculate the relative levels of gene expression, using day 0 or control cell (MLO-Y4 cells alone) expression levels as a control.

Protein quantification
Protein levels of tumor necrosis factor (TNF)-α, interleukin (IL)-6, IL-1β, soluble receptor activator of nuclear factor kappa-B ligand (RANKL), and osteoprotegerin (OPG) in RAW264.7 macrophage conditioned medium preparations and MLO-Y4 supernatants was determined by enzyme-linked immunosorbent assay (ELISA) (R&D Systems, Minneapolis, USA). Prostaglandin E_2 (PGE₂) was measured in conditioned media and supernatant samples as a measure of cyclooxygenase-2 (COX-2) enzyme activity using the PGE₂ EIA Kit (Cayman Chemical, Ann Arbor, USA).

TNF-α and COX-2 inhibition experiments
For TNF-α blocking experiments, 5 μg/mL TNF-α neutralizing antibody (monoclonal rat IgG1, clone MP6-XT22) or IgG1 isotype control (both from R&D Systems) was added to MLO-Y4 cells for 1 h prior to the addition of RAW264.7 macrophage conditioned medium for 24 h. The concentration of TNF-α neutralizing antibody was chosen based on optimization experiments whereby three different concentrations (0.5, 2.5, and 5 μg/mL) of neutralizing antibody was added to MLO-Y4 cells prior to the addition of 4 ng/mL TNF-α for 24 h. The addition of 5 μg/mL TNF-α neutralizing antibody suppressed TNF-α-induced expression of COX-2, IL-11, and RANKL genes by MLO-Y4 cells (data not shown).

For COX-2 blocking experiments, 1 μM COX-2-specific inhibitor (SC-236, Sigma-Aldrich) was added to MLO-Y4 cells for 1 h prior to the addition of RAW264.7 macrophage conditioned medium for 24 h.

Histology of joint samples affected by gout
Human joint samples (two each from finger proximal and distal interphalangeal joints, and one each from the knee, mid-foot, and a big toe interphalangeal joint) were obtained from two patients with gout undergoing orthopedic surgery and three cadaveric donors with microscopically proven gout. Cadaveric samples were transferred to 70% ethanol immediately after collection and all samples were demineralized at room temperature in 10% formic acid for 1 week prior to paraffin embedding. Slides were prepared and stained with toluidine blue as previously described [17] or used for immunohistochemistry. The spatial relationship between osteocytes, macrophages, and MSU crystals in joint samples was examined using polarizing light microscopy. Immunohistochemistry was used to identify CD68[+] macrophage cells and COX-2 expression.

Immunohistochemistry for CD68 and COX-2

Sections were dewaxed for 12 min in Safsolvent (Ajax Finechem Pty Ltd., Melbourne, Australia) and rehydrated through graded ethanol solutions for 5 min each. Once hydrated, sections were immersed in 0.5% pepsin for 14 min at 37 °C (CD68) or pH 9.0 Dako Target Retrieval Solution (Produktionsvej, Denmark) for 20 min at 96 °C (COX-2). To block endogenous peroxidase activity, sections were incubated in Dual Endogenous Enzyme-Blocking Reagent (Dako, Produktionsvej, Denmark) for 20 min (CD68) or 3% hydrogen peroxide in methanol for 15 min (COX-2). To block nonspecific binding, sections were incubated in 10% goat serum for 30 min (CD68) or 3% bovine serum albumin (MP Biomedicals New Zealand, Auckland, New Zealand) for 30 min (COX-2). Sections were incubated with primary antibody (1:200 dilution of anti-human CD68 clone PG-M1, Dako; 1:100 dilution of anti-human COX-2, clone SP21, Thermo Fisher Scientific) at 4 °C overnight. After washing with phosphate-buffered saline (PBS), slides were incubated with the Dako Dual link system peroxidase secondary antibody for 30 min (CD68) or 2 h (COX-2). After further washing, the Impact DAB Substrate Kit (Vector Laboratories, Burlingame, CA) was used to detect staining according to the manufacturer's instructions. Slides were briefly counterstained with Hematoxylin QS counter stain (Vector Laboratories) and dehydrated through graded ethanol solutions and xylol. Slides were mounted with DPX (BDH, Poole, UK) and analyzed by light microscopy.

Statistical analysis

Data were analyzed using SAS Software (SAS Institute, Cary, USA) and GraphPad Prism Software (v7, GraphPad Software, San Diego, USA). For all experiments, data were pooled from three to five biological repeats. Data were analyzed using one-way or two-way analysis of variance (ANOVA) with post-hoc Dunnett's or Sidak's multiple comparison tests in the case of more than two groups, or by two-tailed paired t test in the case of two groups.

Results

MSU crystals directly reduce MLO-Y4 cell and primary mouse osteocyte cell viability over time

The higher concentrations of MSU crystals (0.3–0.5 mg/mL) reduced the viability of MLO-Y4 cells and primary mouse osteocytes after 24 h as assessed by alamarBlue® assays, with a further reduction in viability observed at the 48 h time point (Fig. 1a). The inhibitory effect was specific to MSU crystals, since soluble urate at the same concentrations (Fig. 1b) and other types of crystals (CPPD, BCP, aluminum) did not reduce MLO-Y4 cell viability (Fig. 1c). The effects on MLO-Y4 cell viability were not altered with different MSU crystal lengths (Additional file 1: Figure S1).

To assess whether MLO-Y4 cell death induced by MSU crystals was consistent throughout the 3D collagen gel, LIVE/DEAD® assays were performed and MLO-Y4 cell death in the top, middle, and bottom layers of the collagen gel were determined. In these assays, significant MLO-Y4 cell death was observed in the top layer of the gel compared with the middle and bottom layers following culture with 0.3 mg/mL MSU crystals for 24 h or 48 h (Fig. 1d).

MSU crystals do not directly alter MLO-Y4 cell expression of bone-related or inflammatory genes

Real-time PCR was used to determine changes in gene expression in MLO-Y4 cells cultured with MSU crystals for 1, 6, and 24 h. MSU crystals alone did not alter the expression of bone-related genes, including E11 (*Pdpn*), connexin 43 (*Gja1*), RANKL (*Tnfsf11*), or OPG (*Tnfrs11b*) (Fig. 2a), or inflammatory genes, including TNF-α (*Tnfa*), COX-2 (*Ptgs2*), IL-6 (*Il6*), and IL-11 (*Il11*) (Fig. 2b). IL-1β (*Il1b*) was not expressed by MLO-Y4 cells.

Conditioned medium from MSU crystal-stimulated RAW264.7 macrophages has no effect on MLO-Y4 cell viability

To assess whether soluble factors released by macrophages in response to MSU crystals indirectly affect osteocyte viability, RAW264.7 cells were cultured with or without 0.5 mg/mL MSU crystals for 24 h, and conditioned medium was harvested. The addition of increasing concentrations of control or MSU crystal-stimulated conditioned medium had no effect on MLO-Y4 cell viability as determined by the alamarBlue® assay after 24 and 48 h (Additional file 2: Figure S2).

Conditioned medium from MSU crystal-stimulated RAW264.7 macrophages alters MLO-Y4 cell expression of bone-related factors and upregulates MLO-Y4 expression of inflammatory mediators

The addition of 40% conditioned medium from MSU crystal-stimulated RAW264.7 macrophages to MLO-Y4 cell cultures led to an approximate two- to fourfold increase in expression of E11 and connexin 43 at the 6 and 24 h time points compared with control conditioned medium. RANKL expression was upregulated approximately sixfold at the 6 and 24 h time points, and OPG expression was reduced at the 6 h time point by approximately twofold (Fig. 3a).

The expression of inflammatory genes by MLO-Y4 cells was also significantly upregulated with the addition of MSU crystal-stimulated conditioned medium, including TNF-α (~ 4-fold) after 1 h, COX-2 (~ 11-fold) after 6 and 24 h, IL-6 after 6 and 24 h (~ 1800-fold and ~ 700-fold, respectively), and IL-11 (~ 200-fold) after 6 and 24 h (Fig. 3b).

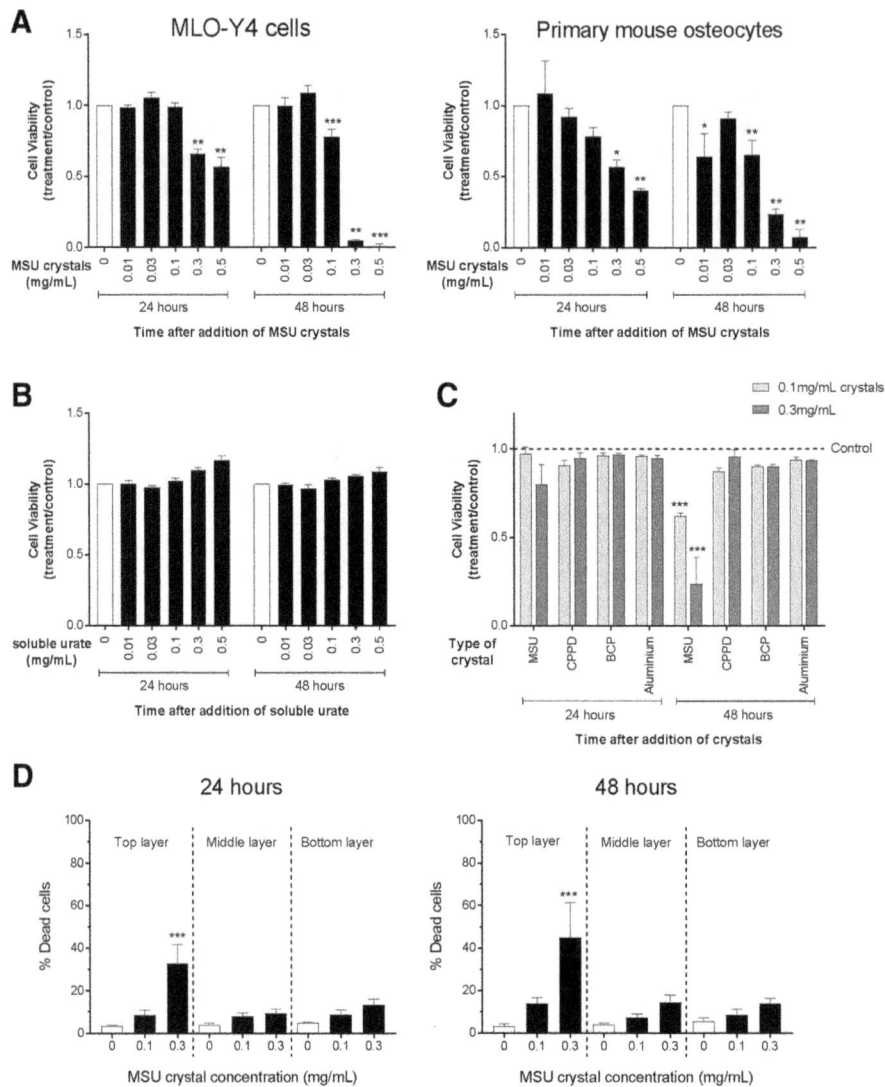

Fig. 1 The direct effects of MSU crystals on osteocyte viability. The alamarBlue® assay was used to determine the viability of **a** MLO-Y4 cells and primary mouse osteocytes cultured with monosodium urate (MSU) crystals for 24 h, **b** MLO-Y4 cells cultured with soluble urate for 24 h, and **c** MLO-Y4 cells cultured with different types of crystals for 24 h. Viability was assessed 24 and 48 h after the addition of crystals or soluble urate. Data shown are pooled from three to four biological repeats and are presented as mean (SEM); by two-way ANOVA **a** $P_{Interaction} < 0.0001$ for MLO-Y4 cells, $P_{Interaction} = 0.026$ for primary mouse osteocytes, **b** $P_{Interaction} = 0.24$, and **c** $P_{Interaction} = 0.057$ at 24 h, $P_{Interaction} < 0.0001$ at 48 h; with post-hoc Dunnett's test $*p < 0.05$, $**p < 0.01$, and $***p < 0.001$ versus control (no crystals or soluble urate) at that time point. **d** The LIVE/DEAD® assay was used to determine the percentage of dead MLO-Y4 cells within three separate layers of the collagen gel following culture with MSU crystals for 24 h or 48 h. Data shown are pooled from four biological repeats and are presented as mean (SEM); one-way ANOVA $p < 0.0001$ at 24 h, $p = 0.004$ at 48 h; with post-hoc Sidak's test $***p < 0.001$ versus control (no MSU crystals) for each layer of the gel. BCP basic calcium phosphate, CPPD calcium pyrophosphate dehydrate

To assess changes at the protein level, MLO-Y4 cell supernatants were harvested and protein concentrations were measured in the MLO-Y4 cell supernatants and compared with RAW264.7 macrophage conditioned medium alone (before addition to MLO-Y4 cells). High levels of TNF-α, PGE$_2$, and IL-6 protein were secreted by MLO-Y4 cells in response to conditioned medium from RAW264.7 macrophages cultured with MSU crystals (Fig. 4a–c). OPG protein levels were unchanged

(Fig. 4d) and soluble RANKL was not detected in any conditioned media or supernatant samples.

The inflammatory response induced in MLO-Y4 cells by conditioned medium from MSU crystal-stimulated RAW264.7 macrophages is suppressed with inhibition of COX-2

The concentration of candidate inflammatory mediators and bone factors in conditioned medium collected from

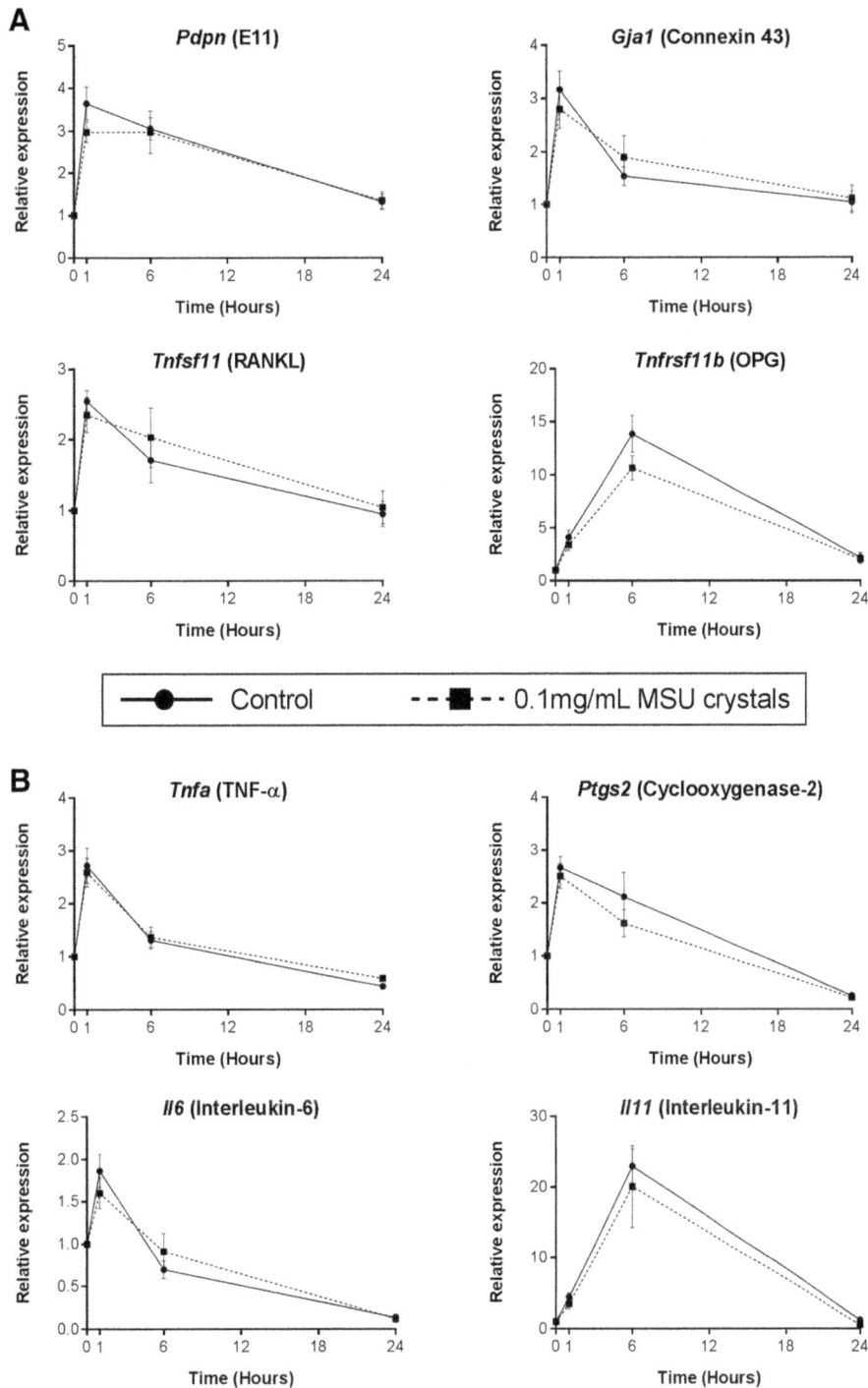

Fig. 2 Direct effects of MSU crystals on MLO-Y4 cell expression of bone-related or inflammatory genes. Real-time PCR was used to determine changes in the relative mRNA expression levels of **a** bone-related and **b** inflammatory genes in MLO-Y4 cells, following culture with 0.1 mg/mL monosodium urate (MSU) crystals for 0, 1, 6, and 24 h. Data shown are pooled from three biological repeats and are presented as mean (SEM); two-way ANOVA $P_{Interaction} > 0.1$ for all genes. OPG osteoprotegerin, RANKL receptor activator of nuclear factor kappa-B ligand, TNF tumor necrosis factor

RAW264.7 macrophages was measured using ELISA. The addition of MSU crystals to RAW264.7 macrophages led to significantly increased secretion of TNF-α protein and PGE₂ compared with control cells (without MSU crystals) (Additional file 3: Figure S3). There was no change in IL-1β or OPG release, and IL-6 and soluble

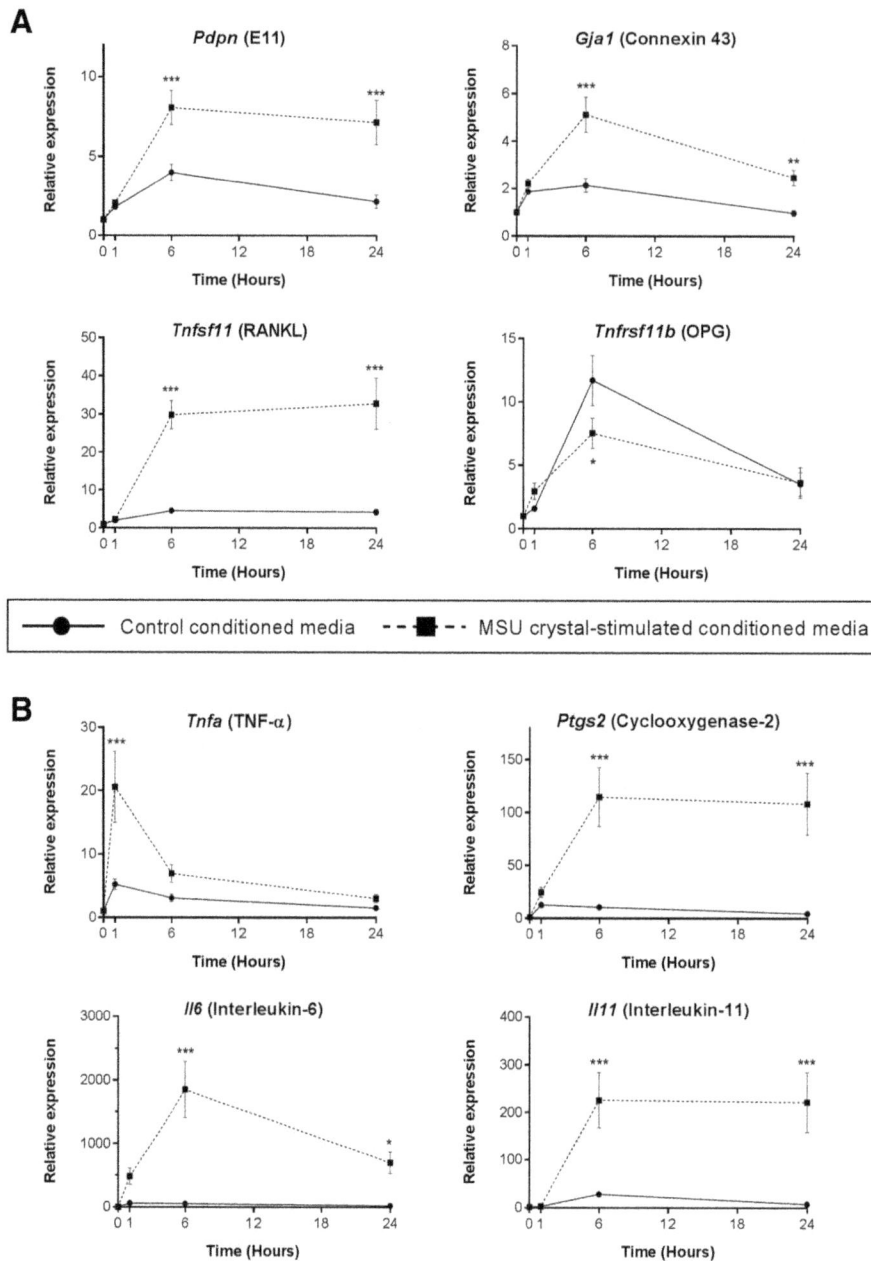

Fig. 3 Indirect effects of MSU crystal-stimulated RAW264.7 macrophage conditioned medium on MLO-Y4 cell gene expression. RAW264.7 macrophages were cultured with or without 0.5 mg/mL monosodium urate (MSU) crystals for 24 h for preparation of MSU crystal-stimulated conditioned medium and control conditioned medium, respectively. Conditioned medium preparations were added to MLO-Y4 cells (40% final concentration in a well) for 0, 1, 6, and 24 h. MLO-Y4 cells were harvested and real-time PCR was used to determine changes in the relative mRNA expression levels of **a** bone-related and **b** inflammatory genes. Data shown are pooled from three biological repeats and are presented as mean (SEM); two-way ANOVA $P_{Interaction} = 0.007$ for $Tnfrsf11b$, $P_{Interaction} = 0.0005$ for $Tnfa$, $P_{Interaction} < 0.0001$ for all other genes; with post-hoc Sidak's test $*p < 0.05$, $**p < 0.01$, and $***p < 0.001$ versus control conditioned medium at that time point. OPG osteoprotegerin, RANKL receptor activator of nuclear factor kappa-B ligand, TNF tumor necrosis factor

RANKL protein were undetected in both control conditioned medium and MSU crystal-stimulated conditioned medium (Additional file 3: Figure S3).

The addition of TNF-α neutralizing antibody did not significantly change the induced expression of COX-2, IL-6, IL-11, and RANKL genes by MLO-Y4 cells

following culture with MSU crystal-stimulated conditioned medium (Additional file 4: Figure S4). In contrast, addition of a COX-2 inhibitor to MLO-Y4 cell cultures prior to the addition of MSU crystal-stimulated conditioned medium led to a significant reduction in IL-6, IL-11, and RANKL gene expression (Fig. 5a), and PGE$_2$

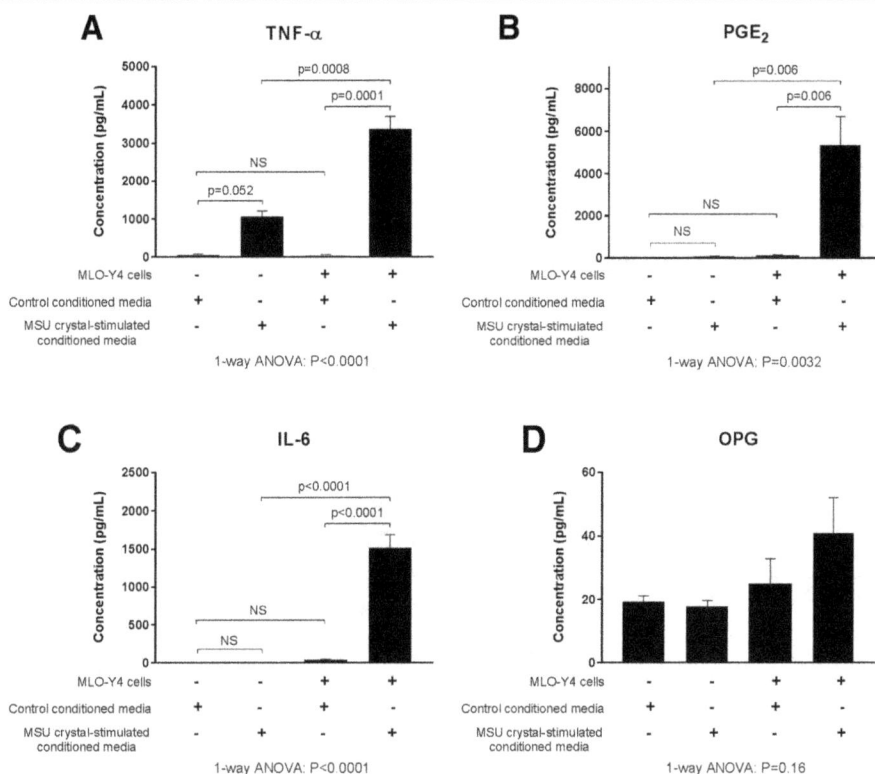

Fig. 4 Secretion of proinflammatory mediators by MLO-Y4 cells in response to MSU crystal-stimulated RAW264.7 macrophages. RAW264.7 macrophages were cultured with or without 0.5 mg/mL monosodium urate (MSU) crystals for 24 h for preparation of MSU crystal-stimulated conditioned medium and control conditioned medium, respectively. Conditioned medium preparations were added to MLO-Y4 cells (40% final concentration in a well) for 24 h and supernatants harvested. The concentrations of **a** tumor necrosis factor (TNF)-α, **b** prostaglandin E$_2$ (PGE$_2$), **c** interleukin (IL)-6, and **d** osteoprotegerin (OPG) protein in the RAW264.7 macrophage conditioned medium samples (control and MSU crystal-stimulated) and the MLO-Y4 cell supernatants were measured by ELISA. Data shown are pooled from three biological repeats and are presented as mean (SEM); one-way analysis of variance (ANOVA) with post-hoc Sidak's test between groups as indicated. NS no significant difference

and IL-6 protein expression (Fig. 5b). TNF-α gene expression was slightly increased following COX-2 inhibition (Fig. 5a); however, there was no difference at the protein level (Fig. 5b). MLO-Y4 cell gene expression of OPG and COX-2 was unchanged (Fig. 5a); however, PGE$_2$ levels were significantly decreased with the addition of COX-2 inhibitor (Fig. 5b). Soluble RANKL protein was undetected in the MLO-Y4 cell supernatants.

MSU crystals and macrophages are observed in close proximity to bone, and COX-2 is also expressed in human joints affected by tophaceous gout

The clinical relevance of our in-vitro results was assessed by examining the relationship between MSU crystals, inflammatory cells, and bone in human joint tissue affected by gout. In joint samples from people with tophaceous gout, collections of MSU crystals were observed both immediately adjacent to the bone (direct contact) and also distant from the bone, separated from the bone surface by a rim of inflammatory tissue (Fig. 6a, b). Multiple CD68[+] macrophages were identified within tophi adjacent to the bone (Fig. 6c). In addition, COX-2

expression was observed in both mononucleated and multinucleated cells within the corona zone of tophi and in cells close to the bone in joints affected by tophaceous gout (Fig. 6d).

Discussion

This study shows that MSU crystals have significant inhibitory effects on osteocyte viability, but no direct effect on osteocyte gene expression in vitro. In contrast, in conditioned media experiments, factors released by macrophages in response to MSU crystals have profound effects on the expression profile of osteocytes, with upregulated expression of inflammatory cytokines and mediators, and altered expression of factors involved in bone remodeling. The shift in osteocyte function towards a proinflammatory and proresorptive state is effectively suppressed with COX-2 inhibition.

Our in-vitro assays demonstrate that MSU crystals directly reduce the viability of osteocytes embedded within 3D collagen gels over time. Although the alamarBlue® results showed that direct cell-crystal contact was not necessarily required for this effect, the increased level of

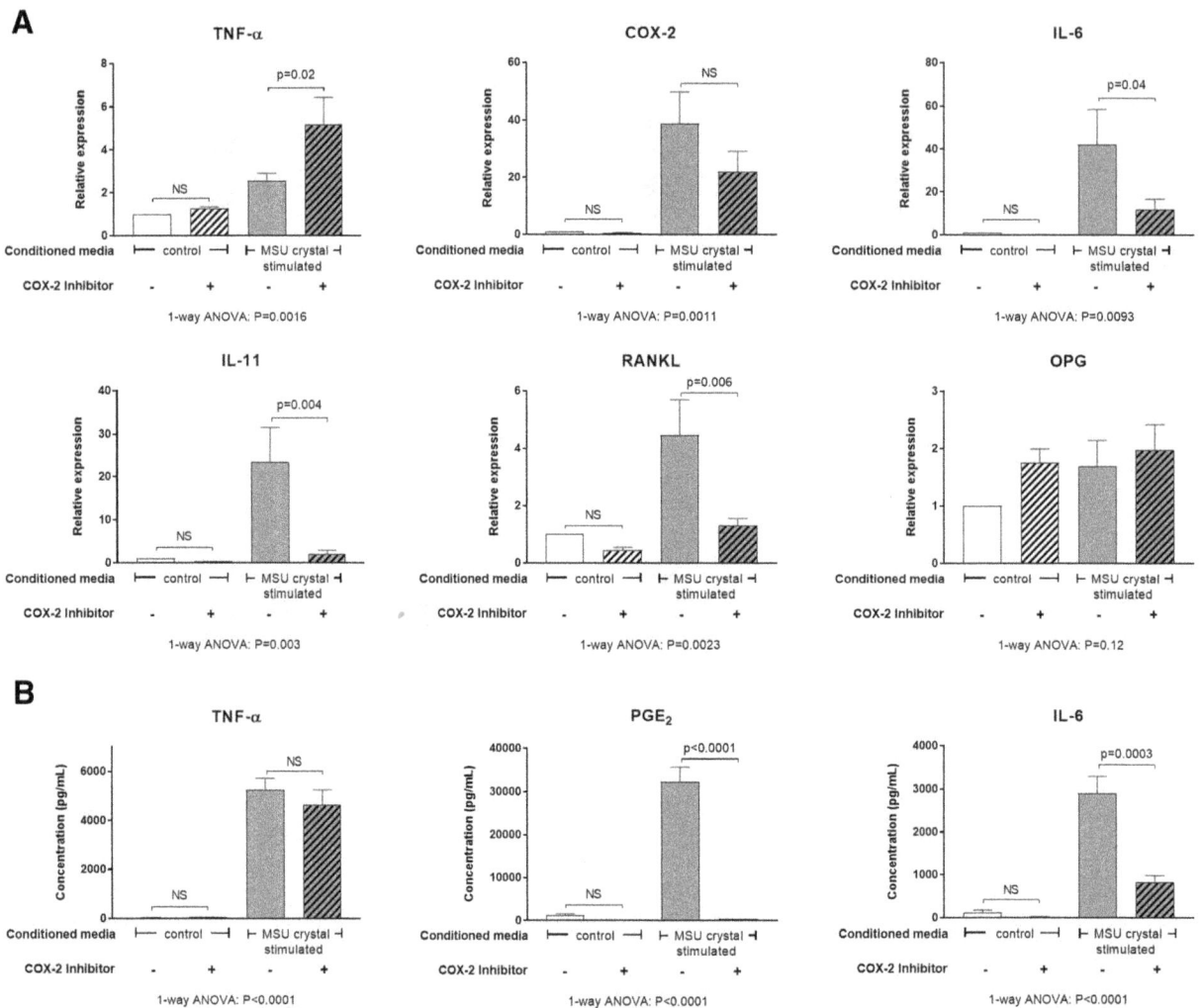

Fig. 5 Effects of COX-2 inhibition on MLO-Y4 cell responses to MSU crystal-stimulated RAW264.7 macrophage conditioned medium. RAW264.7 macrophages were cultured with or without 0.5 mg/mL monosodium urate (MSU) crystals for 24 h for preparation of MSU crystal-stimulated conditioned medium and control conditioned medium, respectively. A cyclooxygenase-2 (COX-2)-specific inhibitor (SC-236) was added to MLO-Y4 cells for 1 h prior to the addition of 40% conditioned medium for 24 h. MLO-Y4 cells were then harvested for mRNA gene expression analysis and supernatants harvested for protein quantification. **a** Changes in mRNA expression of inflammatory genes: tumor necrosis factor (TNF)-α, COX-2, interleukin (IL)-6, and IL-11; and bone-related genes: receptor activator of nuclear factor kappa-B ligand (RANKL) and osteoprotegerin (OPG). **b** Changes in TNF-α, prostaglandin E_2 (PGE$_2$), and IL-6 protein levels in MLO-Y4 cell supernatants. Data shown are pooled from five biological repeats and are presented as (SEM); one-way analysis of variance (ANOVA) with post-hoc Sidak's test between groups as indicated. NS no significant difference

cell death observed in the top layer of the gel in the LIVE/DEAD® assays suggests that direct cell-crystal contact may enhance MSU crystal-induced osteocyte death. Osteocyte cell death is associated with increased osteoclastogenesis and loss of bone [18], with dying osteocytes and their neighboring cells thought to send signals which recruit osteoclast precursors to areas of bone damage [19, 20]. In patients with tophaceous gout, large numbers of osteoclasts are present at the bone-tophus interface at the site of bone erosion [4]. Increased osteocyte death in the presence of MSU crystals may further amplify osteoclast precursor cell recruitment, osteoclastogenesis, and bone resorption at these sites.

MSU crystals did not directly alter MLO-Y4 gene expression in our 3D in-vitro cell culture model and, while direct interaction of MSU crystals with cells in the deeper layers of the gels may have been limited, this model is more representative of osteocytes in vivo which are embedded within a 3D matrix. The histology analysis confirmed that, while MSU crystals are in direct contact with surface bone cells, there is often a rim of macrophages and inflammatory tissue observed between MSU crystals and osteocytes within the bone. Interactions between nearby MSU crystals and macrophages and the resulting inflammation may also influence osteocyte regulation of bone remodeling in joints affected by tophaceous

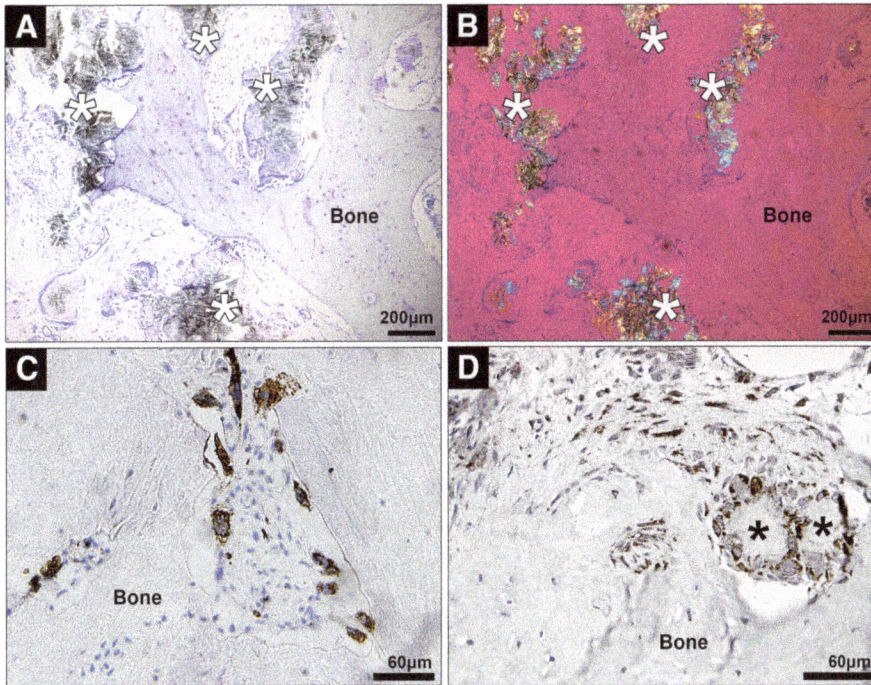

Fig. 6 Histological analysis of human joint tissue affected by tophaceous gout. **a,b** Representative photomicrographs of joint samples affected by tophaceous gout, showing both MSU crystals (indicated by asterisks) and associated inflammatory tissue in close proximity to bone (**a**, toluidine blue staining viewed using light microscopy; **b**, viewed using polarizing light microscopy with a red compensator). Immunohistochemistry staining for **c** CD68+ cells (macrophages) and **d** COX-2 expression in human joint tissue affected by tophaceous gout

gout. The addition of conditioned medium from macrophages cultured with MSU crystals to MLO-Y4 cells led to upregulated expression of genes involved in osteocyte communication (connexin 43 and E11), indicating that the cells may be responding to the external stress [21, 22]. In addition, cytokines and factors known to increase osteoclastogenesis and bone resorption were also upregulated in the MLO-Y4 cell cultures, including TNF-α [23], IL-6 [24], IL-11 [25], and RANKL [26]. COX-2 gene expression was also upregulated in response to MSU crystal-stimulated conditioned medium. Induction of COX-2 leads to the synthesis of prostaglandins, such as PGE_2. In the same experiments, PGE_2 levels were significantly increased in response to MSU crystal-stimulated conditioned medium. PGE_2 has important effects on bone metabolism and can promote both bone resorption and formation [27, 28]. IL-6 and IL-11 are also known to have roles in promoting bone formation under conditions of increased bone turnover [29, 30]. Of note, pathological new bone formation is observed in patients with advanced gout and is more frequently observed in joints with tophi [31]. Thus, osteocytes exposed to MSU crystal-induced inflammation may contribute to both aspects of disordered bone remodeling in gout: pathological bone formation and increased bone resorption.

The addition of MSU crystals to RAW264.7 cells in vitro led to increased secretion of TNF-α and PGE_2 and,

although TNF-α was secreted at higher concentrations, the downstream proinflammatory response evoked in MLO-Y4 osteocytes is unlikely to be dependent on TNF-α since neutralization of TNF-α had no major effect on the induced inflammatory response. In contrast, inhibition of COX-2 activity in MLO-Y4 cells did suppress the induced expression of IL-6, IL-11, RANKL, and PGE_2. The molecular mechanism by which COX-2 inhibition blocked MLO-Y4 cell expression of cytokines and inflammatory mediators in response to MSU crystal-induced inflammation was not further investigated in this study. However, other studies using stromal cells, such as fibroblasts and epithelial cells, have shown a link between COX-2 activation, PGE_2 release, and the subsequent expression of IL-6 in response to inflammatory stimuli [32, 33]. In these studies, COX-2 inhibition decreased downstream IL-6 gene and protein expression [32, 33] by inhibiting PGE_2 activation of NF-κβ and C/EBPβ transcription factors [33]. Other research has demonstrated that addition of exogenous PGE_2 directly induces IL-6 expression in osteoblasts and fibroblasts [24, 34]. In the current study, COX-2 inhibition did not significantly change MLO-Y4 gene expression of COX-2 but did significantly reduce MLO-Y4 production of PGE_2, indicating that increased COX-2 activity is important for the downstream inflammatory response. In tophaceous joint samples, COX-2 protein expression was observed near sites of bone erosion. These results suggest that upregulated COX-2 activity and PGE_2 production at sites affected by tophaceous gout may be important for driving the shift in osteocyte phenotype towards a proinflammatory and proresorptive state in response to MSU crystal-induced inflammation. COX-2 has also been implicated in bone resorption in other forms of inflammatory arthritis. In animal models of rheumatoid arthritis, COX-2 inhibition can reduce inflammatory bone erosion [35, 36]. For current gout management, COX-2 inhibitors are used as anti-inflammatory agents for treatment and prevention of gout flares. Our results raise the possibility that COX-2 inhibition may also inhibit the cellular processes contributing to pathological bone remodeling in tophaceous gout.

IL-1β plays a key role in initiation of the acute gout flare [37, 38]. In our in-vitro model of MSU crystal-induced inflammation by macrophages, IL-1β secretion was not upregulated in RAW264.7 macrophage cells cultured with MSU crystals. This is consistent with previous in-vitro studies where MSU crystals alone did not induce IL-1β release in human or murine macrophages without additional priming of cells with either lipopolysaccharide or phorbol 12-myristate 13-acetate [39, 40]. Activation of the inflammasome and release of IL-1β is critical for initiating the intense acute inflammatory response in the gout flare [37]. However, tophi are not typically acutely inflamed. Therefore, we believe that the indirect experiments using macrophage conditioned medium represent a relevant in-vitro model to examine how interactions between MSU crystals and macrophages affect osteocyte-regulated bone remodeling in tophaceous gout.

Conclusions

In summary, MSU crystals directly reduce osteocyte viability but have no direct effects on osteocyte gene expression. In contrast, interactions between MSU crystals and macrophages indirectly promote osteocyte expression of proinflammatory mediators and factors involved in bone remodeling, particularly proresorptive factors; these effects can be suppressed with COX-2 inhibition in osteocytes. These interactions may contribute to disordered bone remodeling in tophaceous gout.

Additional files

Additional file 1: Figure S1. The effect of different sizes of MSU crystals on MLO-Y4 cell viability. The alamarBlue® assay was used to determine the viability of MLO-Y4 cells cultured with different sizes of MSU crystals for 24 h. Viability was assessed 24 and 48 h after the addition of MSU crystals. Data shown are pooled from three biological repeats and are presented as mean (SEM), two-way ANOVA: $P_{Interaction} = 0.86$; $P_{MSU\ crystal\ size} = 0.96$; and $P_{MSU\ crystal\ concentration} = 0.0001$ for the 24 h time point; and $P_{Interaction} = 0.13$; $P_{MSU\ crystal\ size} = 0.21$; and $P_{MSU\ crystal\ concentration} < 0.0001$ for the 48 h time

Additional file 2: Figure S2. Indirect effects of MSU crystal-stimulated RAW264.7 macrophage conditioned medium on MLO-Y4 cell viability. RAW264.7 macrophages were cultured with or without 0.5 mg/mL MSU crystals for 24 h for preparation of MSU crystal-stimulated conditioned medium and control conditioned medium, respectively. Conditioned medium preparations were added to MLO-Y4 cells at different concentrations (5%, 20%, and 40% final concentration in a well) for 24 h. The alamarBlue® assay was used to determine MLO-Y4 cell viability 24 h and 48 h after the addition of conditioned medium. Data shown are pooled from three biological repeats and are presented as mean (SEM), two-way ANOVA: $P_{interaction} = 0.16$; $P_{Time} = 0.74$; and $P_{Conditioned\ media\ concentration} = 0.17$.

Additional file 3: Figure S3. RAW264.7 macrophage expression of TNF-α and PGE_2 in response to MSU crystals. RAW264.7 macrophages were cultured with or without 0.5 mg/mL MSU crystals for 24 h for preparation of MSU crystal-stimulated conditioned medium and control conditioned medium, respectively. The concentration of TNF-α, PGE2, IL-1β, IL-6, RANKL, and OPG in conditioned medium samples were measured by ELISA. IL-6 and RANKL were undetected in all samples. Data shown are pooled from three biological repeats and are presented as mean (SEM), two-tailed paired

Additional file 4: Figure S4. The effect of neutralizing TNF-α on MLO-Y4 cell inflammation induced by MSU crystal-stimulated RAW264.7 macrophages. RAW264.7 macrophages were cultured with or without 0.5 mg/mL MSU crystals for 24 h for preparation of MSU crystal-stimulated conditioned medium and control conditioned medium, respectively. Conditioned medium and either 5 µg/mL neutralizing TNF-α antibody or 5 µg/mL IgG isotype control were added to MLO-Y4 cells for 24 h and MLO-Y4 cells were then harvested and mRNA extracted for analysis of gene expression by real-time PCR. Data shown are pooled from four biological repeats and are presented as mean (SEM), one-way ANOVA with post-hoc Sidak's test between groups as indicated. NS no significant difference.

Abbreviations

3D: Three-dimensional; ANOVA: Analysis of variance; BCP: Basic calcium phosphate; COX-2: Cyclooxygenase-2; CPPD: Calcium pyrophosphate dehydrate; ELISA: Enzyme-linked immunosorbent assay; FBS: Fetal bovine serum; IL: Interleukin; MSU: Monosodium urate; NF-κβ: Nuclear factor kappa-B; OPG: Osteoprotegerin; PCR: Polymerase chain reaction; PGE_2: Prostaglandin E_2; RANKL: Receptor activator of nuclear factor kappa-B ligand; TNF: Tumor necrosis factor

Acknowledgments

The authors wish to acknowledge Peter Riordan and Satya Amirapu from the Department of Anatomy and Medical Imaging, University of Auckland, New Zealand, for assistance with collection of cadaveric specimens and histological processing, respectively.

Funding

This study was funded by the Auckland Medical Research Foundation (Project grant 9101/3709989) and The University of Auckland (FRDF grant 9101/3704255). AC was funded by a Royal Society of New Zealand Rutherford Foundation Post-Doctoral Research Fellowship (grant 9101/3709428).

Authors' contributions

ND (the guarantor) accepts full responsibility for the work and the conduct of the study, had access to the data, and controlled the decision to publish. Design of study protocol: AC, DM, DN, GM, SM, JC, and ND. Acquisition of study data: AC, BP, KEC, and MLT. Data analysis: AC and ND. Interpretation of data: AC, DN, and ND. Drafting of manuscript: AC and ND. Final approval of manuscript: all authors.

Consent for publication
Not applicable.

Competing interests
ND has received consulting fees, speaker fees, or grants from Takeda, Teijin, Menarini, Pfizer, Ardea, AstraZeneca, Cymabay, Amgen, Abbvie, and Horizon outside the submitted work. The remaining authors declare that they have no competing interests.

Author details
[1]Department of Medicine, Bone & Joint Research Group, University of Auckland, Auckland, New Zealand. [2]Department of Rheumatology, Mater Misericordiae University Hospital, Dublin, Ireland. [3]Department of Anatomy and Medical Imaging, University of Auckland, Auckland, New Zealand. [4]Department of Medicine, Faculty of Medical and Health Sciences, University of Auckland, 85 Park Rd, Grafton, Auckland, New Zealand.

References

1. Dalbeth N, Clark B, Gregory K, Gamble G, Sheehan T, Doyle A, McQueen FM. Mechanisms of bone erosion in gout: a quantitative analysis using plain radiography and computed tomography. Ann Rheum Dis. 2008;8:1290–5.
2. Dalbeth N, Pool B, Gamble GD, Smith T, Callon KE, McQueen FM, Cornish J. Cellular characterization of the gouty tophus: a quantitative analysis. Arthritis Rheum. 2010;62(5):1549–56.
3. Sapsford M, Gamble GD, Aati O, Knight J, Horne A, Doyle AJ, Dalbeth N. Relationship of bone erosion with the urate and soft tissue components of the tophus in gout: a dual energy computed tomography study. Rheumatology. 2016;1:129–33.
4. Dalbeth N, Smith T, Nicolson B, Clark B, Callon K, Naot D, Haskard DO, McQueen FM, Reid IR, Cornish J. Enhanced osteoclastogenesis in patients with tophaceous gout: urate crystals promote osteoclast development through interactions with stromal cells. Arthritis Rheum. 2008;58(6):1854–65.
5. Lee SJ, Nam KI, Jin HM, Cho YN, Lee SE, Kim TJ, Lee SS, Kee SJ, Lee KB, Kim N, et al. Bone destruction by receptor activator of nuclear factor kappaB ligand-expressing T cells in chronic gouty arthritis. Arthritis Res Ther. 2011; 13(5):R164.
6. Chhana A, Callon KE, Pool B, Naot D, Watson M, Gamble GD, McQueen FM, Cornish J, Dalbeth N. Monosodium urate monohydrate crystals inhibit osteoblast viability and function: implications for development of bone erosion in gout. Ann Rheum Dis. 2011;9:1684–91.
7. Nakashima T, Hayashi M, Fukunaga T, Kurata K, Oh-hora M, Feng JQ, Bonewald LF, Kodama T, Wutz A, Wagner EF, et al. Evidence for osteocyte regulation of bone homeostasis through RANKL expression. Nat Med. 2011; 17(10):1231–4.
8. Kramer I, Halleux C, Keller H, Pegurri M, Gooi JH, Weber PB, Feng JQ, Bonewald LF, Kneissel M. Osteocyte Wnt/beta-catenin signaling is required for normal bone homeostasis. Mol Cell Biol. 2010;30(12):3071–85.
9. Bonewald LF. The amazing osteocyte. J Bone Miner Res. 2011;26(2):229–38.
10. Chhana A, Aati O, Gamble GD, Callon KE, Doyle AJ, Roger M, McQueen FM, Horne A, Reid IR, Cornish J, et al. Path analysis identifies receptor activator of nuclear factor-kappaB ligand, osteoprotegerin, and sclerostin as potential mediators of the tophus-bone erosion relationship in gout. J Rheumatol. 2016;43(2):445–9.
11. Kato Y, Windle JJ, Koop BA, Mundy GR, Bonewald LF. Establishment of an osteocyte-like cell line, MLO-Y4. J Bone Miner Res. 1997;12(12):2014–23.
12. Yellowley CE, Li Z, Zhou Z, Jacobs CR, Donahue HJ. Functional gap junctions between osteocytic and osteoblastic cells. J Bone Miner Res. 2000;15(2):209–17.
13. Stern AR, Stern MM, Van Dyke ME, Jahn K, Prideaux M, Bonewald LF. Isolation and culture of primary osteocytes from the long bones of skeletally mature and aged mice. Biotechniques. 2012;52(6):361–73.
14. Matthews BG, Naot D, Callon KE, Musson DS, Locklin R, Hulley PA, Grey A, Cornish J. Enhanced osteoblastogenesis in three-dimensional collagen gels. Bonekey Rep. 2014;3:560.
15. Denko CW, Whitehouse MW. Experimental inflammation induced by naturally occurring microcrystalline calcium salts. J Rheumatol. 1976;3(1):54–62.
16. Evans RW, Cheung HS, McCarty DJ. Cultured human monocytes and fibroblasts solubilize calcium phosphate crystals. Calcif Tissue Int. 1984;1: 645–50.
17. Chhana A, Callon KE, Dray M, Pool B, Naot D, Gamble GD, Coleman B, McCarthy G, McQueen FM, Cornish J, et al. Interactions between tenocytes and monosodium urate monohydrate crystals: implications for tendon involvement in gout. Ann Rheum Dis. 2014;73(9):1737–41.
18. Tatsumi S, Ishii K, Amizuka N, Li M, Kobayashi T, Kohno K, Ito M, Takeshita S, Ikeda K. Targeted ablation of osteocytes induces osteoporosis with defective mechanotransduction. Cell Metab. 2007;5(6):464–75.
19. Verborgt O, Gibson GJ, Schaffler MB. Loss of osteocyte integrity in association with microdamage and bone remodeling after fatigue in vivo. J Bone Miner Res. 2000;15(1):60–7.
20. Kennedy OD, Herman BC, Laudier DM, Majeska RJ, Sun HB, Schaffler MB. Activation of resorption in fatigue-loaded bone involves both apoptosis and active pro-osteoclastogenic signaling by distinct osteocyte populations. Bone. 2012;50(5):1115–22.
21. Zhang K, Barragan-Adjemian C, Ye L, Kotha S, Dallas M, Lu Y, Zhao S, Harris M, Harris SE, Feng JQ, et al. E11/gp38 selective expression in osteocytes: regulation by mechanical strain and role in dendrite elongation. Mol Cell Biol. 2006;26(12):4539–52.
22. Cherian PP, Siller-Jackson AJ, Gu S, Wang X, Bonewald LF, Sprague E, Jiang JX. Mechanical strain opens connexin 43 hemichannels in osteocytes: a novel mechanism for the release of prostaglandin. Mol Biol Cell. 2005;16(7): 3100–6.
23. Bertolini DR, Nedwin GE, Bringman TS, Smith DD, Mundy GR. Stimulation of bone resorption and inhibition of bone formation in vitro by human tumour necrosis factors. Nature. 1986;319(6053):516–8.
24. Ishimi Y, Miyaura C, Jin CH, Akatsu T, Abe E, Nakamura Y, Yamaguchi A, Yoshiki S, Matsuda T, Hirano T. IL-6 is produced by osteoblasts and induces bone resorption. J Immunol. 1990;145(10):3297–303.
25. Sims NA, Jenkins BJ, Nakamura A, Quinn JMW, Li R, Gillespie MT, Ernst M, Robb L, Martin TJ. Interleukin-11 receptor signaling is required for normal bone remodeling. J Bone Miner Res. 2005;20(7):1093–102.
26. Kong YY, Yoshida H, Sarosi I, Tan HL, Timms E, Capparelli C, Morony S, Oliveira-dos-Santos AJ, Van G, Itie A, et al. OPGL is a key regulator of osteoclastogenesis, lymphocyte development and lymph-node organogenesis. Nature. 1999;397(6717):315–23.
27. Klein DC, Raisz LG. Prostaglandins: stimulation of bone resorption in tissue culture. Endocrinology. 1970;86(6):1436–40.
28. Nefussi JR, Baron R. PGE2 stimulates both resorption and formation of bone in vitro: differential responses of the periosteum and the endosteum in fetal rat long bone cultures. Anat Rec. 1985;211(1):9–16.
29. Sims NA, Jenkins BJ, Quinn JMW, Nakamura A, Glatt M, Gillespie MT, Ernst M, Martin TJ. Glycoprotein 130 regulates bone turnover and bone size by distinct downstream signaling pathways. J Clin Invest. 2004;113(3):379–89.
30. Takeuchi Y, Watanabe S, Ishii G, Takeda S, Nakayama K, Fukumoto S, Kaneta Y, Inoue D, Matsumoto T, Harigaya K, et al. Interleukin-11 as a stimulatory factor for bone formation prevents bone loss with advancing age in mice. J Biol Chem. 2002;277(50):49011–8.
31. Dalbeth N, Milligan A, Doyle AJ, Clark B, McQueen FM. Characterization of new bone formation in gout: a quantitative site-by-site analysis using plain radiography and computed tomography. Arthritis Res Ther. 2012;14(4):R165.
32. Bukata SV, Gelinas J, Wei X, Rosier RN, Puzas JE, Zhang X, Schwarz EM, Song XR, Griswold DE, O'Keefe RJ. PGE2 and IL-6 production by fibroblasts in response to titanium wear debris particles is mediated through a cox-2 dependent pathway. J Orthop Res. 2004;22(1):6–12.
33. Zhao Y, Usatyuk PV, Gorshkova IA, He D, Wang T, Moreno-Vinasco L, Geyh AS, Breysse PN, Samet JM, Spannhake EW, et al. Regulation of COX-2 expression and IL-6 release by particulate matter in airway epithelial cells. Am J Respir Cell Mol Biol. 2009;40(1):19–30.
34. Inoue H, Takamori M, Shimoyama Y, Ishibashi H, Yamamoto S, Koshihara Y. Regulation by PGE(2) of the production of interleukin-6, macrophage colony stimulating factor, and vascular endothelial growth factor in human synovial fibroblasts. Br J Pharmacol. 2002;136(2):287–95.
35. Noguchi M, Kimoto A, Sasamata M, Miyata K. Micro-CT imaging analysis for the effect of celecoxib, a cyclooxygenase-2 inhibitor, on inflammatory bone destruction in adjuvant arthritis rats. J Bone Miner Metab. 2008;26(5):461–8.
36. Katagiri M, Ogasawara T, Hoshi K, Chikazu D, Kimoto A, Noguchi M, Sasamata M, Harada S, Akama H, Tazaki H, et al. Suppression of adjuvant-induced arthritic bone destruction by cyclooxygenase-2 selective agents

with and without inhibitory potency against carbonic anhydrase II. J Bone Miner Res. 2006;21(2):219–27.

37. Martinon F, Petrilli V, Mayor A, Tardivel A, Tschopp J. Gout-associated uric acid crystals activate the NALP3 inflammasome. Nature. 2006;440(7081):237–41.

38. Chen C-J, Shi Y, Hearn A, Fitzgerald K, Golenbock D, Reed G, Akira S, Rock KL. MyD88-dependent IL-1 receptor signaling is essential for gouty inflammation stimulated by monosodium urate crystals. J Clin Invest. 2006; 116(8):2262–71.

39. Joosten LA, Netea MG, Mylona E, Koenders MI, Malireddi RK, Oosting M, Stienstra R, van de Veerdonk FL, Stalenhoef AF, Giamarellos-Bourboulis EJ, et al. Engagement of fatty acids with toll-like receptor 2 drives interleukin-1beta production via the ASC/caspase 1 pathway in monosodium urate monohydrate crystal-induced gouty arthritis. Arthritis Rheum. 2010;62(11): 3237–48.

40. Giamarellos-Bourboulis EJ, Mouktaroudi M, Bodar E, van der Ven J, Kullberg BJ, Netea MG, van der Meer JW. Crystals of monosodium urate monohydrate enhance lipopolysaccharide-induced release of interleukin 1 beta by mononuclear cells through a caspase 1-mediated process. Ann Rheum Dis. 2009;68(2):273–8.

6

A five-year prospective study of spinal radiographic progression and its predictors in men and women with ankylosing spondylitis

Anna Deminger[1]* ⓘ, Eva Klingberg[1], Mats Geijer[2,3], Jan Göthlin[4], Martin Hedberg[5], Eva Rehnberg[6], Hans Carlsten[1], Lennart T. Jacobsson[1] and Helena Forsblad-d'Elia[1,7]

Abstract

Background: Knowledge about predictors of new spinal bone formation in patients with ankylosing spondylitis (AS) is limited. AS-related spinal alterations are more common in men; however, knowledge of whether predictors differ between sexes is lacking. Our objectives were to study spinal radiographic progression in patients with AS and investigate predictors of progression overall and by sex.

Methods: Swedish patients with AS, age (mean ± SD) 50 ± 13 years, were included in a longitudinal study. At baseline and at 5-year follow up, spinal radiographs were graded according to the modified Stoke Ankylosing Spondylitis Spine Score (mSASSS). Predictors were assessed by questionnaires, spinal mobility tests and blood samples.

Results: Of 204 patients included, 166 (81%) were re-examined and 54% were men. Men had significantly higher mean mSASSS at baseline and higher mean increase in mSASSS than women (1.9 ± 2.8 vs. 1.2 ± 3.3; $p = 0.005$) More men than women developed new syndesmophytes (30% vs. 12%; $p = 0.007$). Multivariate logistic regression analyses with progression ≥ 2 mSASSS units over 5 years or development of new syndesmophytes as the dependent variable showed that presence of baseline AS-related spinal radiographic alterations and obesity (OR 3.78, 95% CI 1.3 to 11.2) were independent predictors of spinal radiographic progression in both sexes. High C-reactive protein (CRP) was a significant predictor in men, with only a trend seen in women. Smoking predicted progression in men whereas high Bath Ankylosing Spondylitis Metrology Index (BASMI) and exposure to bisphosphonates during follow up (OR 4.78, 95% CI 1.1 to 20.1) predicted progression in women.

Conclusion: This first report on sex-specific predictors of spinal radiographic progression shows that predictors may partly differ between the sexes. New predictors identified were obesity in both sexes and exposure to bisphosphonates in women. Among previously known predictors, baseline AS-related spinal radiographic alterations predicted radiographic progression in both sexes, high CRP was a predictor in men (with a trend in women) and smoking was a predictor only in men.

Keywords: Ankylosing spondylitis, Outcomes research, Treatment, Inflammation, Longitudinal study, Radiography

* Correspondence: anna.deminger@vgregion.se
[1]Department of Rheumatology and Inflammation Research, Sahlgrenska Academy at University of Gothenburg, Box 480, 405 30 Gothenburg, Sweden
Full list of author information is available at the end of the article

Background

Ankylosing spondylitis (AS) is a chronic, inflammatory disease mainly affecting the sacroiliac joints and the spine, where it is characterized by pathological new bone formation and development of syndesmophytes. The new bone formation and spinal inflammation can lead to spinal stiffness and loss of mobility [1]. The ratio of men to women with AS is estimated to be 2–3 to 1 [2].

Conventional x-ray is still considered the gold standard for assessing chronic spinal alterations in AS, with the modified Stoke Ankylosing Spondylitis Spine Score (mSASSS) considered as the most valid method for quantifying these changes [3]. AS-related spinal alterations evaluated by different methods have been shown to be more severe in men [4–6] and longitudinal studies have shown faster radiographic progression in men [6, 7].

There is still limited knowledge on predictors of spinal radiographic progression in AS. The strongest predictor is the presence of syndesmophytes at baseline [5, 8–10]. Higher disease activity measured by the Ankylosing Spondylitis Disease Activity Score (ASDAS) has been associated with more spinal radiographic progression in AS and early axial spondyloarthritis (SpA) [11, 12]. Inflammation measured by erythrocyte sedimentation rate (ESR) or C-reactive protein (CRP) and smoking has been shown to predict radiographic progression in early SpA [10]. Previous studies have largely been in men and knowledge about what predicts radiographic progression in women is scarce.

The objectives of this longitudinal study were to assess spinal radiographic progression in patients with AS and to investigate predictors for progression overall and by sex.

Methods

Patients

The patients were recruited at baseline in 2009 from the rheumatology clinics at Sahlgrenska University Hospital in Gothenburg and the hospitals at Borås and Alingsås, Sweden [13]. The inclusion criterion was AS according to the modified New York criteria [14]. Exclusion criteria were psoriasis, inflammatory bowel disease, dementia, pregnancy and difficulties in understanding the Swedish language. A total of 204 patients completed the baseline protocol and were invited to participate in the 5-year follow up. Written informed consent was obtained from the participants and approval by the regional ethics committee in Gothenburg was obtained both at baseline and at 5-year follow up.

Physical examination and questionnaires

The same questionnaires and physical examinations, including the Bath AS Metrology Index (BASMI) [15] were applied at baseline and at the 5-year follow up. Patients were examined by one physician at baseline (EK)

and one physician at follow up (AD). Questionnaires included medical history, medication, occupation and smoking and the Bath AS Disease Activity Index (BASDAI), the Bath AS Functional Index (BASFI) and the Bath AS Patient Global score (BAS-G) [16–18]. The ASDAS based on CRP (ASDAS_CRP) was calculated [19]. Type of occupation was divided into "blue-collar" work, generally involving manual labor and physical tasks, and "white-collar" work, usually requiring less physical activity and more formal education [20]. Body mass index (BMI) was grouped in categories: 1 = normal (BMI 18.5 to 24.9 kg/m^2), 2 = overweight (BMI 25.0 to 29.9), 3 = obese (BMI ≥ 30) [21]. Data about non-steroidal anti-inflammatory drug (NSAID) consumption during follow up was collected according to the Assessment of SpondyloArthritis international Society (ASAS) recommendations [22]. All patients were invited to undergo transthoracic echocardiography at baseline as previously described [23].

Radiography

Conventional radiographs of the spine were obtained at baseline and at the 5-year follow up and scored according to the mSASSS. With mSASSS, each anterior corner of the cervical spine (from the lower corner of vertebra C2 to the upper corner of T1) and the lumbar spine (from the lower corner of T12 to the upper corner of S1) on lateral radiographs is evaluated with a score between 0 and 3 (0 = no abnormality, 1 = erosion, sclerosis or squaring, 2 = syndesmophyte, 3 = bridging syndesmophyte), with the total score ranging from 0 to 72 [24]. All radiographs were scored simultaneously by the same musculoskeletal radiologist (MG) blinded to the clinical data but with known chronological order. At baseline, 0.3% of the vertebral corners (VC) were not assessable and 0% were not assessable at follow up. Missing VC was handled according to Ramiro et al. [7] where missing baseline VC was replaced by the score from the next observation with the mean progression sum of the segment subtracted from that score. Missing follow-up VC was replaced by the score of the previous observation with the mean progression score of the segment added to that score. No patient had missing VC at both baseline and follow up. Definite radiographic progression was defined either as an increase in mSASSS over 5 years by ≥ 2 points [25] or as development of a new syndesmophyte, defined as mSASSS of at least 2 at a vertebral level with a score of 0 or 1 at baseline [5].

Laboratory tests

Blood samples were analyzed by standard laboratory techniques. The time-averaged ESR and CRP for the last 5 years before follow up were obtained from the medical records, and calculated using the first recorded test for each year unless the patient had a recorded infection at that time point, in which case the ESR/CRP was replaced by the subsequent test.

Statistics

Statistical analyses were performed using IBM SPSS Statistics 22 (IBM, Armonk, NY, USA). Descriptive statistics are presented as means with standard deviations (SD) and frequencies with percentages. To compare measurements in men and women the t test for normally distributed data or the Mann-Whitney U test for not normally distributed data were used for continuous data, and the chi^2 test or Fisher's exact test, when appropriate, was used for categorical data. The Wilcoxon signed rank test was used to compare mSASSS at baseline and at follow up. Radiographs of 40 randomly selected patients were re-scored by the same reader for calculations of reliability data. Intra-reader agreement for status scores and change scores was evaluated with an intraclass correlation coefficient (ICC) two-way mixed-effect model, with single measurement and absolute agreement. Values < 0.5 indicate poor agreement, 0.5–0.75 moderate agreement, 0.75–0.90 good agreement and > 0.90 excellent agreement [26]. The smallest detectable change (SDC), the progression reliably detected above the measurement error, was calculated as proposed by Bruynesteyn et al. [27].

Univariate and multivariate (backward method) logistic regression analyses were performed to find predictors for progression of ≥ 2 mSASSS units over 5 years and the development of new syndesmophytes. Variables with p values ≤ 0.2 in the univariate analyses were entered into the multivariate logistic regression model for the total group. Because of fewer observations in the subgroups, a p value < 0.1 was used for sex-stratified analyses. Variables were entered manually into the multivariate model and if there was multicollinearity (BASMI and BASFI), the variable with the lowest p value in the univariate analyses was kept in the model. The same principle was used for highly correlated variables: age and duration of symptoms and BASMI and lateral spinal flexion (as lateral spinal flexion is a part of BASMI) but for CRP, time-averaged CRP, ESR and time-averaged ESR the baseline variable was prioritized. For mSASSS and BASMI and mSASSS and lateral flexion (highly correlated in the total group and in men), the mSASSS was chosen. Interactions between the main effect variables from the multiple logistic analyses were tested, and if a significant interaction (p ≤ 0.05) was identified, the estimates for progression in the subgroups were analyzed.. Goodness of fit was assessed with the Hosmer-Lemeshow test.

To consider covariates that affect receiving bisphosphonates or tumor necrosis factor inhibitor (TNFi), propensity scores (PS) for the probabilities of being exposed to bisphosphonates, being exposed to TNFi or being treated with TNFi for ≥ 2 years during follow up, respectively, were calculated. Variables included in the PS were sex, HLA-B27, baseline CRP, BASDAI, mSASSS, smoking pack-years, BMI categories, use of NSAID, symptom duration and age of onset of symptoms. The PS and the treatment variable were used as covariates in standard binary logistic regression analyses with either definition of progression as the dependent variable. In order to evaluate any interaction between NSAID and TNFi-exposure, three categorical groups were formed: high NSAID (NSAID index ≥ 50) and TNFi+/–, low NSAID (NSAID index < 50) and TNFi+/– and no NSAID and TNFi+/–. Each group was used as a covariate either in univariate or together with the PS for exposure to TNFi in multivariate logistic regression analyses for radiographic progression, as aforementioned. All tests were two-tailed and p ≤ 0.05 was considered statistically significant.

Results

Patients

Of the 204 patients included at baseline, 169 (83%) completed all examinations at the 5-year follow up: 4 patients died during follow up. Three men with maximum mSASSS at baseline were excluded from the analyses, resulting in 166 (81%) completers, including 89 men (54%) and 77 women (46%) (Fig. 1). The 166 completers did not differ in baseline age or mSASSS compared to the non-completers; the non-completers included patients coming to follow up with baseline mSASSS = 72 and those not coming to follow up (50 ± 13 vs. 50 ± 14 years). There was a trend towards more men in the non-completers vs. the completers (71% vs. 54%, p = 0.078), and there was no significant difference when analyzing only patients who were still alive at follow-up (p = 0.19).

Characteristics and medication use in the total group and a comparison between men and women at baseline are shown in Table 1. There were some significant differences between men and women; more men were HLA-B27-positive, men had lower ESR, higher time-averaged CRP during follow up, and a trend toward lower disease activity measured by the BASDAI. Men had higher mean (SD) mSASSS at baseline than women (20.3 (21.9) vs. 6.4 (9.6), p < 0.001) and 57% of the men had syndesmophytes compared with 33% of the women (p = 0.002). At baseline, 78% of the patients reported using NSAIDs and 20% had treatment with TNFi, with no significant differences between sexes. Bisphosphonates were used by a smaller proportion of men than women (1% vs. 8%, p = 0.050).

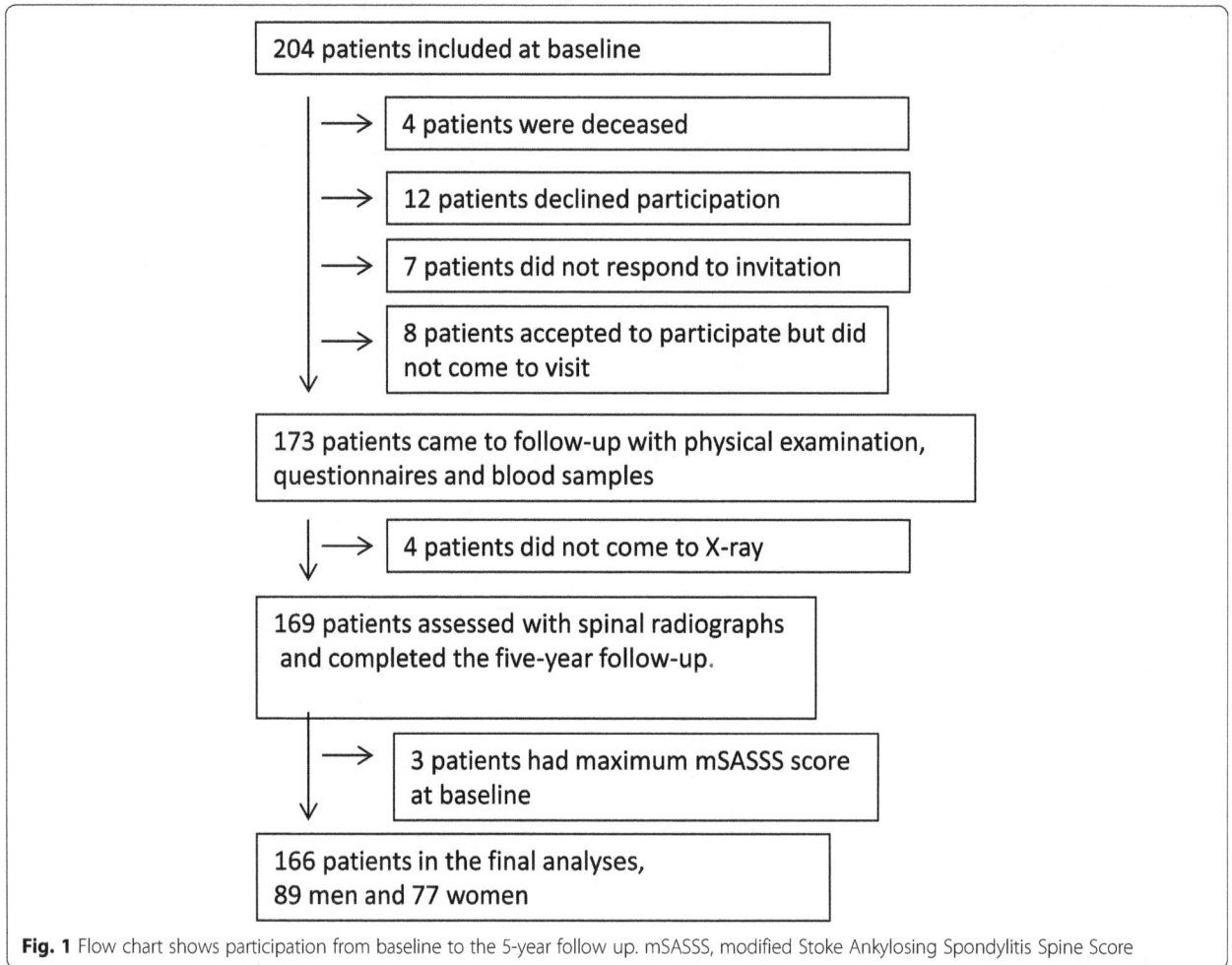

Fig. 1 Flow chart shows participation from baseline to the 5-year follow up. mSASSS, modified Stoke Ankylosing Spondylitis Spine Score

Spinal radiographic progression

In the total group, mSASSS progressed from mean (SD) 13.9 (18.6) units to 15.4 (19.6) units. The mean progression was 1.6 (3.3) mSASSS units over 5 years ($p < 0.001$), with more progression in men compared to women (1.9 (2.8) vs 1.2 (3.3), $p = 0.005$) (Fig. 2). The mSASSS ranged from 0 to 70 in men at baseline and from 0 to 72 at follow up. In women the range was 0–46 at baseline and 0–57 at follow up. Five of the completers had baseline mSASSS > 65. One of these patients reached a maximum mSASSS of 72 at follow up. This patient fulfilled both definitions of progression. The ICC for status scores were 0.98 (95% CI 0.96 to 0.99) for both baseline and follow-up scores and 0.62 (95% CI 0.36 to 0.78) for change scores. The SDC was 2.65.

Progression ≥ 2 mSASSS units over 5 years was seen in 47 patients (28%), more frequently in men than in women, with 32 men (36%) vs. 15 women (20%) ($p = 0.029$). The development of new syndesmophytes was seen in 36 patients (22%), with 27 men (30%) and 9 women (12%) ($p = 0.007$).

Predictors of progression defined as increase of ≥ 2 mSASSS units or new syndesmophyte development over 5 years in univariate analyses (Tables 2 and 3)

Whole study population: several predictors were the same for both definitions of progression. Demographic variables that predicted progression were male sex, older age, and being overweight or obese. Disease-BRS81665 related variables and medication that predicted progression were history of anterior uveitis, high BASMI, reduced lateral spinal flexion, presence of syndesmophytes at baseline and exposure to bisphosphonates during follow up. Inflammation measured by CRP predicted progression of ≥ 2 mSASSS units over 5 years.

Sex-stratified analyses: obesity predicted progression in men according to both definitions. Ever-smoking and high CRP during follow up predicted progression of ≥ 2 mSASSS units over 5 years. Older age and being overweight predicted development of new syndesmophytes. In women exposure to bisphosphonates predicted progression according to both definitions. Shared predictors in both men and women were disease-related variables such as high BASMI, reduced lateral spinal flexion and

Table 1 Baseline characteristics and medication at baseline and during follow up in 166 patients with ankylosing spondylitis

	Total group	Men (n = 89)	Women (n = 77)	p value
Demographic variables				
Age, years	50 (13)	49 (12)	51 (13)	0.45
Current smokers	17 (10)	8 (9)	9 (12)	0.75
Ever-smokers	72 (43)	41 (46)	31 (40)	0.55
BMI category: normal/overweight/obese	85 (51)/	41 (46)/	44 (57)/	0.36
	56 (34)/	33 (37)/	23 (30)/	
	25 (15)	15 (17)	10 (13)	
Blue-collar worker[a]	40 (33)	21 (33)	19 (33)	1.00
Time between x-rays, months	66 (3)	65 (3)	67 (1)	0.003
Disease-related variables				
Duration of symptoms, years	24 (13)	23 (13)	24 (13)	0.58
History of anterior uveitis	85 (51)	50 (56)	35 (46)	0.22
History of peripheral arthritis	95 (57)	47 (53)	48 (62)	0.28
History of coxitis	13 (8)	7 (8)	6 (8)	1.00
BASMI, score	3.0 (1.5)	3.2 (1.8)	2.9 (1.2)	0.61
BASFI, score	2.5 (2.0)	2.3 (1.9)	2.7 (2.1)	0.25
BASDAI, score	3.4 (2.1)	3.1 (2.1)	3.7 (2.0)	0.056
ASDAS_CRP, score	2.1 (0.9)	2.1 (0.9)	2.1 (0.8)	0.53
CRP, mg/L	5.4 (8.5)	6.5 (10.5)	4.2 (5.1)	0.26
Time-averaged CRP during follow up, mg/L	5.8 (5.9)	6.5 (6.4)	4.9 (5.0)	0.043
ESR, mm/h	14.2 (11.2)	12.7 (11.5)	15.9 (10.6)	0.003
Time-averaged ESR during follow-up, mm/h	12.2 (8.4)	10.9 (7.8)	13.8 (8.9)	0.009
HLA-B27 positive	143 (86)	82 (92)	61 (79)	0.030
Aortic insufficiency[b]	25 (16)	13 (16)	12 (17)	0.98
mSASSS, score	13.9 (18.6)	20.3 (21.9)	6.4 (9.6)	< 0.001
Presence of syndesmophyte	76 (46)	51 (57)	25 (33)	0.002
Medications				
Patients on NSAIDs baseline	129 (78)	66 (74)	63 (82)	0.32
NSAID index during follow up, 0–100	34 (38)	39 (39)	29 (33)	0.31
Patients on TNFi at baseline	33 (20)	22 (25)	11 (14)	0.14
Patients exposed to TNFi during follow up	49 (30)	30 (34)	19 (25)	0.27
Patients on bisphosphonate at baseline	7 (4)	1 (1)	6 (8)	0.050
Patients exposed to bisphosphonate during follow-up	30 (18)	11 (12)	19 (25)	0.064

Values are means (SD) or numbers of patients (%)

ASDAS_CRP Ankylosing Spondylitis Disease Activity Score_C-reactive protein, *BASDAI* Bath Ankylosing Spondylitis Disease Activity Index, *BASFI* Bath Ankylosing Spondylitis Functional Index, *BASMI* Bath Ankylosing Spondylitis Metrology Index, *BMI* body mass index, *CRP* C-reactive protein, *ESR* erythrocyte sedimentation rate, *HLA-B27* human leukocyte antigen B27, *mSASSS* modified Stoke Ankylosing Spondylitis Spine Score, *NSAID* non-steroidal anti-inflammatory drug, *TNFi* tumor necrosis factor inhibitor

[a] n = 120 for total group, 63 men and 57 women
[b] n = 153 for total group, 83 men and 70 women

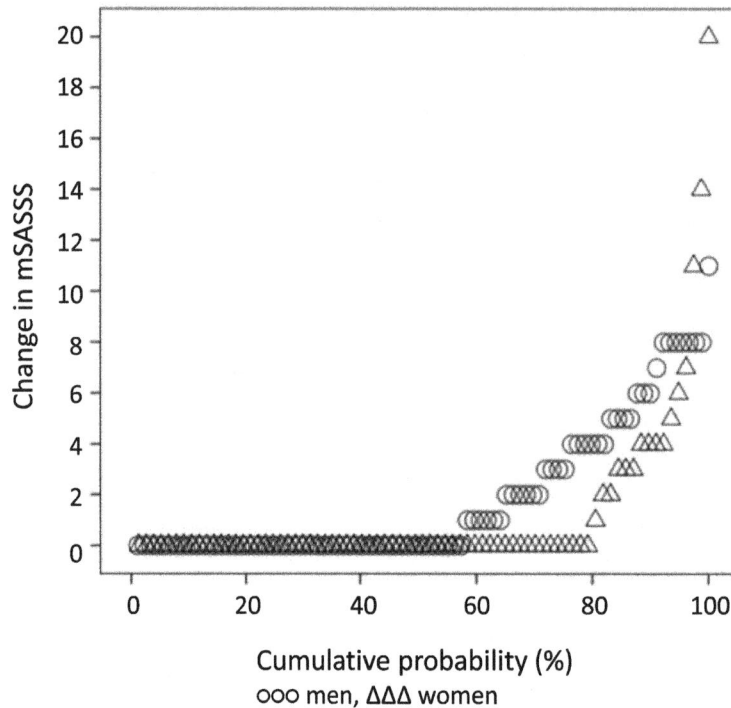

Fig. 2 Cumulative probability for the change in modified Stoke Ankylosing Spondylitis Spine Score (mSASSS) from baseline to follow up in 89 men and 77 women with ankylosing spondylitis

presence of syndesmophytes at baseline (according to both definitions for progression).

Predictors of progression defined as increase of ≥ 2 mSASSS units or new syndesmophyte development over 5 years in multivariate analyses (Figs. 3 and 4)

Whole study population: in multivariate analyses exposure to bisphosphonates during follow up was associated with progression according to both definitions. Obesity, high baseline CRP and male sex predicted progression of ≥ 2 mSASSS units over 5 years. Baseline syndesmophytes and older age predicted development of new syndesmophytes. For development of new syndesmophytes, the point estimates in the model were similar irrespective of whether baseline CRP or time-averaged CRP were included in the model.

Sex-stratified analyses: in men, ever-smoking, obesity and high baseline CRP predicted progression defined as ≥2 mSASSS units over 5 years. Current smoking and presence of baseline syndesmophytes predicted development of new syndesmophytes. In women, exposure to bisphosphonates was independently associated with progression according to both definitions. Baseline mSASSS predicted progression defined as ≥ 2 mSASSS over 5 years whereas there was only a trend for baseline CRP. Obesity and high BASMI predicted development of new syndesmophytes. BASMI also remained significant if the

model was corrected for baseline mSASSS instead of baseline syndesmophytes.

A significant interaction was identified for age and exposure to bisphosphonates on the development of new syndesmophytes. When stratifying by median age (≥ 50 vs. < 50 years), the estimates for exposure to bisphosphonates for the respective group was not significant (OR 1.34 95% CI 0.49 to 3.66 vs. OR 4.56 95% CI 0.72 to 28.95).

Effect of treatment with bisphosphonates in PS-adjusted analyses in the whole study population

Of the 30 patients exposed to bisphosphonates during follow up, 7 patients had used bisphosphonates at baseline. The remaining 23 patients started the medication soon after inclusion, at mean (SD) 7 (0.5) months. The PS for the probability of being exposed to bisphosphonates during follow up was calculated as described in "Methods". In the logistic regression model with the PS included, exposure to bisphosphonates was still a significant predictor for development of new syndesmophytes (OR 2.96, 95% CI 1.02 to 8.62), but was not statistically significant for progression of ≥ 2 mSASSS units over 5 years (Table 4).

Effect of treatment with TNFi in PS-adjusted analyses in the whole study population

Exposure to TNFi during follow up was not significant (*p* value >0.2) in the univariate analyses of association with radiographic progression (Tables 2 and 3) and was

Table 2 Univariate logistic regression analyses for progression of ≥ 2 mSASSS units over 5 years

	Total group, n = 166			Men, n = 89			Women, n = 77		
	OR	95% CI	p value	OR	95% CI	p value	OR	95% CI	p value
Demographic variables									
Male sex	2.32	1.14 to 4.72	**0.020**	NA			NA		
Age, years	1.03	1.01 to 1.06	**0.021**	1.03	1.00 to 1.07	0.078	1.05	1.00 to 1.10	0.075
BMI: overweight (reference, normal)	2.40	1.09 to 5.26	**0.029**	2.62	0.95 to 7.21	0.062	1.76	0.47 to 6.54	0.40
obese (reference, normal)	5.06	1.93 to 13.24	**0.001**	5.33	1.50 to 19.0	**0.010**	4.22	0.91 to 19.51	0.065
Ever-smoker	1.74	0.88 to 3.44	0.11	3.53	1.42 to 8.77	**0.007**	0.47	0.14 to 1.65	0.24
Current smoker	1.44	0.50 to 4.14	0.50	3.33	0.74 to 15.00	**0.12**	0.48	0.06 to 4.18	0.51
Blue-collar work[a]	1.31	0.55 to 3.12	0.55	1.00	0.31 to 3.19	1.00	1.91	0.50 to 7.29	0.35
Time between x-rays, months	0.92	0.81 to 1.05	0.21	0.96	0.83 to 1.11	0.57	1.15	0.66 to 2.00	0.63
Disease-related variables									
Duration of symptoms, years	1.02	0.99 to 1.04	0.24	1.01	0.98 to 1.05	0.57	1.03	0.99 to 1.08	0.17
HLA-B27 positive	1.50	0.52 to 4.30	0.45	1.44	0.26 to 7.90	0.67	1.06	0.26 to 4.33	0.93
History of coxitis	0.74	0.20 to 2.83	0.66	0.27	0.03 to 2.39	0.24	2.23	0.37 to 13.51	0.38
History of uveitis	2.33	1.16 to 4.71	**0.018**	2.28	0.92 to 5.66	0.076	2.08	0.66 to 6.56	0.21
BASMI, score	1.65	1.29 to 2.10	**< 0.001**	1.43	1.10 to 1.86	**0.008**	2.58	1.42 to 4.69	**0.002**
Lateral spinal flexion, cm	0.89	0.84 to 0.96	**0.001**	0.91	0.84 to 0.98	**0.014**	0.83	0.71 to 0.96	**0.012**
BASFI, score	1.15	0.97 to 1.36	0.10	1.13	0.90 to 1.42	0.28	1.27	0.96 to 1.67	0.089
BASDAI, score	0.98	0.83 to 1.15	0.80	0.93	0.76 to 1.15	0.52	1.17	0.87 to 1.56	0.30
ASDAS_CRP, score	1.14	0.78 to 1.68	0.51	1.12	0.70 to 1.80	0.64	1.24	0.63 to 2.46	0.54
CRP, mg/L	1.06	1.02 to 1.11	**0.008**	1.05	1.00 to 1.10	0.051	1.09	0.99 to 1.21	0.083
Time-averaged CRP, mg/L	1.08	1.02 to 1.14	**0.010**	1.09	1.01 to 1.17	**0.035**	1.05	0.95 to 1.16	0.36
ESR, mm/h	1.02	0.99 to 1.05	0.19	1.02	0.98 to 1.06	0.39	1.04	0.99 to 1.09	0.10
Time-averaged ESR, mm/h	1.03	0.99 to 1.07	0.11	1.05	0.99 to 1.11	0.097	1.04	0.98 to 1.10	0.21
Syndesmophytes at baseline	6.46	2.98 to 14.03	**< 0.001**	5.55	1.98 to 15.54	**0.001**	6.27	1.85 to 21.24	**0.003**
mSASSS baseline, units	1.04	1.02 to 1.05	**< 0.001**	1.02	1.00 to 1.04	**0.046**	1.11	1.04 to 1.19	**0.001**
Aortic insufficiency[b]	1.20	0.48 to 3.03	0.70	1.20	0.35 to 4.06	0.77	1.28	0.30 to 5.46	0.74
Medication									
NSAID index, 0–100	1.01	1.00 to 1.01	0.26	1.00	0.99 to 1.02	0.52	1.00	0.99 to 1.02	0.62
Exposure to TNFi	1.17	0.56 to 2.43	0.67	0.84	0.33 to 2.12	0.71	1.71	0.50 to 5.85	0.39
Exposure to bisphosphonates	2.29	1.01 to 5.21	**0.047**	1.57	0.44 to 5.63	0.49	5.30	1.59 to 17.69	**0.007**

ORs reflect a change in one unit for continuous variables. All variables are baseline values except for time-averaged variables and medications. Significant p values are shown in bold typeface

ASDAS_CRP Ankylosing Spondylitis Disease Activity Score_C-reactive protein, *BASDAI* Bath Ankylosing Spondylitis Disease Activity Index, *BASFI* Bath Ankylosing Spondylitis Functional Index, *BASMI* Bath Ankylosing Spondylitis Metrology Index, *BMI* body mass index, *CRP* C-reactive protein, *ESR* erythrocyte sedimentation rate, *HLA-B27* Human leukocyte antigen B27, *mSASSS* modified Stoke Ankylosing Spondylitis Spine Score, *NSAID* non-steroidal anti-inflammatory drug, *TNFi* tumor necrosis factor inhibitor

n = 120 for total group, n = 63 for men, n = 57 for women

‡n = 153 for total group, n = 83 for men and n = 70 for women

thus not included in the multivariate models. To further study associations between TNFi and spinal radiographic progression, the PS for exposure to TNFi or use of TNFi for ≥ 2 years during follow up was calculated as described in "Methods". In the logistic regression model with the PS included, exposure to TNFi (n = 49) or use of TNFi for ≥ 2 years during follow up (n = 38) was still not significantly associated with radiographic progression (Table 4).

To analyze if concomitant use of NSAID and TNFi could have an impact on spinal progression, the patients were grouped according to NSAID and TNFi use during follow up as described in "Methods". There was no significant relationship between dose of NSAID and concomitant use of TNFi in these regression analyses (Table 5). However, only 10 patients had a combination of high-dose NSAID and exposure to TNFi.

Table 3 Univariate logistic regression analyses for development of new syndesmophytes over 5 years

	Total group, n = 166			Men, n = 89			Women, n = 77		
	OR	95% CI	p value	OR	95% CI	p value	OR	95% CI	p value
Demographic variables									
Male sex	3.29	1.44 to 7.54	**0.005**	NA			NA		
Age, years	1.05	1.02 to 1.09	**0.003**	1.06	1.02 to 1.10	**0.007**	1.06	0.99 to 1.13	0.082
BMI: overweight (reference, normal)	2.46	1.04 to 5.85	**0.042**	3.16	1.08 to 9.22	**0.036**	0.95	0.16 to 5.63	0.96
obese (reference, normal)	4.49	1.62 to 12.44	**0.004**	4.25	1.16 to 15.60	**0.029**	4.29	0.78 to 23.43	0.093
Ever-smoker	1.22	0.58 to 2.56	0.60	1.73	0.70 to 4.31	0.24	0.38	0.07 to 1.99	0.25
Current smoker	2.16	0.74 to 6.32	0.16	4.47	0.99 to 20.29	0.052	0.94	0.10 to 8.51	0.95
Blue-collar work[a]	1.18	0.45 to 3.10	0.74	1.47	0.44 to 4.87	0.53	0.78	0.14 to 4.43	0.78
Time between x-rays	0.82	0.71 to 0.94	**0.004**	0.88	0.75 to 1.02	0.083	0.75	0.36 to 1.56	0.44
Disease-related variables									
Duration of symptoms, years	1.02	0.99 to 1.05	0.13	1.02	0.99 to 1.06	0.26	1.04	0.98 to 1.09	0.18
HLA-B27 positive	1.00	0.34 to 2.90	1.00	0.55	0.12 to 2.65	0.46	0.91	0.17 to 4.86	0.91
History of coxitis	1.09	0.28 to 4.19	0.90	0.36	0.04 to 3.14	0.35	4.57	0.71 to 29.61	0.11
History of uveitis	2.26	1.04 to 4.91	**0.039**	1.88	0.73 to 4.81	0.19	2.69	0.62 to 11.66	0.19
BASMI, score	1.57	1.22 to 2.01	**< 0.001**	1.29	1.00 to 1.68	0.053	4.39	**1.77 to 10.84**	**0.001**
Lateral spinal flexion, cm	0.89	0.83 to 0.96	**0.002**	0.92	0.85 to 1.00	**0.036**	0.71	0.55 to 0.91	**0.006**
BASFI, score	1.14	0.95 to 1.36	0.16	1.11	0.88 to 1.40	0.40	1.35	0.97 to 1.87	0.072
BASDAI, score	1.01	0.85 to 1.21	0.91	1.01	0.82 to 1.26	0.90	1.14	0.81 to 1.61	0.45
ASDAS_CRP	1.23	0.81 to 1.86	0.34	1.19	0.73 to 1.95	0.48	1.44	0.63 to 3.32	0.39
CRP, mg/L	1.02	0.99 to 1.06	0.24	1.02	0.98 to 1.06	0.46	1.01	0.89 to 1.15	0.86
Time-averaged CRP, mg/L	1.06	1.00 to 1.12	0.060	1.05	0.98 to 1.13	0.15	1.03	0.91 to 1.16	0.65
ESR, mm/h	0.99	0.95 to 1.02	0.43	1.00	0.96 to 1.04	0.83	0.99	0.92 to 1.06	0.69
Time-averaged ESR, mm/h	0.99	0.94 to 1.03	0.60	1.00	0.94 to 1.06	0.94	1.00	0.93 to 1.09	0.93
Syndesmophytes at baseline	5.98	2.52 to 14.17	**< 0.001**	5.01	1.68 to 14.92	**0.004**	5.16	1.17 to 22.74	**0.030**
Aortic insufficiency[b]	1.53	0.58 to 4.04	0.40	1.11	0.31 to 4.02	0.87	2.89	0.61 to 13.69	0.18
Medication									
NSAID index, 0–100	1.01	1.00 to 1.02	0.11	1.01	1.00 to 1.02	0.11	1.00	0.97 to 1.02	0.72
Exposure to TNFi	1.07	0.48 to 2.38	0.88	0.59	0.22 to 1.62	0.31	2.83	0.67 to 11.86	0.16
Exposure to bisphosphonates	2.57	1.09 to 6.08	**0.031**	2.12	0.59 to 7.67	0.25	8.46	1.87 to 38.38	**0.006**

ORs reflect a change in one unit for continuous variables. All variables are baseline values except for time-averaged variables and medications. Significant p values are shown in bold typeface

ASDAS_CRP Ankylosing Spondylitis Disease Activity Score_C-reactive protein, *BASDAI* Bath Ankylosing Spondylitis Disease Activity Index, *BASFI* Bath Ankylosing Spondylitis Functional Index, *BASMI* Bath Ankylosing Spondylitis Metrology Index, *BMI* body mass index, *CRP* C-reactive protein, *ESR* erythrocyte sedimentation rate, *HLA-B27* Human leukocyte antigen B27, *mSASSS* modified Stoke Ankylosing Spondylitis Spine Score, *NSAID* non-steroidal anti-inflammatory drug, *TNFi* tumor necrosis factor inhibitor

[a] n = 120 for total group, n = 63 for men, n = 57 for women
[b] n = 153 for total group, n = 83 for men and n = 70 for women

Discussion

In the present study, we investigated spinal radiographic progression and its predictors in men and women separately and demonstrated a higher occurrence and development of syndesmophytes in men. Shared predictors of progression in both sexes were the presence of baseline AS-related spinal radiographic alterations and obesity, whereas exposure to smoking may be a more important predictor in men and exposure to bisphosphonates may be more important in women.

The higher occurrence of AS-related spinal alterations in men has also been shown in other studies [4, 6]. Ramiro et al. also identified faster progression in men [7]. Since AS-related spinal radiological changes are more common in men, predictors should be studied separately for men and women in the same setting. To our knowledge, this has not been done previously. In one prior study in women with AS, older age, longer disease duration, severe sacroiliitis, elevated CRP and baseline syndesmophytes were predictors of the development of

Covariates	OR (95%CI)	Exposure to covariates, (no.) Progression ≥ 2 mSASSS, (YES/NO)	
Total group		**YES**, n=47	**NO**, n=119
BMI: overweight	2.16 (0.92 to 5.11)	19	37
obese	**5.83 (2.04 to 16.64)**	13	12
Exposure to bisphosphonates	**3.15 (1.19 to 8.32)**	13	17
Male sex	**2.39 (1.05 to 5.42)**	32	57
CRP at baseline, mg/L	**1.05 (1.01 to 1.10)**	4.0 (1.0-12.0)	2.0 (0.5-5.0)
History of uveitis	1.97 (0.90 to 4.30)	31	54
Men		**YES**, n=32	**NO**, n=57
BMI: overweight	2.43 (0.80 to 7.37)	14	19
obese	**6.62 (1.66 to 26.37)**	9	6
Ever smoker	**3.52 (1.29 to 9.58)**	21	20
CRP at baseline, mg/L	**1.06 (1.01 to 1.11)**	4.5 (1.25-13.5)	2.0 (0.75-5.0)
Women		**YES**, n=15	**NO**, n=65
Exposure to bisphosphonates	**4.72 (1.14 to 19.47)**	8	11
mSASSS at baseline, unit	**1.10 (1.03 to 1.18)**	12.0 (3.0-24.0)	0.0 (0.0-5.3)
CRP at baseline	1.11 (0.99 to 1.24)	3.0 (1.0-10.0)	2.0 (0.5-4.25)

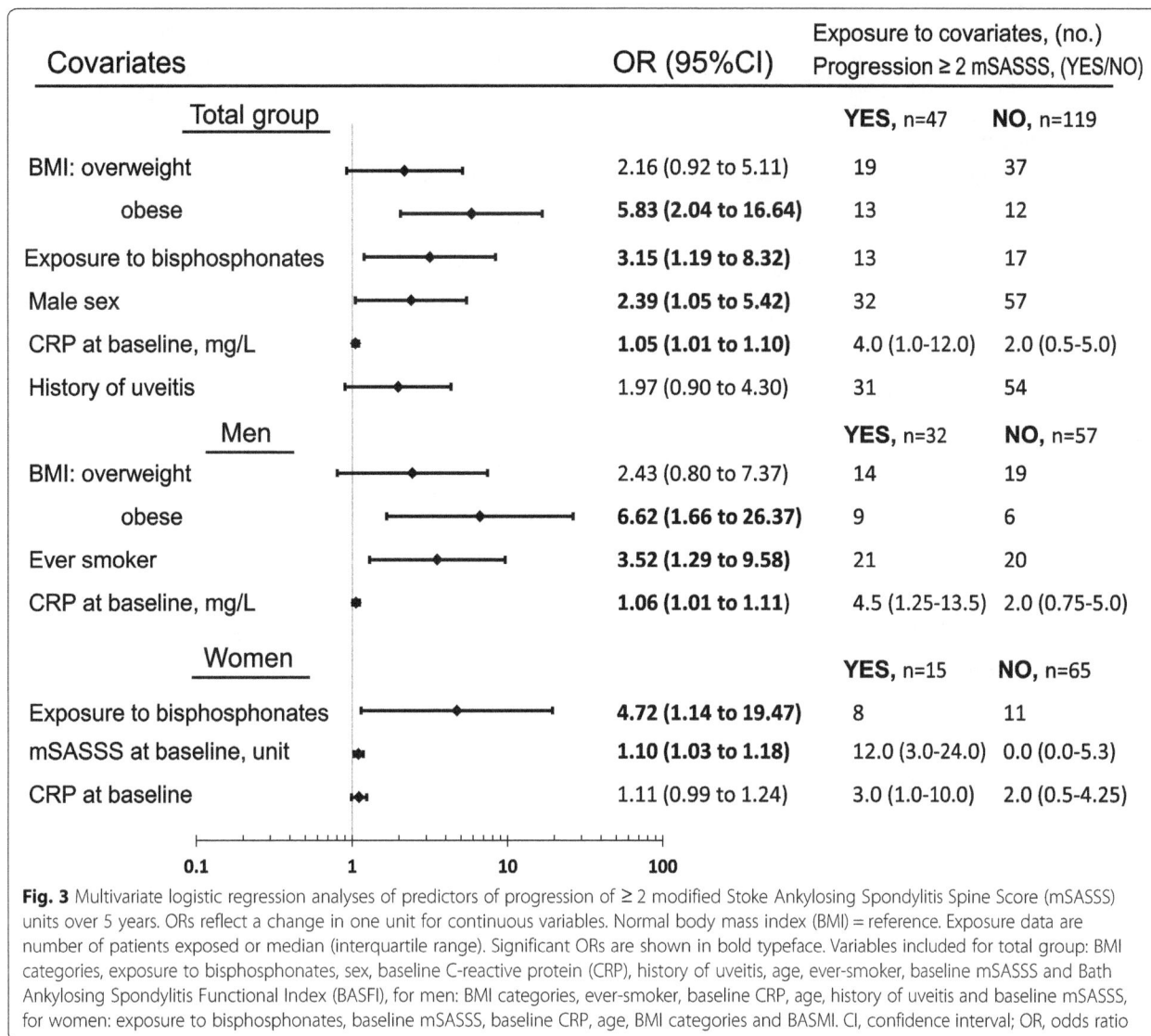

Fig. 3 Multivariate logistic regression analyses of predictors of progression of ≥ 2 modified Stoke Ankylosing Spondylitis Spine Score (mSASSS) units over 5 years. ORs reflect a change in one unit for continuous variables. Normal body mass index (BMI) = reference. Exposure data are number of patients exposed or median (interquartile range). Significant ORs are shown in bold typeface. Variables included for total group: BMI categories, exposure to bisphosphonates, sex, baseline C-reactive protein (CRP), history of uveitis, age, ever-smoker, baseline mSASSS and Bath Ankylosing Spondylitis Functional Index (BASFI), for men: BMI categories, ever-smoker, baseline CRP, age, history of uveitis and baseline mSASSS, for women: exposure to bisphosphonates, baseline mSASSS, baseline CRP, age, BMI categories and BASMI. CI, confidence interval; OR, odds ratio

new syndesmophytes in the lumbar spine over 2 years in univariate analyses. Multivariate analysis was not done due to the small sample size [28]. Several longitudinal studies on mixed gender cohorts have reported, similar to the current study, preexisting syndesmophytes as a predictor in both long-standing AS and early SpA [5, 9, 10, 25]. Elevated CRP or ESR, smoking and high disease activity over time measured by ASDAS_CRP have been independently associated with spinal radiographic progression [11, 29, 30]. Of these, high CRP and smoking were predictors of radiographic progression in men in the current Swedish cohort. The non-significant result for high CRP as a predictor in women might be due to the small sample size whereas the fact that the univariate ORs estimate indicates a negative effect of smoking on radiographic progression in men and a positive effect in women, may imply a real difference between sexes. Based on previous observations a larger sample size

would, however, have been required to have the statistical power to detect any significant difference between sexes in the effect of smoking [29]. Intriguingly, exposure to bisphosphonates during follow up was found to be a predictor of spinal radiographic progression in women. Bisphosphonates have been studied as disease-modifying drugs in AS [31–33]. One of these trials explored spinal radiographic progression and observed no difference in mSASSS progression over 2 years in patients randomized to alendronate compared with placebo [33]. However, in that study, few patients on alendronate were women and not all patients were radiographed. Our results are based on few observations and should be interpreted with caution, and our finding needs confirmation in a larger study with more women. Neither NSAID nor TNFi treatment was associated with spinal radiographic progression but the study was not designed to evaluate treatment effects. Few patients were

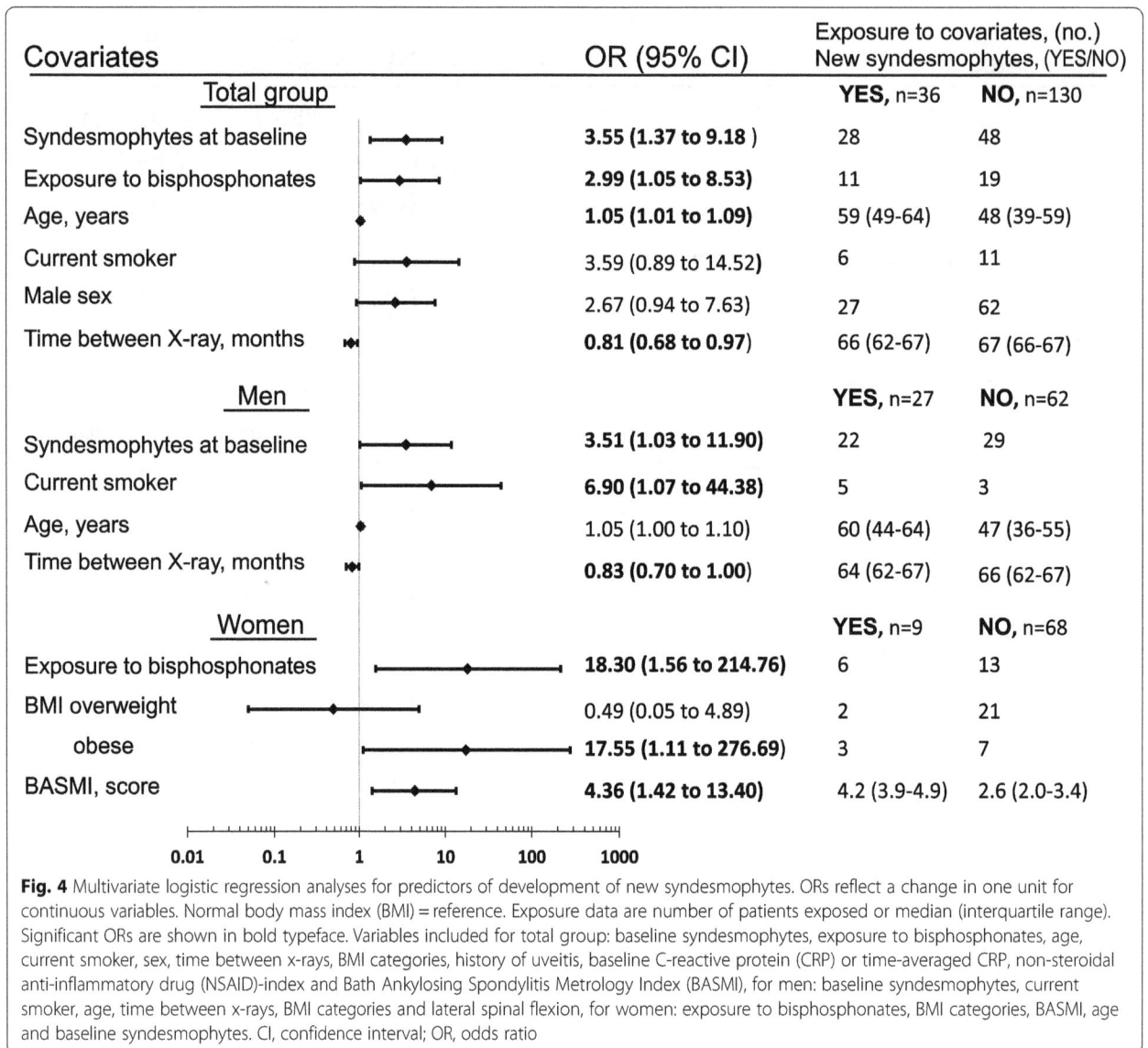

Fig. 4 Multivariate logistic regression analyses for predictors of development of new syndesmophytes. ORs reflect a change in one unit for continuous variables. Normal body mass index (BMI) = reference. Exposure data are number of patients exposed or median (interquartile range). Significant ORs are shown in bold typeface. Variables included for total group: baseline syndesmophytes, exposure to bisphosphonates, age, current smoker, sex, time between x-rays, BMI categories, history of uveitis, baseline C-reactive protein (CRP) or time-averaged CRP, non-steroidal anti-inflammatory drug (NSAID)-index and Bath Ankylosing Spondylitis Metrology Index (BASMI), for men: baseline syndesmophytes, current smoker, age, time between x-rays, BMI categories and lateral spinal flexion, for women: exposure to bisphosphonates, BMI categories, BASMI, age and baseline syndesmophytes. CI, confidence interval; OR, odds ratio

Table 4 Effect of bisphosphonates and TNFi, respectively, on spinal radiographic progression in propensity score-adjusted logistic regression analyses

	Progression ≥ 2 mSASSS units		New syndesmophytes	
	OR (95% CI)	p value	OR (95% CI)	p value
Exposure to bisphosphonates	2.47 (0.89 to 6.86)	0.083	2.96 (1.02 to 8.62)	**0.046**
Propensity score, 0–1	0.32 (0.03 to 3.65)	0.36	0.41 (0.03 to 5.59)	0.51
Exposure to TNFi	0.91 (0.40 to 2.08)	0.83	1.05 (0.43 to 2.52)	0.92
Propensity score, 0–1	6.26 (0.78 to 49.89)	0.084	1.18 (0.12 to 11.30)	0.89
TNFi for ≥ 2 years	0.86 (0.35 to 2.09)	0.73	0.81 (0.30 to 2.21)	0.68
Propensity score, 0–1	3.78 (0.41 to 34.593)	0.24	0.69 (0.06 to 8.46)	0.77

Significant p value is shown in bold typeface
mSASSS modified Stoke Ankylosing Spondylitis Spinal Score, TNFi tumor necrosis factor inhibitor

Table 5 Effect of TNFi on spinal radiographic progression according to NSAID use, with and without propensity score adjustment

	Univariate OR (95% CI)	p value	OR (95% CI) with PS[a]	p value
Progression ≥ 2 mSASSS units				
TNFi vs. no TNFi and no NSAID	3.33 (0.46 to 24.05)	0.23	3.06 (0.27 to 34.70)	0.37
TNFi vs. no TNFi and low NSAID	1.24 (0.46 to 3.38)	0.67	1.16 (0.40 to 3.40)	0.79
TNFi vs. no TNFi and high NSAID	0.74 (0.17 to 3.31)	0.70	0.48 (0.09 to 2.48)	0.38
New syndesmophytes				
TNFi vs. no TNFi and no NSAID	1.25 (0.14 to 10.94)	0.84	2.51 (0.17 to 38.18)	0.51
TNFi vs. no TNFi and low NSAID	1.26 (0.42 to 3.81)	0.67	1.44 (0.44 to 4.70)	0.55
TNFi vs. no TNFi and high NSAID	1.04 (0.23 to 4.69)	0.96	0.84 (0.17 to 4.21)	0.83

BASDAI Bath Ankylosing Spondylitis Disease Activity Index, *BMI* body mass index, *CRP* C-reactive protein, *HLA-B27* Human leucocyte antigen B27, *mSASSS* modified Stoke Ankylosing Spondylitis Spine Score, *NSAID* non-steroidal anti-inflammatory drug, *PS* propensity score, *TNFi* tumor necrosis factor inhibitor
[a]Variables included in PS are sex, HLA-B27, baseline CRP, BASDAI, mSASSS, smoking pack-years, BMI category, symptom duration and age of onset of symptoms

treated with TNFi, with substantial variation in treatment duration and different starting points. The PS for TNFi treatment was also based on baseline variables as variables at other starting points were not available.

Obesity was found to be a predictor of spinal radiographic progression in both sexes. A previous cross-sectional study identified higher BMI in patients with syndesmophytes, which is in line with our findings [34]. whereas a recently published longitudinal study found no association with being overweight or obese and radiographic progression [35]. Obesity is associated with higher bone mineral density (BMD) in the general population, this being attributed to greater mechanical loading and hormones. Also, adipokines secreted by adipose tissue have an effect on BMD, although has not yet been fully elucidated [36]. Adipokines also have an effect on immune functions and inflammatory processes in the body [37] but the knowledge of the role of adipokines in AS is limited and conflicting. Two cross-sectional studies found elevated leptin to be associated with the presence of syndesmophytes [34, 38], whereas one longitudinal study demonstrated a protective effect of leptin against spinal radiographic progression [39] and another found elevated visfatin at baseline to predict spinal progression [40]. Mechanical loading has been shown to result in new bone formation in mice, an effect that is not yet proven in humans [41]. Ramiro et al. used a physically demanding occupation as a proxy for "life time mechanical stress" on the spine and found that blue-collar work amplified the effect of inflammation on radiographic progression [42]. Doran et al., on the other hand, found no association between AS-related radiological changes and occupational activity level in a retrospective study of patients with AS [43]. In the current study there was no association between occupation at baseline and radiographic progression.

High BASMI independently predicted the development of new syndesmophytes in women. The BASMI has to our knowledge not been studied as a predictor of spinal radiographic progression before, but could be an interesting predictor as it is clinically more feasible than, for example, radiographic examinations. The BASMI is correlated with the mSASSS but the variables are not interchangeable [44]. Impaired spinal mobility is more influenced by inflammation in early AS and by spinal radiographic changes later in the disease [45].We do not believe that high BASMI causes the progression but rather that it follows from a high mSASSS.

Progression of mSASSS varied considerably between patients. However, the mean progression of 1.6 mSASSS units over 5 years in the current study was lower than in previous reports on patients with long-standing AS. For instance, previous studies in three different AS cohorts with 100%, 20% and 0% of the patients treated with TNFi showed a progression of mean 1.3 mSASSS units per 2 years [46], 2.0 mSASSS units per 2 years [7, 11] and 1.3 mSASSS units per year [9], respectively. The reason for the modest mSASSS increase in the current study is not obvious, especially since the radiographic alterations at baseline were similar to those in the OASIS cohort [7, 11]. Possibly, it could be explained by differences in the selection of patients. Another factor could be the smaller proportion of men in this Swedish cohort, but not even the progression in men of 1.9 mSASSS units over 5 years was on a level with the previously reported progression rates. Osteo-proliferative changes in the present study were scored with knowledge of the serial order of acquisition of the radiographs, and reading in serial order is more sensitive to change, hence, progression should not have been underestimated [47].

The patients in the current study were recruited from rheumatology clinics and may have more severe disease. However, 70 patients (42%) among the completers had been referred to a general practitioner during follow up due to inactive disease and the percentage of patients using TNFi at baseline was similar to that in Swedish patients with AS in a nationwide register-based report from the same year (20% in our cohort vs 17% in all

Swedish patients with AS) [48]. At baseline, the patients with AS were somewhat older in the current study than the patients that declined participation, as reported previously [49]. At follow up, the completers did not differ in age or mSASSS compared with non-completers, but there was a trend toward there being more women among the completers. Even if we cannot exclude the possibility that there has been some selection bias towards older patients and women in this study, we believe that our patients are representative of patients with AS in our region.

In order to decrease radiographic progression in the spine we propose the supporting of weight loss in obese patients, counseling on the hazardous effect of smoking and treatment of active inflammation. In addition, further and larger studies on the effect of bisphosphonates on radiographic progression in the spine are needed.

One limitation of the present study is the relatively small number of patients in the subgroups, especially of women among whom few have spinal radiographic progression, and in particular the development of new syndesmophytes. This reduces the statistical power as displayed by the large confidence intervals in the results for women. Thus, the results for the subgroups, and in particular for women, need to be interpreted with caution and confirmed in a larger cohort with more women. Another limitation is the use of only one reader of the radiographs. Strengths of this study are the long follow-up time, the prospective longitudinal design with well-characterized patients and many variables identified and analyzed that have potential association with osteo-proliferation. It is also the first study reporting sex-specific predictors of spinal radiographic progression in AS.

Conclusion

Over 5 years, men had greater spinal radiographic progression than women and predictors of progression differed partly between sexes. New predictors identified were obesity in both sexes and exposure to bisphosphonates and impairment of spinal mobility in women. Among previously known predictors, baseline spinal radiographic alterations was a predictor in both sexes, high CRP was a predictor in men, with a trend in women too, whereas smoking predicted progression in men.

Abbreviations
AS: Ankylosing spondylitis; ASAS: Assessment of SpondyloArthritis international Society; ASDAS: Ankylosing Spondylitis Disease Activity Score; ASDAS_CRP: Ankylosing Spondylitis Disease Activity Score based on C-reactive protein; BASDAI: Bath Ankylosing Spondylitis Disease Activity Index; BASFI: Bath Ankylosing Spondylitis Functional Index; BAS-G: Bath Ankylosing Spondylitis Patient Global Score; BASMI: Bath Ankylosing Spondylitis Metrology Index; BMI: Body mass index; CI: Confidence interval; CRP: C-reactive protein; ESR: Erythrocyte sedimentation rate; HLA-B27: Human leukocyte antigen B27; ICC: Intraclass correlation coefficient; mSASSS: modified Stoke Ankylosing Spondylitis Spine Score;

NSAID: Non-steroid anti-inflammatory drug; OR: Odds ratio; PS: Propensity score; SD: Standard deviation; SDC: Smallest detectable change; SpA: Spondyloarthritis; TNFi: Tumor necrosis factor inhibitor

Acknowledgements
We wish to thank all the patients who participated in the study. We are grateful to the research nurses Vera Börjesson and Kerstin Larsson at Sahlgrenska University Hospital for their assistance with the patients. We also want to thank Tony Jurkiewich and Berit Kluft at the radiology department for help with the radiographs.

Funding
This study was supported by grants from the Health and Medical Care Executive Board of the Västra Götaland, Rune and Ulla Amlövs foundation for Rheumatology Research, Göteborg's Association Against Rheumatism, The Swedish Rheumatism association, The Swedish Society of Medicine, The Göteborg Medical Society, the Region Västra Götaland (agreement concerning research and education of doctors), Controlling Chronic Inflammatory Diseases with Combined Efforts (COMBINE), and the Margareta Rheuma research foundation.

Authors' contributions
AD participated in acquisition, analysis and interpretation of data and drafting the manuscript. EK participated in the design of the study and acquisition, analysis and interpretation of data. MG and JG participated in acquisition and interpretation of data. MH and ER participated in acquisition of data. HC participated in the conception and design of the work. LTJ participated in drafting the manuscript and interpretation of data. HFd'E participated in the conception and design of the work, acquisition, analysis and interpretation of data and drafting the manuscript. All authors critically reviewed the manuscript and approved the final version to be published.

Consent for publication
Not applicable.

Competing interests
MG has received consultancy fees from Pfizer and Novartis, outside the submitted work.
LTJ has received Advisory Board Fees from Novartis, Celgene and MSD, outside the submitted work.
HFd'E has received Advisory Board Fees from Sandoz, Novartis and Abbvie and an unrestricted grant from Novartis, outside the submitted work.
AD, EK, JG, MH, ER and HC report no competing interests.

Author details
Department of Rheumatology and Inflammation Research, Sahlgrenska Academy at University of Gothenburg, Box 480, 405 30 Gothenburg, Sweden. [2]Department of Radiology, Skåne University Hospital, 221 85 Lund, Sweden. [3]Faculty of Medicine, Lund University, Box 117, 221 00 Lund, Sweden. [4]Department of Radiology, Sahlgrenska University Hospital, Mölndal, 431 80 Mölndal, Sweden. [5]Section of Rheumatology, Södra Älvsborg Hospital, 501 82 Borås, Sweden. [6]Section of Rheumatology, Alingsås Hospital, 441 33 Alingsås, Sweden. [7]Department of Public Health and Clinical Medicine, Rheumatology, 901 87 Umeå University, Umeå, Sweden.

References
1. Braun J, Sieper J. Ankylosing spondylitis. Lancet. 2007;369(9570):1379–90.
2. Lee W, Reveille JD, Weisman MH. Women with ankylosing spondylitis: a review. Arthritis Care Res (Hoboken). 2008;59(3):449–54.
3. Wanders AJ, Landewe RB, Spoorenberg A, Dougados M, van der Linden S, Mielants H, et al. What is the most appropriate radiologic scoring method for ankylosing spondylitis? A comparison of the available methods based on the Outcome Measures in Rheumatology Clinical Trials filter. Arthritis Rheum. 2004;50(8):2622–32.
4. Lee W, Reveille JD, Davis JC Jr, Learch TJ, Ward MM, Weisman MH. Are there gender differences in severity of ankylosing spondylitis? Results from the PSOAS cohort. Ann Rheum Dis. 2007;66(5):633–8.

5. van Tubergen A, Ramiro S, van der Heijde D, Dougados M, Mielants H, Landewe R. Development of new syndesmophytes and bridges in ankylosing spondylitis and their predictors: a longitudinal study. Ann Rheum Dis. 2012;71(4):518–23.

6. Webers C, Essers I, Ramiro S, Stolwijk C, Landewe R, van der Heijde D, et al. Gender-attributable differences in outcome of ankylosing spondylitis: long-term results from the outcome in ankylosing spondylitis international study. Rheumatology (Oxford). 2016;55(3):419–28.

7. Ramiro S, Stolwijk C, van Tubergen A, van der Heijde D, Dougados M, van den Bosch F, et al. Evolution of radiographic damage in ankylosing spondylitis: a 12 year prospective follow-up of the OASIS study. Ann Rheum Dis. 2015;74(1):52–9.

8. Baraliakos X, Listing J, Rudwaleit M, Haibel H, Brandt J, Sieper J, et al. Progression of radiographic damage in patients with ankylosing spondylitis: defining the central role of syndesmophytes. Ann Rheum Dis. 2007;66(7):910–5.

9. Baraliakos X, Listing J, von der Recke A, Braun J. The natural course of radiographic progression in ankylosing spondylitis - evidence for major individual variations in a large proportion of patients. J Rheumatol. 2009; 36(5):997–1002.

10. Poddubnyy D, Haibel H, Listing J, Marker-Hermann E, Zeidler H, Braun J, et al. Baseline radiographic damage, elevated acute-phase reactant levels, and cigarette smoking status predict spinal radiographic progression in early axial spondylarthritis. Arthritis Rheum. 2012;64(5):1388–98.

11. Ramiro S, van der Heijde D, van Tubergen A, Stolwijk C, Dougados M, van den Bosch F, et al. Higher disease activity leads to more structural damage in the spine in ankylosing spondylitis: 12-year longitudinal data from the OASIS cohort. Ann Rheum Dis. 2014;73(8):1455–61.

12. Poddubnyy D, Protopopov M, Haibel H, Braun J, Rudwaleit M, Sieper J. High disease activity according to the ankylosing spondylitis disease activity score is associated with accelerated radiographic spinal progression in patients with early axial spondyloarthritis: results from the GErman SPondyloarthritis inception cohort. Ann Rheum Dis. 2016;75(12):2114–8.

13. Klingberg E, Lorentzon M, Mellstrom D, Geijer M, Gothlin J, Hilme E, et al. Osteoporosis in ankylosing spondylitis - prevalence, risk factors and methods of assessment. Arthritis Res Ther. 2012;14(3):12.

14. van der Linden S, Valkenburg HA, Cats A. Evaluation of diagnostic criteria for ankylosing spondylitis. A proposal for modification of the New York criteria. Arthritis Rheum. 1984;27(4):361–8.

15. Jenkinson TR, Mallorie PA, Whitelock HC, Kennedy LG, Garrett SL, Calin A. Defining spinal mobility in ankylosing spondylitis (AS). The Bath AS Metrology Index. J Rheumatol. 1994;21(9):1694–8.

16. Garrett S, Jenkinson T, Kennedy LG, Whitelock H, Gaisford P. Calin a. A new approach to defining disease status in ankylosing spondylitis: the bath ankylosing spondylitis disease activity index. J Rheumatol. 1994; 21(12):2286–91.

17. Calin A, Garrett S, Whitelock H, Kennedy LG, O'Hea J, Mallorie P, et al. A new approach to defining functional ability in ankylosing spondylitis: the development of the bath ankylosing spondylitis functional index. J Rheumatol. 1994;21(12):2281–5.

18. Jones SD, Steiner A, Garrett SL, Calin A. The bath ankylosing spondylitis patient global score (BAS-G). Br J Rheumatol. 1996;35(1):66–71.

19. Lukas C, Landewe R, Sieper J, Dougados M, Davis J, Braun J, et al. Development of an ASAS-endorsed disease activity score (ASDAS) in patients with ankylosing spondylitis. Ann Rheum Dis. 2009;68(1):18–24.

20. Niknian M, A LL, Lasater TM, Carleton RA. Use of population-based data to assess risk factor profiles of blue and white collar workers. J Occup Environ Med. 1991;33(1):29–36.

21. Seidell JC, Flegal KM. Assessing obesity: classification and epidemiology. Br Med Bull. 1997;53(2):238–52.

22. Dougados M, Simon P, Braun J, Burgos-Vargas R, Maksymowych WP, Sieper J, et al. ASAS recommendations for collecting, analysing and reporting NSAID intake in clinical trials/epidemiological studies in axial spondyloarthritis. Ann Rheum Dis. 2011;70(2):249–51.

23. Klingberg E, Svealv BG, Tang MS, Bech-Hanssen O, Forsblad-d'Elia H, Bergfeldt L. Aortic regurgitation is common in ankylosing spondylitis: time for routine echocardiography evaluation? Am J Med. 2015;128(11):1244–1250.e1241.

24. Creemers MC, Franssen MJ, van't Hof MA, Gribnau FW, van de Putte LB, van Riel PL. Assessment of outcome in ankylosing spondylitis: an extended radiographic scoring system. Ann Rheum Dis. 2005;64(1):127–9.

25. Baraliakos X, Listing J, Rudwaleit M, Haibe H, Sieper J, Braun J. Progression of radiographic damage in patients with ankylosing spondylitis - defining the central role of syndesmophytes. Ann Rheum Dis. 2007;66:85.

26. Koo TK, Li MY. A guideline of selecting and reporting Intraclass correlation coefficients for reliability research. J Chiropr Med. 2016;15(2):155–63.

27. Bruynesteyn K, Boers M, Kostense P, van der Linden S, van der Heijde D. Deciding on progression of joint damage in paired films of individual patients: smallest detectable difference or change. Ann Rheum Dis. 2005; 64(2):179–82.

28. Kang KY, Kwok SK, Ju JH, Park KS, Park SH, Hong YS. The predictors of development of new syndesmophytes in female patients with ankylosing spondylitis. Scand J Rheumatol. 2015;44(2):125–8.

29. Poddubnyy D, Haibel H, Listing J, Marker-Hermann E, Zeidler H, Braun J, et al. Cigarette smoking has a dose-dependent impact on progression of structural damage in the spine in patients with axial spondyloarthritis: results from the GErman SPondyloarthritis inception cohort (GESPIC). Ann Rheum Dis. 2013;72(8):1430–2.

30. Poddubnyy D, Halibel H, Listing J, Märker-Hermann E, Zeidler H, Braun J et al. Cigarette smoking has a dose-dependent impact on progression of structural damage in the spine in patients with axial spondyloarthritis: results from the GErman SPondyloarthritis Inception Cohort (GESPIC). Ann Rheum Dis. 2013;72(8):1430–2.

31. Maksymowych WP, Jhangri GS, Fitzgerald AA, LeClercq S, Chiu P, Yan A, et al. A six-month randomized, controlled, double-blind, dose-response comparison of intravenous pamidronate (60 mg versus 10 mg) in the treatment of nonsteroidal antiinflammatory drug-refractory ankylosing spondylitis. Arthritis Rheum. 2002;46(3):766–73.

32. Viapiana O, Gatti D, Idolazzi L, Fracassi E, Adami S, Troplini S, et al. Bisphosphonates vs infliximab in ankylosing spondylitis treatment. Rheumatology (Oxford). 2014;53(1):90–4.

33. Coates L, Packham JC, Creamer P, Hailwood S, Bhalla AS, Chakravarty K, et al. Clinical efficacy of oral alendronate in ankylosing spondylitis: a randomised placebo-controlled trial. Clin Exp Rheumatol. 2017;35(3):445–51.

34. Kim KJ, Kim JY, Park SJ, Yoon H, Yoon CH, Kim WU, et al. Serum leptin levels are associated with the presence of syndesmophytes in male patients with ankylosing spondylitis. Clin Rheumatol. 2012;31(8):1231–8.

35. Molnar C, Scherer A, Baraliakos X, de Hooge M, Micheroli R, Exer P, et al. TNF blockers inhibit spinal radiographic progression in ankylosing spondylitis by reducing disease activity: results from the Swiss clinical quality management cohort. Ann Rheum Dis. 2018;77(1):63–9.

36. Shapses SA, Sukumar D. Bone metabolism in obesity and weight loss. Annu Rev Nutr. 2012;32:287–309.

37. Tilg H, Moschen AR. Adipocytokines: mediators linking adipose tissue, inflammation and immunity. Nat Rev Immunol. 2006;6(10):772–83.

38. Gonzalez-Lopez L, Fajardo-Robledo NS, Miriam Saldana-Cruz A, Moreno-Sandoval IV, Bonilla-Lara D, Zavaleta-Muniz S, et al. Association of adipokines, interleukin-6, and tumor necrosis factor-alpha concentrations with clinical characteristics and presence of spinal syndesmophytes in patients with ankylosing spondylitis: a cross-sectional study. J Int Med Res. 2017;45(3):1024–35.

39. Hartl A, Sieper J, Syrbe U, Listing J, Hermann KG, Rudwaleit M, et al. Serum levels of leptin and high molecular weight adiponectin are inversely associated with radiographic spinal progression in patients with ankylosing spondylitis: results from the ENRADAS trial. Arthritis Res Ther. 2017;19(1):140.

40. Syrbe U, Callhoff J, Conrad K, Poddubnyy D, Haibel H, Junker S, et al. Serum adipokine levels in patients with ankylosing spondylitis and their relationship to clinical parameters and radiographic spinal progression. Arthritis & rheumatology (Hoboken, NJ). 2015;67(3):678–85.

41. Jacques P, Lambrecht S, Verheugen E, Pauwels E, Kollias G, Armaka M, et al. Proof of concept: enthesitis and new bone formation in spondyloarthritis are driven by mechanical strain and stromal cells. Ann Rheum Dis. 2014; 73(2):437–45.

42. Ramiro S, Landewé R, van Tubergen A, Boonen A, Stolwijk C, Dougados M et al. Lifestyle factors may modify the effect of disease activity on radiographic progression in patients with ankylosing spondylitis: a longitudinal analysis. RMD Open. 2015;1:e000153.

43. Doran MF, Brophy S, MacKay K, Taylor G, Calin A. Predictors of longterm outcome in ankylosing spondylitis. J Rheumatol. 2003;30(2):316–20.

44. Wanders A, Landewe R, Dougados M, Mielants H, van der Linden S, van der Heijde D. Association between radiographic damage of the spine and spinal mobility for individual patients with ankylosing spondylitis: can assessment of spinal mobility be a proxy for radiographic evaluation? Ann Rheum Dis. 2005;64(7):988–94.

45. Machado P, Landewé R, Braun J, Hermann K-GA, Baker D, van der Heijde D. Both structural damage and inflammation of the spine contribute to impairment of spinal mobility in patients with ankylosing spondylitis. Ann Rheum Dis. 2010;69(8):1465–70.

46. Maas F, Spoorenberg A, Brouwer E, Bos R, Efde M, Chaudhry RN, et al. Spinal radiographic progression in patients with ankylosing spondylitis treated with TNF-alpha blocking therapy: a prospective longitudinal observational cohort study. PLoS One. 2015;10(4):e0122693.

47. Wanders A, Landewe R, Spoorenberg A, de Vlam K, Mielants H, Dougados M, et al. Scoring of radiographic progression in randomised clinical trials in ankylosing spondylitis: a preference for paired reading order. Ann Rheum Dis. 2004;63(12):1601–4.

48. Exarchou S, Lindstrom U, Askling J, Eriksson JK, Forsblad-d'Elia H, Neovius M, et al. The prevalence of clinically diagnosed ankylosing spondylitis and its clinical manifestations: a nationwide register study. Arthritis Res Ther. 2015; 17:118.

49. Klingberg E, Geijer M, Gothln J, Mellstrom D, Lorentzon M, Hilme E, et al. Vertebral fractures in ankylosing spondylitis are associated with lower bone mineral density in both central and peripheral skeleton. J Rheumatol. 2012; 39(10):1987–95.

7

Interaction between CD177 and platelet endothelial cell adhesion molecule-1 downregulates membrane-bound proteinase-3 (PR3) expression on neutrophils and attenuates neutrophil activation induced by PR3-ANCA

Hui Deng[1,2,3,4], Nan Hu[1,2,3,4], Chen Wang[1,2,3,4], Min Chen[1,2,3,4*] and Ming-Hui Zhao[1,2,3,4]

Abstract

Background: A recent study found that CD177 served as a receptor of membrane-bound proteinase-3 (mPR3) in a subset of neutrophils. Furthermore, CD177 has been identified as a high-affinity heterophilic binding partner for the endothelial cell platelet endothelial cell adhesion molecule-1 (PECAM-1). The current study aimed to investigate whether the interaction between PECAM-1 and CD177 could influence mPR3 expression as well as PR3-antineutrophil cytoplasmic antibody (ANCA)-induced neutrophil activation and glomerular endothelial cell (GEnC) injury.

Methods: The effect of interaction between CD177 and PECAM-1 on mPR3 expression was explored by enzyme-linked immunosorbent assay (ELISA) and flow cytometry. The effect of PECAM-1 on neutrophil activation and GEnC injury induced by PR3-ANCA-positive immunoglobulin (Ig)Gs was evaluated by dihydrorhodamine (DHR) assay and ELISA. CD177-negative neutrophils were selected by magnetic cell sorting (MACS), and the inhibitory effect of PECAM-1 on CD177-negative and mixed neutrophils was explored by measuring neutrophil degranulation.

Results: The level of specific interaction between CD177 and PECAM-1 was elevated with increasing CD177 concentration. The expression of mPR3 significantly decreased in neutrophils preincubated with PECAM-1 in a dose-dependent manner. Consistently, the levels of respiratory burst and degranulation induced by PR3-ANCA-positive IgGs in recombinant human tumor necrosis factor-alpha (TNF-α)-primed neutrophils was significantly reduced by preincubation with PECAM-1 (440.6 ± 123.0 vs. 511.4 ± 95.5, $p < 0.05$; and 3155.0 ± 1733.0 ng/ml vs. 5903.0 ± 717.5 ng/ml, $p < 0.05$, respectively). In CD177-negative neutrophils incubated with PR3-ANCA-positive IgGs, the level of degranulation was not significantly changed by preincubation with PECAM-1. However, in mixed neutrophils, PECAM-1 significantly decreased the level of degranulation induced by PR3-ANCA-positive IgGs ($1015.9 \pm 229.2\%$ vs. $1725.2 \pm 412.4\%$, $p < 0.01$). Furthermore, with preincubation of TNF-α-primed neutrophils with PECAM-1, the level of soluble intercellular cell adhesion molecule-1 (sICAM-1), a marker of endothelial cell activation and injury, in the supernatant of GEnCs treated with primed neutrophils plus PR3-ANCA-positive IgGs was significantly attenuated (112.7 ± 24.2 pg/ml vs. 167.5 ± 27.7 pg/ml, $p < 0.05$).

(Continued on next page)

* Correspondence: chenmin74@sina.com
[1]Renal Division, Department of Medicine, Peking University First Hospital, Peking University Institute of Nephrology, Beijing 100034, China
[2]Key Laboratory of Renal Disease, Ministry of Health of China, Beijing 100034, China
Full list of author information is available at the end of the article

(Continued from previous page)

Conclusions: PECAM-1 can decrease the level of mPR3 expression on neutrophils, resulting in attenuation of neutrophil activation and subsequent GEnC injury induced by PR3-ANCA-positive IgGs.

Keywords: ANCA, Proteinase-3, CD177, Platelet endothelial cell adhesion molecule-1

Background

Antineutrophil cytoplasmic antibody (ANCA)-associated vasculitis (AAV) consists of granulomatosis with polyangiitis (GPA, previously named Wegener's granulomatosis), microscopic polyangiitis (MPA), and eosinophilic granulomatosis with polyangiitis (EGPA) [1]. The kidney is one of the most commonly involved organs in AAV. ANCAs, the serological markers for primary small vessel vasculitis, are involved in inducing and amplifying endothelial injury in AAV [2]. Proteinase-3 (PR3) and myeloperoxidase (MPO) are the two main target antigens of ANCA in AAV [3, 4]. During the priming process of neutrophils by proinflammatory cytokines such as tumor necrosis factor-alpha (TNF-α), membrane-bound PR3 (mPR3) is upregulated in a subset of neutrophils [5]. PR3-ANCA may recognize mPR3 and lead to degranulation and reactive oxygen species (ROS) production in neutrophils, causing massive injury to endothelial cells, in particular glomerular endothelial cells (GEnCs) [5, 6].

CD177 is a neutrophil surface molecule that was identified in 1971 as the target of alloimmune antibodies associated with fetal neutropenia [7]. Its expression is restricted to a subset of neutrophils and the percentage of CD177-positive neutrophils ranges from 0% to 100% in an individual, with a mean percentage of 45–65% [8–10]. The function of CD177 is largely unknown. Recently, CD177 has been identified as a high-affinity heterophilic binding partner for platelet endothelial cell adhesion molecule-1 (PECAM-1)/CD31 on endothelial cells [11]. PECAM-1 is highly expressed on endothelial cells and is a major constituent of the endothelial cell intercellular junction in confluent vascular beds [12, 13]. Interaction of CD177 and PECAM-1 has indicated its role as an adhesion molecule in neutrophil adhesion and transmigration.

As previously mentioned, in the pathogenesis of endothelium injury in AAV, PR3-ANCA recognizes mPR3 and triggers degranulation and respiratory burst of neutrophils, which in turn causes necrosis of endothelial cells [14]. CD177 and mPR3 are colocalized on the neutrophil membrane, and CD177 is probably the receptor for mPR3 [15–17]. Therefore, it is of interest to investigate the role of CD177 as the receptor of mPR3, and its binding partner PECAM-1, in the process of neutrophil activation. We hypothesized that the interaction of CD177 and PECAM-1 may influence the binding of mPR3 to CD177 on the neutrophil membrane. Furthermore, PR3-ANCA-mediated neutrophil activation and endothelial injury may also be affected by the interaction between CD177 and PECAM-1 on neutrophils.

Methods

Reagents

Recombinant PECAM-1, junctional adhesion molecule-1 (JAM-1), and CD177 were purchased from Sino Biological Inc. (Beijing, China). Fluorochrome dihydrorhodamine (DHR), phorbol myristate acetate (PMA), and normal human immunoglobulin (Ig)G were purchased from Sigma (St Louis, USA). For indirect enzyme-linked immunosorbent assay (ELISA), mouse anti-human CD177 antibody was purchased from Sino Biological Inc. and horseradish peroxidase (HRP)-conjugated goat anti-mouse IgG was purchased from Abcam (Cambridge, UK). For flow cytometry analysis, phycoerythrin (PE)-conjugated mouse monoclonal antibody against human CD177 and the isotype control mouse IgG1 were purchased from BioLegend (San Diego, CA, USA). Fluorescein isothiocyanate (FITC)-conjugated mouse monoclonal antibody against human PR3 and the isotype control mouse IgG1 were purchased from Abcam. For magnetic neutrophil sorting, anti-PE microbeads and separation columns were purchased from Miltenyi Biotech (Bergisch-Gladbach, Germany). For Western blot, antibodies against SHP-1 (C14H6) and phosphor-SHP-1 (Tyr564) were purchased from Cell Signaling Technology (Boston, MA, USA), and mouse anti-human GAPDH antibody was purchased from Santa Cruz Biotech (Santa Cruz, CA, USA).

Cell culture

Primary human renal GEnCs (ScienCell Research Laboratories, San Diego, CA, USA) were cultured in endothelial cell basal medium (ECM) (ScienCell) with the addition of 5% fetal bovine serum (FBS), 1% penicillin/streptomycin, and 1% endothelial cell growth factor for the formation of a confluent endothelial cell monolayer. The flasks for cell subculture were bio-coated with human plasma fibronectin (Millipore, Billerica, USA) beforehand according to the manufacturer's recommendations. For synchronization of the cell cycle, GEnC monolayers were starved in basal medium without serum and endothelial cell growth factor for 12 h without bio-coating. All experiments were performed using GEnCs at passage 3–5. All cultures were incubated at 37 °C in 5% CO_2.

Interaction between CD177 and PECAM-1

The interaction between CD177 and PECAM-1 was detected by ELISA with recombinant soluble PECAM-1 (sPECAM-1) at 2 µg/ml as the solid-phase antigen. sPECAM-1 in a coating buffer (0.05 M bicarbonate buffer, pH 9.6) was used to coat the wells of half of a polystyrene microtiter plate (Nunc-Immuno plate; Nunc, Roskilde, Denmark) and was incubated overnight at 4 °C. The other half of the plate was coated with coating buffer alone to establish antigen-free wells. The wells were blocked with 3% bovine serum albumin (BSA) in phosphate-buffered saline (PBS) and incubated with CD177 at various concentrations for 1 h at 37 °C. After washing three times with PBS-tween 20 (PBS-T), the wells were incubated with mouse anti-human CD177 antibody (1:1000; Sino Biological) for 1 h at 37 °C, and HRP-conjugated goat anti-mouse IgG (1:1000) was used as the secondary antibody. Tetramethylbenzidine (TMB; Sigma, St. Louis, MO) was used as the substrate and the reaction was stopped by the addition of sulfuric acid 0.5 mol/L (Carl Roth GmbH, Germany). Optical densities of formed complexes were measured at 450 nm using a microplate reader (Bio-Rad, Tokyo, Japan).

Isolation and priming of neutrophils

Neutrophils were isolated as described previously [18]. In brief, venous human blood for neutrophil isolation was obtained from healthy donors by venipuncture and anticoagulated with ethylenediaminetetraacetic acid (EDTA). Neutrophils were isolated by density gradient centrifugation on Lymphoprep (Nycomed, Oslo, Norway). Erythrocytes were lysed with ice-cold red cell lysis buffer (Tiangen Biotech, Beijing, China), and then neutrophils were washed in PBS without Ca^{2+}/Mg^{2+} ($PBS^{-/-}$; Chemical reagents, Beijing, China) and suspended in $PBS^{-/-}$ to a concentration of 1×10^6 cells/ml and used for further analysis. The trypan blue staining technique was used as an index of the proportion of viable cells in a cell population. Where indicated, cells were primed with 2 ng/ml recombinant TNF-α (Sigma, USA) at 37 °C for 15 min, and untreated cells were incubated with control medium under the same conditions.

Magnetic neutrophil sorting

CD177-negative neutrophils were separated with negative selection by magnetic cell sorting (MACS) separation columns (Miltenyi Biotech, Bergisch-Gladbach, Germany) according to the manufacture's manual, as described previously [19]. All steps were carried out on ice. Freshly isolated neutrophils were stained with PE-conjugated monoclonal antibody to CD177 (MEM166). Subsequently, the cells were labeled with anti-PE microbeads (Miltenyi Biotech) and loaded on MACS LD columns (Miltenyi Biotech). The flow-through containing the nonlabeled CD177-negative neutrophils was collected. The purity of CD177-negative neutrophils was $86.4 \pm 8.5\%$ as assessed by flow cytometry.

Preparation of PR3-ANCA-positive IgGs

PR3-ANCA-positive IgGs were prepared from plasma exchange liquid of patients with active PR3-ANCA-positive primary small vessel vasculitis using a High-Trap-protein G column on an AKTA-FPLC system (GE Biosciences, South San Francisco, CA, USA). The preparation of IgGs was performed according to methods described previously [20]. In brief, plasma exchange liquid was filtered through a 0.2-µm syringe filter (Schleicher & Schuell, Duesseldorf, Germany) and applied to a High-Trap-protein G column on an AKTA-FPLC system (GE Biosciences). The column was treated with equal volume of 20 mmol/l Tris-HCl buffer, pH 7.2 (binding buffer), and IgG was eluted with 0.1 mol/l glycine-HCl buffer, pH 2.7 (elution buffer). After the antibodies emerged from the column, the pH value of the eluent was adjusted to pH 7.0 using 2 mol/l Tris-HCl (pH 9.0) immediately. The protein concentration of the antibodies was measured using the Nanodrop-1000 (Pierce, Rockford, IL, USA), and the level of PR3-ANCA IgG was measured by an ELISA kit (EUROIMMUN, Lubeck, Germany). We obtained written informed consent from the participants involved in our study. The research was in compliance with the Declaration of Helsinki and was approved by the clinical research ethics committee of the Peking University First Hospital.

Detection of mPR3 expression on neutrophils and PR3 in supernatant after incubation with PECAM-1

Expression of mPR3 on neutrophils was detected by flow cytometry. Primed neutrophils were incubated with PECAM-1 at serial concentrations (Fig. 1b). There was a dose-dependent response of PECAM-1 in inducing mPR3 downregulation. In further experiments, neutrophils were incubated with PECAM-1 at a concentration of 30 µg/ml or buffer control for 2 h at 37 °C. Since PECAM-1 and JAM-1 are both members of the immunoglobulin superfamily of adhesion molecules with many similarities in their expression profiles and functions [21, 22], JAM-1 was used as the control. Levels of PR3 in the supernatant were tested using commercially available ELISA kits (Elabscience, Wuhan, China). The assay was conducted according to the manufacturer's instructions. All further steps of mPR3 detection on neutrophils were performed on ice, and washing steps were performed using PBS. TruStain FcR Solution (BioLegend, San Diego, CA, USA) was used in all samples prior to the addition of antibodies to block nonspecific binding. Next, cells were stained with a saturating dose of FITC-conjugated mouse monoclonal antibody directed against human PR3 (Abcam, Cambridge, UK) or with

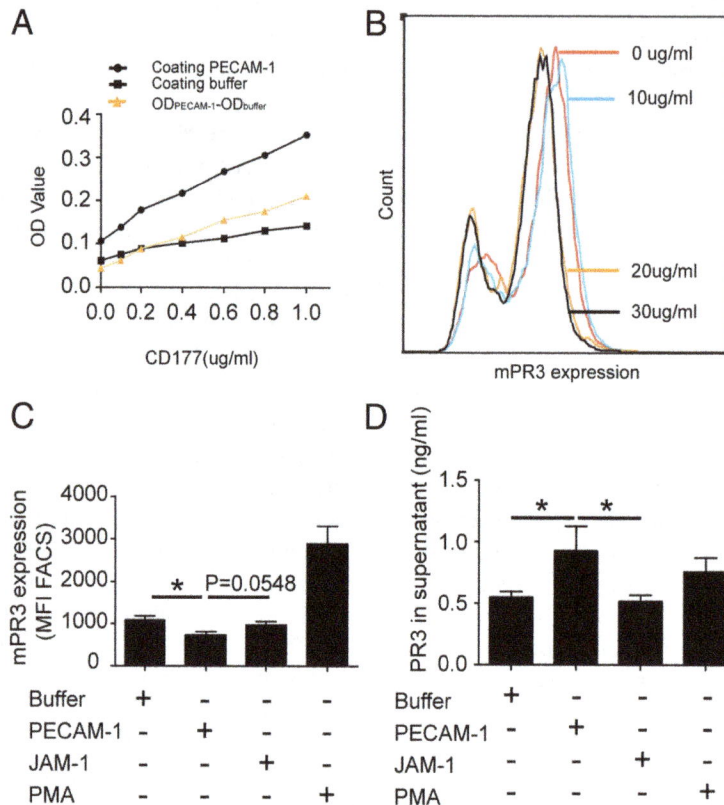

Fig. 1 Downregulation of mPR3 after treating neutrophils with PECAM-1. **a** interaction between platelet endothelial cell adhesion molecule-1 (PECAM-1) and CD177 at various concentrations. **b** Representative histogram of the effect of PECAM-1 on membrane-bound proteinase-3 (mPR3) expression in a dose-dependent manner. **c** Incubation of TNF-α-primed neutrophils with PECAM-1 at 30 µg/ml significantly decreased mPR3 expression. Bars denote means ± SD of mPR3 expression (mean fluorescence intensity; MFI). **d** Incubation of TNF-α-primed neutrophils with PECAM-1 at 30 µg/ml significantly increased proteinase-3 (PR3) levels in the supernatant. Bars denote means ± SD of PR3 concentration (ng/ml). Neutrophils treated with phorbol myristate acetate (PMA) were employed as positive control. *$p < 0.05$. FACS fluorescence-activated cell sorting, JAM-1 junctional adhesion molecule-1, OD optical density

isotype antibody for 20 min in the dark. Fluorescence intensity of FITC was analyzed using flow cytometry. Samples were analyzed using a FACScan (BD, Biosciences, USA). Neutrophils were gated in forward/sideward scatter (FSC/SSC) and data were collected from 10,000 cells per sample. Data were analyzed using FlowJo software (TreeStar, Ashland, Oregon, USA).

Evaluation of neutrophil respiratory burst by DHR assay

We assessed the generation of ROS using DHR as described previously [23]. This method is based on the fact that reactive oxygen radicals cause an oxidation of the nonfluorescent DHR to the green fluorescent rhodamine. In brief, isolated neutrophils suspended in Hanks' balanced salt solution (HBSS) were incubated with 0.05 mM DHR123 (Sigma-Aldrich, Louis, USA) for 30 min at 37 °C. Sodium azide (NaN$_3$; 2 mM) was added to prevent intracellular breakdown of H$_2$O$_2$ by catalase. The neutrophils were then primed with TNF-α (2 ng/ml) for 15 min at 37 °C. After incubating with PECAM-1 (30 µg/ml) or JAM-1 (30 µg/ml) as described

above, patient-derived ANCA-positive IgGs (5 RU/ml) or normal IgG were added. After incubation at 37 °C for 1 h, the reaction was stopped by the addition of 1 ml ice-cold 1% BSA in HBSS. Samples were kept on ice and analyzed using a FACScan. Neutrophils were gated in FSC/SSC and mean fluorescence intensity (MFI; representing the level of neutrophil activation) were collected from 10,000 cells per sample. Data were analyzed using FlowJo software (TreeStar, Ashland, Oregon, USA).

Measurement of neutrophil degranulation by lactoferrin quantification

Lactoferrin, an iron-binding multifunctional glycoprotein, is an abundant component of the specific granules of neutrophils [24, 25]. Lactoferrin is considered as a biomarker of neutrophil degranulation [26–28]. Neutrophils were primed with TNF-α (2 ng/ml) at 37 °C for 15 min, and then were incubated with PECAM-1 or JAM-1 (30 µg/ml) at 37 °C for 2 h followed by stimulation with patient-derived ANCA-positive IgGs or normal IgG for 1 h. Lactoferrin in the supernatant was tested by

ELISA using a commercial kit (Abcam, Cambridge, UK). The ELISA procedure for measuring lactoferrin was performed according to the manufacturer's instructions, as described previously [27].

SHP-1 phosphorylation detected by Western blot

To detect phosphor-SHP-1, isolated neutrophils were primed with TNF-α (2 ng/ml) or PBS at 37 °C for 15 min, and then were incubated with or without PECAM-1 (30 μg/ml) for 1 h. The cells were then incubated on ice in cell lysis buffer (Beyotime Biotechnology, Beijing, China) supplemented with proteinase inhibitors (Sigma, St. Louis, MO, USA) and phosphatase inhibitors (Roche, Mannheim, Germany) for 30 min. The insoluble material was pelleted, and samples were boiled with reduced loading buffer and run in 8% sodium dodecyl sulfate-polyacrylamide gel electrophoresis (SDS-PAGE) gels. Protein was transferred to polyvinylidene difluoride (PVDF) membranes (Millipore, Bedford, MA, USA), and detected by rabbit anti-human SHP-1 antibody (1:1000), rabbit anti-human phosphor-SHP-1 antibody (1:1000), and mouse anti-human GAPDH antibody (1:500) overnight at 4 °C. Finally, the strips were incubated with HRP-conjugated goat anti-mouse (1:5000) or goat anti-rabbit secondary antibodies (1:5000) for 1 h at room temperature with gentle agitation and then revealed on autoradiographic film using the ECL Plus Western Blotting Detection System (GE Healthcare, Piscataway, NJ, USA).

GEnC activation and injury indicated by soluble intercellular cell adhesion molecule-1

Soluble intercellular cell adhesion molecule-1 (sICAM-1) is considered as one of the markers of endothelial cell activation and injury [29]. To explore the role of PECAM-1 in PR3-ANCA-induced endothelial cell injury, the isolated neutrophils were incubated with PECAM-1, JAM-1, or control buffer at 37 °C for 1 h after priming with TNF-α. After incubation, neutrophils were added to GEnC monolayers with patient-derived PR3-ANCA-positive IgGs or normal IgG. After incubation for 4 h at 37 °C, the cell culture supernatant was collected for the ICAM-1 assays. Samples were tested using the human ICAM-1/CD54 ELISA kit (R&D, Abingdon, UK). The assay was conducted according to the manufacturer's instructions as described previously [20]. In brief, samples were added to the microtiter plate coated with capture antibody and incubated for 2 h at room temperature, followed by detection antibody incubation for another 2 h. Then HRP-conjugated streptavidin was added. After 20 min of incubation avoiding direct light, the plate was washed, and substrate solution was added to the wells. After adding the stop solution, the absorption measurements were obtained at 450 nm (with a correction of 570 nm to eliminate

optical imperfections in the plate) using a microtiter plate reader (Bio-Rad iMark™ Microplate Reader). All samples and standards were performed in duplicate.

Statistical analysis

The Shapiro-Wilk test was used to examine whether the data were normally distributed. Quantitative data are expressed as mean ± SD for data that was normally distributed or the median and range for data that was not normally distributed. Differences in quantitative parameters between groups were assessed using one-way analysis of variance (ANOVA) for data that was normally distributed or the Mann-Whitney U test for data that was not normally distributed, as appropriate. Differences were considered significant if $p < 0.05$. Analysis was performed with SPSS statistical software package (version 13.0, Chicago, IL, USA).

Results

Interaction between CD177 and PECAM-1

To explore the interaction between CD177 and PECAM-1, indirect ELISA was performed using soluble PECAM-1 (sPECAM-1) and CD177 at various concentrations. As shown in Fig. 1a, the level of specific interaction between CD177 and PECAM-1, indicated by $OD_{PECAM1} - OD_{buffer}$, elevated with increasing CD177 concentration in a dose-dependent manner.

Downregulation of mPR3 induced by the interaction between PECAM-1 and CD177 on neutrophils

Neutrophils were preincubated with serial concentrations of sPECAM-1 (0, 10, 20, and 30 μg/ml) after priming. Expression of mPR3 on neutrophils was analyzed using flow cytometry. The level of mPR3 gradually decreased with increased concentration of sPECAM-1 (Fig. 1b). After priming with TNF-α, mPR3 expression significantly decreased by treating with sPECAM-1 at 30 μg/ml (730.1 ± 228.8 vs. 1082.0 ± 267.4, $p < 0.05$). Treating neutrophils with JAM-1, another adhesion molecule on endothelial cells, at 30 μg/ml did not significantly affect mPR3 expression (970.4 ± 229.8 vs. 1082.0 ± 267.4, $p = 0.38$). Neutrophils activated by PMA showed high levels of mPR3, which was used as the positive control (Fig. 1c).

PR3 in the supernatant was detected by ELISA. In primed neutrophils treated with sPECAM-1, the concentration of PR3 in supernatant was significantly higher than that treated with JAM-1 (0.93 ± 0.60 ng/ml vs. 0.52 ± 0.21 ng/ml, $p < 0.05$). However, the PR3 concentration was comparable between neutrophils treated with buffer and JAM-1 (0.55 ± 0.17 ng/ml vs. 0.52 ± 0.21 ng/ml, $p = 0.6143$) (Fig. 1d).

PECAM-1 attenuated the ANCA-induced respiratory burst of neutrophils

Compared with TNF-α-primed neutrophils, the MFI value of rhodamine was significantly higher in TNF-α-primed neutrophils treated with PR3-ANCA-positive IgGs (511.4 ± 95.5 vs. 356.7 ± 2.3, $p < 0.05$) (Fig. 2), and the MFI value in TNF-α-primed neutrophils was comparable with neutrophils treated with normal IgG (372.0 ± 11.8 vs. 356.7 ± 2.3, $p = 0.0916$) (Fig. 2). In the presence of PR3-ANCA-positive IgGs, the level of oxygen radical production significantly decreased in neutrophils preincubated with PECAM-1 (440.6 ± 123.0 vs. 511.4 ± 95.5, $p < 0.05$), while it did not significantly change by preincubation with JAM-1 (535.2 ± 134.1 vs. 511.4 ± 95.5, $p = 0.7547$) (Fig. 2).

PECAM-1 decreased ANCA-induced degranulation of neutrophils

ANCA-induced neutrophil degranulation was determined by measuring the concentration of lactoferrin in the supernatant. Compared with TNF-α-primed neutrophils, the concentration of lactoferrin in the supernatant significantly increased in TNF-α-primed neutrophils treated with PR3-ANCA-positive IgGs (5903.0 ± 717.5 ng/ml vs. 3382 ± 233.0 ng/ml, $p < 0.05$), while the elevation of lactoferrin concentration was significantly inhibited by preincubation with PECAM-1 (3155.0 ± 1733.0 ng/ml vs. 5903.0 ± 717.5 ng/ml, $p < 0.05$) (Fig. 3).

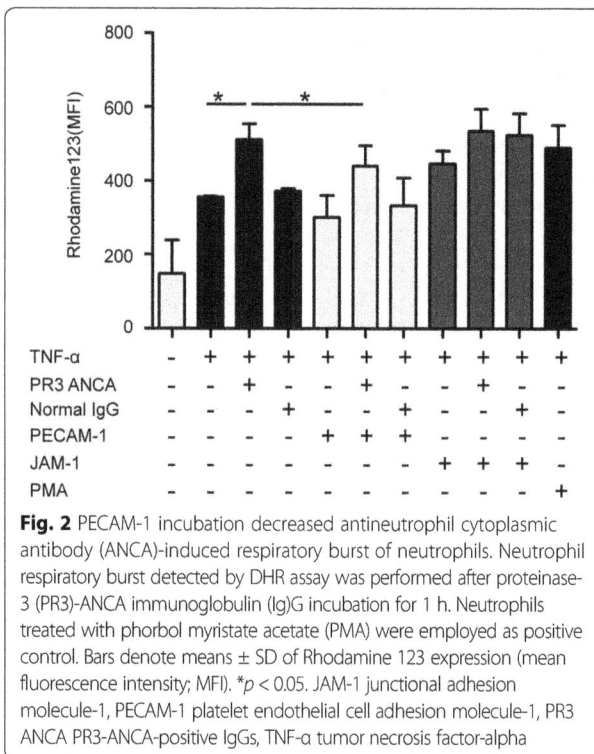

Fig. 3 PECAM-1 incubation decreased antineutrophil cytoplasmic antibody (ANCA)-induced degranulation of neutrophils. Lactoferrin is considered as a biomarker of neutrophil degranulation and was detected after proteinase-3 (PR3)-ANCA immunoglobulin (Ig)G incubation for 1 h. Neutrophils treated with phorbol myristate acetate (PMA) were employed as positive control. Bars denote means ± SD of lactoferrin concentration (ng/ml). *$p < 0.05$. JAM-1 junctional adhesion molecule-1, PECAM-1 platelet endothelial cell adhesion molecule-1, PR3 ANCA PR3-ANCA-positive IgGs, TNF-α tumor necrosis factor-alpha

Effect of PECAM-1 on ANCA-induced degranulation in CD177-negative neutrophils

It has been reported that PECAM-1 has two immunoreceptor tyrosine-based inhibitory motifs (ITIMs). The homophilic interaction between PECAM-1 on neutrophils and endothelial cells could induce ITIM phosphorylation, resulting in inhibitory signal pathway activation, including the protein-tyrosine phosphatase SHP-1 phosphorylation [30, 31]. In our study, phosphor-SHP-1 was detected in neutrophils incubated with PECAM-1 (Fig. 4a), indicating the existence of a homophilic interaction of PECAM-1. We speculated that the detected inhibitory effect of PECAM-1 on neutrophil activation not only resulted from the heterophilic interaction between CD177 and sPECAM-1, but also from the homophilic interaction between transmembrane PECAM-1 and sPECAM-1. CD177-negative neutrophils were acquired by negative selection to test the effect of homophilic interaction of PECAM-1. The initial isolated mixed neutrophils without selection were assessed in parallel for comparison, and the samples contained on average 72.7 ± 10.7% CD177-positive neutrophils. In CD177-negative neutrophils incubated with PR3-ANCA, the level of degranulation did not significantly change by preincubation with PECAM-1, suggesting that the homophilic interaction of PECAM-1 has little, if any, inhibitory effect on neutrophil activation induced by PR3-ANCA. However, in mixed neutrophils, the level of degranulation induced by

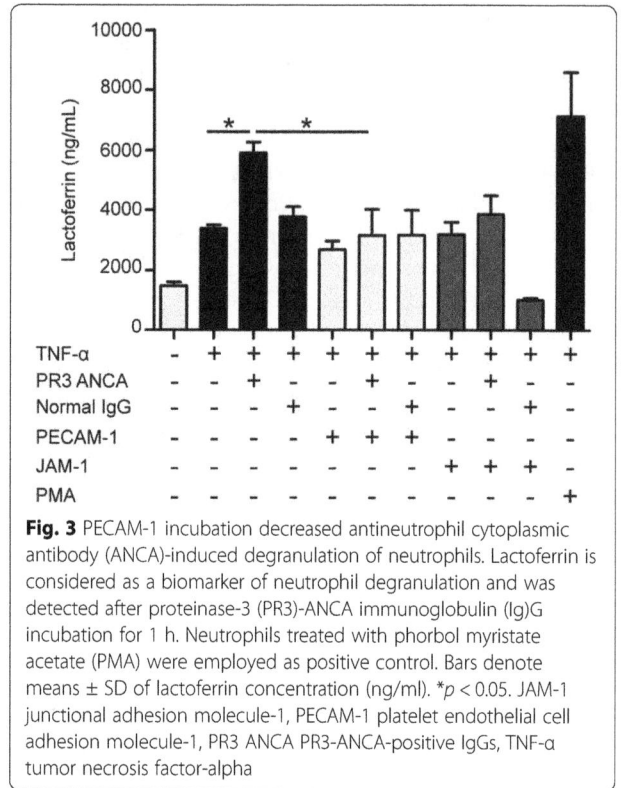

Fig. 2 PECAM-1 incubation decreased antineutrophil cytoplasmic antibody (ANCA)-induced respiratory burst of neutrophils. Neutrophil respiratory burst detected by DHR assay was performed after proteinase-3 (PR3)-ANCA immunoglobulin (Ig)G incubation for 1 h. Neutrophils treated with phorbol myristate acetate (PMA) were employed as positive control. Bars denote means ± SD of Rhodamine 123 expression (mean fluorescence intensity; MFI). *$p < 0.05$. JAM-1 junctional adhesion molecule-1, PECAM-1 platelet endothelial cell adhesion molecule-1, PR3 ANCA PR3-ANCA-positive IgGs, TNF-α tumor necrosis factor-alpha

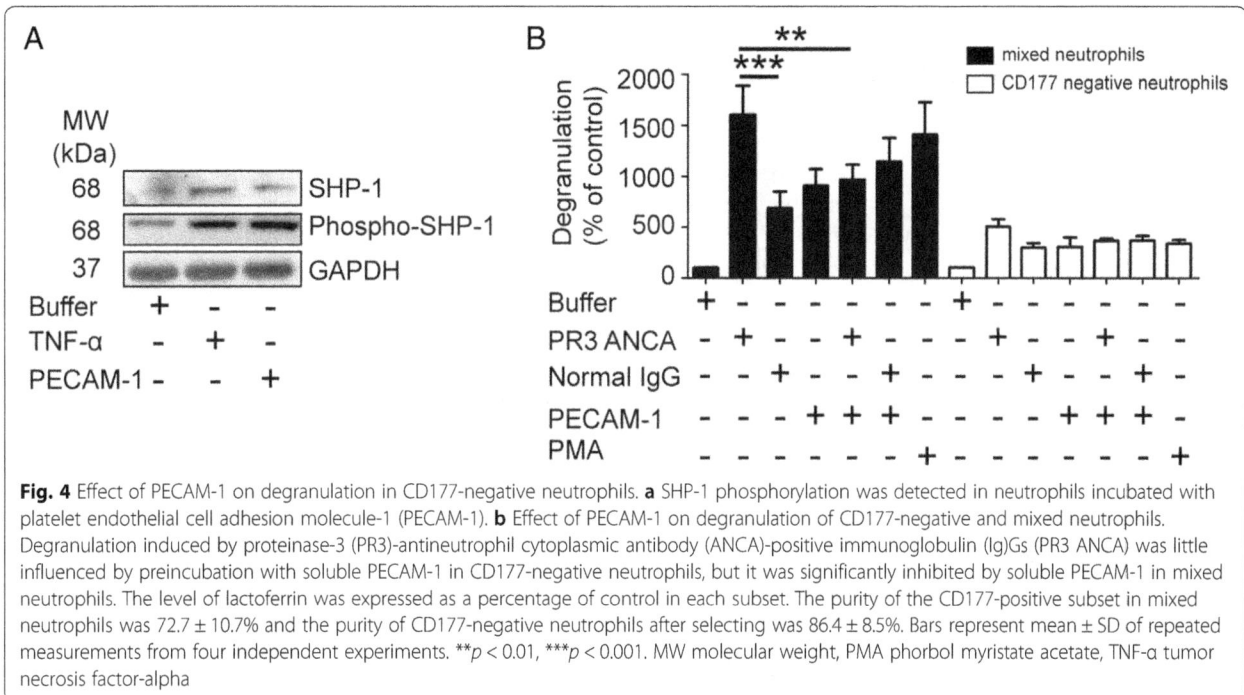

Fig. 4 Effect of PECAM-1 on degranulation in CD177-negative neutrophils. **a** SHP-1 phosphorylation was detected in neutrophils incubated with platelet endothelial cell adhesion molecule-1 (PECAM-1). **b** Effect of PECAM-1 on degranulation of CD177-negative and mixed neutrophils. Degranulation induced by proteinase-3 (PR3)-antineutrophil cytoplasmic antibody (ANCA)-positive immunoglobulin (Ig)Gs (PR3 ANCA) was little influenced by preincubation with soluble PECAM-1 in CD177-negative neutrophils, but it was significantly inhibited by soluble PECAM-1 in mixed neutrophils. The level of lactoferrin was expressed as a percentage of control in each subset. The purity of the CD177-positive subset in mixed neutrophils was $72.7 \pm 10.7\%$ and the purity of CD177-negative neutrophils after selecting was $86.4 \pm 8.5\%$. Bars represent mean $\pm$ SD of repeated measurements from four independent experiments. $**p < 0.01$, $***p < 0.001$. MW molecular weight, PMA phorbol myristate acetate, TNF-α tumor necrosis factor-alpha

PR3-ANCA-positive IgGs was significantly higher than that induced by normal IgG (expressed as percentages of control in each subset, $1725.2 \pm 412.4\%$ vs. $878.4 \pm 309.3\%$, $p < 0.001$). Preincubation with PECAM-1 significantly decreased the level of degranulation induced by PR3-ANCA-positive IgGs ($1015.9 \pm 229.2\%$ vs. $1725.2 \pm 412.4\%$, $p < 0.01$) (Fig. 4b). The inhibition rate of PECAM-1 to degranulation induced by PR3-ANCA was significantly higher in mixed neutrophils than that in CD177-negative neutrophils ($38.5 \pm 6.3\%$ vs. $15.0 \pm 13.0\%$, $p < 0.05$). These results indicated that the heterophilic interaction between CD177 and PECAM-1 contributed to the dominant inhibitory effect on neutrophil activation induced by PR3-ANCA.

PECAM-1 decreased GEnC activation and injury induced by neutrophils plus patient-derived PR3-ANCA-positive IgGs

Soluble ICAM-1 is considered as one of the typical markers of endothelial cell activation and injury. Compared with GEnCs treated with TNF-α-primed neutrophils, the levels of sICAM-1 increased significantly in the supernatant of GEnCs treated with TNF-α-primed neutrophils plus patient-derived PR3-ANCA-positive IgGs (167.5 ± 27.7 pg/ml vs. 46.4 ± 14.5 pg/ml, $p < 0.05$). However, preincubation of neutrophils with PECAM-1 significantly decreased the level of sICAM-1 in the

supernatant of GEnCs treated with primed neutrophils plus PR3-ANCA-positive IgGs (112.7 ± 24.2 pg/ml vs. 167.5 ± 27.7 pg/ml, $p < 0.05$) (Fig. 5).

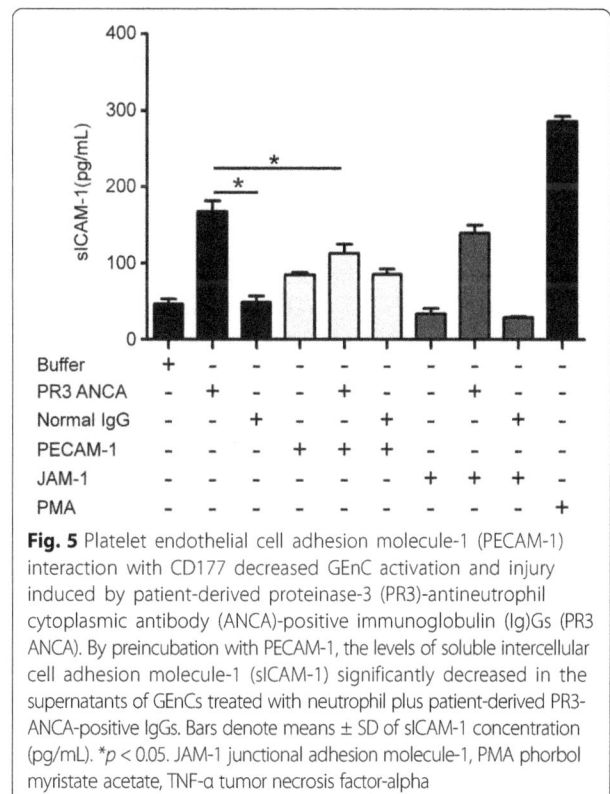

Fig. 5 Platelet endothelial cell adhesion molecule-1 (PECAM-1) interaction with CD177 decreased GEnC activation and injury induced by patient-derived proteinase-3 (PR3)-antineutrophil cytoplasmic antibody (ANCA)-positive immunoglobulin (Ig)Gs (PR3 ANCA). By preincubation with PECAM-1, the levels of soluble intercellular cell adhesion molecule-1 (sICAM-1) significantly decreased in the supernatants of GEnCs treated with neutrophil plus patient-derived PR3-ANCA-positive IgGs. Bars denote means $\pm$ SD of sICAM-1 concentration (pg/mL). $*p < 0.05$. JAM-1 junctional adhesion molecule-1, PMA phorbol myristate acetate, TNF-α tumor necrosis factor-alpha

Discussion

Neutrophil transendothelial migration is a critical event in the inflammatory cascade, during which the heterophilic interaction between endothelial cell PECAM-1 and neutrophil CD177 plays an important role. PR3 can locate on neutrophils by binding to CD177, and it has been demonstrated that PR3-ANCA triggers degranulation and a respiratory burst of neutrophils by recognizing mPR3 and subsequently causes necrosis of endothelial cells [14]. The binding of CD177 with PR3 might be affected by the heterophilic interaction between endothelial cell PECAM-1 and neutrophil CD177. In this study, we demonstrated that sPECAM-1 could decrease mPR3 expression on neutrophils. We also found that PR3-ANCA-induced neutrophil activation and endothelial cell injury were alleviated by preincubation with PECAM-1. Therefore, role of CD177, the receptor of mPR3 on the neutrophil membrane, should be further depicted in the pathogenesis of AAV.

Besides its expression on endothelial cells as a major constituent of the endothelial cell intercellular junction, PECAM-1 could also be expressed on most cells of the hematopoietic lineage, including neutrophils [32]. During the process of neutrophil migration, endothelial PECAM-1 could interact with both PECAM-1 and CD177 on neutrophils. In the current study, sPECAM-1 was used to simulate endothelial PECAM-1 and to eliminate the influence from other adhesion molecules, e.g., selectins, on neutrophils and endothelial cells. Based on dissociation constants, the heterophilic interaction between CD177 and PECAM-1 is approximately 15 times stronger than the PECAM-1 homophilic interactions [11, 33], and the heterophilic interaction was further confirmed in our study. Considering the downregulating effect of sPECAM-1 on mPR3, we assumed that interaction of CD177 with its binding partner PECAM-1 may affect PR3 anchoring to the neutrophil membrane. However, the mechanism of the binding between CD177 and PR3 is not yet fully clear.

PR3-ANCA could bind and cross-link with mPR3 causing neutrophil activation [34, 35], which then contributes to necrotizing vasculitis. As reported, neutrophils with a higher level of mPR3 respond more strongly to PR3-ANCA in vitro, and the level of mPR3 expression correlates with disease severity [19, 36]. As detected in the current study, the level of mPR3 could be downregulated by the heterophilic interaction between CD177 and PECAM-1. Neutrophils with downregulated levels of mPR3 exhibited significantly lower levels of respiratory burst and degranulation in the presence of PR3-ANCA-positive IgGs. However, CD177 is a glycosylphosphatidylinositol (GPI)-anchored molecule that lacks an intracellular domain [10]; thus, intracellular signals could not be induced directly by CD177. As reported, CD177 could modulate neutrophil transmigration through activating CD11b/CD18 (Mac-1) [37], and neutrophil activation induced by PR3-ANCA

could be attenuated by blocking CD177 or Mac-1 [38]. Therefore, PECAM-1 might attenuate PR3-ANCA-induced neutrophil activation by downregulating mPR3 as well as by inhibiting CD177 cross-linking with Mac-1.

In addition, SHP-1 phosphorylation was detected in neutrophils incubated with PECAM-1, indicating that both homophilic and heterophilic interaction might exist on neutrophils. However, the level of neutrophil activation induced by PR3-ANCA-positive IgGs was not obviously influenced by preincubation with sPECAM-1 in CD177-negative neutrophils, while it was significantly inhibited by sPECAM-1 in unsorted neutrophils. The results suggested that the inhibitory effect of PECAM-1 on neutrophil degranulation mainly resulted from the heterophilic interaction between CD177 and PECAM-1.

In AAV, endothelial cell injury is the result of the synergistic effect of several factors, including complement activation, neutrophil respiratory burst and degranulation, and neutrophil extracellular traps (NETs) release [14]. In our study, we demonstrated a protective effect of sPECAM-1 on endothelial cell injury by reducing neutrophil respiratory burst and degranulation in the presence of PR3-ANCA in vitro. However, PECAM-1 incubation could also elevate the level of free PR3 in the supernatant. Free PR3 could be acquired by endothelial cells, resulting in endothelial cytoskeleton disruption and subsequent apoptosis [39] which leads to a damaging effect on endothelial cells. Whether the protective effect outweighs the damaging effect of PR3 release in vivo is not clear.

Conclusions

In conclusion, during the migration of neutrophils, PECAM-1 may interact with CD177 and decrease mPR3 expression on neutrophils, which results in attenuation of neutrophil activation and endothelial injury induced by PR3-ANCA. The current findings may have therapeutic implications in neutrophil-mediated PR3-ANCA vasculitis.

Abbreviations

AAV: Antineutrophil cytoplasmic antibody-associated vasculitis; ANCA: Antineutrophil cytoplasmic antibody; BSA: Bovine serum albumin; DHR: Dihydrorhodamine; ECM: Endothelial cell basal medium; EDTA: Ethylenediaminetetraacetic acid; EGPA: Eosinophilic granulomatosis with polyangiitis; ELISA: Enzyme-linked immunosorbent assay; FITC: Fluorescein isothiocyanate; FSC: Forward scatter; GEnC: Glomerular endothelial cell; GPA: Granulomatosis with polyangiitis; HBSS: Hanks' balanced salt solution; HRP: Horseradish peroxidase; Ig: Immunoglobulin; ITIM: Immunoreceptor tyrosine-based inhibitory motif; JAM-1: Junctional adhesion molecule-1; MACS: Magnetic cell sorting; MFI: Mean fluorescence intensity; MPA: Microscopic polyangiitis; MPO: Myeloperoxidase; mPR3: Membrane-bound proteinase-3; NaN₃: Sodium azide; PBS: Phosphate-buffered saline; PE: Phycoerythrin; PECAM-1: Platelet endothelial cell adhesion molecule-1; PMA: Phorbol myristate acetate; PR3: Proteinase-3; ROS: Reactive oxygen species; sICAM-1: Soluble intercellular cell adhesion molecule-1; SSC: Side scatter; TNF-α: Tumor necrosis factor-alpha

Funding
This study was supported by a grant from the National Key Research and Development Program (2016YFC0906102), four grants from the National Natural Science Fund (81501392, 81700623, 81425008, and 81621092), and a grant from the University of Michigan Health System and Peking University Health Sciences Center Joint Institute for Translational and Clinical Research.

Authors' contributions
HD carried out cell culture, IgG preparation, measurement of neutrophil activation, GEnC injury detection, and data analysis, and was a major contributor in writing the manuscript. NH participated in the study design and helped to draft the article. CW participated in sample collection and data analysis. MC and M-HZ approved the final manuscript. All authors read and approved the final manuscript.

Consent for publication
Not applicable.

Competing interests
The authors declare that they have no competing interests.

Author details
[1]Renal Division, Department of Medicine, Peking University First Hospital, Peking University Institute of Nephrology, Beijing 100034, China. [2]Key Laboratory of Renal Disease, Ministry of Health of China, Beijing 100034, China. [3]Key Laboratory of Chronic Kidney Disease Prevention and Treatment, Ministry of Education, Peking University, Beijing 100034, China. [4]Peking-Tsinghua Center for Life Sciences, Beijing 100034, China.

References
1. Jennette JC, Falk RJ, Bacon PA, Basu N, Cid MC, Ferrario F, et al. 2012 Revised international Chapel Hill consensus conference nomenclature of vasculitides. Arthritis Rheum. 2013;65:1–11.
2. Jennette JC, Falk RJ, Hu P, Xiao H. Pathogenesis of antineutrophil cytoplasmic autoantibody-associated small-vessel vasculitis. Annu Rev Pathol. 2013;8:139–60.
3. Kallenberg CG, Heeringa P, Stegeman CA. Mechanisms of disease: pathogenesis and treatment of ANCA-associated vasculitides. Nat Clin Pract Rheumatol. 2006;2: 661–70.
4. Jennette JC, Falk RJ. Small-vessel vasculitis. N Engl J Med. 1997;337:1512–23.
5. Kallenberg CG. Pathogenesis of PR3-ANCA associated vasculitis. J Autoimmun. 2008;30:29–36.
6. Rarok AA, Limburg PC, Kallenberg CG. Neutrophil-activating potential of antineutrophil cytoplasm autoantibodies. J Leukoc Biol. 2003;74:3–15.
7. Lalezari P, Murphy GB, Allen FJ. NB1, a new neutrophil-specific antigen involved in the pathogenesis of neonatal neutropenia. J Clin Invest. 1971;50:1108–15.
8. Stroncek DF, Shankar RA, Noren PA, Herr GP, Clement LT. Analysis of the expression of NB1 antigen using two monoclonal antibodies. Transfusion. 1996;36:168–74.
9. Matsuo K, Lin A, Procter JL, Clement L, Stroncek D. Variations in the expression of granulocyte antigen NB1. Transfusion. 2000;40:654–62.
10. Stroncek DF, Caruccio L, Bettinotti M. CD177: a member of the Ly-6 gene superfamily involved with neutrophil proliferation and polycythemia vera. J Transl Med. 2004;2:8.
11. Sachs UJ, Andrei-Selmer CL, Maniar A, Weiss T, Paddock C, Orlova VV, et al. The neutrophil-specific antigen CD177 is a counter-receptor for platelet endothelial cell adhesion molecule-1 (CD31). J Biol Chem. 2007;282:23603–12.
12. Muller WA, Ratti CM, McDonnell SL, Cohn ZA. A human endothelial cell-restricted, externally disposed plasmalemmal protein enriched in intercellular junctions. J Exp Med. 1989;170:399–414.
13. Newman PJ. The biology of PECAM-1. J Clin Invest. 1997;99:3–8.
14. Chen M, Jayne DRW, Zhao M. Complement in ANCA-associated vasculitis: mechanisms and implications for management. Nat Rev Nephrol. 2017;13: 359–67.
15. Bauer S, Abdgawad M, Gunnarsson L, Segelmark M, Tapper H, Hellmark T. Proteinase 3 and CD177 are expressed on the plasma membrane of the same subset of neutrophils. J Leukoc Biol. 2007;81:458–64.
16. von Vietinghoff S, Tunnemann G, Eulenberg C, Wellner M, Cristina Cardoso M, Luft FC, et al. NB1 mediates surface expression of the ANCA antigen proteinase 3 on human neutrophils. Blood. 2007;109:4487–93.
17. Jerke U, Marino SF, Daumke O, Kettritz R. Characterization of the CD177 interaction with the ANCA antigen proteinase 3. Sci Rep. 2017;7:43328.
18. Hao J, Huang YM, Zhao MH, Chen M. The interaction between C5a and sphingosine-1-phosphate in neutrophils for antineutrophil cytoplasmic antibody mediated activation. Arthritis Res Ther. 2014;16:R142.
19. Schreiber A, Luft FC, Kettritz R. Membrane proteinase 3 expression and ANCA-induced neutrophil activation. Kidney Int. 2004;65:2172–83.
20. Deng H, Wang C, Chang DY, Hu N, Chen M, Zhao MH. High mobility group box-1 contributes to anti-myeloperoxidase antibody-induced glomerular endothelial cell injury through a moesin-dependent route. Arthritis Res Ther. 2017;19:125.
21. Vestweber D. Adhesion and signaling molecules controlling the transmigration of leukocytes through endothelium. Immunol Rev. 2007;218:178–96.
22. Nourshargh SF, Krombach F, Dejana E. The role of JAM-A and PECAM-1 in modulating leukocyte infiltration in inflamed and ischemic tissues. J Leukoc Biol. 2006;80:714–8.
23. Reumaux D, Vossebeld PJ, Roos D, Verhoeven AJ. Effect of tumor necrosis factor-induced integrin activation on fc gamma receptor II-mediated signal transduction: relevance for activation of neutrophils by anti-proteinase 3 or anti-myeloperoxidase antibodies. Blood. 1995;86:3189–95.
24. Baker EN, Baker HM. Molecular structure, binding properties and dynamics of lactoferrin. Cell Mol Life Sci. 2005;62:2531–9.
25. Lonnerdal B, Iyer S. Lactoferrin: molecular structure and biological function. Annu Rev Nutr. 1995;15:93–110.
26. Hoenderdos K, Lodge KM, Hirst RA, Chen C, Palazzo SG, Emerenciana A, et al. Hypoxia upregulates neutrophil degranulation and potential for tissue injury. Thorax. 2016;71:1030–8.
27. Franssen CF, Huitema MG, Muller KA, Oost-Kort WW, Limburg PC, Tiebosch A, et al. In vitro neutrophil activation by antibodies to proteinase 3 and myeloperoxidase from patients with crescentic glomerulonephritis. J Am Soc Nephrol. 1999;10:1506–15.
28. van der Veen BS, Chen M, Muller R, van Timmeren MM, Petersen AH, Lee PA, et al. Effects of p38 mitogen-activated protein kinase inhibition on anti-neutrophil cytoplasmic autoantibody pathogenicity in vitro and in vivo. Ann Rheum Dis. 2011;70:356–65.
29. Page AV, Liles WC. Biomarkers of endothelial activation/dysfunction in infectious diseases. Virulence. 2013;4:507–16.
30. Newman PJ, Newman DK. Signal transduction pathways mediated by PECAM-1: new roles for an old molecule in platelet and vascular cell biology. Arterioscler Thromb Vasc Biol. 2003;23:953–64.
31. Woodfin A, Voisin MB, Nourshargh S. PECAM-1: a multi-functional molecule in inflammation and vascular biology. Arterioscler Thromb Vasc Biol. 2007;27:2514–23.
32. Privratsky JR, Newman DK, Newman PJ. PECAM-1: conflicts of interest in inflammation. Life Sci. 2010;87:69–82.
33. Newton JP, Hunter AP, Simmons DL, Buckley CD, Harvey DJ. CD31 (PECAM-1) exists as a dimer and is heavily N-glycosylated. Biochem Biophys Res Commun. 1999;261:283–91.
34. Kettritz R, Jennette JC, Falk RJ. Crosslinking of ANCA-antigens stimulates superoxide release by human neutrophils. J Am Soc Nephrol. 1997;8: 386–94.
35. Kettritz R. How anti-neutrophil cytoplasmic autoantibodies activate neutrophils. Clin Exp Immunol. 2012;169:220–8.
36. Witko-Sarsat V, Lesavre P, Lopez S, Bessou G, Hieblot C, Prum B, et al. A large subset of neutrophils expressing membrane proteinase 3 is a risk factor for vasculitis and rheumatoid arthritis. J Am Soc Nephrol. 1999;10:1224–33.
37. Bai M, Grieshaber-Bouyer R, Wang J, Schmider AB, Wilson ZS, Zeng L, et al. CD177 modulates human neutrophil migration through activation-mediated integrin and chemoreceptor regulation. Blood. 2017;130:2092–100.
38. Jerke U, Rolle S, Dittmar G, Bayat B, Santoso S, Sporbert A, et al. Complement receptor mac-1 is an adaptor for NB1 (CD177)-mediated PR3-ANCA neutrophil activation. J Biol Chem. 2011;286:7070–81.
39. Jerke U, Hernandez DP, Beaudette P, Korkmaz B, Dittmar G, Kettritz R. Neutrophil serine proteases exert proteolytic activity on endothelial cells. Kidney Int. 2015;88:764–75.

8

Arhalofenate acid inhibits monosodium urate crystal-induced inflammatory responses through activation of AMP-activated protein kinase (AMPK) signaling

Charles McWherter[1], Yun-Jung Choi[1], Ramon L. Serrano[2,3], Sushil K. Mahata[2,3], Robert Terkeltaub[2,3] and Ru Liu-Bryan[2,3]* (iD)

Abstract

Background: Arhalofenate acid, the active acid form of arhalofenate, is a non-agonist peroxisome proliferator-activated receptor γ (PPARγ) ligand, with uricosuric activity via URAT1 inhibition. Phase II studies revealed decreased acute arthritis flares in arhalofenate-treated gout compared with allopurinol alone. Hence, we investigated the anti-inflammatory effects and mechanisms of arhalofenate and its active acid form for responses to monosodium urate (MSU) crystals.

Methods: We assessed in-vivo responses to MSU crystals in murine subcutaneous air pouches and in-vitro responses in murine bone marrow-derived macrophages (BMDMs) by enzyme-linked immunosorbent assay (ELISA), SDS-PAGE/Western blot, immunostaining, and transmission electron microscopy analyses.

Results: Oral administration of arhalofenate (250 mg/kg) blunted total leukocyte ingress, neutrophil influx, and air pouch fluid interleukin (IL)-1β, IL-6, and CXCL1 in response to MSU crystal injection ($p < 0.05$ for each). Arhalofenate acid (100 μM) attenuated MSU crystal-induced IL-1β production in BMDMs via inhibition of NLRP3 inflammasome activation. In addition, arhalofenate acid dose-dependently increased activation (as assessed by phosphorylation) of AMP-activated protein kinase (AMPK). Studying AMPKα1 knockout mice, we elucidated that AMPK mediated the anti-inflammatory effects of arhalofenate acid. Moreover, arhalofenate acid attenuated the capacity of MSU crystals to suppress AMPK activity, regulated expression of multiple downstream AMPK targets that modulate mitochondrial function and oxidative stress, preserved intact mitochondrial cristae and volume density, and promoted anti-inflammatory autophagy flux in BMDMs.

Conclusions: Arhalofenate acid is anti-inflammatory and acts via AMPK activation and its downstream signaling in macrophages. These effects likely contribute to a reduction of gout flares.

Keywords: Gout, Inflammation, AMPK, Mitochondria, Autophagy flux

* Correspondence: ruliu@ucsd.edu
[2]VA San Diego Healthcare System, 111K, 3350 La Jolla Village Drive, San Diego, CA 92161, USA
[3]University of California San Diego, La Jolla, California, USA
Full list of author information is available at the end of the article

Background

Anti-inflammatory prevention and treatment of attacks of gouty arthritis remain challenging, in part because many patients have incomplete responses or contraindications to one or more of the primary oral anti-inflammatory therapies (colchicine, nonsteroidal anti-inflammatory drugs (NSAIDs), and corticosteroids) [1, 2]. Moreover, gout flares often increase in frequency in the initial phase of urate-lowering therapy (ULT), thereby contributing to poor adherence to ULT and lack of improvement in health-related quality of life [1, 2]. Arhalofenate is a non-agonist ligand of peroxisome proliferator-activated receptor γ (PPARγ) with weak transactivation but robust transrepression activity [3]. It was first developed as an insulin sensitizer for type 2 diabetes mellitus [3]. Subsequently, arhalofenate was demonstrated to have uricosuric activity, as an inhibitor of URAT1, organic anion transporter 4 (OAT4) and OAT10 [4]. In a recent phase II trial in gout patients, which assessed acute gout flare as the primary endpoint, arhalofenate significantly reduced the risk of acute gouty arthritis in comparison with allopurinol alone, whereas there was no significant difference compared with allopurinol in combination with prophylactic colchicine [5]. The risk for urate-lowering therapy-induced gout flares depends on the degree of serum urate lowering [2]. Hence, this study was performed to directly test and characterize the anti-inflammatory effects of arhalofenate pertinent to gout.

Acute gouty arthritis is a characteristically severe phenotypic inflammatory response to deposits of monosodium urate (MSU) crystals which induce expression of NF-κB-dependent proinflammatory cytokines including pro-interleukin (IL)-1β and multiple chemokines [6, 7]. MSU crystals also stimulate activation of the NLRP3 inflammasome, with consequent maturation and release of IL-1β [6, 7]. This is a central driver of the gouty inflammation cascade which involves recruitment and activation of phagocytes [6, 7]. Core factors that modulate activation of the NLRP3 inflammasome, and experimental gout-like inflammation, include mitochondrial function, autophagy, and AMP-activated protein kinase (AMPK) [8, 9].

Mitochondrial reactive oxygen species (ROS) and oxidized mitochondrial DNA (mtDNA) promote inflammation [10–12], mediated by activation of NF-κB [10–12] and activation of the NLRP3 inflammasome via dysregulated balance between thioredoxins (TRXs) and thioredoxin-interacting protein (TXNIP) [13]. TRX1 and TRX2, mainly located in the cytoplasm and mitochondria, respectively, control cellular ROS by reduction of disulfides to thiol groups [14]. TXNIP directly binds to TRX and inhibits the reducing activity of TRX through disulfide exchange [14]. However, ROS triggers disassociation of TXNIP from TRX1, promoting direct physical interaction between TXNIP and NLRP3 that leads to activation of caspase-1 and release of mature IL-1β [13].

Autophagy mediates cellular homeostasis by degrading damaged proteins and organelles, including mitochondria [15–17]. Although MSU crystals promote autophagosome formation, the crystals also induce impairment of proteasomal degradation leading to accumulation of p62 [17]. As a selective autophagy receptor adaptor protein [17], p62 interacts with LC3-II to facilitate autophagic degradation [17], and also is involved in MSU crystal-induced caspase-1 activation and IL-1β release [18]. One of the major factors promoting autophagy is serine/threonine kinase AMPK [19].

AMPK is a nutritional biosensor that maintains cellular energy balance [19, 20], but nutritional excesses and other factors, including stimulation by MSU crystals and IL-1β, decrease AMPK activity [9]. Significantly, AMPK functions as an NF-κB and NLRP3 inflammasome inhibitor and promotes anti-inflammatory macrophage polarization, and markedly decreases the inflammatory response to MSU crystals in cultured macrophages [21, 22]. Moreover, AMPK transduces colchicine anti-inflammatory effects in vitro [22]. Pharmacologic AMPK activation markedly limits experimental gouty inflammation in the mouse in vivo using the subcutaneous air pouch model [22]. Conversely, MSU crystal-induced inflammation is prominently potentiated in AMPKα1 knockout (KO) mice [22].

Thiazolidinedione PPARγ agonists have been shown to cause phosphorylation and activation of AMPK [23–25]. Downstream targets of activated AMPK result in anti-inflammatory and cellular stress resistance effects that include PPARγ co-activator 1α (PGC-1α), the latter being a master regulator of mitochondrial biogenesis [26], as well as sirtuin 1 (SIRT1), which is a nicotinamide adenine dinucleotide (NAD)-dependent deacetylase [20, 26]. AMPK stimulates SIRT1 activity and phosphorylates the PGC-1α protein, which allows SIRT1 to deacetylate and activate PGC-1α [20, 26]. Activation of PGC-1α not only increases mitochondrial biogenesis by promoting expression of mitochondrial transcription factor A (TFAM), but also increases mitochondrial antioxidant capacity by upregulating expression of antioxidant enzymes [20, 26]. Here, we characterized anti-inflammatory effects of arhalofenate in vivo and the in-vitro mechanisms of action of arhalofenate acid (the circulating active acid form of arhalofenate) in MSU crystal-induced macrophage activation. Our results implicate AMPK through its downstream signaling actions in impacting mitochondria, TRX and TXNIP, and autophagy as a central mediator of the anti-inflammatory activity of arhalofenate.

Methods

Reagents

All chemical reagents were from Sigma-Aldrich (St. Louis, MO) unless otherwise stated. Arhalofenate acid (MBX-102 acid), the active form of arhalofenate, was used for in-vitro studies. Arhalofenate (MBX-102) was used for in-vivo studies. MSU crystals were prepared as described previously [22], suspended at 25 mg/mL in sterile, endotoxin-free phosphate-buffered saline (PBS), and verified to be free of detectable lipopolysaccharide contamination by Limulus lysate assay (Lonza, Walkersville, MD). A-769662 was from LC laboratories (Woburn, MA). Antibodies to phospho-AMPKα (Thr172) and total AMPKα (recognizing both AMPKα isoforms), SIRT1, TFAM, TRX1, TRX2, and TXNIP were from Cell Signaling Technology (Danvers, MA). Antibodies to pro-caspase-1 and cleaved caspase-1 (p10) were from Biovision (Milpitas, CA) and Santa Cruz Biotechnology (Santa Cruz, CA), respectively.

Subcutaneous air pouch model and flow cytometry analysis

C57BL/6 mice ($n = 8$–10/group) were subcutaneously injected under the skin adjacent to the back of the neck with sterile air (day 1, 5 mL; day 4, 3 mL) to form air pouches as described previously [22]. On day 4, mice were dosed daily with vehicle (1% carboxymethylcellulose/2% Tween-80), arhalofenate (at a loading dose of 250 mg/kg per oral), or dexamethasone (20 mg/kg intraperitoneally) for 3 days. On day 7, 30 min after the last dose, MSU crystals (20 mg in 5 mL saline) were injected into the air pouch to elicit an acute immune response. After 4 h, the mice were sacrificed and 5 mL of heparinized saline was injected into the air pouch to collect the exudates.

Exudates were centrifuged and resuspended in PBS. The cell suspension was incubated with phycoerythrin (PE)-conjugated rat anti-mouse CD45+ antibody (diluted 1:100; MCA1031PE; AbD Serotech) for all leucocyte staining, and fluorescein isothiocyanate (FITC)-conjugated rat anti-mouse Ly-6B.2 alloantigen (diluted 1:100; #MCA771FB; AbD Serotech) for neutrophil staining according to the manufacturer's protocol. Propidium iodide staining solution (BD Pharmingen™; #556463) was added to the cell suspension to exclude non-viable cells. All live cells were further gated based on CD45 expression for leukocytes. BD™ Compbeads (BD Biosciences; #552845) were used for nonspecific binding of antibodies to optimize fluorescence compensation settings. Counting beads (Spherotech Accuount fluorescent particles; #ACFP-100-3) were added to the stained cells to obtain absolute cell number. FACS analysis was performed on a BD LSR II flow cytometer using Diva software (v6.1.2, Becton Dickinson) and analyzed using FlowJo software (v9.5.3, Tree Star Inc.).

Cell culture

Bone marrow-derived macrophages (BMDMs) were generated as described previously [22]. Briefly, bone marrow cells were cultured in complete RPMI media containing 10% fetal bovine serum (FBS), penicillin (100 U/mL), and streptomycin (100 µg/mL) in the presence of macrophage colony-stimulating factor (M-CSF; 20 ng/mL; Gemini Bio-products, West Sacramento, CA). After 5–7 days, the M-CSF-derived macrophages were re-plated onto 24-well (5×10^5/well) or six-well (2×10^6/well) plates and primed with 20 ng/mL granulocyte-macrophage colony-stimulating factor (GM-CSF; Gemini Bio-products, West Sacramento, CA) for 24 h in complete RPMI medium before treatment with the indicated reagents in fresh RPMI containing only 1% FBS.

Western blot

Cells were lysed in RIPA buffer with 2 mM sodium vanadate and protease inhibitor cocktails (Roche, Mannheim, Germany). Cell lysates (10–15 µg) were separated by gradient 4–20% SDS-PAGE and transferred onto nitrocellulose membranes (Bio-Rad, Hercules, CA), probed with antibodies, exposed to SuperSignal West Pico Chemiluminescent Substrate (Thermo Scientific, Waltham, MA), and visualized by radiography.

Cytokine analyses

Mouse IL-1β and CXCL1 (KC) were measured using DuoSet enzyme-linked immunosorbent assay (ELISA; R&D Systems, Minneapolis, MN).

Fluorescence microscopy

BMDMs were incubated with MitoSOX Red reagent (Thermo Scientific) reagent (1 µM) to examine mitochondrial ROS generation which was visualized by fluorescence microscopy. Cells were also incubated with 10 nM MitoTracker Green (which is insensitive to ROS) to confirm the localization of MitoSOX Red to mitochondria. Immunofluorescence microscopy was carried out to visually identify p62 puncta and lysosomes and to determine co-localization of p62 and lysosomal-associated membrane protein 1 (LAMP1), which indicates autophagosome and lysosome fusion (i.e., activated autophagy). In brief, cells were fixed and permeabilized with cold methanol. Immunocytochemical staining of cells used rabbit anti-p62 monoclonal antibody (Cell Signaling, #23214) or rabbit anti-LAMP1 antibody (Abcam, #ab24210). Alexa Fluor 488 goat anti-rabbit IgG (Thermo Scientific) and Alexa Flour 555 goat anti-rabbit IgG (Thermo Scientific) secondary antibodies were used to detect p62 and LAMP1, respectively. Imaging was acquired via a confocal microscope (Zeiss LSM 880 Confocal with FAST Airyscan).

Transmission electron microscopy (TEM)

Cells were fixed with 2.5% glutaraldehyde in 0.15 M cacodylate buffer, and postfixed in 1% OsO_4 in 0.1 M cacodylate buffer for 1 h on ice, followed by staining en bloc with 2–3% uranyl acetate for 1 h on ice. The cells were dehydrated in a graded series of washes with ethanol (20–100%) on ice followed by one wash with 100% ethanol and two washes with acetone (15 min each) and embedded with Durcupan. Ultrathin (50–60 nm) sections were cut on a Leica UCT ultramicrotome, and picked up on Formvar and carbon-coated copper grids. Sections were stained with 2% uranyl acetate for 5 min and Sato's lead stain for 1 min. Grids were viewed using a JEOL JEM1400-plus TEM (JEOL, Peabody, MA). TEM images were taken using a Gatan One-View digital camera with 4 k × 4 k resolution (Gatan, Pleasanton, CA). Mitochondrial area was determined using the free-hand tool in ImageJ and manually tracing around the mitochondrial outer membrane. The area of each crista membrane was also calculated in the same manner. The sum of the areas of the total complement of cristae was then divided by the sum of the mitochondrial area to obtain the cristae volume density as described previously [27].

Statistical analyses

Data are presented as either mean values ± standard deviation (SD) or mean ± standard error of the mean (SEM) as indicated. Statistical analyses were performed by one-way or two-way analysis of variance with Bonferroni post-hoc testing using GraphPad Prism software, version 6. p values less than 0.05 were considered significant.

Results

Arhalofenate attenuated MSU crystal-induced inflammation in mice in vivo

In the murine subcutaneous air pouch model of acute gouty inflammation, arhalofenate significantly inhibited leukocyte or neutrophil infiltration and production of IL-1β, IL-6, and CXCL1 induced by MSU crystals (Fig. 1). The effects of arhalofenate in this model were comparable with those of the positive control dexamethasone, and indicated the capacity of arhalofenate to limit MSU crystal-induced inflammation. Of note, arhalofenate or dexamethasone alone did not exhibit any toxicity effect (data not shown).

Arhalofenate acid suppressed MSU crystal-induced NLRP3 inflammasome activation

Arhalofenate acid (100 μM) inhibited MSU crystal-induced IL-1β release in cultured murine BMDMs (Fig. 2a). Partial inhibition of MSU crystal-induced IL-1β release was observed with lower doses at 25 and 50 μM (data not shown). No cytotoxicity of arhalofenate at the concentrations

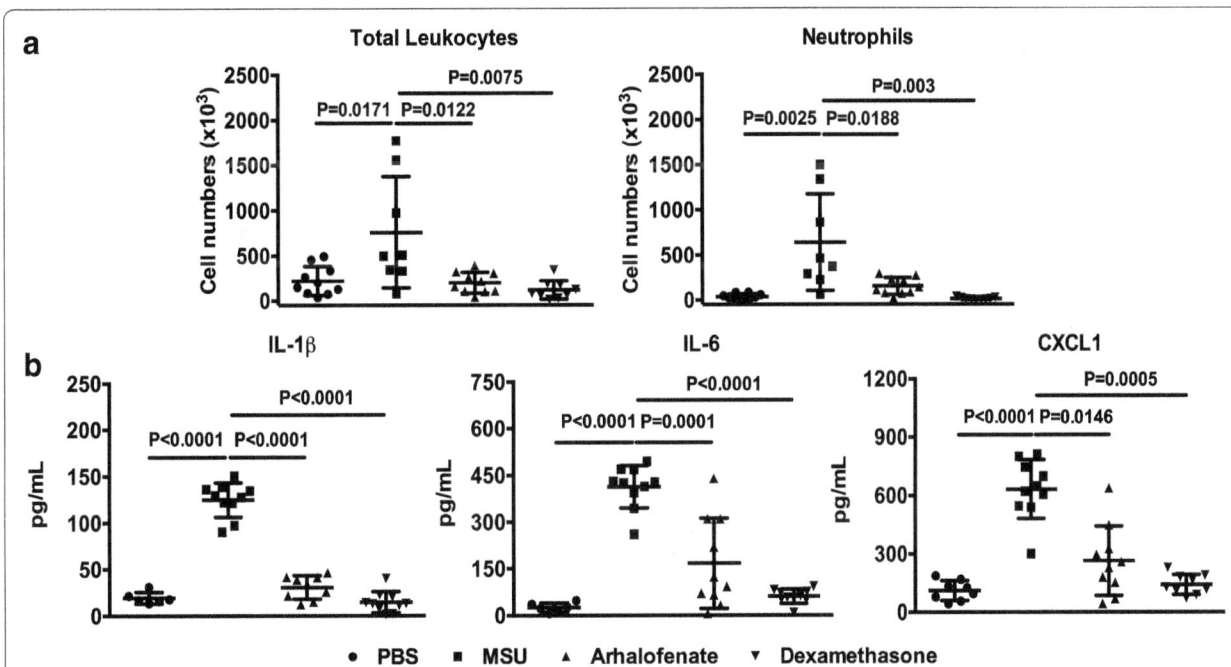

Fig. 1 Arhalofenate attenuates MSU crystal-induced inflammation in mice in vivo. Air pouches were created in normal C57BL/6 mice, and mice were subsequently dosed with arhalofenate orally for 3 days prior to the introduction of monosodium urate (MSU) crystals into the air pouch as described in the Methods section. The acute inflammatory response to crystal injection was determined by measuring the number of total infiltrating leukocytes or neutrophils (a), and production of interleukin (IL)-1β, IL-6 and CXCL1 (b) in the air pouch exudate 4 h post-dose. Dexamethasone served as the anti-inflammatory control agent. Data are shown as the mean ± SEM (n = 8–10 mice per group). The p values represent comparisons between MSU crystals alone and the phosphate-buffered saline (PBS) control, or between MSU crystals alone and MSU crystals plus arhalofenate or dexamethasone

a

IL-1β Release

b

Fig. 2 Arhalofenate acid attenuates MSU crystal-induced IL-1β release by inhibiting NLRP3 inflammasome activation in BMDMs in vitro. BMDMs were pretreated with arhalofenate acid at a concentration of 100 μM for 1 h before being stimulated with monosodium urate (MSU) crystals (0.2 mg/mL) in RPMI containing 1% FBS for 18 h. The conditioned media was used for ELISA for interleukin (IL)-1β (**a**), and the cell lysates were subjected to Western blot analysis (**b**) for expression of NLRP3, pro-caspase 1, and cleaved caspase 1 (p10). Data in **a** are the mean ± SD of three individual experiments, and p values represent comparisons between none and MSU crystals alone, or between MSU crystal alone and MSU crystals plus arhalofenate acid. Data in **b** are representative of three individual experiments

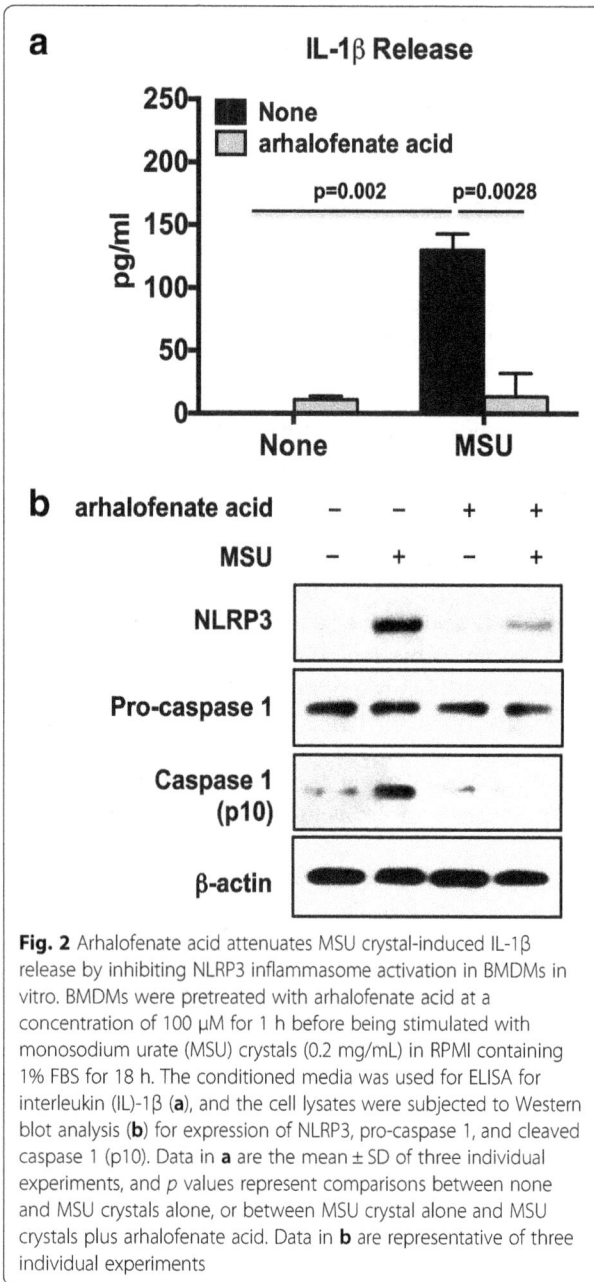

studied was observed (data not shown). Western blot analysis showed that the level of NLRP3 protein expression increased in response to MSU crystals, an effect reduced by arhalofenate acid (Fig. 2b). Similarly, MSU crystal-induced expression of cleaved caspase-1 was diminished by arhalofenate acid, indicating inhibition of MSU crystal-induced NLRP3 inflammasome activation (Fig. 2b).

Arhalofenate acid induced functionally important AMPK activation

Arhalofenate acid enhanced phosphorylation of AMPKα and expression of SIRT1 in a dose-dependent manner (Fig. 3a). Notably, the basal level of SIRT1 expression

was reduced in AMPKα1KO BMDMs, and arhalofenate acid failed to enhance SIRT1 expression in AMPKα1KO BMDMs (Fig. 3b). These results indicated that SIRT1 was a downstream target of AMPK, and that arhalofenate acid-induced increase in SIRT1 expression was dependent on AMPK. Arhalofenate acid inhibited the capacity of MSU crystals to reduce AMPK activity (Fig. 4a), and correlated with suppressed IL-1β release (Fig. 4b) in wild-type BMDMs. However, arhalofenate acid failed to significantly limit IL-1β release in AMPKα1KO BMDMs (Fig. 4b).

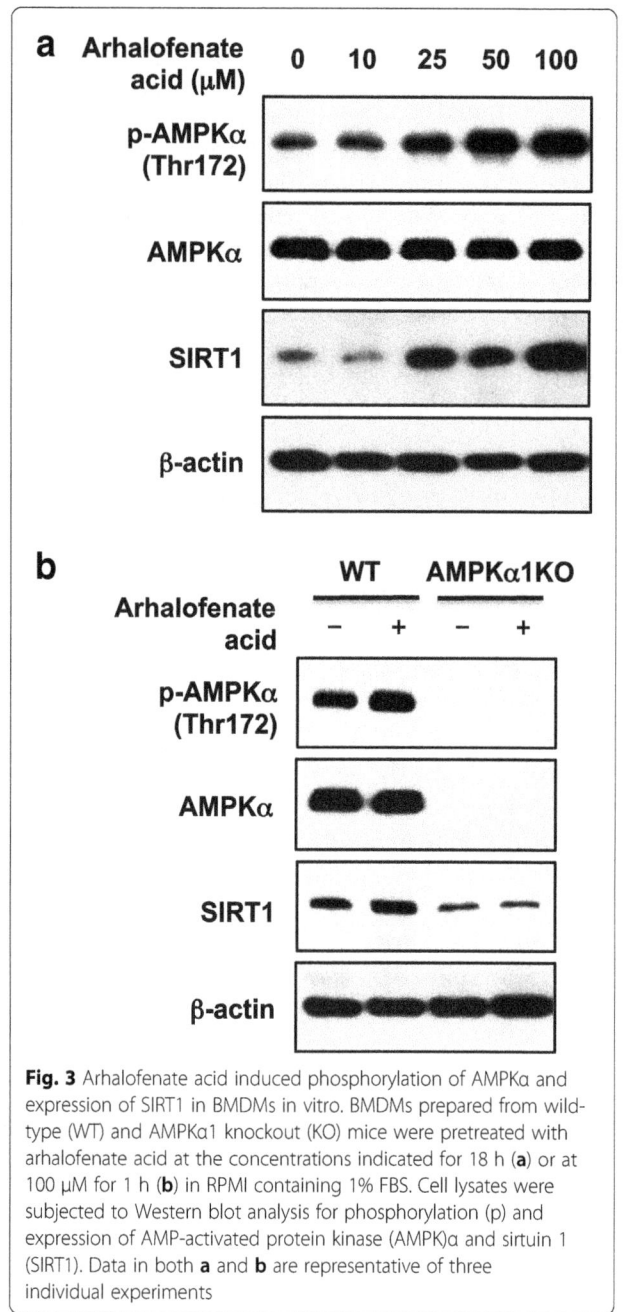

a

b

Fig. 3 Arhalofenate acid induced phosphorylation of AMPKα and expression of SIRT1 in BMDMs in vitro. BMDMs prepared from wild-type (WT) and AMPKα1 knockout (KO) mice were pretreated with arhalofenate acid at the concentrations indicated for 18 h (**a**) or at 100 μM for 1 h (**b**) in RPMI containing 1% FBS. Cell lysates were subjected to Western blot analysis for phosphorylation (p) and expression of AMP-activated protein kinase (AMPK)α and sirtuin 1 (SIRT1). Data in both **a** and **b** are representative of three individual experiments

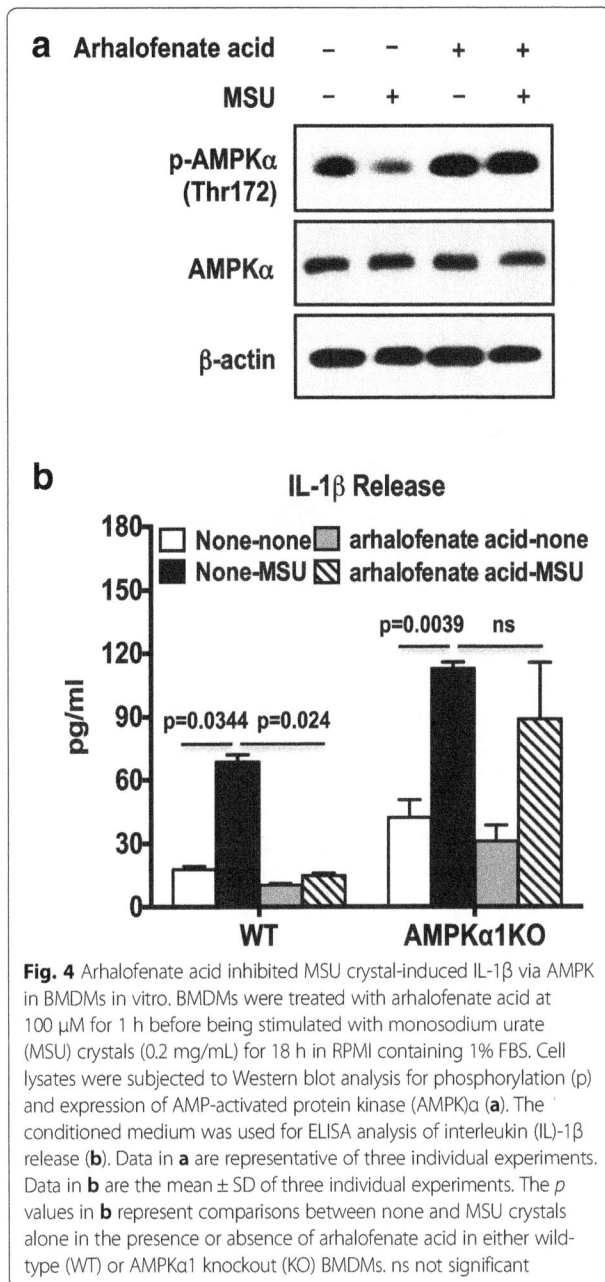

Fig. 4 Arhalofenate acid inhibited MSU crystal-induced IL-1β via AMPK in BMDMs in vitro. BMDMs were treated with arhalofenate acid at 100 μM for 1 h before being stimulated with monosodium urate (MSU) crystals (0.2 mg/mL) for 18 h in RPMI containing 1% FBS. Cell lysates were subjected to Western blot analysis for phosphorylation (p) and expression of AMP-activated protein kinase (AMPK)α (**a**). The conditioned medium was used for ELISA analysis of interleukin (IL)-1β release (**b**). Data in **a** are representative of three individual experiments. Data in **b** are the mean ± SD of three individual experiments. The *p* values in **b** represent comparisons between none and MSU crystals alone in the presence or absence of arhalofenate acid in either wild-type (WT) or AMPKα1 knockout (KO) BMDMs. ns not significant

Arhalofenate acid modulated AMPK-regulated downstream mitochondrial targets and ultrastructure

MSU crystals concurrently reduced AMPK activity (assessed by phosphorylation of AMPKα) and the expression of SIRT1, PGC-1α, and TFAM, with all of these effects limited by arhalofenate acid (Fig. 5a). In addition, arhalofenate acid also enhanced basal levels of SIRT1, PGC-1α, and TFAM, with similar results seen with treatment with the selective AMPK activator A-769662 (Additional file 1). Moreover, MSU crystals induced mitochondrial ROS generation, evidenced by prominent Mito-SOX Red staining (Fig. 5b). MitoTracker Green staining confirmed the localization of MitoSOX Red to

mitochondria (Fig. 5b). Notably, arhalofenate acid was able to inhibit this effect (Fig. 5b). TEM studies revealed that macrophages stimulated with MSU crystals exhibited broken cristae with a consequent decrease in cristae volume density. Interestingly, arhalofenate prevented MSU crystal-induced loss of intact mitochondrial cristae, the folds in the inner membrane of mitochondria that provide the high surface area for oxidative phosphorylation (OXPHOS) for generation of ATP (Fig. 5c). The protective effects of arhalofenate acid on mitochondrial respiratory function were associated with preservation of mitochondrial ultrastructure, supported by the ability of arhalofenate acid to maintain cristae volume density (Fig. 5d). Since AMPK activation has been shown to inhibit TXNIP expression [28, 29], we next assessed the effects of arhalofenate acid on expression of TRX and TXNIP. As seen in Fig. 5a, MSU crystals decreased the expression of TRX1 and TRX2 isoforms, and induced the expression of TXNIP. These effects were inhibited by arhalofenate acid, suggesting an ability of arhalofenate acid for maintaining the balance between the TRX isoforms and TXNIP. Interestingly, the levels of TRX2 expression were noticeably higher in cells treated with MSU crystals in the presence of arhalofenate acid compared with cells treated with arhalofenate acid alone.

Arhalofenate acid prevented MSU crystal-induced p62 accumulation by promoting autophagy flux

We first confirmed [18] that MSU crystals increased the expression of LC3-II, the lipidated form of LC3, indicating autophagosome formation at both 2 and 6 h in BMDMs (Fig. 6a). Expression of p62 was also induced at 2 h and greatly enhanced at 6 h by MSU crystals. Bafilomycin, a known inhibitor of the late phase of autophagy that prohibits phagosome and lysosome fusion and thereby inhibits autophagy flux, caused accumulation of LC3-II and p62 regardless of the presence or absence of MSU crystals and arhalofenate acid. Notably, arhalofenate acid had a minimal effect on MSU-induced expression of LC3-II at 2 and 6 h, and markedly decreased MSU crystal-induced p62 expression at 6 h, but not at 2 h (Fig. 6a). A similar result was observed with A-769662 (Additional file 1). Immunofluorescence analysis of p62 (green color) and LAMP1 (red color) showed significantly less yellow punctae (co-localization of p62 and LAMP1) in MSU crystal-treated cells in the presence of arhalofenate acid in comparison with the cells treated with MSU crystals alone (Additional file 2). TEM analysis demonstrated that cells treated with MSU crystals alone at 6 h had large amounts of electron dense material within the phagosomes, which were considerably less abundant when arhalofenate acid was also present (Fig. 6b). In addition, the number of autophagosomes containing dense debris was significantly smaller

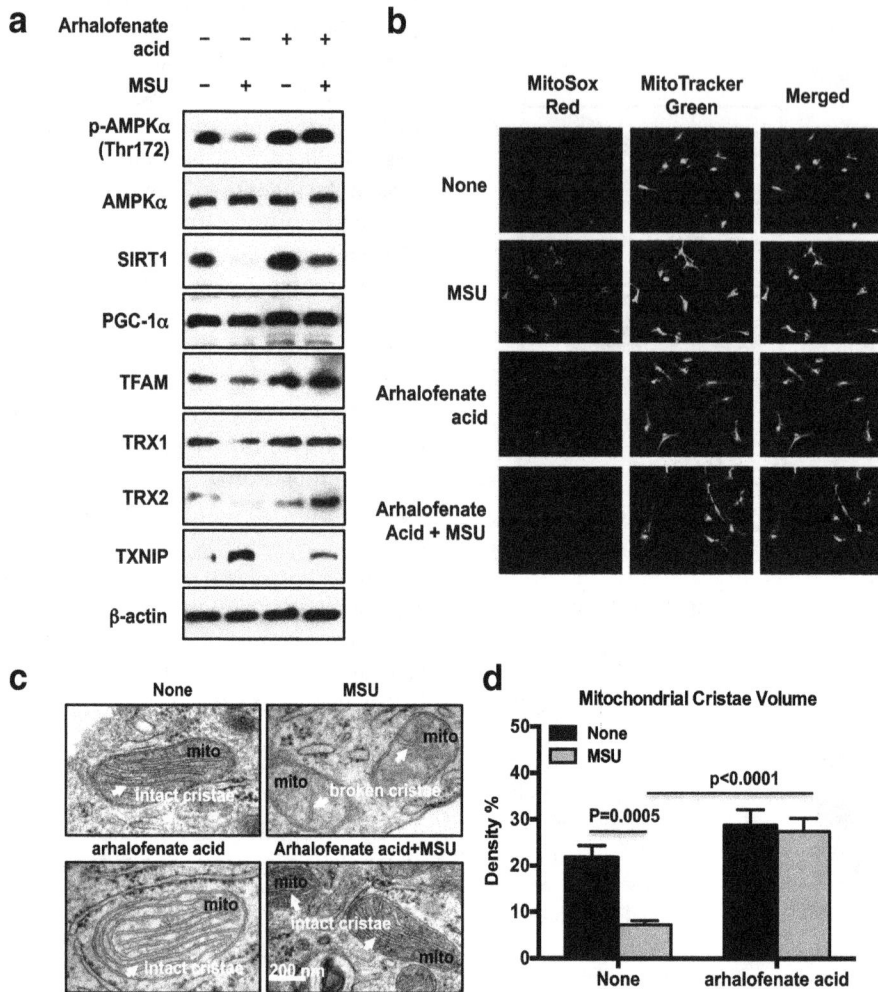

Fig. 5 Arhalofenate acid activated AMPK downstream targets involved in regulation of mitochondrial function and maintained mitochondrial cristae area. BMDMs were treated with arhalofenate acid (100 μM) for 1 h before stimulation with monosodium urate (MSU) crystals (0.2 mg/mL) for 1 h or 18 h in RPMI containing 1% FBS. Cell lysates prepared from 18-h treatment samples were subjected to Western blot analysis of phosphorylation (p) and expression of AMP-activated protein kinase (AMPK)α, expression of sirtuin 1 (SIRT1), peroxisome proliferator-activated receptor γ co-activator 1α (PGC-1α), and mitochondrial transcription factor A (TFAM), and expression of thioredoxin (TRX)1, TRX2, and thioredoxin-interacting protein (TXNIP) (**a**). Cells from 1-h treatment were then stained with MitoSOX Red and MitoTracker Green and visualized by fluorescence microscopy (**b**, magnification 20×). TEM analysis was performed to examine mitochondrial cristae (the folds of inner mitochondrial membrane indicated by white arrows in **c**), and the cristae volume density are presented (**d**). Data in **a** and **b** are representative of three individual experiments. Data in **c** are representative of 30 cells examined for each condition. Data in **d** are the mean ± SEM of 30 cells. The p values represent comparisons between none and MSU crystals alone, or between MSU crystals alone and MSU crystals plus arhalofenate acid

under the same conditions with arhalofenate acid treatment (Fig. 6c). Collectively, the results pointed to the capacity of arhalofenate acid to promote autophagy flux, thereby preventing accumulation of p62 induced by MSU crystals.

Discussion

This study demonstrated that the uricosuric arhalofenate (and its active acid form) has anti-inflammatory effects, and it also characterized the molecular mechanism of action for these activities of MSU crystal-induced inflammation. We discovered that arhalofenate acid

inhibited MSU crystal-induced inflammatory responses through activation of AMPK and AMPK downstream signaling. This enabled cellular resistance to stresses induced by MSU crystals, largely by maintaining mitochondrial function and cellular quality control through autophagy.

We confirmed that arhalofenate attenuated MSU crystal-induced inflammatory responses in a murine air pouch model in vivo, and that arhalofenate acid mitigated MSU crystal-induced IL-1β production by inhibiting NLRP3 inflammasome activation in macrophages in vitro. Moreover, we found that arhalofenate acid, which is a

A

B

C

Fig. 6 Arhalofenate acid prevented prolonged accumulation of p62 by promoting autophagy flux in response to MSU crystals. BMDMs were treated with arhalofenate acid (100 μM) for 1 h before stimulated with monosodium urate (MSU) crystals (0.2 mg/mL) for 2 h in the presence or absence of bafilomycin (Baf; 100 nM) and for 6 h in RPMI containing 1% FBS. Cell lysates were subjected to Western blot analysis of LC3 and p62 (**a**). TEM was performed to examine autophagosomes (indicated by black arrows in **b**), and the numbers of autophagosomes containing electron dense material per μm^2 are presented (**c**). Data in **a** and **b** are representative of three individual experiments. Data in **c** are the mean ± SEM of 30 cells. The p values represent comparisons between none and MSU crystals alone, or between MSU crystals alone and MSU crystals plus arhalofenate acid

non-agonist ligand of PPARγ, induced phosphorylation of AMPKα in a dose-dependent manner in macrophages. It is known that PPARγ agonists (e.g., thiazolidinedione drugs) can activate AMPK by phosphorylation of AMPKα [30]. Furthermore, we have previously demonstrated that activation of AMPK attenuated MSU crystal-induced inflammatory responses through inhibition of NLRP3 inflammasome activation [22]. The hypothesis that

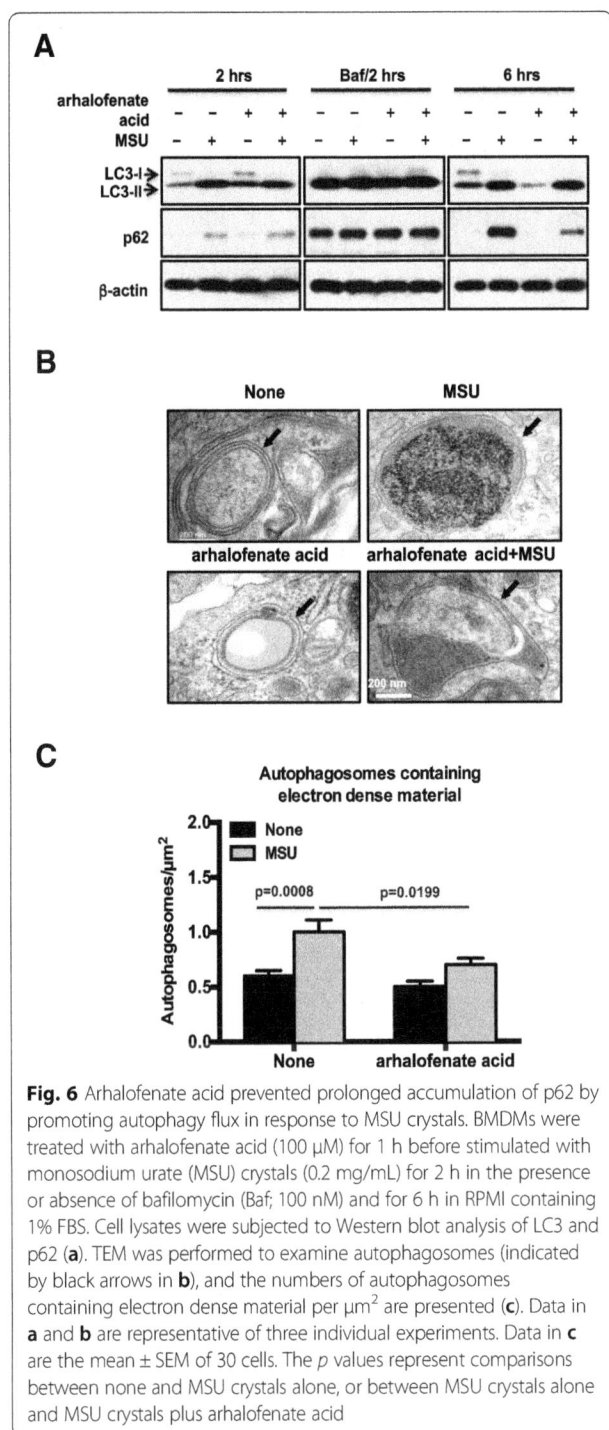

arhalofenate acid was acting in an AMPK-dependent manner to exert anti-inflammatory effects was strongly supported by the data that arhalofenate acid was no longer able to significantly inhibit MSU crystal-induced IL-1β release in macrophages deficient in AMPKα1, the predominant α isoform of AMPK in macrophages.

In this study, arhalofenate acid, and similarly the AMPK selective activator A-769662, prevented MSU crystal-induced decrease in phosphorylation of AMPKα, and the expression of SIRT1, PGC-1α, and TFAM. In addition, we found that arhalofenate acid prohibited the loss of mitochondrial cristae induced by MSU crystals. As such, arhalofenate acid was demonstrated to have the ability to regulate mitochondrial function not only via AMPK and downstream signaling, but also by preserving mitochondrial ultrastructure. The significance of our findings stems partly from the recent emergence of mitochondria as central regulators of NLRP3 inflammasome activation [10–12]. The NLRP3 inflammasome can sense danger-associated signals that are induced by defective mitochondria including mitochondrial ROS and oxidized mtDNA [10–12]. The major function of mitochondria is to generate ATP through the process of OXPHOS. Defects in the electron transport chain (the transport system that generates the major amount of ATP through OXPHOS) are usually detrimental to the host. Our TEM analysis clearly demonstrated that MSU crystals induced the breakdown of mitochondrial cristae in macrophages, with a consequent decrease in cristae volume density, and that the cristae are known to provide a large surface area in the inner membrane of the mitochondria for OXPHOS to generate ATP. Inhibition of mitochondrial complex-I by rotenone or complex-III by antimycin A induces robust ROS production by mitochondria [31, 32]. This enhanced ROS production is sufficient to drive NLRP3 inflammasome activation [10–12]. The oxidized mtDNA released from damaged mitochondria directly binds NLRP3 to activate the inflammasome [10–12]. Activation of AMPK is known to promote the oxidative metabolism and mitochondrial biogenesis via the downstream targets SIRT1 and PGC-1α [20]. Activation of PGC-1α leads to increased expression of the mitochondrial transcription factor TFAM, which in turn stimulates mitochondrial DNA replication [26].

Increased TRX1 and decreased TXNIP are beneficial for preventing hyperinflammation, neurodegeneration, and the progression of diabetes [14]. In this study, we found that arhalofenate acid, similar to the effects of A-769662, increased basal levels of expression of TRX1 and TRX2 and restrained MSU crystals from reducing the expression of TRX1 and TRX2 and inhibited MSU crystal-induced TXNIP expression. We observed that the levels of TRX2 expression were even higher in cells treated with MSU crystals in the presence of arhalofenate acid compared with cells treated with arhalofenate acid alone. The mechanism responsible for this paradoxically higher TRX2 expression in response to the combination of MSU crystals and arhalofenate remains to be determined and was beyond the scope of this study. TXNIP has been shown to translocate to the mitochondria where it binds to oxidized TRX2 leading to increasing ROS accumulation and mitochondrial dysfunction [14]. TRX2 binds to apoptosis signaling regulating kinase 1 (Ask1). Increasing binding of TXNIP to TRX2 reduces the interaction between TRX2 and Ask1, and induces Ask1 activation for apoptosis [14]. Although dysregulation of the balance between TRX1 and TXNIP is involved in NLRP3 inflammasome activation in a redox-dependent manner [13], the functions of TRX2 and TXNIP in regulating the NLRP3 inflammasome are unclear. We speculate that arhalofenate acid regulates the expression of TRX and TXNIP through AMPK signaling. In this context, metformin increases TRX expression through activation of AMPK [33], and it also inhibits TXNIP expression [34]. Moreover, AMPK mediates nutrient regulation of TXNIP expression [28].

In this study, we showed that arhalofenate acid prevented the prolonged accumulation of p62 induced by MSU crystals, indicating that arhalofenate acid may inhibit MSU crystal-induced NLRP3 inflammasome activation partly by improving autophagy flux. Autophagy is a fundamental cellular process that is required for clearance of damaged and dysfunctional organelles, such as mitochondria [15–17]. Incomplete clearance of damaged mitochondria can trigger aberrant inflammasome activation and promote a variety of human inflammatory diseases [15–17]. In macrophages, autophagy blockade increases the production of mitochondrial ROS that induces mitochondrial damage, in turn activating the inflammasome [12]. Autophagy consists of four essential steps: initiation of autophagosome formation, elongation and closure of autophagic membrane, fusion between autophagosome and lysosome, and degradation [35]. MSU crystals induce autophagosome formation and lipidation of LC3 (conversion from LC3-I to LC3-II) [18]. However, MSU crystals also induce accumulation of p62, a selective autophagy adaptor for degradation of ubiquitinated substrates [18]. Since p62 has an LC3-binding motif, p62 binds with LC3 on the autophagosome and facilitates autophagic degradation [36]. Levels of p62 usually inversely correlate with autophagic degradation in later stages of autophagy [36]. Although studies have shown that p62 is increased and translocated to damaged mitochondria in NLRP3 inflammasome-activated cells, the detailed molecular mechanism on the link between the NLRP3 inflammasome and autophagy, especially mitophagy, is not yet fully understood. Interestingly, recent studies reported that, on stimulation of

macrophages with NLRP3 inflammasome activators, p62, whose expression is induced via NF-κB, LC3-II, and Parkin, were recruited to the damaged mitochondria, initiating organelle clearance via mitophagy [36, 37]. This "NF-κB-p62-mitophagy" signaling axis represents a key macrophage-intrinsic regulatory mechanism that keeps NLRP3 inflammasome activation in check [37, 38]. Further studies on how arhalofenate acid controls MSU crystal-induced NLRP3 inflammation related to mitophagy will be of interest.

Conclusion

Arhalofenate acid, the active acid form of arhalofenate, exerts anti-inflammatory effects in MSU crystal-treated macrophages. These effects were mediated to a large degree by inducing AMPK activation, and at least in part by associated maintenance of mitochondrial function through activation of AMPK and its downstream signaling and preservation of mitochondrial cristae surface area, and by increasing cellular quality control by promoting autophagy. The results of this study identify basic mechanisms by which arhalofenate treatment decreases acute flares in patients with gout [5].

Abbreviations
AMPK: AMP-activated protein kinase; Ask1: Apoptosis signaling regulating kinase 1; BMDM: Bone marrow-derived macrophage; FBS: Fetal bovine serum; GM-CSF: Granulocyte-macrophage colony-stimulating factor; IL: Interleukin; KO: Knockout; LAMP1: Lysosomal-associated membrane protein 1; M-CSF: Macrophage colony-stimulating factor; MSU: Monosodium urate; mtDNA: Mitochondrial DNA; NAD: Nicotinamide adenine dinucleotide; OXPHOS: Oxidative phosphorylation; PBS: Phosphate-buffered saline; PGC-1α: Peroxisome proliferator-activated receptor γ co-activator 1α; PPARγ: Peroxisome proliferator-activated receptor γ; ROS: Reactive oxygen species; SIRT1: Sirtuin 1; TEM: Transmission electron microscopy; TFAM: Mitochondrial transcription factor A; TRX: Thioredoxin; TXNIP: Thioredoxin-interacting protein

Funding
The study was supported by the Department of Veterans Affairs Merit Review grants I01BX002234 (to RLB) and I01BX001660 (to RT), and NIH grant P50 AR060772-6 Project 1 (to RT).

Authors' contributions
CM, RT, and RLB conceived of and designed the study. YJC, RLS, SKM, and RLB acquired the data and performed data analysis. All authors contributed to data interpretation. CM, RT, and RLB wrote and revised the manuscript. All authors read and approved the final manuscript.

Ethics approval
The handing of mice and experimental procedures were in accordance with requirements of the Institutional Animal Care and Use Committee and this study was granted permission by the CymaBay Research Oversight Committee.

Competing interests
RT has received research support jointly from Ardea/Astra-Zeneca and Ironwood, and has received payment as a consultant to SOBI, Selecta, and Horizon, and has a consulting agreement with CymaBay Therapeutics, Inc. RLB has received research funding from by CymaBay Therapeutics, Inc. The remaining authors declare that they have no competing interests.

Author details

[1]CymaBay Therapeutics, Inc., Newark, California, USA. [2]VA San Diego Healthcare System, 111K, 3350 La Jolla Village Drive, San Diego, CA 92161, USA. [3]University of California San Diego, La Jolla, California, USA.

References

1. Zhu Y, Pandya BJ, Choi HK. Prevalence of gout and hyperuricemia in the US general population: the National Health and nutrition examination survey 2007–2008. Arthritis Rheum. 2011;63:3136–41.

2. Keenan RT, O'Brien WR, Lee KH, Crittenden DB, Fisher MC, et al. Prevalence of contraindications and prescription of pharmacologic therapies for gout. Am J Med. 2011;124:155–63.

3. Gregoire FM, Zhang F, Clarke HJ, Gustafson TA, Sears DD, et al. MBX-102/JNJ39659100, a novel peroxisome proliferator-activated receptor-ligand with weak transactivation activity retains antidiabetic properties in the absence of weight gain and edema. Mol Endocrinol. 2009;23:975–88.

4. Lavan BE, McWherter C, Choi YJ. Arhalofenate, a novel uricosuric agent, is an inhibitor of human uric acid transporters [abstract]. Ann Rheum Dis. 2013;71(Suppl 3):450–1.

5. Poiley J, Steinberg AS, Choi YJ, Davis CS, Martin RL, et al. Arhalofenate flare study investigators. A randomized, double-blind, active- and placebo-controlled efficacy and safety study of arhalofenate for reducing flare in patients with gout. Arthritis Rheum. 2016;68:2027–34.

6. Busso N, So A. Mechanisms of inflammation in gout. Arthritis Res Ther. 2010;12:206.

7. Cronstein BN, Sunkureddi P. Mechanistic aspects of inflammation and clinical management of inflammation in acute gouty arthritis. J Clin Rheumatol. 2013;19:19–29.

8. Cleophas MC, Crişan TO, Joosten LA. Factors modulating the inflammatory response in acute gouty arthritis. Curr Opin Rheumatol. 2017;29:163–70.

9. Terkeltaub R. What makes gouty inflammation so variable? BMC Med. 2017;15:158.

10. Yu JW, Lee MS. Mitochondria and the NLRP3 inflammasome: physiological and pathological relevance. Arch Pharm Res. 2016;39:1503–18.

11. Gurung P, Lukens JR, Kanneganti TD. Mitochondria: diversity in the regulation of the NLRP3 inflammasome. Trends Mol Med. 2015;21:193–201.

12. Zhou R, Yazdi AS, Menu P, Tschopp J. A role for mitochondria in NLRP3 inflammasome activation. Nature. 2011;469:221–5.

13. Zhou R, Tardivel A, Thorens B, Choi I, Tschopp J. Thioredoxin-interacting protein links oxidative stress to inflammasome activation. Nat Immunol. 2010;11:136–40.

14. Yoshihara E, Masaki S, Matsuo Y, Chen Z, Tian H, et al. Thioredoxin/TXNIP: redoxisome as a redox switch for the pathogenesis of diseases. Front Immunol. 2014;4:514.

15. Jin HS, Suh HW, Kim SJ, Jo EK. Mitochondrial control of innate immunity and inflammation. Immune Netw. 2017;17:77–88.

16. Okamoto K, Kondo-Okamoto N. Mitochondria and autophagy: critical interplay between the two homeostats. Biochim Biophys Acta. 2012;1820:595–600.

17. Rodgers MA, Bowman JW, Liang Q, Jung JU. Regulation where autophagy intersects the inflammasome. Antioxid Redox Signal. 2014;20:495–506.

18. Choe JY, Jung HY, Park KY, Kim SK. Enhanced p62 expression through impaired proteasomal degradation is involved in caspase-1 activation in monosodium urate crystal-induced interleukin-1b expression. Rheumatology (Oxford). 2014;53:1043–53.

19. Carling D. AMPK signalling in health and disease. Curr Opin Cell Biol. 2017;45:31–7.

20. Salminen A, Kaarniranta K. AMP-activated protein kinase (AMPK) controls the aging process via an integrated signaling network. Ageing Res Rev. 2012;11:230–41.

21. Salminen A, Hyttinen JM, Kaarniranta K. AMP-activated protein kinase inhibits NF-κB signaling and inflammation: impact on healthspan and lifespan. J Mol Med (Berl). 2011;89:667–76.

22. Wang Y, Viollet B, Terkeltaub R, Liu-Bryan R. AMP-activated protein kinase suppresses urate crystal-induced inflammation and transduces colchicine effects in macrophages. Ann Rheum Dis. 2016;75:286–94.

23. Zhang J, Zhang Y, Xiao F, Liu Y, Wang J, et al. The peroxisome proliferator-activated receptor γ agonist pioglitazone prevents NF-κB activation in cisplatin nephrotoxicity through the reduction of p65 acetylation via the AMPK-SIRT1/p300 pathway. Biochem Pharmacol. 2016;101:100–11.

24. Osman I, Segar L. Pioglitazone, a PPARγ agonist, attenuates PDGF-induced vascular smooth muscle cell proliferation through AMPK-dependent and AMPK-independent inhibition of mTOR/p70S6K and ERK signaling. Biochem Pharmacol. 2016;101:54–70.

25. Morrison A, Yan X, Tong C, Li J. Acute rosiglitazone treatment is cardioprotective against ischemia-reperfusion injury by modulating AMPK, Akt, and JNK signaling in nondiabetic mice. Am J Physiol Heart Circ Physiol. 2011;301:H895–902.

26. Fernandez-Marcos PJ, Auwerx J. Regulation of PGC-1alpha, a nodal regulator of mitochondrial biogenesis. Am J Clin Nutr. 2011;93:884S–90.

27. Pasqua T, Mahata S, Bandyopadhyay GK, Biswas A, Perkins GA, et al. Impact of chromogranin A on catecholamine storage, catecholamine granule morphology, and chromaffin cell energy metabolism in vivo. Cell Tissue Res. 2016;363:693–712.

28. Shaked M, Ketzinel-Gilad M, Cerasi E, Kaiser N, Leibowitz G. AMP-activated protein kinase (AMPK) mediates nutrient regulation of thioredoxin-interacting protein (TXNIP) in pancreatic beta-cells. PLoS One. 2011;6:e28804.

29. Gao K, Chi Y, Sun W, Takeda M, Yao J. 5'-AMP-activated protein kinase attenuates adriamycin-induced oxidative podocyte injury through thioredoxin-mediated suppression of the apoptosis signal-regulating kinase 1-P38 signaling pathway. Mol Pharmacol. 2014;85:460–71.

30. Lee WH, Kim SG. AMPK-dependent metabolic regulation by PPAR agonists. PPAR Res. 2010;2010. https://doi.org/10.1155/2010/549101.

31. Huang LS, Cobessi D, Tung EY, Berry EA. Binding of the respiratory chain inhibitor antimycin to the mitochondrial BC1 complex: a new crystal structure reveals an altered intramolecular hydrogen-bonding pattern. J Mol Biol. 2005;351:573–97.

32. Li N, Ragheb K, Lawler G, Sturgis J, Rajwa B, et al. Mitochondrial complex I inhibitor rotenone induces apoptosis through enhancing mitochondrial reactive oxygen species production. J Biol Chem. 2003;278:8516–25.

33. Hou X, Song J, Li XN, Zhang L, Wang X, et al. Metformin reduces intracellular reactive oxygen species levels by upregulating expression of the antioxidant thioredoxin via the AMPK-FOXO3 pathway. Biochem Biophys Res Commun. 2010;396:199–205.

34. Chai TF, Hong SY, He H, Zheng L, Hagen T, et al. A potential mechanism of metformin-mediated regulation of glucose homeostasis: inhibition of thioredoxin-interacting protein (TXNIP) gene expression. Cell Signal. 2012;24:1700–5.

35. Kim MJ, Yoon JH, Ryu JH. Mitophagy: a balance regulator of NLRP3 inflammasome activation. BMB Rep. 2016;49:529–35.

36. Lazarou M. Keeping the immune system in check: a role for mitophagy. Immunol Cell Biol. 2015;93:3–10.

37. Zhong Z, Umemura A, Sanchez-Lopez E, Liang S, Shalapour S, et al. NF-κB restricts inflammasome activation via elimination of damaged mitochondria. Cell. 2016;164:896–910.

38. Zhong Z, Sanchez-Lopez E, Karin M. Autophagy, NLRP3 inflammasome and auto-inflammatory/immune diseases. Clin Exp Rheumatol. 2016;34:12–6.

9

What is the value of musculoskeletal ultrasound in patients presenting with arthralgia to predict inflammatory arthritis development?

Rosaline van den Berg[1*] (iD), Sarah Ohrndorf[2,3], Marion C. Kortekaas[2] and Annette H. M. van der Helm-van Mil[1,2]

Abstract

Objective: Musculoskeletal ultrasound (US) is frequently used in several rheumatology practices to detect subclinical inflammation in patients with joint symptoms suspected for progression to inflammatory arthritis. Evaluating the scientific basis for this specific US use, we performed this systematic literature review determining if US features of inflammation are predictive for arthritis development and which US features are of additive value to other, regularly used biomarkers.

Methods: Medical literature databases were systematically searched up to May 2017 for longitudinal studies reporting on the association between greyscale (GSUS) and Power Doppler (PDUS) abnormalities and inflammatory arthritis development in arthralgia patients. Quality of studies was assessed by two independent reviewers using a set of 18 criteria. Studies were marked high quality if scored ≥ 80.6% (which is the median score). Best-evidence synthesis was performed to determine the level of evidence (LoE). Positive and negative likelihood ratios (LR+, LR−) were determined.

Results: Of 3061 unique references, six fulfilled inclusion criteria (three rated high quality), of which two reported on the same cohort. Heterogeneity in arthralgia populations, various US machines and scoring systems hampered the comparability of results. LoE for GSUS as predictor was limited and moderate for PDUS; LoE for the additive value of GSUS and PDUS with other biomarkers was limited to moderate. Estimated LR+ values were mostly < 4 and LR− values > 0.5.

Conclusions: Data on the value of GSUS and PDUS abnormalities for predicting inflammatory arthritis development are sparse. Although a potential benefit is not excluded, current LoE is limited to moderate. Future studies are required, preferably performed in clearly defined, well-described arthralgia populations, using standardized US acquisition protocols and scoring systems.

Keywords: Arthralgia, Ultrasound, Rheumatoid arthritis

* Correspondence: rosalinevandenberg@gmail.com
[1]Department of Rheumatology, Erasmus Medical Center, Rotterdam, The Netherlands
Full list of author information is available at the end of the article

Background

The development of rheumatoid arthritis (RA) is supposed to consist of several stages: a) genetic risk factors for RA; b) environmental risk factors for RA; c) systemic autoimmunity associated with RA; d) symptoms without clinical arthritis; e) unclassified arthritis (UA); f) RA [1]. The phase of arthralgia preceding clinical arthritis (phase d) is of particular interest since it is hypothesized that disease-modifying treatment initiated in this phase might result in better disease outcomes than when initiated in the phases of UA and RA [2]. However, musculoskeletal symptoms such as arthralgia are prevalent, and arthralgia is frequently not related to imminent RA. In order to identify arthralgia patients at risk for RA, different strategies can be undertaken, such as selecting arthralgia patients based on clinical features associated with RA development, using autoantibody tests or imaging to detect subclinical inflammation, or a combination of these.

Musculoskeletal ultrasound (US) is a frequently used imaging modality as it is fast, easy to apply, and readily accessible. Although US is frequently used in patients presenting with arthralgia (as also proposed in an algorithm for the pragmatic use of US [3]) in several rheumatology practices, we questioned what the scientific basis is to use US as a predictor for future inflammatory arthritis development. Therefore, we systematically studied the literature to determine if US features of inflammation are predictive for inflammatory arthritis development and, if so, to determine which US features are of additive value to other regularly used biomarkers, with the ultimate goal of obtaining evidence-based information on the value of US in patients presenting with arthralgia.

Methods

Systematic literature search

The PRISMA guidelines were followed [4]. Search strategies were built in collaboration with an experienced librarian (WB) and executed in electronic medical literature databases (Embase.com, Medline Ovid, Web of Science, Scopus, Cochrane Central, Google Scholar) up to 11 May 2017 (complete searches in Additional file 1: File S1). Reference lists of the included papers were checked for additional papers and unpublished and ongoing trials were identified using the World Health Organization (WHO) International Clinical Trials Registry Platform (ICTRP) search portal (http://apps.who.int/trialsearch/) and ClinicalTrials.gov (http://clinicaltrials.gov).

Selection of studies based on inclusion and exclusion criteria

Two reviewers (SO, RvdB) assessed each title for suitability for inclusion in this review, according to predetermined inclusion and exclusion criteria. Next, abstracts were retrieved for detailed review and, finally, full-text papers were assessed if further information was required. Papers not addressing the topic of interest were excluded and reasons for exclusion recorded.

From the total number of studies identified by the database search, studies were included if the following inclusion criteria were met: 1) investigation of subjects without clinical arthritis, suffering from arthralgia, regardless of rheumatoid factor (RF) and anti-citrullinated protein antibody (ACPA) status or ACPA+ musculoskeletal symptoms; 2) investigation of small hand and/or feet joints of subjects using US; 3) joints and/or tendons were assessed for inflammatory features (GS synovial hypertrophy and/or PDUS); 4) subjects were followed prospectively; 5) development of (persistent) inflammatory arthritis or RA was defined as outcome. Studies about other inflammatory joint conditions, animal studies, reviews, letters to the editor, case reports, case series, commentaries, guidelines, editorials, abstracts, study populations < 18 years of age, and studies in languages other than English, Dutch, and German were excluded.

Data extraction

The two reviewers independently assessed the full texts of the included studies using a predefined sheet to extract data about: 1) study population (number of patients, age, gender, symptom duration); 2) follow-up period; 3) musculoskeletal US equipment (producer, transducer, machine setting, mode (GSUS/PDUS); 4) US acquisition (number and type of examined joints, examined pathology, scoring method, potential used cut-off); 5) longitudinal outcome.

Data from univariable analyses were extracted to answer the first aim; data from multivariable analyses were extracted to answer the second aim on added value.

Quality assessment and analyses

Due to heterogeneity of the studies, it was not possible to perform meta-analyses and calculate pooled effect estimates. Therefore, we performed a best-evidence synthesis based on the guidelines on systemic review of the Cochrane Collaboration Back and Neck (CBN) Group [5], a method summarizing the level of evidence (LoE) in observational studies if study population, outcomes and data analyses are heterogenic (Additional file 1: Table S1). LoE is based on presence of statistical significance, which depends on sample sizes, taking into account the quality of the studies. Quality of the studies was evaluated by the two reviewers individually, using a set of 18 criteria based on previous systematic reviews in prognostic factors in the field of musculoskeletal disorders [2, 6]. This list included seven criteria specifically for the use of US, of which three were considered mandatory (Additional file 1: Table S2). A study was considered high quality if all three mandatory criteria were fulfilled and the total score was ≥ 80.6% (median of quality scores obtained in this review).

Positive and negative likelihood ratios (LR+ and LR–, respectively) and positive and negative predictive values (PPV and NPV, respectively) were calculated based on presented data regarding outcome (using the presented follow-up duration (Table 1)) to evaluate the predictive accuracy. Also, due to heterogeneity, no summary estimates were calculated.

Results
Selection and inclusion of articles
In total, 5028 titles were identified and, after removing duplicates, 3061 unique references were screened (Additional file 1: Figure S1). After detailed review, six full-text papers fulfilled the inclusion and exclusion criteria (Table 1) [7–12], of which two studies reported on the same cohort [10, 11]. One of them reports on dichotomous PDUS results only and the other presents PDUS and GS synovial hypertrophy results for various cut-offs.

Quality assessment
The two reviewers rated 108 items and agreed on 98 (91.6%); disagreement on items was solved by discussion (Additional file 1: Table S3). All six included studies fulfilled the three mandatory criteria. Median quality score was 80.6% (range 61.1–83.3%). Two of the three high-quality papers described the same cohort [8, 10, 11].

Study characteristics
The number of included patients varied between 80 and 379; the majority were female (69–83%) aged > 50 years. None of the studies had stringent inclusion criteria with respect to symptom constitution. The cohort described in the papers by Nam et al. [10] and Rakieh et al. [11] included ACPA+ patients with new onset musculoskeletal symptoms from primary care physician clinics and the rheumatology early arthritis clinic in Leeds. In the study of Van der Ven et al. [8], patients with inflammatory joint complaints involving at least two joints in the hands, feet, or shoulders for < 1 year which could not be explained by other conditions were included if they had also at least two of the following criteria: morning stiffness for > 1 h, unable to clench a fist in the morning, pain when shaking someone's hand, pins and needles in the fingers, difficulties wearing rings or shoes, family history of RA, and/or unexplained fatigue. In the paper by Zufferey et al. [7], ACPA- and RF-negative patients with polyarthralgia for > 6 weeks with an inflammatory or mixed (mechanical and inflammatory) character referred by their general practitioner or rheumatologist were included. Van de Stadt et al. [12] recruited ACPA+ and/or RF+ patients with arthralgia, defined as "non-traumatic

pain in any joint", at rheumatology clinics in Amsterdam after referral by their general practitioner. Patients presenting with new-onset arthralgia to the Newcastle Early Arthritis Clinic were included in the study by Pratt et al. [9], but no description of arthralgia was provided.

Symptom duration at inclusion varied between 6 weeks and 23 months (Table 1). Patients were followed for > 12 months in all studies (range 12–28 months). Three studies included only ACPA+ and/or RF+ patients [10–12]; one study only ACPA- and RF-negative patients [7] and the remaining studies included both ACPA+ and/or RF+ and arthralgia negative patients [8, 9].

Acquisition of ultrasound
US specifications are presented in Table 2. Three studies used a transducer with 12 or 13 MHz as maximum [7, 9, 12]. Various US machines were used, various scoring systems with various definitions of pathology were used to grade synovitis [13–20], and the number of examined joints varied (range 16–32). In one study only tender joints were scanned [12]. Four studies reported on both GS synovial hypertrophy and PDUS [8–10, 12], one only on GS synovial hypertrophy [7], and one only on PDUS [11]. Only one study scored the presence of tenosynovitis (GSUS) [12]. All studies except one [10] used a cut-off to define a positive "inflammation US score", yet the definitions varied (Table 2).

Two studies reported on inter-observer reliability, which was moderate (kappa = 0.56 for GS synovial hypertrophy) to substantial (kappa = 0.64 for PDUS) [9] in one study, and fair (kappa = 0.22 for effusion) to moderate (kappa = 0.47 for synovitis) and substantial (kappa = 0.67 for PDUS) in another study [12], yet good in terms of overall percentage agreement (88–92%).

Outcome
Outcome was defined as RA (ACR/EULAR 2010 criteria [21]) in one study and (persistent) (inflammatory) arthritis in the remaining five. Outcome was reached in 8.8–50.0% of patients; frequency was lowest in ACPA-/RF-negative populations and highest in ACPA+/RF+ populations. Duration until outcome was reached varied between 7.9 and 18.3 months and was not specified in two studies (Table 1).

LoE of GSUS and PDUS abnormalities as predictor for arthritis development
The prevalence of different US features varied per patient group and cut-off used. For GS synovial hypertrophy it ranged from 11.6 (GSUS ≥ 2 in patients without arthritis development) to 77.2% (GSUS ≥ 2 in patients that developed arthritis); for PDUS from 6.3 (PDUS = 2 in patients without arthritis development) to 44.0% (PDUS ≥ 1 in patients that developed arthritis)

Table 1 Overview of selected studies

Study	Study population	N	Female (%)	Age (years; mean (±SD) or median (IQR))	Symptom duration at inclusion (mean (±SD) or median (IQR))	Outcome of relevance	Mean follow-up duration (months; mean (±SD) or median (IQR))	N (%) patients with outcome	Duration until diagnosis/outcome (months)	Univariable	Adjustment factors	Multivariable
Rakieh et al. 2015 [11]	**ACPA+ patients with MSK symptoms (primary and secondary care)**	**100**	**69**	**51.2 ± 11.9**	**22.7 (8.2–42.4) months**	**IA**	**19.8 (7.6–34.4)**	**50 (50.0)**	**7.9 (3.2–14.5)**	**PDUS≥ 1: HR 1.88 (1.07–3.29)**	**Tenderness small joints** / **Morning stiffness ≥ 30 min** / **High ++ RF and/or ACPA**	**PDUS ≥ 1: HR 1.51 (0.83–2.74)¥**
Nam et al. 2016 [10]	ACPA+ patients with MSK symptoms (primary and secondary care)	136	73.7	51.3 ± 12.4	17.2 (7.0–33.4) months	IA	28.1 (range 4.7–79.6) for non-progressors	57 (41.9)	18.3 (range 0.1–79.6)	GSUS ≥ 2: HR 2.8 (0.4–20.3) / PDUS ≥ 1: HR 1.6 (0.9–3.2)	None	ND
van der Ven et al. 2017 [8]	**Inflammatory arthralgia in > = 2 painful joints (hands, feet, shoulders), plus 2 additional criteria* (secondary care)**	**174**	**83**	**45.0 ± 11.3**	**7.0 ± 3.1 months**	**IA**	**12**	**31 (17.8)**	**Within 1 year; not specified**	**GSUS ≥ 2 and/or PDUS ≥ 1⁺: OR 3.03 (1.69–5.41) / PDUS ≥ 1: OR 3.12 (1.61–6.03)**	**GSUS ≥ 2 and/or PDUS ≥ 1⁺: Age / Morning stiffness > 30 min / ACPA ; PDUS ≥ 1: Age / Morning stiffness > 30 min**	**GSUS ≥ 2 and/or PDUS ≥ 1⁺: OR 2.65 (1.44–4.88) / PDUS ≥ 1: OR 3.44 (1.71–6.95)**
van de Stadt et al. 2010 [12]	Arthralgia with RF+ and/or ACPA+ (secondary care)	192	72	47 ± 11	12 (9–36) months	Arthritis	26 (range 6–54)	45 (23.4)	11 ± 9	Synovitis: OR 1.41 (0.54–3.65) / PDUS: OR 1.54 (0.67–3.54) / Effusion: OR 2.05 (0.80–5.27) / Tenosynovitis: OR 1.50 (0.44–5.11)	None	ND
Pratt et al. 2013 [9]	Inflammatory arthralgia (secondary care)	379	72	51 (36–66)	20 (10–34) weeks	Persistent IA‡	27 (range 12–44)	162 (42.7)	NP	NP	Age / Symptom duration / Swollen joint count / CRP / ACPA / ESR	Grade 1 GSUS synovitis in ≥ 3/16 joints: OR 4.91 (2.32–10.4)
Zufferey et al. 2017 [7]	ACPA- and RF- inflammatory polyarthralgia > 6 weeks (secondary care)	80	77	51 ± 14	NP	RA	18 ± 7	7 (8.8)	18	NP	Gender / Elevated CRP	SONAR > 8/22*: OR 7.45 (1.19–42.8) / US score ≥ 2 joints with grade ≥ 2 synovitis*: OR 10.1 (1.1–49)

Studies marked in bold are scored as high-quality (high-quality study > 80% (which is the median of all quality scores))

GSUS greyscale ultrasound, NA not applicable, ND not done, NP not presented, NPV negative predictive value, PPV positive predictive value, PDUS power Doppler ultrasound, IA inflammatory arthritis, MSK musculoskeletal

*Morning stiffness for more than 1 h, unable to clench a fist in the morning, pain when shaking someone's hand, pins and needles in the fingers, difficulty wearing rings or shoes, family history of RA and/or unexplained fatigue for < 1 year

‡Persistent IA was defined as RA, psoriatic arthritis, enteropathic arthritis, ankylosing spondylitis, undifferentiated spondyloarthritis, connective tissue disease, "self-limiting inflammatory/reactive arthritis" warranting DMARD treatment and other inflammatory arthritides

¥In the PDUS model corrected for tenderness small joints, morning stiffness ≥ 30 min, high ++ RF and/or ACPA

§One or more swollen joint on physical examination

*See Table 2 for a detailed description of the cut-offs and thresholds used to define a positive US

Table 2 Specification of US in selected study

Study	Machine	Probe	Mode	Synovitis (scoring method)	Tenosynovitis (scoring method)	Erosion	Locations scanned	One side (1)/both sides (2)	Total number of joints	Volar/dorsal side	Cut-off/threshold def. "inflammation US score"	Positive "inflammation US score", % total group (progressors, non-progressors)
Rakieh et al. 2015 [11]	**Philips ATL HDI 5000**	**12-5 MHz and 8-15 MHz**	**PDUS**	**Yes (0-3) [16, 19]**	**ND**	**ND**	**Wrist MCP I-V PIP I-V**	**2**	**22**	**NP**	**PDUS ≥ 1**	**33.0 (44.0, 22.0)**
Nam et al. 2016 [10]	**Philips ATL HDI 5000 and General Electric S7**	5-12 and 8-15 MHz (Philips); 6-15 MHz (GE)	GSUS and PDUS	Yes (0-3; for both GSUS and PDUS) [22]	ND	Yes (0/1)	Wrist MCP I-V PIP I-V MTP I-V	2	32	Dorsal	None	GSUS = 0: 4.4 (1.8, 6.3) GSUS = 1: 27.9 (21.1, 32.9) GSUS ≥ 2: 67.6 (77.2, 60.8) PDUS = 0: 66.9 (50.9, 78.5) PDUS = 1: 18.4 (22.8, 15.2) PDUS = 2: 14.7 (26.3, 6.3) ERO = 0: 79.4 (64.9, 89.9) ERO = 1: 20.6 (35.1, 10.1)
van der Ven et al. 2017 [8]	**Mylab 60 (Esaote, Genoa, Italy)**	10-18 MHz	GSUS and PDUS	Yes (0-3; for both GSUS and PDUS) [15]	ND	ND	Wrist MCP II-V PIP I-V MTP II-V	2	26	Dorsal	**a.** Positive synovitis: GSUS ≥ 2 and/or PDUS ≥ 1 **b.** PDUS score: ≥ 1	**a.** 35.6 (54.8, 31.5) **b.** 14.9 (29.0, 11.9)
van de Stadt et al. 2010 [12]	Acuson Antares, premium edition (Siemens, Malvern, PA, USA)	5-13 MHz	GSUS and PDUS	Yes (0-3; for both GSUS and PDUS) [13]	Yes (0-3)	ND	Only tender joints*	2	NA	Volar	PDUS ≥ 1 Joint effusion, synovitis, tenosynovitis ≥ 2	GSUS synovitis ≥ 2: 12.5 (15.6, 11.6) GSUS effusion ≥ 2: 11.5 (17.7, 9.5) PDUS ≥ 1: 17.2 (22.2, 15.6) Tenosynovitis ≥ 2: 6.8 (8.9, 6.1)
Pratt et al. 2013 [9]	Aplio Diagnostic Ultrasound System (Toshiba Medical Systems Corporation, Tochigi-Ken, Japan)	12 MHz	GSUS and PDUS	Yes (0-3; for both GSUS and PDUS) [13-15, 20]	ND	Yes (0-3)	MCP II-IV PIP II-IV MTP I-II	2	16	Dorsal and volar	GSUS: a. sum score ≥ 2; b. sum score/ 6 joints (worst hand) ≥ 2; c. number of joints ≥ 1: ≥ 3. PDUS: d. sum score ≥ 1; e. number of joints ≥ 1: ≥ 2	a. 35.1 (56.2, 19.4) b. 29.6 (48.8, 15.0) c. 30.1 (50.6, 14.7) d. 29.0 (46.9, 15.7) e. 16.9 (29.6, 7.4)
Zufferey et al. 2017 [7]	Philips HD 11	7-13 MHz	GSUS	Yes (0-3) [17, 18]	ND	ND	Wrist MCP II-V PIP II-V Elbows Knees	2	22	NP	a. B-mode score > 8 (of total possible score of 66). b. ≥ 2 joints (of total number of 22 joints) with grade ≥ 2 synovitis [18]	a. 21.3 (57.1, 17.8) b. 25.0 (71.4, 20.5)

Studies marked in bold are scored as high-quality (high-quality study > 80% (which is the median of all all quality scores))

ERO erosions, *GSUS* greyscale ultrasound, *MCP* metacarpophalangeal joint, *MHz* megahertz, *MTP* metatarsophalangeal joint, *NA* not applicable, *ND* not done, *NP* not presented, *PIP* proximal interphalangeal joint, *PDUS* power Doppler, *US* ultrasound

*Tender joints at physical examination were scanned, otherwise joints that were painful by history were scanned. For MCP, PIP, and MTP joints the directly adjacent joints in the same joint group as the painful joints were scanned

(Table 2). The prevalence of tenosynovitis ranged from 6.1 (GSUS ≥ 2 in patients without arthritis development) to 8.9% (GSUS ≥ 2 in patients with arthritis development).

GS synovial hypertrophy

One high-quality and one low-quality study reported a non-statistically significant association between GS synovial hypertrophy and arthritis development (HR 2.8 [95% CI 0.4–20.3] and (OR 1.41 [95% CI 0.54–3.65], respectively) [10, 12]. One other high-quality study reported a statistically significant association (OR 3.03 [95% CI: 1.69–5.41]) for a "positive US" defined as GSUS ≥ 2 and/or PDUS ≥ 1 [8]. Hence, LoE with regard to the predictive value of GSUS is limited.

PDUS synovitis

Two high-quality studies reported a statistically significant association between PDUS and arthritis development (OR 3.12 [95% CI 1.61–6.03] [8], HR 1.88 [95% CI 1.07–3.29] [11]). The third high-quality study (performed in the same cohort as [11]) reported a non-statistically significant association (HR 1.6 [95% CI 0.9–3.2]) [10]; thus the statistically significant association found in the first 100 patients was lost after inclusion of additional patients. A low-quality study reported a non-significant association as well (OR 1.54 [95% CI 0.67–3.54]) [12]. Hence, LoE with regard to the predictive value of PDUS is moderate.

Tenosynovitis

One low-quality study evaluated tenosynovitis and found no statistically significant association with arthritis development (OR 1.50 [95% CI 0.44–5.11]) [12]. Hence, LoE with regard to the predictive value of tenosynovitis is insufficient.

LoE of GSUS and PDUS abnormalities being additive to other biomarkers

Three studies investigated the association of GS synovial hypertrophy with arthritis development, correcting for different biomarkers (Table 1). Two low-quality studies reported statistically significant associations of GS synovial hypertrophy and arthritis development (OR 4.91 [95% CI 2.32–10.4]), OR 7.45 [95% CI 1.19–42.8], and OR 10.1 [95% CI 1.1–49] [7, 9]. One high-quality study reported a statistically significant association of a "positive US" (GSUS ≥ 2 and/or PDUS ≥ 1; OR 2.65 [95% CI 1.44–4.88]) [8]. Hence, LoE with regard to the question of whether GS synovial hypertrophy may have value in predicting arthritis development, additive to regularly assessed biomarkers, is moderate.

Likewise, two studies performed multivariable analysis with PDUS. After correction for (different) biomarkers

(Table 1), one high-quality study reported a statistically significant association (OR 3.44 [95% CI 1.71–6.95]) [8]. The other high-quality study reported a non-significant association (HR 1.51 [95% CI 0.83–2.74]) [11]. Hence, LoE of the value of PDUS in addition to other biomarkers is limited.

The value of tenosynovitis (GS/PD) in addition to other biomarkers was not investigated.

Positive and negative likelihood ratios and absolute risks

Calculated LRs varied and confidence intervals (CIs) were wide. For GS synovial hypertrophy, LR+ ranged from 1.27–3.48 and LR– ranged from 0.36–0.95. For PDUS, LR+ ranged from 1.42–4.16 and LR– ranged from 0.63–0.92 (Fig. 1 and Additional file 1: Table S4).

Predictive values are directly proportional to disease prevalence. Percentages of patients that developed arthritis varied between 8.8 and 50%; thus, prior risks for not progressing were 50–91.2%. We calculated the increase in the absolute risks of inflammatory arthritis provided by US-detected abnormalities by comparing PPV and NPV with prior risks (Additional file 1: Table S4). Overall, PPVs were low or moderate (23.5–71.9% for GS synovial hypertrophy; 30.3–75% for PDUS) and the increase in absolute risks in US-positive patients ranged from 5.8–29.2% (GS synovial hypertrophy) and 6.9–33.1% (PDUS). NPVs were higher (68.9–96.7% for GS synovial hypertrophy; 58.2–85.1% for PDUS), but the gain in relation to prior risk of not progressing to arthritis was relatively small (0.8–12.5% for GS synovial hypertrophy; 2.9–13.9% for PDUS). Thus, NPVs were largely explained by prior risks of not developing inflammatory arthritis.

Discussion

The aim of this systematic literature review was to determine if US features of inflammation are predictive for inflammatory arthritis development and, if so, which US features are of additive value to other regularly used biomarkers. LoE for GS synovial hypertrophy as predictor for arthritis was limited and moderate for PDUS. LoE for the additive value of GS synovial hypertrophy and PDUS with other regularly used biomarkers was limited to moderate. Additionally, there was insufficient data on the value of US-detected tenosynovitis. Thus, there is a discrepancy between the frequent use of US in arthralgia patients to search for subclinical inflammation (which, if present, is generally considered a sign of imminent RA) in several rheumatology practices and the absence of strong scientific evidence on its prognostic value.

The limited/moderate LoE might be explained by relatively low number of studies and the presence of different types of heterogeneity. Only six studies were included in this systematic literature review, of which two described the same cohort. The number of included

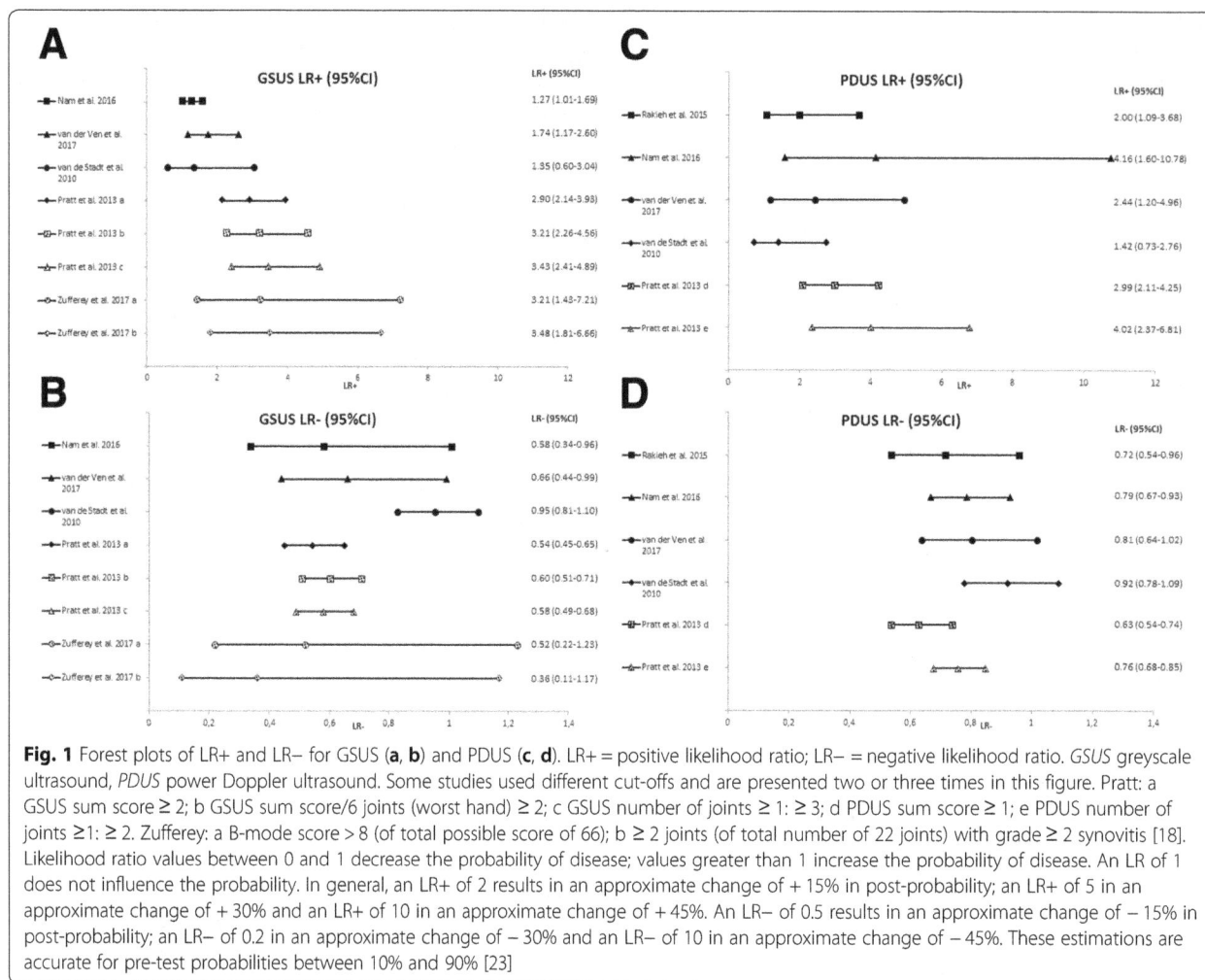

Fig. 1 Forest plots of LR+ and LR– for GSUS (**a**, **b**) and PDUS (**c**, **d**). LR+ = positive likelihood ratio; LR– = negative likelihood ratio. *GSUS* greyscale ultrasound, *PDUS* power Doppler ultrasound. Some studies used different cut-offs and are presented two or three times in this figure. Pratt: a GSUS sum score ≥ 2; b GSUS sum score/6 joints (worst hand) ≥ 2; c GSUS number of joints ≥ 1: ≥ 3; d PDUS sum score ≥ 1; e PDUS number of joints ≥1: ≥ 2. Zufferey: a B-mode score > 8 (of total possible score of 66); b ≥ 2 joints (of total number of 22 joints) with grade ≥ 2 synovitis [18]. Likelihood ratio values between 0 and 1 decrease the probability of disease; values greater than 1 increase the probability of disease. An LR of 1 does not influence the probability. In general, an LR+ of 2 results in an approximate change of + 15% in post-probability; an LR+ of 5 in an approximate change of + 30% and an LR+ of 10 in an approximate change of + 45%. An LR– of 0.5 results in an approximate change of − 15% in post-probability; an LR– of 0.2 in an approximate change of − 30% and an LR– of 10 in an approximate change of − 45%. These estimations are accurate for pre-test probabilities between 10% and 90% [23]

patients per study was rather low, influencing the power to achieve statistical significance. Furthermore, heterogeneous arthralgia populations (seropositive arthralgia, seronegative arthralgia, ACPA+ patients with unspecific musculoskeletal (MSK) symptoms) were studied in different settings (primary and/or secondary care), with slightly differently defined outcomes ((persistent) (inflammatory) arthritis, RA), contributing to the various ranges of frequencies of outcome (8.8–50%).

Moreover, the US acquisition protocol, definitions of pathology, and scoring systems varied, although all followed internationally recognized recommendations and scoring systems [13–20]. Only very recently, EULAR/ OMERACT published a standardized, consensus-based semi-quantitative scoring system for GS synovial hypertrophy and PDUS (separately and combined) [24, 25], but this was not available when the studies included in this review were executed.

Other sources of heterogeneity were the selection of assessed joints, whether they were scanned from a volar or dorsal aspect, and the fact that different machines were

used. It is known that the diverse machines have a wide variation in sensitivity to pick up inflammation, especially with regard to Doppler modalities [26]. Three studies used a transducer with 12 or 13 MHz as maximum, while higher frequencies are recommended especially for scanning small hand joints. Ideally, in order to arrive at a higher LoE, future studies should be performed in more homogeneous arthralgia populations (e.g., fulfilling the EULAR definition of arthralgia at risk for RA [27]), using the same scan and scorings protocols (e.g., EULAR/ OMERACT [24, 25]).

Another issue is the definition of a "positive US". Different cut-offs were applied and none of the studies included information on US findings in healthy volunteers. It has been shown that a cut-off incorporating such findings increased the prognostic value for the use of MRI in arthralgia patients [28]. Also US "inflammatory features" can be detected in healthy volunteers, especially in certain joints and increasing with age [29–36]. Whether incorporating age-dependent US reference values might increase the predictive value of US remains to be determined.

There was insufficient data to determine whether US-detected tenosynovitis is an (important) predictor of arthritis development, which is the case for MRI-detected subclinical tenosynovitis (which is an even stronger predictor than MRI-detected subclinical synovitis or bone marrow edema) [37]. Therefore, the potential of US-detected tenosynovitis requires further investigation.

We sought to explore the value of US abnormalities in addition to other frequently used predictors of arthritis development. Some studies performed multivariable analyses but adjusted for different variables; hence, the results of these multivariable analyses could not be directly compared. Further studies on this subject are needed, also using methods such as net reclassification index.

Best-level evidence synthesis focuses on statistical significance. Since this is not directly applicable for clinical practice, we also expressed prognostic accuracy using LRs. Estimated LR+ values were mostly < 4 and LR− values > 0.5, some with wide CIs, indicating that the post-test probability was altered to only a small degree. This was also observed when we calculated increases in absolute risks (comparing pre-test with observed post-test risks). Although absolute NPVs were higher than PPVs, and seemingly more informative, this was caused by the prior risks, which were relatively low. Our comparison of pre-test and post-test risks suggested that US is slightly more helpful in "ruling in" than "ruling out" imminent inflammatory arthritis.

Conclusions

US is frequently used in arthralgia patients in several rheumatologic practices, and although some studies have suggested a potential benefit of US, the current LoE is limited to moderate at best, due to heterogeneity of studies and lack of replication. Yet, there is a strong need for validation of results in future US studies, preferably performed in clearly defined, well-described arthralgia patients. The EULAR definition of arthralgia suspicious for progression to RA might be used to this end.

Abbreviations
ACPA: Anti-citrullinated protein antibody; ACR: American College of Rheumatology; CI: Confidence interval; EULAR: European League Against Rheumatology; GS: Greyscale; GSUS: Greyscale ultrasound; HR: Hazard ratio; ICTRP: International Clinical Trials Registry Platform; LoE: Level of evidence; LR−: Negative likelihood ratio; LR+: Positive likelihood ratio; MHz: Megahertz; MRI: Magnetic resonance imaging; NPV: Negative predictive value; OMERACT: Outcome measures in rheumatology; OR: Odds ratio; PD: Power Doppler; PDUS: Power Doppler ultrasound; PPV: Positive predictive value; RA: Rheumatoid arthritis; RF: Rheumatoid factor; UA: Unclassified arthritis; US: Ultrasound; WHO: World Health Organization

Acknowledgements
We would like to thank Wichor Bramer from the Medical Library of the Erasmus Medical Center for helping us to build the search strategies.

Funding
This work was supported by the Dutch Arthritis Foundation.
The work of Sarah Ohrndorf was supported by the Articulum fellowship grant from Pfizer (Vienna, Austria) and by the BMBF (German ministry for education and research) funded project 'ArthroMark'.

Authors' contributions
RvdB, SO, MCK, and AHMvdH-vM contributed to the conception and design of the review. RvdB performed the literature search. RvdB and SO assessed all papers and performed the data extraction and quality assessment. RvdB performed the analyses. RvdB and AHMvdH-vM drafted the paper. MCK and SO revised the article for important intellectual content. All authors gave final approval of the version to be published.

Consent for publication
NA

Competing interests
The authors declare that they have no competing interests.

Author details
[1]Department of Rheumatology, Erasmus Medical Center, Rotterdam, The Netherlands. [2]Department of Rheumatology, Leiden University Medical Center, Leiden, The Netherlands. [3]Department of Rheumatology and Clinical Immunology, Charité – Universitätsmedizin Berlin, Berlin, Germany.

References
1. Gerlag DM, Raza K, van Baarsen LG, et al. EULAR recommendations for terminology and research in individuals at risk of rheumatoid arthritis: report from the Study Group for Risk Factors for Rheumatoid Arthritis. Ann Rheum Dis. 2012;71:638–41.
2. van Nies JA, Krabben A, Schoones JW, et al. What is the evidence for the presence of a therapeutic window of opportunity in rheumatoid arthritis? A systematic literature review. Ann Rheum Dis. 2014;73:861–70.
3. D'Agostino MA, Terslev L, Wakefield R, et al. Novel algorithms for the pragmatic use of ultrasound in the management of patients with rheumatoid arthritis: from diagnosis to remission. Ann Rheum Dis. 2016;75:1902–8.
4. Moher D, Liberati A, Tetzlaff J, et al. Preferred reporting items for systematic reviews and meta-analyses: the PRISMA statement. J Clin Epidemiol. 2009;62:1006–12.
5. Furlan AD, Malmivaara A, Chou R, et al. 2015 Updated method guideline for systematic reviews in the Cochrane Back and Neck Group. Spine (Phila Pa 1976). 2015;40:1660–73.
6. Kwok WY, Plevier JW, Rosendaal FR, et al. Risk factors for progression in hand osteoarthritis: a systematic review. Arthritis Care Res (Hoboken). 2013;65:552–62.
7. Zufferey P, Rebell C, Benaim C, et al. Ultrasound can be useful to predict an evolution towards rheumatoid arthritis in patients with inflammatory polyarthralgia without anticitrullinated antibodies. Joint Bone Spine. 2017;84:299–303.
8. van der Ven M, van der Veer-Meerkerk M, Ten Cate DF, et al. Absence of ultrasound inflammation in patients presenting with arthralgia rules out the development of arthritis. Arthritis Res Ther. 2017;19:202.
9. Pratt AG, Lorenzi AR, Wilson G, et al. Predicting persistent inflammatory arthritis amongst early arthritis clinic patients in the UK: is musculoskeletal ultrasound required? Arthritis Res Ther. 2013;15:R118.

10. Nam JL, Hensor EM, Hunt L, et al. Ultrasound findings predict progression to inflammatory arthritis in anti-CCP antibody-positive patients without clinical synovitis. Ann Rheum Dis. 2016;75:2060–7.

11. Rakieh C, Nam JL, Hunt L, et al. Predicting the development of clinical arthritis in anti-CCP positive individuals with non-specific musculoskeletal symptoms: a prospective observational cohort study. Ann Rheum Dis. 2015; 74:1659–66.

12. van de Stadt LA, Bos WH, Meursinge Reynders M, et al. The value of ultrasonography in predicting arthritis in auto-antibody positive arthralgia patients: a prospective cohort study. Arthritis Res Ther. 2010;12:R98.

13. Szkudlarek M, Court-Payen M, Jacobsen S, et al. Interobserver agreement in ultrasonography of the finger and toe joints in rheumatoid arthritis. Arthritis Rheum. 2003;48:955–62.

14. Szkudlarek M, Klarlund M, Narvestad E, et al. Ultrasonography of the metacarpophalangeal and proximal interphalangeal joints in rheumatoid arthritis: a comparison with magnetic resonance imaging, conventional radiography and clinical examination. Arthritis Res Ther. 2006;8:R52.

15. Wakefield RJ, Balint PV, Szkudlarek M, et al. Musculoskeletal ultrasound including definitions for ultrasonographic pathology. J Rheumatol. 2005;32:2485–7.

16. Torp-Pedersen ST, Terslev L. Settings and artefacts relevant in colour/power Doppler ultrasound in rheumatology. Ann Rheum Dis. 2008;67:143–9.

17. Mandl P, Naredo E, Wakefield RJ, et al. A systematic literature review analysis of ultrasound joint count and scoring systems to assess synovitis in rheumatoid arthritis according to the OMERACT filter. J Rheumatol. 2011;38:2055–62.

18. Zufferey P, Moller B, Brulhart L, et al. Persistence of ultrasound synovitis in patients with rheumatoid arthritis fulfilling the DAS28 and/or the new ACR/EULAR RA remission definitions: results of an observational cohort study. Joint Bone Spine. 2014;81:426–32.

19. Naredo E, Collado P, Cruz A, et al. Longitudinal power Doppler ultrasonographic assessment of joint inflammatory activity in early rheumatoid arthritis: predictive value in disease activity and radiologic progression. Arthritis Rheum. 2007;57:116–24.

20. Scheel AK, Hermann KG, Kahler E, et al. A novel ultrasonographic synovitis scoring system suitable for analyzing finger joint inflammation in rheumatoid arthritis. Arthritis Rheum. 2005;52:733–43.

21. Aletaha D, Neogi T, Silman AJ, et al. 2010 rheumatoid arthritis classification criteria: an American College of Rheumatology/European League Against Rheumatism collaborative initiative. Ann Rheum Dis. 2010;69:1580–8.

22. D'Agostino MA, Wakefield RJ, Filippucci E, et al. Intra- and inter-observer reliability of ultrasonography for detecting and scoring synovitis in rheumatoid arthritis: a report of a EULAR ECSISIT task force [abstract]. Ann Rheum Dis. 2005;64(Supplement III):62.

23. McGee S. Simplifying likelihood ratios. J Gen Intern Med. 2002;17:647–50.

24. D'Agostino MA, Terslev L, Aegerter P, et al. Scoring ultrasound synovitis in rheumatoid arthritis: a EULAR-OMERACT ultrasound taskforce-Part 1: definition and development of a standardised, consensus-based scoring system. RMD Open. 2017;3:e000428.

25. Terslev L, Naredo E, Aegerter P, et al. Scoring ultrasound synovitis in rheumatoid arthritis: a EULAR-OMERACT ultrasound taskforce-Part 2: reliability and application to multiple joints of a standardised consensus-based scoring system. RMD Open. 2017;3:e000427.

26. Torp-Pedersen S, Christensen R, Szkudlarek M, et al. Power and color Doppler ultrasound settings for inflammatory flow: impact on scoring of disease activity in patients with rheumatoid arthritis. Arthritis Rheumatol. 2015;67:386–95.

27. van Steenbergen HW, Aletaha D, Beaart-van de Voorde LJ, et al. EULAR definition of arthralgia suspicious for progression to rheumatoid arthritis. Ann Rheum Dis. 2017;76:491–6.

28. Boer AC, Burgers LE, Mangnus L, et al. Using a reference when defining an abnormal MRI reduces false-positive MRI results-a longitudinal study in two cohorts at risk for rheumatoid arthritis. Rheumatology (Oxford). 2017;56: 1700–6.

29. Padovano I, Costantino F, Breban M, et al. Prevalence of ultrasound synovial inflammatory findings in healthy subjects. Ann Rheum Dis. 2016;75:1819–23.

30. Ellegaard K, Torp-Pedersen S, Holm CC, et al. Ultrasound in finger joints: findings in normal subjects and pitfalls in the diagnosis of synovial disease. Ultraschall Med. 2007;28:401–8.

31. Millot F, Clavel G, Etchepare F, et al. Musculoskeletal ultrasonography in healthy subjects and ultrasound criteria for early arthritis (the ESPOIR cohort). J Rheumatol. 2011;38:613–20.

32. Kitchen J, Kane D. Greyscale and power Doppler ultrasonographic evaluation of normal synovial joints: correlation with pro- and anti-inflammatory cytokines and angiogenic factors. Rheumatology (Oxford). 2015;54:458–62.

33. Fodor D, Felea I, Popescu D, et al. Ultrasonography of the metacarpophalangeal joints in healthy subjects using an 18 MHz transducer. Med Ultrason. 2015;17:185–91.

34. Machado FS, Furtado RN, Takahashi RD, et al. Sonographic cutoff values for detection of abnormalities in small, medium and large joints: a comparative study between patients with rheumatoid arthritis and healthy volunteers. Ultrasound Med Biol. 2015;41:989–98.

35. Machado FS, Natour J, Takahashi RD, et al. Sonographic assessment of healthy peripheral joints: evaluation according to demographic parameters. J Ultrasound Med. 2014;33:2087–98.

36. Hiraga M, Ikeda K, Shigeta K, et al. Sonographic measurements of low-echoic synovial area in the dorsal aspect of metatarsophalangeal joints in healthy subjects. Mod Rheumatol. 2015;25:386–92.

37. van Steenbergen HW, Mangnus L, Reijnierse M, et al. Clinical factors, anticitrullinated peptide antibodies and MRI-detected subclinical inflammation in relation to progression from clinically suspect arthralgia to arthritis. Ann Rheum Dis. 2016;75:1824–30.

10

T-cell transcriptomics from peripheral blood highlights differences between polymyositis and dermatomyositis patients

Miranda Houtman[1][*] [iD], Louise Ekholm[1], Espen Hesselberg[1], Karine Chemin[1], Vivianne Malmström[1], Ann M. Reed[2], Ingrid E. Lundberg[1] and Leonid Padyukov[1]

Abstract

Background: Polymyositis (PM) and dermatomyositis (DM) are two distinct subgroups of idiopathic inflammatory myopathies, a chronic inflammatory disorder clinically characterized by muscle weakness and inflammatory cell infiltrates in muscle tissue. In PM, a major component of inflammatory cell infiltrates is CD8+ T cells, whereas in DM, CD4+ T cells, plasmacytoid dendritic cells, and B cells predominate. In this study, with the aim to differentiate involvement of CD4+ and CD8+ T-cell subpopulations in myositis subgroups, we investigated transcriptomic profiles of T cells from peripheral blood of patients with myositis.

Methods: Total RNA was extracted from CD4+ T cells (PM = 8 and DM = 7) and CD8+ T cells (PM = 4 and DM = 5) that were isolated from peripheral blood mononuclear cells via positive selection using microbeads. Sequencing libraries were generated using the Illumina TruSeq Stranded Total RNA Kit and sequenced on an Illumina HiSeq 2500 platform, yielding about 50 million paired-end reads per sample. Differential gene expression analyses were conducted using DESeq2.

Results: In CD4+ T cells, only two genes, *ANKRD55* and *S100B*, were expressed significantly higher in patients with PM than in patients with DM (false discovery rate [FDR] < 0.05, model adjusted for age, sex, *HLA-DRB1*03* status, and RNA integrity number [RIN]). On the contrary, in CD8+ T cells, 176 genes were differentially expressed in patients with PM compared with patients with DM. Of these, 44 genes were expressed significantly higher in CD8+ T cells from patients with PM, and 132 genes were expressed significantly higher in CD8+ T cells from patients with DM (FDR < 0.05, model adjusted for age, sex, and RIN). Gene Ontology analysis showed that genes differentially expressed in CD8+ T cells are involved in lymphocyte migration and regulation of T-cell differentiation.

Conclusions: Our data strongly suggest that CD8+ T cells represent a major divergence between PM and DM patients compared with CD4+ T cells. These alterations in the gene expression in T cells from PM and DM patients might advocate for distinct immune mechanisms in these subphenotypes of myositis.

Keywords: Idiopathic inflammatory myopathies, Polymyositis, Dermatomyositis, T cells, CD4+ T cells, CD8+ T cells, Differential gene expression, RNA sequencing

* Correspondence: miranda.houtman@ki.se
[1]Division of Rheumatology, Department of Medicine, Karolinska Institutet,
Karolinska University Hospital, Stockholm, Sweden
Full list of author information is available at the end of the article

Background

Polymyositis (PM) and dermatomyositis (DM) are chronic inflammatory disorders clinically characterized by skeletal muscle weakness and muscle inflammation [1]. Other organs, such as the skin, joints, and lungs, are frequently involved in these disorders. Although the etiology of PM and DM is unknown, certain environmental and genetic factors are important. The major risk factor for these disorders in Caucasian populations is *HLA-DRB1*03:01* [2–4]. In addition, autoantibodies are found in more than 80% of the PM and DM patients, supporting a role for the adaptive immune system in the pathogenesis of these disorders [5].

In both PM and DM patients, inflammatory cell infiltrates are commonly found in the affected tissues [6, 7]. In PM, the cellular infiltrates are located mainly in the endomysium surrounding muscle fibers and typically dominated by CD8+ T cells [8, 9]. In contrast, in patients with DM, the inflammatory cell infiltrates are located mainly in the perimysium and in perivascular areas, and the infiltrates are predominated by CD4+ T cells with occasional plasmacytoid dendritic cells and B cells [6]. Further phenotyping of T cells in muscle tissue has led to the observation that the muscle-infiltrating T cells in both PM and DM are predominantly of the CD8+CD28^{null} and CD4+CD28^{null} phenotypes, which both have cytotoxic properties [10, 11]. Interestingly, these subpopulations of T cells can also be detected in peripheral blood of patients with myositis [10, 12]. Still, the differences in the tissue location of inflammatory cell infiltrates suggest that the underlying immune mechanisms may vary between PM and DM.

In this study, we aimed to investigate whole-genome transcriptomes of CD4+ and CD8+ T cells from peripheral blood in different subsets of patients with idiopathic inflammatory myopathies (IIMs). We used RNA sequencing to identify differentially expressed genes between PM and DM, as well as in patients with both types of IIM, considering *HLA-DRB1*03* alleles.

Methods

Patient recruitment

Initially, 33 consecutive adult individuals with PM or DM (not drug-free) from the Karolinska Hospital Rheumatology Clinic were selected for the study on the basis of diagnosis (PM and DM) and *HLA-DRB1*03* status (positive and negative). Patients with myositis visited the clinic between January 21 and April 23, 2014, and were fully validated according to the new European League Against Rheumatism/American College of Rheumatology classification criteria [13]. Thirty-one of the 33 patients also satisfied the Bohan and Peter criteria [14, 15]. Extensive clinical data, including disease phenotypes and treatment regimen, were collected from clinical records by experienced rheumatologists. All patients gave written consent for their participation in the study. The study was approved by the Stockholm regional ethics board.

Autoantibody detection

Patient sera were analyzed by RNA and protein immunoprecipitation for the presence of autoantibodies against Jo1, PL12, PL7, OJ, EJ, KS, Mi-2, MDA5, TIF-1γ, SRP, PM-Scl, Ro52, Ro60, U1RNP, and Ku. Sera collected after 2013 were screened using a validated line immunoassay system (EUROLINE myositis panel 4; EUROIMMUN AG, Lübeck, Germany) according to the manufacturer's instructions or by enzyme-linked immunosorbent assays for the presence of myositis-specific autoantibodies or myositis-associated autoantibodies.

HLA typing

HLA typing was performed by sequence-specific primer PCR (HLA-DR low-resolution kit; Olerup SSP, Stockholm, Sweden) and analyzed by agarose gel electrophoresis [16]. An interpretation table was used to determine the specific genotype according to the manufacturer's instructions.

Blood sampling and cell sorting

Patients' blood was collected in heparin tubes (40–50 ml in total), and peripheral blood mononuclear cells (PBMCs) were isolated by density gradient centrifugation using Ficoll density gradient medium (GE Healthcare Bio-Sciences AB, Uppsala, Sweden). CD4+ cells and CD8+ cells were isolated from the PBMCs via positive selection using CD4 or CD8 MicroBeads on an autoMACS® Pro Separator (Miltenyi Biotec Norden AB, Lund, Sweden). Flow cytometry was used to determine the purity of some of the sorted T-cell samples, and over 90% of CD45+ cells expressed CD4 ($n = 5$) or CD8 ($n = 5$). The following antibodies were used: CD45 (HI30; BioLegend, San Diego, CA, USA), CD4 (OKT4; BioLegend), and CD8 (SK1; BD Biosciences, Stockholm, Sweden).

RNA sequencing

Total RNA was extracted with the RNeasy Mini Kit (Qiagen AB, Sollentuna, Sweden) according to the manufacturer's instructions. Samples were treated with DNase (Qiagen) for 20 minutes at room temperature to avoid contamination with genomic DNA. The quality of each RNA sample was characterized using a RNA 6000 Nano Chip (Agilent Technologies Sweden AB, Kista, Sweden) on the Agilent Bioanalyzer 2100. Fifteen CD4+ T-cell samples and nine CD8+ T-cell samples met the RNA quality criteria (RNA integrity number [RIN] > 4) and were sequenced. The RNA was fragmented and prepared into sequencing libraries using the TruSeq Stranded Total RNA Sample Preparation Kit (Illumina, San Diego, CA, USA) with ribosomal depletion using Ribo-Zero (2×125 bp; Illumina) and analyzed on an

Illumina HiSeq 2500 sequencer (SNP&SEQ Technology Platform, Uppsala, Sweden). On average, 50 million reads were produced per sample. Raw read quality was evaluated using FastQC. Prefiltering on quality of reads using cutadapt (version 1.9.1) was applied (–q 30 -a AGATCGG AAGAGCACACGTCTGAACTCCAGTCAC -A AGATC GGAAGAGCGTCGTGTAGGGAAAGAGTGTAGATCT CGGTGGTCGCCGTATCATT -m 40). Filtered reads were aligned to the hg38 assembly and quantified using STAR (version 2.5.1b) [17] with default settings.

Cell-type enrichment analysis

The xCell tool [18] was used to identify cellular heterogeneity in the CD4+ and CD8+ T-cell subsets from gene expression data. xCell uses the expression levels ranking (transcripts per million), and these were obtained using Salmon (version 0.8.2) [19].

Differential gene expression analysis

Raw expression counts were adjusted for library size using the R package DESeq2 (version 1.16.1) [20]. Prefiltering of low-count genes was performed to keep only genes that have at least 50 reads in total. Principal component analysis (PCA) was used to identify outliers. For each sample, the first five principal components (PCs) were extracted and correlated with available clinical and technical data. For the CD4+ T-cell subset, age group (< 60 and ≥ 60 years), sex, HLA-DRB1*03 status (positive and negative), and RIN value were used as covariates in the analyses. The formula used for defining the model was the following:

$$Gene\,expression \sim age\,group + sex \\ + HLA-DRB1*03\,status \\ + RIN\,value + diagnosis$$

For the CD8+ T-cell subset, sex, age group (< 60 and ≥ 60 years), and RIN value were used as covariates in the analyses. The formula used for defining the model was the following:

$$Gene\,expression \sim age\,group + sex + RIN\,value \\ + diagnosis$$

Owing to possible contamination of samples with other cell types, differential gene expression analyses were performed in two stages. The analyses were performed first on all samples and second on a subset of samples excluding potential outliers. The differentially expressed genes that overlapped between the two analyses were taken as robust evidence for significant findings in order to exclude false-positive findings due to heterogeneity in the CD4+ and CD8+ T-cell subsets.

Table 1 Clinical characteristics of patients with myositis at time of blood sampling

Patient	CD4	CD8	Age (years)	Sex	Diagnosis	Autoantibodies	HLA-DRB1*03 status (genotype)	Prednisone	Other treatment
CEL-004	×		76	Female	PM, prob	PM-Scl	Positive (*03/*07)	Yes	MTX
CEL-005	×		48	Male	DM, def	SSA	Negative (*11/*11)	Yes	AZA, TAC
CEL-006	×		60	Male	PM, pos	SRP	Positive (*03/*15)	Yes	–
CEL-008	×	×	47	Male	DM, prob	MDA5	Negative (*11/*16)	Yes	AZA, ABT
CEL-009		×	80	Male	PM, def	Jo1	Positive (*03/*13)	Yes	–
CEL-010	×		74	Female	PM, prob	None	Positive (*03/*10)	No	IVIg
CEL-011	×	×	55	Female	DM, def	Mi-2	Negative (*07/*16)	Yes	MTX
CEL-014		×	74	Male	DM, def	SSA	Negative (*07/*11)	No	–
CEL-016	×		78	Male	DM, def	None	Positive (*03/*11)	Yes	MMF
CEL-017	×	×	80	Female	PM, def	None	Positive (*03/*13)	Yes	MTX
CEL-019	×		46	Female	DM, def	PM-Scl	Positive (*03/*04)	No	MTX
CEL-020	×		61	Female	PM, def	PM-Scl	Positive (*01/*03)	Yes	MMF
CEL-023	×		58	Male	DM, def	TIF1γ	Negative (*04/*07)	Yes	AZA, RIX
CEL-024	×	×	63	Female	PM, def	SSA	Positive (*03/*08)	Yes	AZA, CsA
CEL-027		×	65	Male	PM, def	Jo1	Positive (*03/*08)	Yes	–
CEL-030	×		40	Female	PM, def	Jo1	Positive (*03/*03)	Yes	–
CEL-031	×	×	68	Female	DM, def	TIF1γ	Negative (*01/*11)	Yes	–
CEL-033		×	42	Male	DM, def	MDA5	Negative (*04/*07)	Yes	MTX
CEL-034	×		56	Female	PM, def	Jo1, SSA, SSB	Negative (*11/*16)	Yes	MTX

Abbreviations: ABT Abatacept, AZA Azathioprine, CsA Cyclosporine A, Def Definite, DM Dermatomyositis, IVIg Intravenous immunoglobulin, MMF Mycophenolate mofetil, MTX Methotrexate, PM Polymyositis, Pos Possible, Prob Probable, RIX Rituximab, SRP Signal recognition particle, TAC Tacrolimus
Demographic and clinical characteristics of patients with myositis in the CD4+ (n = 15) and CD8+ T-cell subsets (n = 9) at time of blood sampling. The patients were classified according to the new European League Against Rheumatism/American College of Rheumatology classification criteria [13]

The default DESeq2 options were used, including log fold change shrinkage. We considered differentially expressed genes when the Benjamini-Hochberg adjusted p value (false discovery rate [FDR]) was < 0.05.

Functional enrichment analysis

To further understand the biological relevance and associated pathways of the differentially expressed genes, functional enrichment analysis was performed using the Gene Ontology (GO) database (released on 2 February 2018). Fisher's exact test with FDR correction (< 0.05) was used to determine significantly enriched GO biological processes.

Results

Differential gene expression in CD4+ T cells of PM and DM patients

The clinical characteristics of patients with myositis in the CD4+ T-cell subset are summarized in Table 1. No significant differences were found in patients with PM compared with patients with DM regarding disease activity measures and laboratory data (Additional file 1: Table S1 and S2).

Because PM and DM represent two similar but clinically distinct diseases, we searched for differentially expressed genes in CD4+ T cells in PM versus DM

patients. First, the whole-genome expression pattern in CD4+ T cells of PM and DM patients was examined by PCA. The first two PCs did not significantly separate between PM and DM (Fig. 1a), suggesting that, in general, the overall gene expression in CD4+ T cells from patients with PM or DM is similar. At the first analytical stage, we performed differential gene expression analysis using DESeq2 with sex, age group, *HLA-DRB1*03* status, and RIN value as covariates. Based on the cutoff criteria of Benjamini-Hochberg based FDR correction of < 0.05, 13 genes were found to be differentially expressed. Among these genes, six were expressed higher in PM patients and seven were expressed higher in DM patients (Fig. 1b and Additional file 2: Table S6).

The PCA plot shown in Fig. 1a indicates three potential outliers with a PC1 score lower than − 20. These three samples represent higher gene expression levels related to monocytes according to the xCell tool (Additional file 3: Figure S1). To exclude the possibility that the differentially expressed genes were obtained because of a difference in cell composition, at the second analytical stage, we removed the three potential outliers from the analysis. This did not affect clustering of PM and DM samples in PCA (Fig. 2a). Using the same covariates as above, four genes were found to be differentially expressed in CD4+ T cells comparing PM patients with

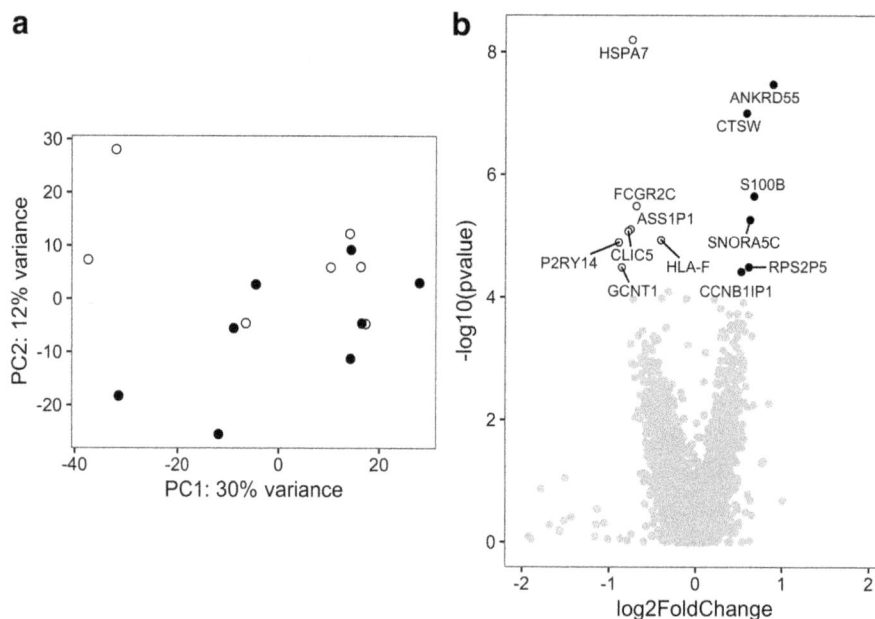

Fig. 1 Gene expression profile in CD4+ T cells of polymyositis (PM) and dermatomyositis (DM) patients. **a** Principal components (PCs) 1 and 2 plotted according to the diagnosis of the patients in a dataset of 21,008 genes ($n = 15$). Samples from patients with PM are represented by *filled circles*, and those from DM patients are represented by *open circles*. **b** Differential genome-wide transcriptomic profile for the contrast between PM and DM in CD4+ T cells. The fold changes ($\log_2$) are shown on the x-axis, and the p values ($-\log_{10}$) are shown on the y-axis. The genes that are expressed significantly higher in PM are shown as *filled circles*, and the genes expressed significantly higher in DM are shown as *open circles*. A false discovery rate threshold of 5% based on the method of Benjamini-Hochberg was used to identify significant differentially expressed genes

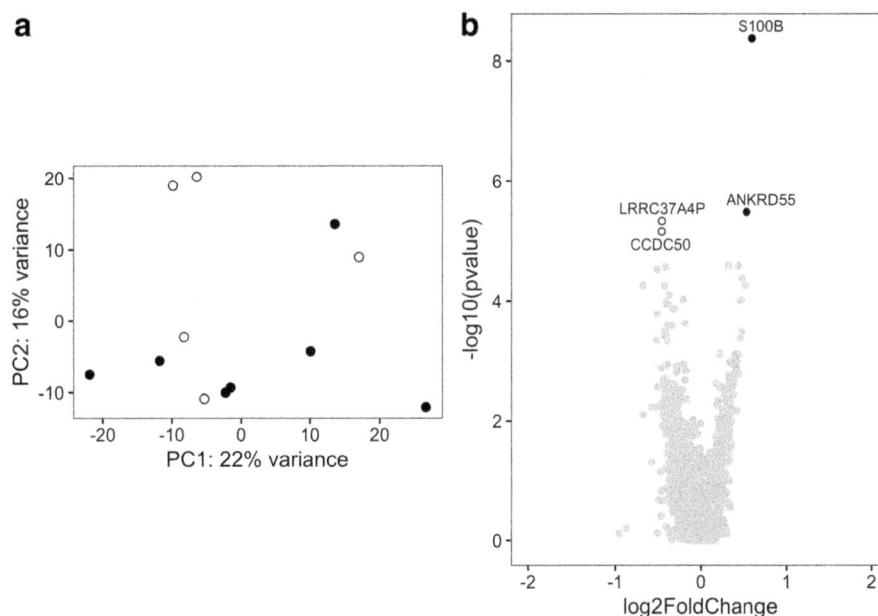

Fig. 2 Gene expression profile in CD4+ T cells of polymyositis (PM) and dermatomyositis (DM) patients excluding potential outliers. **a** Principal components (PCs) 1 and 2 plotted according to the diagnosis of the patients in a dataset of 20,091 genes ($n = 12$). Samples from patients with PM are represented by *filled circles*, and those from patients with DM are represented by *open circles*. **b** Differential genome-wide transcriptomic profile for the contrast between PM and DM in CD4+ T cells. The fold changes ($\log_2$) are shown on the x-axis, and the p values ($-\log_{10}$) are shown on the y-axis. The genes that are expressed significantly higher in PM are shown by *filled circles*, and the genes expressed significantly higher in DM are shown by *open circles*. A false discovery rate threshold of 5% based on the method of Benjamini-Hochberg was used to identify significant differentially expressed genes

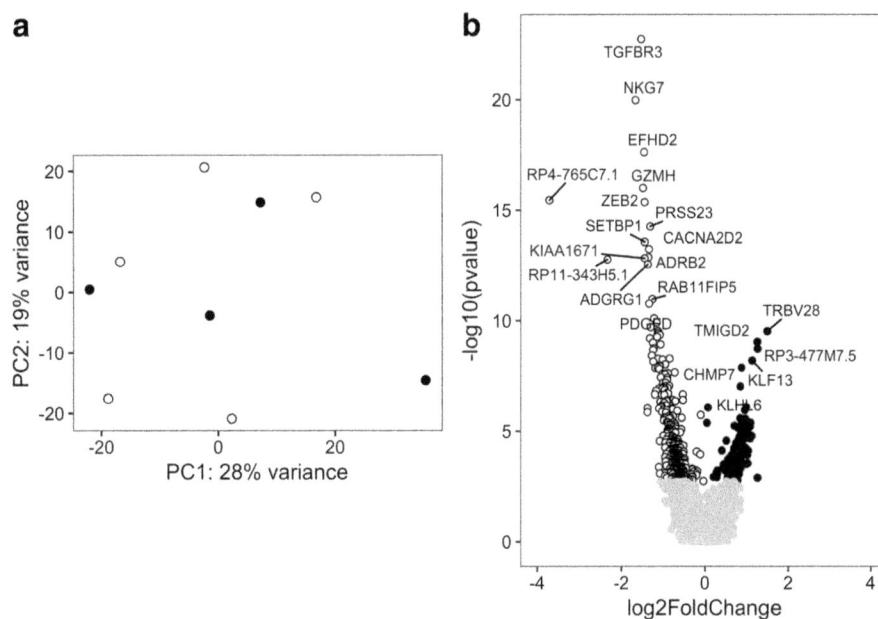

Fig. 3 Gene expression profile in CD8+ T cells of polymyositis (PM) and dermatomyositis (DM) patients. **a** Principal components (PCs) 1 and 2 plotted according to the diagnosis of the patients in a dataset of 18,696 genes ($n = 9$). Samples from patients with PM are represented by *filled circles*, and those from patients with DM are represented by *open circles*. **b** Differential genome-wide transcriptomic profile for the contrast between PM and DM in CD8+ T cells. The fold changes ($\log_2$) are shown on the x-axis, and the p values ($-\log_{10}$) are shown on the y-axis. The genes that are expressed significantly higher in PM are shown by *filled circles*, and the genes expressed significantly higher in DM are shown by *open circles*. A false discovery rate threshold of 5% based on the method of Benjamini-Hochberg was used to identify significant differentially expressed genes. The symbols of the differentially expressed genes with an adjusted p value $< 5 \times 10^5$ and $< 5 \times 10^8$ are shown for PM and DM, respectively

DM patients by applying an FDR correction cutoff of < 0.05. Two genes had a higher expression in CD4+ T cells of patients with PM compared with patients with DM, and two genes had a higher expression in CD4+ T cells of patients with DM compared with patients with PM (Fig. 2b and Additional file 2: Table S7). Thus, after accounting for possible contamination of the CD4+ T-cell population with monocytes, we considered only the genes that were found to be differentially expressed at both analytical stages. These analyses indicate that in CD4+ T cells, *ANKRD55* and *S100B* had a higher expression in CD4+ T cells of patients with PM compared with patients with DM.

Differential gene expression in CD8+ T cells of PM and DM patients

The clinical characteristics of patients with myositis in the CD8+ T-cell subset are summarized in Table 1. No significant differences were found in patients with PM compared with patients with DM regarding disease activity measures and laboratory data (Additional file 1: Table S1 and S3).

Another cell type that is commonly found in affected tissues of patients with myositis are CD8+ T cells.

Therefore, we also searched for differentially expressed genes between PM and DM in CD8+ T cells. First, the gene expression pattern in PM and DM was examined by PCA. PCA showed no clustering of PM and DM (Fig. 3a), which suggests that the overall gene expression in PM and DM is similar in CD8+ T cells. To identify genes that are differentially expressed between PM and DM, DESeq2 was used with sex, age group, and RIN value as covariates at the first analytical stage. Upon applying Benjamini-Hochberg-based FDR correction of < 0.05, we found that 588 genes were differentially expressed between PM and DM. Among these genes, 182 had a higher expression in CD8+ T cells of patients with PM patients compared with DM patients, and 406 had a higher expression in CD8+ T cells of patients with DM compared with patients with PM (Fig. 3b and Additional file 4: Table S8).

The PCA plot shown in Fig. 3a indicates one potential outlier with a PC1 score > 20. This sample clustered together with the CD4+ T-cell samples (data not shown) and was removed from the analysis at the second analytical stage. After removing this sample from the analysis, the PCA showed that the overall gene expression remained similar in PM and DM (Fig. 4a). Based on the cutoff criteria of FDR < 0.05, 308 genes were found to be

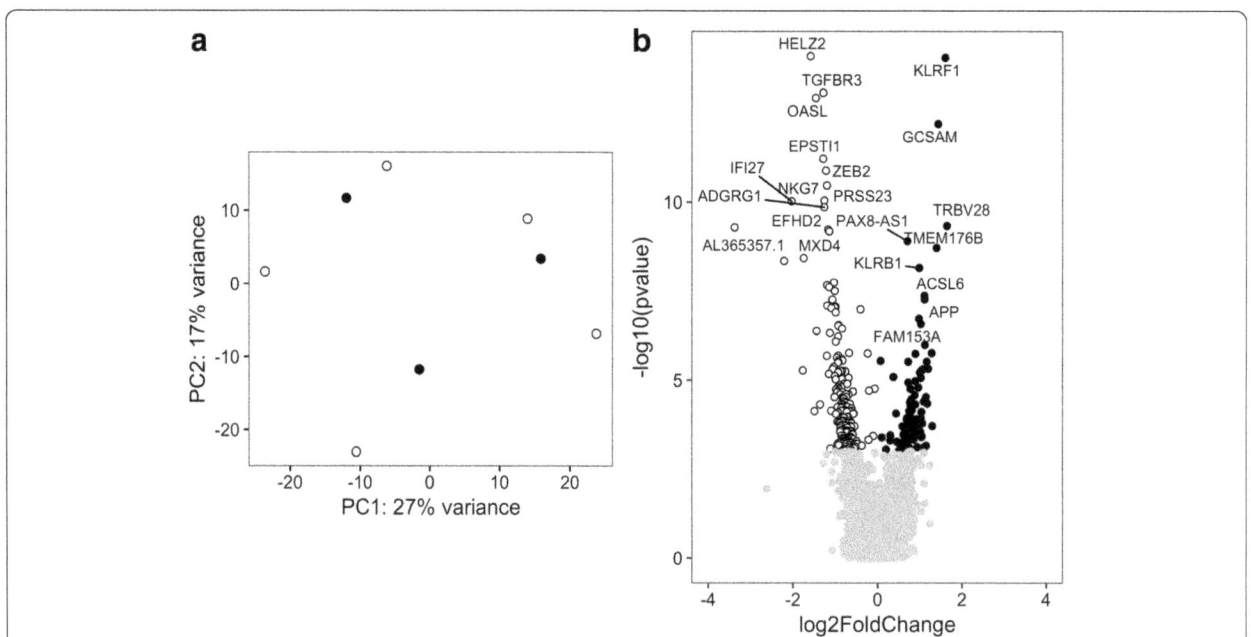

Fig. 4 Gene expression profile in CD8+ T cells of polymyositis (PM) and dermatomyositis (DM) patients excluding potential outliers. **a** Principal components (PCs) 1 and 2 plotted according to the diagnosis of the patients in a dataset of 18,289 genes (*n* = 8). Samples from patients with PM are represented by *filled circles*, and those from patients with DM are represented by *open circles*. **b** Differential genome-wide transcriptomic profile for the contrast between PM and DM in CD8+ T cells. The fold changes (log$_2$) are shown on the *x*-axis, and the *p* values (−log$_{10}$) are shown on the *y*-axis. The genes that are expressed significantly higher in PM are shown by *filled circles*, and the genes expressed significantly higher in DM are shown by *open circles*. A false discovery rate threshold of 5% based on the method of Benjamini-Hochberg was used to identify significant differentially expressed genes. The symbols of the differentially expressed genes with an adjusted *p* value < 1 × 10^4 and < 1 × 10^6 are shown for PM and DM, respectively

differentially expressed in CD8+ T cells comparing PM patients with DM patients. Among these genes, 107 genes had a higher expression in CD8+ T cells of PM patients compared with patients with DM, and 201 genes had a higher expression in CD8+ T cells of DM patients compared with PM patients (Fig. 4b and Additional file 4: Table S9).

Thus, after accounting for heterogeneity in the CD8+ T-cell subset, we considered only the genes that were found to be differentially expressed at both analytical stages. Together, a total of 44 genes were commonly expressed higher in CD8+ T cells of patients with PM compared with patients with DM (Table 2), and 132 genes were commonly expressed higher in CD8+ T cells of patients with DM compared with patients with PM (Table 3).

To identify enriched biological processes and pathways for the 176 genes that were differentially expressed between PM and DM, the GO database was used. Using Fisher's exact test with FDR correction (< 0.05), the enriched GO biological processes included lymphocyte migration and regulation of T-cell differentiation (Table 4 and Additional file 5: Table S10).

Differential gene expression in CD4+ T cells of HLA-DRB1*03-positive and -negative myositis patients

HLA-DRB1*03 haplotype is the major genetic risk factor for myositis. Therefore, we searched for differentially expressed genes between HLA-DRB1*03-positive and -negative myositis patients in CD4+ T cells. No significant differences were found in patients with HLA-DRB1*03-positive and -negative myositis regarding disease activity measures and laboratory data (Table 1 and Additional file 1: Tables S4 and S5). The gene expression pattern in HLA-DRB1*03-positive and -negative myositis was examined by PCA, but the first PCs did not separate HLA-DRB1*03-positive from HLA-DRB1*03-negative myositis patients (Fig. 5a), suggesting that these patients are similar on a high genomic level. At the first analytical stage, we performed differential expression analysis using DESeq2 with sex, age group, diagnosis, and RIN value as covariates. This resulted in eight genes that were differentially expressed between HLA-DRB1*03-positive and -negative myositis (FDR < 0.05). Of these genes, one had a higher expression in HLA-DRB1*03-positive patients with myositis, and seven had a higher expression in HLA-DRB1*03-negative patients with myositis (Fig. 5b and Additional file 6: Table S11).

Excluding the potential outliers, which represent higher gene expression levels linked to monocytes, did not affect the PCA (Fig. 6a). At the second analytical stage, we found that although HLA-DRB1*03-positive and -negative myositis are not separated by the first

PCs, 12 genes were differentially expressed in CD4+ T cells in comparison of myositis patients with different genotypes. Among these, five genes had a higher expression in CD4+ T cells from HLA-DRB1*03-positive patients with myositis, and eight genes had a higher expression in CD4+ T cells from HLA-DRB1*03-negative patients with myositis (Fig. 6b and Additional file 6: Table S12). Finally, we considered only the genes that were found to be differentially expressed at both analytical stages. PI4KAP1 was found to have a higher expression in CD4+ T cells of HLA-DRB1*03-positive patients with myositis, and TRGC2, CTSW, HPCAL4, ZNF683, and GOLGA8B were found to have a higher expression in CD4+ T cells of HLA-DRB1*03-negative patients with myositis.

Discussion

In our study, we observed significantly more differentially expressed genes in the CD8+ T-cell subset than in the CD4+ T-cell subset when comparing PM and DM patients. In CD8+ T cells, we identified 176 genes that were differentially expressed between PM and DM. In contrast, in CD4+ T cells, only two genes, ANKRD55 and S100B, were found to be differentially expressed between PM and DM. To our knowledge, this is the first study comparing transcriptomic profiles of CD4+ and CD8+ T cells between DM and PM patients. Our data align with the understanding that PM and DM have many common features but differ in genetic architecture and immunohistopathological characteristics. Our findings, together with previous observations, suggest that immune mechanisms related to subpopulations of T cells may significantly vary between these subphenotypes of myositis and also emphasize CD8+ T cells as being of interest both in patients with PM and in those with DM [10, 21, 22].

PM and DM have been modeled as subgroups of myositis in which muscle tissues are infiltrated by T cells, mainly CD8+ T cells in PM and CD4+ T cells in DM [6–9]. More recently, we have demonstrated an overlapping phenotype among the muscle-infiltrating T cells, regardless of their CD4 or CD8 lineage, in that they both display a cytotoxic signature in combination with the absence of the costimulatory CD28 receptor [10, 11]. Such differentiated T cells can also be detected in peripheral blood of patients with PM and DM, reflecting the systemic course of autoimmune disorders [10, 12].

In CD8+ T cells of PM and DM patients, 176 genes were differentially expressed. Interestingly, we noted relatively high expression of GZMH and GZMB in CD8 + T cells of DM patients compared with CD8+ T cells of PM patients. The protein encoded by GZMB is granzyme B and its secretion by CD28[null] T cells may cause

Table 2 Genes expressed significantly higher in CD8+ T cells of patients with polymyositis than in those with dermatomyositis

Gene symbol	Gene name
TRBV28	T cell receptor beta variable 28
RP3-477M7.5	
TMIGD2	Transmembrane and immunoglobulin domain containing 2
KLF13	Kruppel like factor 13
CA6	Carbonic anhydrase 6
TMTC1	Transmembrane and tetratricopeptide repeat containing 1
LINC00402	Long intergenic non-protein coding RNA 402
TRBV30	T cell receptor beta variable 30 (gene/pseudogene)
IL6R	Interleukin 6 receptor
EPHA1	EPH receptor A1
XKR9	XK related 9
GABPB1-AS1	GABPB1 antisense RNA 1
LAPTM4B	Lysosomal protein transmembrane 4 beta
EPHA1-AS1	EPHA1 antisense RNA 1
CAMSAP2	Calmodulin regulated spectrin associated protein family member 2
AC012636.1	Uncharacterized LOC101929215
RP11-28F1.2	
CHMP7	Charged multivesicular body protein 7
SYNJ2	Synaptojanin 2
KLHL6	Kelch like family member 6
PRKCQ-AS1	PRKCQ antisense RNA 1
CASP10	Caspase 10
TXK	TXK tyrosine kinase
CD27	CD27 molecule
TBC1D4	TBC1 domain family member 4
CLN5	CLN5, intracellular trafficking protein
JAML	Junction adhesion molecule like
FAM153A	Family with sequence similarity 153 member A
TNFRSF10D	TNF receptor superfamily member 10d
DHX32	DEAH-box helicase 32 (putative)
STRBP	Spermatid perinuclear RNA binding protein
AL034550.2	Uncharacterized LOC101929698
DGKA	Diacylglycerol kinase alpha
COX10-AS1	COX10 antisense RNA 1
GCSAM	Germinal center associated signaling and motility
SLC7A6	Solute carrier family 7 member 6
ACSL6	Acyl-CoA synthetase long chain family

Table 2 Genes expressed significantly higher in CD8+ T cells of patients with polymyositis than in those with dermatomyositis (Continued)

Gene symbol	Gene name
	member 6
AKAP7	A-kinase anchoring protein 7
AP005131.6	
UXS1	UDP-glucuronate decarboxylase 1
PAX8-AS1	PAX8 antisense RNA 1
C21orf33	Chromosome 21 open reading frame 33
RP11-65I12.1	
GSTM1	Glutathione S-transferase mu 1

The table demonstrates the genes that overlap between the two analytical stages and have a significantly higher expression in CD8+ T cells of patients with polymyositis than in those with dermatomyositis. A false discovery rate threshold of 5% based on the method of Benjamini-Hochberg was used to identify significant differentially expressed genes

muscle cell damage [11]. Furthermore, granzyme B cleavage sites have been identified in autoantigens, such as FHL1 and HisRS, targeted in autoimmune disorders, including myositis [23, 24]. Moreover, two T-cell receptor (TCR) beta variable genes, TRBV28 and TRBV30, had a higher expression in CD8+ T cells of patients with PM than in patients with DM. TRBV28 has been found to be one of the most common TCR variable segments in muscle tissue of myositis patients carrying the HLA-DRB1*03 allele [25]. This aligns well with the fact that in our analysis of the CD8+ T-cell subset, all PM patients are HLA-DRB1*03-positive and all DM patients are HLA-DRB1*03-negative (Table 1). The TCR beta variable genes are probably differentially expressed due to the HLA status of these patients and might reflect the expansion of pathogenic T-cell clones in this subset of patients. In addition, TGFB1, ZEB2, and SMAD7 had a higher expression in CD8+ T cells of patients with DM than in those with PM. This may suggest that transforming growth factor-β signaling [26–29] is upregulated in CD8+ T cells of DM patients compared with PM patients.

In CD4+ T cells, two genes, ANKRD55 and S100B, had a higher expression in PM than in DM. ANKRD55 encodes ankyrin repeat domain-containing protein 55, which mediates protein-protein interactions [30]. Interestingly, single-nucleotide polymorphisms in this gene have previously been associated with several autoimmune disorders, including rheumatoid arthritis [31–33], Crohn's disease [34], and multiple sclerosis [35]. A study to reveal the function of this gene in the context of immune function is pending. S100B encodes a member of the S100 protein family and is involved in the calcium-dependent regulation of a variety of intracellular activities [36]. S100B is

Table 3 Genes expressed significantly higher in CD8+ T cells of patients with dermatomyositis than in those with polymyositis

Gene symbol	Gene name
AL365357.1	Ribosomal protein S14 pseudogene 2
AL591846.1	Ribosomal protein S14 pseudogene 1
NKG7	Natural killer cell granule protein 7
TGFBR3	Transforming growth factor beta receptor 3
GZMH	Granzyme H
EFHD2	EF-hand domain family member D2
ZEB2	Zinc finger E-box binding homeobox 2
KIAA1671	KIAA1671
SETBP1	SET binding protein 1
FAM118A	Family with sequence similarity 118 member A
ADGRG1	Adhesion G protein-coupled receptor G1
ADRB2	Adrenoceptor beta 2
CACNA2D2	Calcium voltage-gated channel auxiliary subunit alpha2delta 2
PDGFD	Platelet-derived growth factor D
SH3TC1	SH3 domain and tetratricopeptide repeats 1
PRSS23	Serine protease 23
TBKBP1	TBK1 binding protein 1
AC009951.1	
RAB11FIP5	RAB11 family interacting protein 5
GNAO1	G protein subunit alpha o1
MUC16	Mucin 16, cell surface associated
RP11-107E5.2	
KIF19	Kinesin family member 19
CST7	Cystatin F
SMAD7	SMAD family member 7
LINC02086	Long intergenic non-protein coding RNA 2086
AC040970.1	Uncharacterized LOC101927963
LLGL2	LLGL2, scribble cell polarity complex component
SYNE1	Spectrin repeat containing nuclear envelope protein 1
RAP1GAP2	RAP1 GTPase activating protein 2
FAM53B	Family with sequence similarity 53 member B
TOGARAM2	TOG array regulator of axonemal microtubules 2
FRMPD3	FERM and PDZ domain containing 3
TBX21	T-box 21
SESN2	Sestrin 2
PAX5	Paired box 5
MIDN	Midnolin

Table 3 Genes expressed significantly higher in CD8+ T cells of patients with dermatomyositis than in those with polymyositis *(Continued)*

Gene symbol	Gene name
CCL5	C-C motif chemokine ligand 5
SYTL3	Synaptotagmin like 3
GAB3	GRB2 associated binding protein 3
TTC38	Tetratricopeptide repeat domain 38
LDLR	Low density lipoprotein receptor
CCL4	C-C motif chemokine ligand 4
DMWD	DM1 locus, WD repeat containing
CASZ1	Castor zinc finger 1
LAG3	Lymphocyte activating 3
DYRK1B	Dual specificity tyrosine phosphorylation regulated kinase 1B
GPR153	G protein-coupled receptor 153
MATK	Megakaryocyte-associated tyrosine kinase
SH2D2A	SH2 domain containing 2A
RHBDF2	Rhomboid 5 homolog 2
ADGRG5	Adhesion G protein-coupled receptor G5
UBE2Q2P1	Ubiquitin conjugating enzyme E2 Q2 pseudogene 1
GALNT3	Polypeptide N-acetylgalactosaminyltransferase 3
RUNX3	Runt related transcription factor 3
PLA2G16	Phospholipase A2 group XVI
SLC15A4	Solute carrier family 15 member 4
PPP2R2B	Protein phosphatase 2 regulatory subunit beta
RGS9	Regulator of G protein signaling 9
PATL2	PAT1 homolog 2
C1orf21	Chromosome 1 open reading frame 21
S1PR5	Sphingosine-1-phosphate receptor 5
TMCC3	Transmembrane and coiled-coil domain family 3
TLR3	Toll like receptor 3
GLB1L2	Galactosidase beta 1 like 2
PRELID2	PRELI domain containing 2
ADAP1	ArfGAP with dual PH domains 1
TRGJ2	T cell receptor gamma joining 2
DENND3	DENN domain containing 3
SOX13	SRY-box 13
GZMB	Granzyme B
FGFBP2	Fibroblast growth factor binding protein 2
RAP2A	RAP2A, member of RAS oncogene family
FCRL6	Fc receptor like 6
ITGAL	Integrin subunit alpha L
ABHD17A	Abhydrolase domain containing 17A
CHST12	Carbohydrate sulfotransferase 12
NBEAL2	Neurobeachin like 2

Table 3 Genes expressed significantly higher in CD8+ T cells of patients with dermatomyositis than in those with polymyositis (Continued)

Gene symbol	Gene name
ADAM8	ADAM metallopeptidase domain 8
SLC1A7	Solute carrier family 1 member 7
LTBP4	Latent transforming growth factor beta binding protein 4
CRIP1	Cysteine rich protein 1
RNF166	Ring finger protein 166
MXD4	MAX dimerization protein 4
TNFSF9	TNF superfamily member 9
ZNF683	Zinc finger protein 683
CTD-2377D24.8	
HNRNPLL	Heterogeneous nuclear ribonucleoprotein L like
MPST	mercaptopyruvate sulfurtransferase
ATP1A3	ATPase Na$^+$/K$^+$ transporting subunit alpha 3
IFNLR1	Interferon lambda receptor 1
PTMS	Parathymosin
SLC20A1	Solute carrier family 20 member 1
MVD	Mevalonate diphosphate decarboxylase
SH3RF2	SH3 domain containing ring finger 2
RAPGEF1	Rap guanine nucleotide exchange factor 1
TGFB1	Transforming growth factor beta 1
AL928654.3	
BHLHE40	Basic helix-loop-helix family member e40
MAPKAPK2	Mitogen-activated protein kinase-activated protein kinase 2
PTPRJ	Protein tyrosine phosphatase, receptor type J
DGKQ	Diacylglycerol kinase theta
MYO3B	Myosin IIIB
DUSP8	Dual specificity phosphatase 8
FLNA	Filamin A
NOP14-AS1	NOP14 antisense RNA 1
ITGB2	Integrin subunit beta 2
GNG2	G protein subunit gamma 2
MSC	Musculin
ARHGAP10	Rho GTPase activating protein 10
DNMBP	Dynamin binding protein
MYO1G	Myosin IG
DDN-AS1	DDN and PRKAG1 antisense RNA 1
SIPA1	Signal-induced proliferation-associated 1
AC093616.1	Anaphase-promoting complex subunit 1-like
CTSW	Cathepsin W
PXN	Paxillin
SSBP3	Single-stranded DNA binding protein 3
SLC2A1	Solute carrier family 2 member 1

Table 3 Genes expressed significantly higher in CD8+ T cells of patients with dermatomyositis than in those with polymyositis (Continued)

Gene symbol	Gene name
MCOLN2	Mucolipin 2
NAA50	N(alpha)-acetyltransferase 50, NatE catalytic subunit
RDH10	Retinol dehydrogenase 10
NFATC2	Nuclear factor of activated T cells 2
KDM4B	Lysine demethylase 4B
GALNT10	Polypeptide N-acetylgalactosaminyltransferase 10
DPY19L1P1	DPY19L1 pseudogene 1
INSIG1	Insulin induced gene 1
PLEKHA2	Pleckstrin homology domain containing A2
PROK2	Prokineticin 2
PTP4A2	Protein tyrosine phosphatase type IVA, member 2
GPR27	G protein-coupled receptor 27
LINC00355	Long intergenic non-protein coding RNA 355

The table demonstrates the genes that overlap between the two analytical stages and have a significantly higher expression in CD8+ T cells of patients with dermatomyositis than in those with polymyositis. A false discovery rate threshold of 5% based on the method of Benjamini-Hochberg was used to identify significant differentially expressed genes

detected in CD8+ T cells and natural killer (NK) cells, but not in CD4+ T cells [37]. This, together with low levels of *S100B* observed in CD4+ T cells in our study, may suggest either that *S100B* expression is evidence of contamination by other cell types or that this expression is characteristic of CD4+ T cells in PM. In any scenario, these data will need replication in an independent group of patients.

The *HLA-DRB1*03* haplotype is strongly associated with IIM, especially with PM [2, 38]. We made an effort to investigate how IIM patients with and without this genetic risk factor are different in their transcriptomic profiles in CD4+ T cells. Six genes were differentially expressed in CD4+ T cells of *HLA-DRB1*03*-positive compared with *HLA-DRB1*03*-negative myositis patients. We found that *PI4KAP1* had a higher expression in CD4+ T cells of *HLA-DRB1*03*-positive myositis and that *TRGC2*, *CTSW*, *HPCAL4*, *ZNF683*, and *GOLGA8B* had a higher expression in CD4+ T cells of *HLA-DRB1*03*-negative myositis patients. Interestingly, we found that *ZNF683* also had a higher expression in CD8+ T cells of *HLA-DRB1*03*-negative myositis patients when comparing PM and DM, suggesting that the expression of *ZNF683* is common for both subpopulations of T cells. ZNF683 is upregulated in T cells with cytotoxic characteristics [39] and is involved in the transcriptional regulation of effector functions, such as production of interferon-γ and granzyme B [40, 41]. *CTSW* encodes a protein of the cathepsin family,

Table 4 Significant Gene Ontology (GO) biological processes in CD8+ T cells of polymyositis and dermatomyositis patients

GO biological process complete	Fold enrichment	p value	FDR
Lymphocyte migration (GO:0072676)	11.50	1.05E-04	4.19E-02
Regulation of T-cell differentiation (GO:0045580)	10.10	4.82E-07	2.50E-03
Regulation of lymphocyte differentiation (GO:0045619)	8.31	2.24E-06	3.88E-03
Myeloid leukocyte migration (GO:0097529)	8.17	1.26E-04	4.69E-02
Response to transforming growth factor beta (GO:0071559)	6.73	1.11E-04	4.31E-02
Regulation of leukocyte differentiation (GO:1902105)	5.48	2.05E-05	1.68E-02
Regulation of T cell activation (GO:0050863)	5.26	4.48E-06	6.34E-03
Leukocyte migration (GO:0050900)	5.04	2.79E-06	4.35E-03
Positive regulation of GTPase activity (GO:0043547)	4.42	1.10E-05	1.15E-02
Positive regulation of cell adhesion (GO:0045785)	4.26	3.41E-05	2.41E-02
Positive regulation of MAPK cascade (GO:0043410)	3.85	1.11E-05	1.08E-02
Regulation of GTPase activity (GO:0043087)	3.75	5.71E-05	3.18E-02
Regulation of cell activation (GO:0050865)	3.54	2.88E-05	2.24E-02
Regulation of leukocyte activation (GO:0002694)	3.51	5.87E-05	3.05E-02
Transmembrane receptor protein tyrosine kinase signaling pathway (GO:0007169)	3.47	1.21E-04	4.61E-02
Regulation of MAPK cascade (GO:0043408)	3.42	6.96E-06	8.34E-03
Regulation of cell adhesion (GO:0030155)	3.27	6.93E-05	3.27E-02
Enzyme linked receptor protein signaling pathway (GO:0007167)	3.08	7.94E-05	3.53E-02
Cell migration (GO:0016477)	2.91	3.48E-05	2.35E-02
Positive regulation of immune system process (GO:0002684)	2.88	9.42E-06	1.05E-02
Regulation of immune system process (GO:0002682)	2.75	2.77E-07	2.16E-03
Positive regulation of intracellular signal transduction (GO:1902533)	2.75	4.75E-05	2.84E-02
Regulation of immune response (GO:0050776)	2.70	3.87E-05	2.51E-02
Positive regulation of catalytic activity (GO:0043085)	2.45	3.19E-05	2.36E-02
Immune response (GO:0006955)	2.41	5.32E-06	6.91E-03
Cell surface receptor signaling pathway (GO:0007166)	2.31	5.02E-07	1.95E-03
Positive regulation of signal transduction (GO:0009967)	2.31	6.66E-05	3.24E-02
Positive regulation of molecular function (GO:0044093)	2.24	7.60E-05	3.48E-02
Regulation of intracellular signal transduction (GO:1902531)	2.22	3.92E-05	2.44E-02
Immune system process (GO:0002376)	2.21	8.12E-07	2.11E-03
Regulation of multicellular organismal development (GO:2000026)	2.15	8.34E-05	3.61E-02
Positive regulation of response to stimulus (GO:0048584)	2.14	1.65E-05	1.51E-02
Regulation of catalytic activity (GO:0050790)	2.12	1.83E-05	1.59E-02
Regulation of signal transduction (GO:0009966)	2.01	2.08E-06	4.05E-03
Regulation of developmental process (GO:0050793)	2.00	5.79E-05	3.11E-02
Regulation of signaling (GO:0023051)	2.00	5.40E-07	1.68E-03
Regulation of cell communication (GO:0010646)	1.99	8.44E-07	1.88E-03
Regulation of response to stimulus (GO:0048583)	1.91	2.14E-07	3.33E-03
Regulation of multicellular organismal process (GO:0051239)	1.91	6.12E-05	3.08E-02
Regulation of molecular function (GO:0065009)	1.84	8.55E-05	3.60E-02
Signaling (GO:0023052)	1.58	5.65E-05	3.26E-02
Cell communication (GO:0007154)	1.55	9.36E-05	3.84E-02

GO Gene ontology
Significant GO biological processes for the differentially expressed genes in CD8+ T cells of patients with dermatomyositis and patients with polymyositis. Fisher's exact test with false discovery rate correction (< 0.05) was used to determine significant biological processes. The genes mapped to each GO can be found in Additional file 5: Table S10

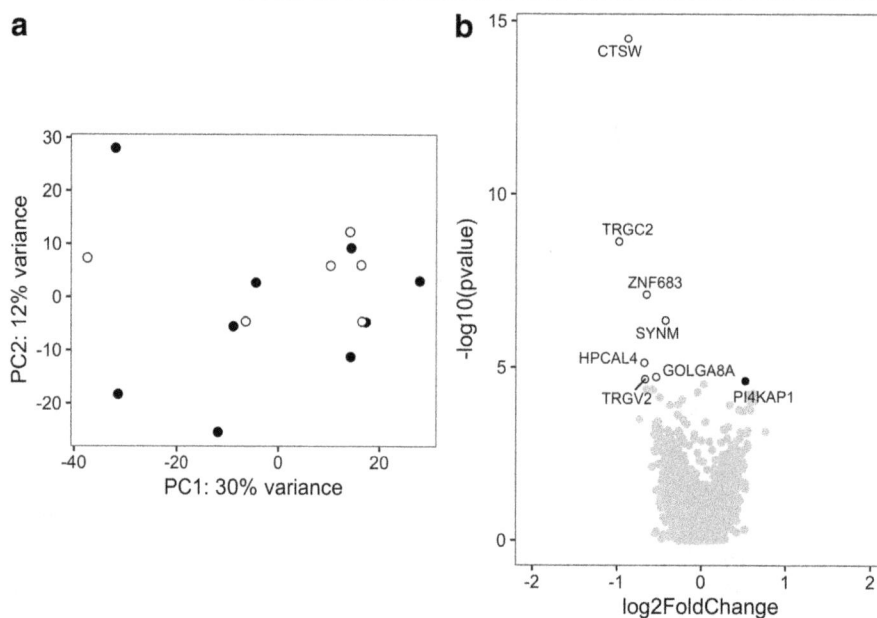

Fig. 5 Gene expression profile in CD4+ T cells of *HLA-DRB1*03*-positive and -negative patients with myositis. **a** Principal components (PCs) 1 and 2 plotted according to the *HLA-DRB1*03* status of the patients in a dataset of 21,008 genes (*n* = 15). Samples from *HLA-DRB1*03*-positive patients with myositis are represented by *filled circles*, and those from *HLA-DRB1*03*-negative patients with myositis are represented by *open circles*. **b** Differential genome-wide transcriptomic profile in CD4+ T cells for the contrast between *HLA-DRB1*03*-positive and -negative patients with myositis. The fold changes (log₂) are shown on the *x*-axis, and the *p* values (−log₁₀) are shown on the *y*-axis. The genes that are expressed significantly higher in *HLA-DRB1*03*-positive myositis are shown by *filled circles*, and the genes expressed significantly higher in *HLA-DRB1*03*-negative myositis are shown by *open circles*. A false discovery rate threshold of 5% based on the method of Benjamini-Hochberg was used to identify significant differentially expressed genes

cathepsin W. Cathepsins are found in antigen-presenting cells and are involved in antigen processing [42]. Cathepsin W has been found to be exclusively expressed in CD8 + T cells and NK cells [43]. However, this does not exclude the possibility of differential expression of the transcript in other cell types.

Evidence of differentially expressed genes in whole blood and muscle tissue between various subphenotypes of myositis has been reported previously [22, 44]. These prior investigators found that several type 1 interferon-induced transcripts and proteins were expressed relatively higher in DM patients than in healthy individuals and PM patients. In our study, we did not find type 1 interferon-inducible transcripts to be differentially expressed between PM and DM patients. However, we measured gene expression levels in CD4+ and CD8+ T cells and not in interferon-producing plasmacytoid dendritic cells. In addition, most of the patients in our study were receiving prednisone and additional immunosuppressive drugs that may significantly suppress the type 1 interferon-inducible signature [45].

The limited number of patients with PM and DM, which is the major weakness of our study, did not allow us to consider contribution of autoantibody positivity in the statistical model. The majority of patients in our study had autoantibodies of different specificities (Table 1). It has been shown that anti-MDA5 antibodies are associated with DM complicated by rapidly progressive interstitial lung disease (ILD) [46]. In addition, anti-TIF1-γ antibodies have been associated with cancer-associated DM [47]. Furthermore, anti-Jo-1 antibodies are strongly associated with a clinical phenotype named anti-synthetase syndrome, characterized by ILD, arthritis, mechanic's hands, and myositis [48]. Further studies with a high number of myositis patients are needed to address correlations between transcriptomic profile and autoantibodies. Moreover, the differences in gene expression levels need to be confirmed at the protein level and in further functional studies.

Conclusions

In the current study, we analyzed, for the first time to our knowledge, the transcriptomic profiles of different subpopulations of T cells in patients with PM or DM and could demonstrate that these two clinical phenotypes differ regarding T-cell phenotypes related to gene

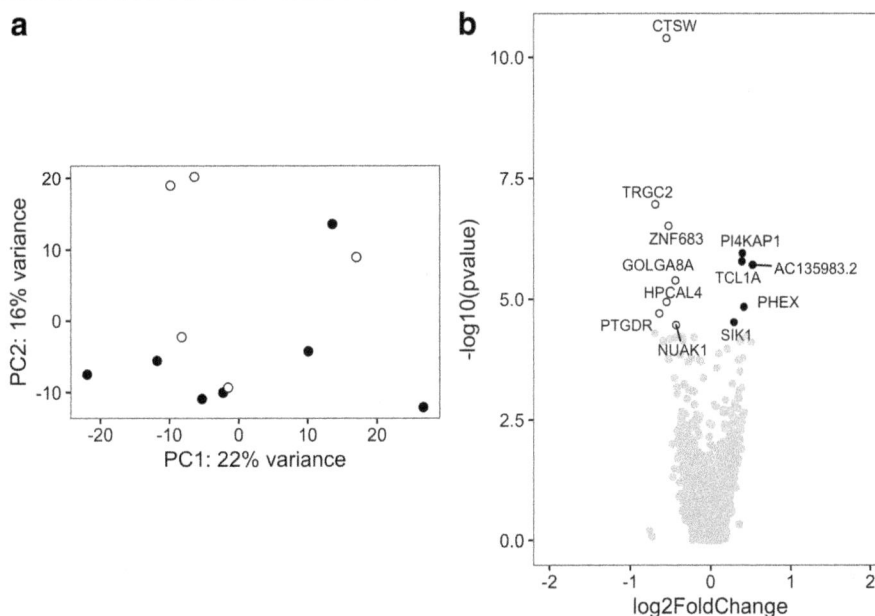

Fig. 6 Gene expression profile in CD4+ T cells of *HLA-DRB1*03*-positive and -negative patients with myositis excluding potential outliers. **a** Principal components (PCs) 1 and 2 plotted according to the *HLA-DRB1*03* status of the patients in a dataset of 20,091 genes (*n* = 12). Samples from *HLA-DRB1*03*-positive patients with myositis are represented by *filled circles*, and those from *HLA-DRB1*03*-negative patients with myositis are represented by *open circles*. **b** Differential genome-wide transcriptomic profile in CD4+ T cells for the contrast between *HLA-DRB1*03*-positive and -negative patients with myositis. The fold changes (log$_2$) are shown on the x-axis, and the *p* values (−log$_{10}$) are shown on the y-axis. The genes that are expressed significantly higher in *HLA-DRB1*03*-positive patients with myositis are shown by *filled circles*, and the genes expressed significantly higher in *HLA-DRB1*03*-negative patients with myositis are shown by *dark open circles*. A false discovery rate threshold of 5% based on the method of Benjamini-Hochberg was used to identify significant differentially expressed genes

expression. It is evident that these differences are more profound for CD8+ T cells when comparing PM patients with DM patients. Although the differentially expressed genes will need to be confirmed in a larger group of patients, these alterations in the transcriptomes of PM and DM patients suggest different immune mechanisms involved in different subphenotypes of IIM.

Additional files

Additional file 1: Additional clinical characteristics of patients included in this study. Tables S1–S3 provide additional clinical characteristics of patients included in this study regarding PM and DM. Table S1 includes all patients, whereas, Tables S2 and S3 contain the data for the CD4+ and CD8+ T-cell subsets, respectively. Tables S4 and S5 provide additional clinical characteristics of patients included in this study regarding *HLA-DRB1*03* status. Table S4 includes all patients, whereas Table S5 contains

Additional file 2: Differentially expressed genes for CD4+ T cells of PM and DM patients. Table S6 and S7 provide differentially expressed genes for CD4+ T cells of PM and DM patients at analytical stage 1 (including potential outliers) and analytical stage 2 (excluding potential outliers),

Additional file 3: Clustering heat map showing cellular heterogeneity in CD4+ and CD8+ T-cell subsets. Figure S1 shows a clustering heat map indicating cellular heterogeneity in CD4+ and CD8+ T-cell subsets, which indicates minor contamination of other cell types in these subsets.

Additional file 4: Differentially expressed genes for CD8+ T cells of PM and DM patients. Tables S8 and S9 provide differentially expressed genes for CD8+ T cells of PM and DM patients at analytical stage 1 (including potential outliers) and analytical stage 2 (excluding potential outliers),

Additional file 5: Gene Ontology biological processes for the differentially expressed genes in CD8+ T cells of PM and DM patients. Table S10 shows the genes mapped to the enriched GO biological processes for the differentially expressed genes in CD8+ T cells of PM

Additional file 6: Differentially expressed genes in CD4+ T cells of *HLA-DRB1*03*-positive and -negative myositis patients. Table S11 and S12 provide differentially expressed genes for CD4+ T cells of *HLA-DRB1*03*-positive and -negative myositis patients at analytical stage 1 (including potential outliers) and analytical stage 2 (excluding potential outliers),

Abbreviations
DM: Dermatomyositis; FDR: False discovery rate; GO: Gene Ontology; IIM: Idiopathic inflammatory myopathy; ILD: Interstitial lung disease; NK: Natural killer; PBMC: Peripheral blood mononuclear cell; PC: Principal component; PCA: Principal component analysis; PM: Polymyositis; RIN: RNA integrity number; SNP: Single-nucleotide polymorphism; TCR: T-cell receptor; TGF: Transforming growth factor

Acknowledgements
We are very thankful to Dr. Yvonne Sundström, Dr. Danika Schepis, and Dr. Louise Berg for running flow cytometry on sorted cell populations. We thank Dr. Z. E. Betteridge (RNA and protein immunoprecipitation) and Prof. J. Rönnelid (line immunoassay) for their collaboration in autoantibody detection. Transcriptomic profiling was performed by the SNP&SEQ Technology Platform in Uppsala. This facility is part of the National Genomics

Infrastructure (NGI) Sweden and Science for Life Laboratory. The SNP&SEQ Technology Platform is also supported by the Swedish Research Council and the Knut and Alice Wallenberg Foundation. The computations were performed on resources provided by SNIC through Uppsala Multidisciplinary Center for Advanced Computational Science (UPPMAX), supported by NGI Sweden.

Funding
This study was supported by a collaborative grant between the Mayo Clinic and Karolinska Institutet, the Swedish Research Council, the Swedish Rheumatism Association, King Gustaf V's 80-year foundation, and the regional agreement on medical training and clinical research (ALF) between Stockholm County Council and Karolinska Institutet.

Authors' contributions
MH, LE, AMR, IEL, and LP were involved with the conception and design of the present study. LE and IEL provided clinical data. MH and EH performed the experiments. MH analyzed and interpreted the data. LE, KC, VM, IEL, and LP contributed to the interpretation of the results. MH and LP drafted the manuscript. All authors reviewed and edited the manuscript. All authors read and approved the final manuscript.

Consent for publication
Not applicable.

Competing interests
The authors declare that they have no competing interests.

Author details
[1]Division of Rheumatology, Department of Medicine, Karolinska Institutet, Karolinska University Hospital, Stockholm, Sweden. [2]Department of Pediatrics, Duke Children's Hospital, Duke University Medical Center, Durham, USA.

References
1. Dalakas MC, Hohlfeld R. Polymyositis and dermatomyositis. Lancet. 2003;362: 971–82.
2. Rothwell S, Cooper RG, Lundberg IE, Miller FW, Gregersen PK, Bowes J, et al. Dense genotyping of immune-related loci in idiopathic inflammatory myopathies confirms HLA alleles as the strongest genetic risk factor and suggests different genetic background for major clinical subgroups. Ann Rheum Dis. 2016;75:1558–66.
3. Hirsch TJ, Enlow RW, Bias WB, Arnett FC. HLA-D related (DR) antigens in various kinds of myositis. Hum Immunol. 1981;3:181–6.
4. O'Hanlon TP, Carrick DM, Arnett FC, Reveille JD, Carrington M, Gao X, et al. Immunogenetic risk and protective factors for the idiopathic inflammatory myopathies: distinct HLA-A, -B, -Cw, -DRB1 and -DQA1 allelic profiles and motifs define clinicopathologic groups in Caucasians. Medicine. 2005;84: 338–49.
5. Ghirardello A, Bassi N, Palma L, Borella E, Domeneghetti M, Punzi L, et al. Autoantibodies in polymyositis and dermatomyositis. Curr Rheumatol Rep. 2013;15:335.
6. Arahata K, Engel AG. Monoclonal antibody analysis of mononuclear cells in myopathies. I: quantitation of subsets according to diagnosis and sites of accumulation and demonstration and counts of muscle fibers invaded by T cells. Ann Neurol. 1984;16:193–208.
7. Engel AG, Arahata K. Monoclonal antibody analysis of mononuclear cells in myopathies. II: phenotypes of autoinvasive cells in polymyositis and inclusion body myositis. Ann Neurol. 1984;16:209–15.
8. Goebels N, Michaelis D, Engelhardt M, Huber S, Bender A, Pongratz D, et al. Differential expression of perforin in muscle-infiltrating T cells in polymyositis and dermatomyositis. J Clin Invest. 1996;97:2905 10.
9. Orimo S, Koga R, Goto K, Nakamura K, Arai M, Tamaki M, et al. Immunohistochemical analysis of perforin and granzyme a in inflammatory myopathies. Neuromuscul Disord. 1994;4:219–26.
10. Fasth AER, Dastmalchi M, Rahbar A, Salomonsson S, Pandya JM, Lindroos E, et al. T cell infiltrates in the muscles of patients with dermatomyositis and polymyositis are dominated by CD28[null] T cells. J Immunol. 2009;183:4792–9.
11. Pandya JM, Venalis P, Al-Khalili L, Hossain MS, Stache V, Lundberg IE, et al. CD4[+] and CD8[+] CD28[null] T cells are cytotoxic to autologous muscle cells in patients with polymyositis. Arthritis Rheumatol. 2016;68:2016–26.
12. Benveniste O, Chérin P, Maisonobe T, Merat R, Chosidow O, Mouthon L, et al. Severe perturbations of the blood T cell repertoire in polymyositis, but not dermatomyositis patients. J Immunol. 2001;167:3521–9.
13. Lundberg IE, Tjärnlund A, Bottai M, Werth VP, Pilkington C, de Visser M, et al. 2017 European League Against Rheumatism/American College of Rheumatology classification criteria for adult and juvenile idiopathic inflammatory myopathies and their major subgroups. Ann Rheum Dis. 2017; 76:1955–64.
14. Bohan A, Peter JB. Polymyositis and dermatomyositis (first of two parts). N Engl J Med. 1975;292:344–7.
15. Bohan A, Peter JB. Polymyositis and dermatomyositis (second of two parts). N Engl J Med. 1975;292:403–7.
16. Olerup O, Zetterquist H. HLA-DR typing by PCR amplification with sequence-specific primers (PCR-SSP) in 2 hours: an alternative to serological DR typing in clinical practice including donor-recipient matching in cadaveric transplantation. Tissue Antigens. 1992;39:225–35.
17. Dobin A, Davis CA, Schlesinger F, Drenkow J, Zaleski C, Jha S, et al. STAR: ultrafast universal RNA-seq aligner. Bioinformatics. 2013;29:15–21.
18. Aran D, Hu Z, Butte AJ. xCell: digitally portraying the tissue cellular heterogeneity landscape. Genome Biol. 2017;18:220.
19. Patro R, Duggal G, Love MI, Irizarry RA, Kingsford C. Salmon: fast and bias-aware quantification of transcript expression using dual-phase inference. Nat Methods. 2017;14:417–9.
20. Love MI, Huber W, Anders S. Moderated estimation of fold change and dispersion for RNA-seq data with DESeq2. Genome Biol. 2014;15:550.
21. Szodoray P, Alex P, Knowlton N, Centola M, Dozmorov I, Csipo I, et al. Idiopathic inflammatory myopathies, signified by distinctive peripheral cytokines, chemokines and the TNF family members B-cell activating factor and a proliferation inducing ligand. Rheumatology (Oxford). 2010;49:1867–77.
22. Greenberg SA, Sanoudou D, Haslett JN, Kohane IS, Kunkel LM, Beggs AH, et al. Molecular profiles of inflammatory myopathies. Neurology. 2002;59:1170–82.
23. Albrecht I, Wick C, Hallgren Å, Tjärnlund A, Nagaraju K, Andrade F, et al. Development of autoantibodies against muscle-specific FHL1 in severe inflammatory myopathies. J Clin Invest. 2015;125:4612–24.
24. Levine Stuart M, Raben N, Xie D, Askin Frederic B, Tuder R, Mullins M, et al. Novel conformation of histidyl–transfer RNA synthetase in the lung. Arthritis Rheum. 2007;56:2729–39.
25. Englund P, Wahlström K, Fathi M, Rasmussen E, Grunewald J, Tornling G, et al. Restricted T cell receptor BV gene usage in the lungs and muscles of patients with idiopathic inflammatory myopathies. Arthritis Rheum. 2007;56: 372–83.
26. Confalonieri P, Bernasconi P, Cornelio F, Mantegazza R. Transforming growth factor-β1 in polymyositis and dermatomyositis correlates with fibrosis but not with mononuclear cell infiltrate. J Neuropathol Exp Neurol. 1997;56:479–84.
27. Dominguez CX, Amezquita RA, Guan T, Marshall HD, Joshi NS, Kleinstein SH, et al. The transcription factors ZEB2 and T-bet cooperate to program cytotoxic T cell terminal differentiation in response to LCMV viral infection. J Exp Med. 2015;212:2041–56.
28. Omilusik KD, Best JA, Yu B, Goossens S, Weidemann A, Nguyen JV, et al. Transcriptional repressor ZEB2 promotes terminal differentiation of CD8+ effector and memory T cell populations during infection. J Exp Med. 2015; 212:2027–39.
29. Verschueren K, Remacle JE, Collart C, Kraft H, Baker BS, Tylzanowski P, et al. SIP1, a novel zinc finger/homeodomain repressor, interacts with Smad

proteins and binds to 5'-CACCT sequences in candidate target genes. J Biol Chem. 1999;274:20489–98.

30. Li J, Mahajan A, Tsai MD. Ankyrin repeat: a unique motif mediating protein-protein interactions. Biochemistry. 2006;45:15168–78.

31. Stahl EA, Raychaudhuri S, Remmers EF, Xie G, Eyre S, Thomson BP, et al. Genome-wide association study meta-analysis identifies seven new rheumatoid arthritis risk loci. Nat Genet. 2010;42:508–14.

32. Okada Y, Wu D, Trynka G, Raj T, Terao C, Ikari K, et al. Genetics of rheumatoid arthritis contributes to biology and drug discovery. Nature. 2014;506:376–81.

33. Eyre S, Bowes J, Diogo D, Lee A, Barton A, Martin P, et al. High density genetic mapping identifies new susceptibility loci for rheumatoid arthritis. Nat Genet. 2012;44:1336–40.

34. Jostins L, Ripke S, Weersma RK, Duerr RH, McGovern DP, Hui KY, et al. Host-microbe interactions have shaped the genetic architecture of inflammatory bowel disease. Nature. 2012;491:119–24.

35. Alloza I, Otaegui D, de Lapuente AL, Antigüedad A, Varadé J, Núñez C, et al. ANKRD55 and DHCR7 are novel multiple sclerosis risk loci. Genes Immun. 2011;13:253–7.

36. Zimmer DB, Cornwall EH, Landar A, Song W. The S100 protein family: history, function, and expression. Brain Res Bull. 1995;37:417–29.

37. Steiner J, Marquardt N, Pauls I, Schiltz K, Rahmoune H, Bahn S, et al. Human CD8+ T cells and NK cells express and secrete S100B upon stimulation. Brain Behav Immun. 2011;25:1233–41.

38. Miller FW, Chen W, O'Hanlon TP, Cooper RG, Vencovsky J, Rider LG, et al. Genome-wide association study identifies HLA 8.1 ancestral haplotype alleles as major genetic risk factors for myositis phenotypes. Genes Immun. 2015;16:470–80.

39. Oja AE, Vieira Braga FA, Remmerswaal EBM, Kragten NAM, Hertoghs KML, Zuo J, et al. The transcription factor Hobit identifies human cytotoxic CD4+ T cells. Front Immunol. 2017;8:325.

40. Mackay LK, Minnich M, Kragten NAM, Liao Y, Nota B, Seillet C, et al. Hobit and Blimp1 instruct a universal transcriptional program of tissue residency in lymphocytes. Science. 2016;352:459–63.

41. van Gisbergen KPJM, Kragten NAM, Hertoghs KML, Wensveen FM, Jonjic S, Hamann J, et al. Mouse Hobit is a homolog of the transcriptional repressor Blimp-1 that regulates NKT cell effector differentiation. Nat Immunol. 2012; 13:864–71.

42. Hsing L C, Rudensky AY. The lysosomal cysteine proteases in MHC class II antigen presentation. Immunol Rev. 2005;207:229–41.

43. Stoeckle C, Gouttefangeas C, Hammer M, Weber E, Melms A, Tolosa E. Cathepsin W expressed exclusively in CD8+ T cells and NK cells, is secreted during target cell killing but is not essential for cytotoxicity in human CTLs. Exp Hematol. 2009;37:266–75.

44. Walsh RJ, Kong SW, Yao Y, Jallal B, Kiener PA, Pinkus JL, et al. Type I interferon–inducible gene expression in blood is present and reflects disease activity in dermatomyositis and polymyositis. Arthritis Rheum. 2007; 56:3784–92.

45. de Jong TD, Vosslamber S, Blits M, Wolbink G, Nurmohamed MT, van der Laken CJ, et al. Effect of prednisone on type I interferon signature in rheumatoid arthritis: consequences for response prediction to rituximab. Arthritis Res Ther. 2015;17:78.

46. Cao H, Pan M, Kang Y, Xia Q, Li X, Zhao X, et al. Clinical manifestations of dermatomyositis and clinically amyopathic dermatomyositis patients with positive expression of anti–melanoma differentiation–associated gene 5 antibody. Arthritis Care Res (Hoboken). 2012;64:1602–10.

47. Trallero-Araguás E, Rodrigo-Pendás Jose Á, Selva-O'Callaghan A, Martínez-Gómez X, Bosch X, Labrador-Horrillo M, et al. Usefulness of anti-p155 autoantibody for diagnosing cancer-associated dermatomyositis: a systematic review and meta-analysis. Arthritis Rheum. 2012;64:523–32.

48. Fathi M, Dastmalchi M, Rasmussen E, Lundberg I, Tornling G. Interstitial lung disease, a common manifestation of newly diagnosed polymyositis and dermatomyositis. Ann Rheum Dis. 2004;63:297–301.

11

Functional intraepithelial lymphocyte changes in inflammatory bowel disease and spondyloarthritis have disease specific correlations with intestinal microbiota

Emilie H. Regner[1,4†], Neha Ohri[2,4†], Andrew Stahly[2], Mark E. Gerich[1,4], Blair P. Fennimore[1,4], Diana Ir[3], Widian K. Jubair[2,4], Carsten Görg[6], Janet Siebert[6], Charles E. Robertson[3], Liron Caplan[2,5], Daniel N. Frank[3] and Kristine A. Kuhn[2,4*] [iD]

Abstract

Background: Dysbiosis occurs in spondyloarthritis (SpA) and inflammatory bowel disease (IBD), which is subdivided into Crohn's disease (CD) and ulcerative colitis (UC). The immunologic consequences of alterations in microbiota, however, have not been defined. Intraepithelial lymphocytes (IELs) are T cells within the intestinal epithelium that are in close contact with bacteria and are likely to be modulated by changes in microbiota. We examined differences in human gut-associated bacteria and tested correlation with functional changes in IELs in patients with axial SpA (axSpA), CD, or UC, and in controls.

Methods: We conducted a case-control study to evaluate IELs from pinch biopsies of grossly normal colonic tissue from subjects with biopsy-proven CD or UC, axSpA fulfilling Assessment of SpondyloArthritis International Society (ASAS) criteria and from controls during endoscopy. IELs were harvested and characterized by flow cytometry for cell surface markers. Secreted cytokines were measured by ELISA. Microbiome analysis was by 16S rRNA gene sequencing from rectal swabs. Statistical analyses were performed with the Kruskal-Wallis and Spearman's rank tests.

Results: The total number of IELs was significantly decreased in subjects with axSpA compared to those with IBD and controls, likely due to a decrease in TCRβ+ IELs. We found strong, significant negative correlation between peripheral lymphocyte count and IEL number. IELs secreted significantly increased IL-1β in patients with UC, significantly increased IL-17A and IFN-γ in patients with CD, and significantly increased TNF-α in patients with CD and axSpA as compared to other cohorts. For each disease subtype, IELs and IEL-produced cytokines were positively and negatively correlated with the relative abundance of multiple bacterial taxa.

Conclusions: Our data indicate differences in IEL function among subjects with axSpA, CD, and UC compared to healthy controls. We propose that the observed correlation between altered microbiota and IEL function in these populations are relevant to the pathogenesis of axSpA and IBD, and discuss possible mechanisms.

Keywords: Inflammatory bowel disease, Ulcerative colitis, Crohn's disease, Spondyloarthritis, Intraepithelial lymphocytes, Microbiome

* Correspondence: kristine.kuhn@ucdenver.edu
†Emilie H. Regner and Neha Ohri contributed equally to this work.
2Division of Rheumatology, Department of Medicine, University of Colorado School of Medicine, Aurora, CO, USA
4Mucosal Inflammation Program, University of Colorado School of Medicine, Aurora, CO, USA
Full list of author information is available at the end of the article

Background

Spondyloarthritis (SpA), characterized by inflammation of vertebral and peripheral joints sometimes progressing to fusion of the sacroiliac joints, affects up to 1% of the population and includes the diseases ankylosing spondylitis (AS), psoriatic arthritis, reactive arthritis, and inflammatory bowel disease (IBD)-related SpA. While symptoms start in the second and third decade of life, there are no disease-specific biomarkers, often causing delays in diagnosis resulting in increased functional impairment and disability [1]. IBD, which is significantly associated with SpA, is characterized by relapsing and remitting intestinal inflammation and can be subdivided into Crohn's disease (CD) and ulcerative colitis (UC). Affecting up to 0.5% of the population, IBD also lacks a disease-specific biomarker and results in substantial morbidity [2]. The clinical overlap of SpA with IBD, and observations of reactive arthritis triggered by intestinal pathogens, suggest a shared pathogenesis between the two diseases, which is likely driven by genetic susceptibility and an environmental trigger provided by intestinal microbes [3].

The most frequently cited genetic susceptibility for SpA is conferred with major histocompatibility complex (MHC) class I allele HLA-B27, which is found in 85% of individuals with axial SpA (axSpA). In non-axial SpA the presence of HLA-B27 positivity is much lower. For example, in those with IBD-associated SpA, 63% are HLA-B27+ [4]. HLA-B27 positivity is thought to result in altered recognition and handling of bacterial antigens [5, 6]. Some evidence also links IL-23 receptor variants to susceptibility risk for both axSpA and IBD. IL-23 acts as a regulator of cellular immunity by promoting a T helper (Th)17 response [7], which develops at the intestinal mucosa in the presence of commensal bacteria [8]. Thus, there appears to be an association between genetic susceptibility, intestinal microbiota, and the mucosal immune response in the pathophysiology of both axSpA and IBD.

In addition to association with genes involved in altered recognition and handling of bacterial antigens, both axSpA [9–11] and IBD [12, 13] have a well-known association with dysbiosis (alteration in microbiota)—a finding that extends to newly diagnosed and untreated patients [14]. However, the effect of dysbiosis on disease onset, progression, and recurrence is unclear [12]. It is possible that dysbiosis-mediated alteration in mucosal immune cell function plays a key role in disease pathogenesis.

We have previously shown that the function of colonic intraepithelial lymphocytes (IELs) is altered by dysbiosis in mice [15]. The epithelium is the most superficial layer of the alimentary tract and as such, would be expected to be affected to the greatest degree by alterations in the microbiome. Thus, IELs serve as prime targets to study how changes in resident bacteria influence immune response. These cells have the contradictory role of tolerating colonization by resident bacteria while still mounting a prompt and robust immune response against invading pathogens [16]. Moreover, intraepithelial lymphocytosis has a well-known association with other immune-mediated diseases of the gut including lymphocytic colitis, celiac disease, autoimmune enteropathy, and allergic colitis [17, 18]. Unlike those in healthy individuals, IELs from patients with IBD do not downregulate proliferative responses of primed allogeneic peripheral blood mononuclear cells on re-challenge with antigens [19]. Thus, dysregulation of IELs may provide new insights into the influence the microbiome has on systemic and mucosal immunity.

In this study, we hypothesized that alterations in microbiota in axSpA and IBD would be associated with functional changes in colonic IELs. Specifically, we examined total number and type of IELs and individual cytokine secretion by IELs, and we completed an exploratory analysis of microbiome interaction with IELs and cytokine secretion. We found unique patterns of IEL phenotype, cytokine expression, and cytokine-microbiome interactions by disease state that begin to elucidate how the microbiome affects immunity.

Methods

Study population and design

This study utilized a case-control study design. Control participants were recruited from the routine endoscopy schedule at the University of Colorado Hospital in Aurora, Colorado from March 2015 to January 2017; these subjects were undergoing colonoscopy for colon cancer screening (at age 50 years or younger if a family history of colon cancer is present) or due to changes in bowel habits. Subjects were included only if they were negative for malignancy and inflammation on biopsies. Patients with IBD (cases) were recruited if undergoing disease activity assessment or colon cancer or dysplasia screening; only those negative for cancer or dysplasia were included in the study. Patients with AxSpA (cases) were recruited to undergo an elective flexible sigmoidoscopy ($n = 4$) or underwent colonoscopy due to symptoms of a change in bowel habits ($n = 2$). Those with change in bowel habits were only included when the endoscopic exam and colonic and ileal biopsies excluded IBD. Fifteen biopsies were taken from endoscopically non-inflamed portions of the left colon (descending, sigmoid, and rectum) so as to avoid the confounding effect of inflammation, as IEL number has previously been shown to increase in active colitis [20]. Patients were eligible if they had biopsy-proven IBD or axSpA fulfilling the 2009 Assessment of SpondyloArthritis International Society (ASAS) criteria [21]; individuals with an overlap of both IBD and

SpA were excluded, to allow for clear discrimination between cohorts. Controls were eligible if they did not have IBD or SpA and did not meet the exclusion criteria. Exclusion criteria for all groups included pregnancy, use of antibiotics within the past 14 days, current colon cancer, celiac disease, diagnosis of any rheumatologic disease (except in the axSpA group in which only a diagnosis of SpA was permitted), chemotherapy or radiation therapy for any malignancy within the past year, daily use of aspirin or non-steroidal anti-inflammatory drugs (NSAIDs) with inability to hold the drug 7 days before and after the procedure, use of anticoagulation, HIV, *Clostridium difficile* infection within the past 3 months, or evidence of inflammatory spinal or axial arthritis (post-inflammatory changes on radiographs or a diagnosis of sacroiliitis) based on chart review (except in the axSpA group).

Information about demographic characteristics, medical history, disease history, and family history were abstracted from charts. All subjects completed a questionnaire inquiring about dietary habits such as meat and fish consumption, fruit and vegetable consumption, and whole grain consumption. Patients (cases) completed questionnaires to obtain the Harvey Bradshaw Index (HBI) in CD, the Simple Clinical Colitis Activity Index (SCCAI) in UC, and the Bath Ankylosing Spondylitis Disease Activity Index (BASDAI) in axSpA. Blood was collected to measure C-reactive protein (CRP) and white blood cell count (WBC) if not measured within the past 30 days, and to test HLA-B27 status if not already performed for routine clinical care. Fecal samples were collected by cotton swab of the rectum and stored at 80 °C until analysis. During endoscopy, 15 pinch biopsies of colonic mucosa were taken from endoscopically normal-appearing colonic tissue, combined in phosphate-buffered saline (PBS) on ice, and taken to the laboratory for further processing.

All clinical investigations were conducted according to the principles expressed in the Declaration of Helsinki. The study protocol was approved by the Colorado Multiple Institutional Review Board. All patients provided written informed consent and authorization for release of personal health information. An independent safety officer was assigned and met every 12 months with the investigators to conduct safety reviews.

Analysis of IELs

IELs were harvested from tissue by vortexing the 15 pinch biopsies together in 10 mL of PBS with 1 mM EDTA for 10 min at room temperature. They were filtered through a 70-μm cell filter, centrifuged, and resuspended in 1 mL of PBS with 5% fetal calf serum. T cells were counted using a hemocytometer then divided: 200 μL for flow cytometry and 800 μl for magnetic

sorting using a modified human T cell isolation kit (StemCell Technologies, Vancouver, BC, Canada). The isolated human epithelial cells from pinch biopsies were mixed with 10 μl of human T cell enrichment cocktail (StemCell Technologies) and 2 μL biotinylated anti-CD236 (1B7, eBiosciences, San Diego, CA, USA) for 10 min at room temperature. The remaining steps of the kit protocol were then followed to complete magnetic separation. The sorted cells were again counted to corroborate with our presorted cell counts in which IELs were quantified using flow cytometry data. The flow cytometry percentages with presort counts were used to calculate IEL numbers except in the few cases (four individuals) in which the flow cytometry data were of poor quality. In those cases, the post-sort counts were used for total IEL numbers, but further T cell subsets could not be quantified.

Post-sorted IELs were mitogen-stimulated with 10 ng/mL of phorbol 12-myristate 13-acetate (PMA) and 1 ng/mL ionomycin overnight. Cytokines IL-1β, IL-6, IL-10, IL-17A, interferon (IFN)-γ, and TNF-α in the culture supernatants were measured by ELISA (Meso Scale Discovery, Rockville, MD, USA).

For flow cytometry, cells were stained for surface markers CD3 (UCHT1), CD45 (HI30), CD4 (RPA-T4), CD8α (RPA-T8), CD8β (SIDI8BEE), CD44 (IM7), CD103 (B-Ly7), TCRβ (WT31), TCRγδ (B1.1), and a viability dye (Ghost Dye™ Violet 510, Tonbo Biosciences, San Diego, CA, USA) and then fixed in 4% paraformaldehyde in PBS. Samples were run on a LSR II (Becton, Dickinson and Company Biosciences, San Jose, CA, USA) and data analyzed with FlowJo version 10.1 (Treestar, San Carlos, CA, USA).

Microbiome analysis

DNA from feces of cases and controls was extracted using a commercial kit (UltraPure Fecal DNA, MO BIO Inc., Carlsbad, CA, USA). Bacterial profiles were determined by broad-range amplification and sequence analysis of 16S rRNA genes following our previously described methods [22–25]. In brief, amplicons were generated using barcoded primers [26] that target approximately 340 base pairs of the V3 V4 variable region of the 16S rRNA gene. Illumina paired-end sequencing was performed on the Miseq platform with versions v2.4 of the Miseq Control Software and of MiSeq Reporter, using a 600 cycle version 3 reagent kit.

Illumina Miseq paired-end reads were aligned to human reference genome hg19 with bowtie2 and matching sequences discarded [27, 28]. As previously described, the remaining non-human paired-end sequences were demultiplexed [24], assembled [29, 30], trimmed (moving window of five nucleotides until average quality was met or exceeded 20), and chimera-checked with

Uchime (usearch6.0.203_i86linux32) [31] using the Schloss [32] Silva reference sequences. Trimmed sequences with more than 1 ambiguity or shorter than 250 nucleotides were discarded. Assembled sequences were aligned and classified with SINA (1.3.0-r23838) [33] using the 418,497 bacterial sequences in Silva 115NR99 [34] as reference configured to yield the Silva taxonomy. Operational taxonomic units (OTUs) were produced by clustering sequences with identical taxonomic assignments. This process generated ~ 6,000,000 high-quality 16S sequences with Goods coverage score ≥ 99% for all samples. Relative abundances for each subject were calculated by dividing the sequence count for each OTU by the total number of 16S rRNA sequences for the subject. The software package Explicet (v2.10.5, www.explicet.org) [35] was used for visualization of the data.

Statistical analysis

A total sample size of 24 was determined to have 80% power to detect an effect size of 0.75 across four groups using one-way analysis of variance (ANOVA) with a two-tailed significance of 0.05 for the primary outcome of differences in IELs between study cohorts. Variables were tested for normality using the Shapiro-Wilk test; those data not normally distributed are presented in the figures using a logarithmic y-axis. Patient demographic comparisons were made using ANOVA or Fisher's exact test to compare patients with CD, UC, and axSpA, and controls, except for medications, which were compared in the CD, UC, and axSpA groups only. The Kruskal-Wallis test with Dunn's post-hoc analysis for pairwise comparisons of significant groups was used to evaluate differences in IEL phenotype and cytokine production. Linear regression was used to test correlation between IEL characteristics and continuous variables including CRP, WBC, duration of disease, disease activity scores, and age. Fisher's exact test was utilized to test associations between IEL secretion and categorical variables such as sex, family history of autoimmunity, smoking history, diet, and TNF inhibitor (TNFi) use. The Kruskal-Wallis test was used to compare relative abundance of OTUs between study groups. Spearman's rank correlation was tested between OTUs and IEL changes that were found to be statistically significantly different between groups. Permutation-based multiple analysis of variance (PERMANOVA) was conducted using the vegan R package (Bray-Curtis Method, 10,000 permutations).

Community diversity was estimated by both the Shannon H index and Simpson inverse diversity indices. Chao1 was used to measure microbial richness and Good's coverage was used to confirm the adequacy of sequencing coverage. All tests of significance were two-sided and a p value < 0.05 was considered statistically significant. Statistical analyses were conducted with the R and SPSS (version 22; IBM, Armonk, NY, USA) statistical packages, while graphics were created using SPSS, GraphPad version 8.2 (GraphPad Software, La Jolla, CA, USA), and Excel Office Professional Plus 2013 (Microsoft, Redmond, WA, USA).

Results

Baseline characteristics

A total of 38 subjects (15 controls, 10 patients with CD, 7 patients with UC, and 6 patients with axSpA) were recruited (Table 1). There were no significant differences in baseline basic demographic features (sex, ethnicity, smoking status, family history of autoimmunity). More patients with CD (50%) or axSpA (83%) were on TNF inhibitors (TNFi) compared to patients with UC (0%, p < 0.01). As expected, patients with axSpA (83%) were more likely to be HLA-B27-positive than patients with IBD (20%) or controls (0%, $p = 0.0001$). Patients with axSpA were noted to have significantly higher leukocyte counts than patients with IBD and controls ($p = 0.02$), although the increased leukocyte count was not outside the normal range determined by the clinical laboratory. Overall, subjects with IBD had long-established disease and low disease activity at the time of their endoscopy. Patients with axSpA also had long-established disease, moderate disease activity, and more TNFi use at the time of their endoscopy.

IEL populations

The total number of IELs was significantly decreased in subjects with axSpA compared to those with IBD and controls ($p = 0.03$; Fig. 1a). When analyzed by T cell subsets, a decrease in T cell receptor (TCR)β+ IELs likely accounted for this difference ($p = 0.06$; Fig. 1b). There were trends toward reduced TCRβ+ subsets of CD4+ and CD8aa+ IELs ($p = 0.074$ and $p = 0.030$, respectively; Additional file 1: Figure S1A), but no significant differences between cohorts in total TCRγδ+ IELs (Fig. 1c) or in CD4+, CD4-CD8-, CD8αα+, and CD8αβ+ subsets of TCRγδ+ IELs (Additional file 1: Figure S1B). Nor were there significant differences between cohorts in the presence of cell markers CD44+, CD103+ (integrin αE, which mediates retention of the IEL at the epithelial surface [36]), or IL-23R (Additional file 1: Figure S1C-E). As the number of IELs could be influenced by the systemic level of lymphocytes, which were significantly higher in subjects with axSpA, we tested for correlation between IELs and peripheral blood absolute lymphocyte count in those with axSpA. To our surprise, we found strong, significant negative correlation between the peripheral lymphocyte count and IEL number in subjects with axSpA ($\rho = -0.94$, $R^2 = 0.89$, $p = 0.0047$; Fig. 1d). We did not, however, observe

Table 1 Demographic and clinical characteristics of study subjects

	Controls ($N = 15$)	CD ($N = 10$)	UC ($N = 7$)	axSpA ($N = 6$)	p value
Age in years	48.4 (9.7)	40.5 (15.2)	39.2 (12.4)	34.4 (3.3)	0.06
Female	9 (60%)	7 (70%)	3 (43%)	1 (17%)	0.18
Non-Hispanic white	15 (100%)	9 (90%)	6 (86%)	6 (100%)	0.29
Former smoker	4 (27%)	5 (50%)	1 (14%)	3 (50%)	0.34
Family history of autoimmunity	6 (40%)	3 (30%)	1 (14%)	2 (33%)	0.53
Disease duration in months	–	127.5 (107.9)	171.7 (153.9)	78.5 (58.1)	0.36
HLA-B27 positivity	0	0	1 (14%)	5 (83%)	**0.0001**[a]
WBC (10^9 cells/L)	7.2 (2.2)	6.6 (2.2)	5.5 (3.2)	9.5 (2.3)	**0.04**
Absolute lymphocytes (10^9 cells/L)	1.9 (0.1)	1.7 (0.2)	0.9 (0.1)	2.6 (0.3)	**0.004**
CRP (mg/L)	2.5 (2.5)	4.2 (3.0)	1.7 (1.7)	5.6 (12.5)	0.5
TNF inhibitor usage	–	5 (50%)	0 (0%)	5 (83%)	**< 0.01**
Prednisone usage	–	2 (20%)	0 (0%)	1 (17%)	0.5
Harvey Bradshaw Index	–	1.9 (0.526)		–	–
Simple Clinical Colitis Activity Index	–	–	0.857 (0.553)	–	–
Bath AS Disease Activity Index	–	–	–	3.96 (1.01)	–

Data are mean (SD) or number (%); p value is based on Fisher's exact test for categorical variables and on one-way analysis of variance for continuous variables.
[a]Bold text indicates significant p-values
HC healthy controls, CD Crohn's disease, UC ulcerative colitis, axSpA axial spondyloarthritis, CRP C-reactive protein, AS ankylosing spondylitis

significant correlation between IEL number and disease activity in any of our cohorts (Additional file 2: Table S1).

Because we hypothesized that subjects with axSpA and IBD would exhibit functional changes in IELs compared to control subjects, we evaluated individual cytokine secretion by IELs obtained from biopsy tissue. A few subjects had dramatically elevated levels of certain cytokines but these were not limited to the same subjects. IELs secreted significantly increased IL-1β in patients with UC as compared to other cohorts (Fig. 2a), significantly increased IL-17A and IFN-γ in patients with CD as compared to other cohorts (Fig. 2b, c), and significantly increased TNF-α in patients with CD and axSpA as compared to other cohorts (Fig. 2d). The data are shown on a logarithmic axis to demonstrate the range of cytokine values. No significant differences in IEL secretion of IL-6, IL-10, or IL-22 was detected between cohorts (Additional file 1: Figure S2).

Sex, age, race, length of disease, disease activity scores, CRP, and family history of autoimmune disease was not associated with the presence or absence of individual cytokine secretion when analyzed using linear regression (Additional file 2: Table S2). Smoking history was negatively associated with secretion of TNF-α ($p = 0.008$), and TNFi use was associated with secretion of TNF-α and IFN-γ ($p = 0.001$ and $p = 0.04$, respectively). Kruskal-Wallis analysis did not identify any significant association between cytokine levels and intake of red meat, fish, whole grains, fruits, or vegetables (Additional file 2: Table S2).

Microbiome associations

Bacterial profiling of subjects' fecal material was of sufficient depth as indicated by Good's coverage > 99% for all subjects. No difference in richness (Chao1) was noted among the three groups (Additional file 1: Figure S3A). Analysis of diversity indices showed no difference in community complexity, as measured by the mean Shannon H index (Additional file 1: Figure S3B), or in community evenness (Additional file 1: Figure S3C).

Our study was primarily powered to evaluate differences in IEL phenotypes across groups. Nevertheless, our exploratory analysis identified appreciable differences in overall microbiota composition between healthy controls and subjects with axSpA (PERMANOVA $p = 0.06$; Fig. 3a). In pairwise comparisons between healthy controls and patients with CD, UC, and axSpA we identified few significant differences as defined by $p < 0.05$ analyzed by the Wilcoxon rank-sum test. In CD there was increased relative abundance of *Carnobacteriaceae* (Fig. 3b). In healthy controls, as compared to patients with UC, the relative abundance of *Bradyrhizobiaceae* was increased (Fig. 3c). In patients with axSpA as compared to healthy controls, the relative abundance of *Rickettsiales* was increased (Fig. 3d).

We next evaluated how IELs related to specific bacteria in the setting of disease. For each subject group, total IEL number or IEL-produced cytokine level (using only those cytokines that were significantly different between subject groups) was correlated with the relative abundance of each OTU.

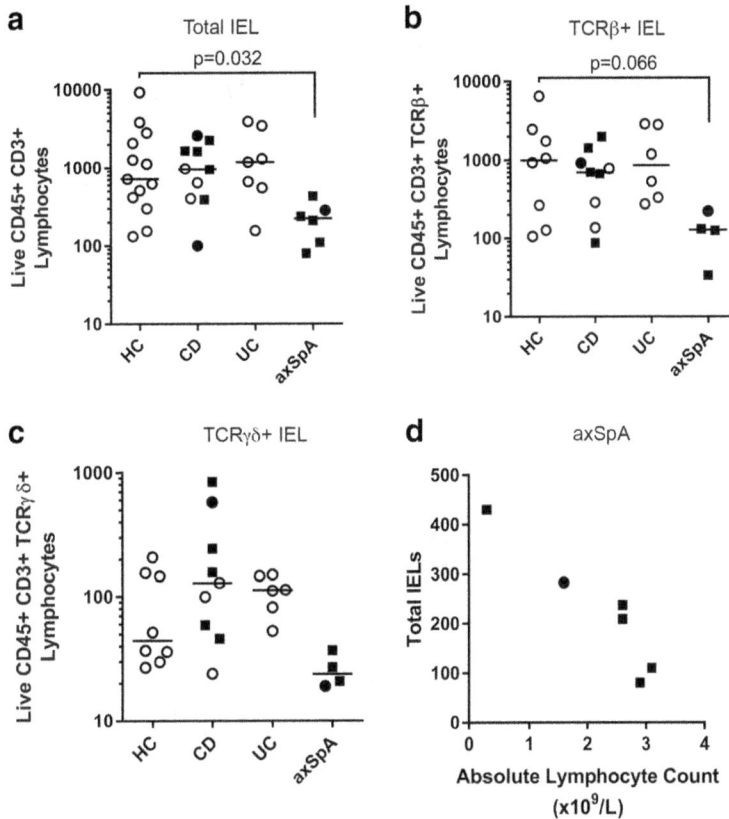

Fig. 1 Colonic intraepithelial lymphocytes (IELs) are significantly decreased in individuals with axial spondyloarthritis (axSpA) and inversely correlate with peripheral blood lymphocyte counts. IELs were obtained from colonic mucosal biopsies as described in "Methods" and evaluated by flow cytometry for the absolute number of total IELs (**a**), T cell receptor (TCR)β+ IELs (**b**), and TCRγδ+ IELs (**c**). Each dot represents an individual within the study group identified on the x-axis. A solid square indicates subjects on a TNF inhibitor, a solid dot indicates the subject was taking steroids, and an open dot indicates the subject was taking neither. Bars are the mean ± SEM. Statistical significance was determined using the Kruskal-Wallis test with Dunn's post-hoc analysis. **d** Total IELs (y-axis) in each individual with axSpA were compared to the absolute lymphocyte count (x-axis) and the Pearson's correlation coefficient was calculated ($\sigma = -0.94$, $R^2 = 0.89$, $p = 0.0047$). HC, healthy controls; CD, Crohn's disease; UC, ulcerative colitis

Within the healthy control group, we identified statistically significant positive correlation between *Eubacteriaceae*, *Victivallaceae*, *Campylobacteraceae*, *Cardiobacteriaceae*, *Neisseriaceae*, and *Pseudomonadales* and IL-17A and between *Alcaligenaceae* and *Neiseriaceae* and IFN-γ (Fig. 4). Also in the healthy control group, we identified statistically significant negative correlation between the abundances of *Deferribacteraceae* and IL-17A; between *Corynebacteriaceae* and TNF-α; and between *Dermabacteraceae*, *Sphingobacteriaceae*, *Aerococcaceae*, *Rhizobiales*, and *Rhodobacteraceae* and IFN-γ (Fig. 4). Within the CD group, there was statistically significant positive correlation between the abundances of *Victivallaceaea* and *Sphingomonadaceae* and IL-1β; between *Staphylococcaceaea* and IL-17A; between *Rikenellaceae* and TNF-α; and between *Staphylococcaceaea* and *Rikenellaceae* and IFN-γ (Fig. 4). Also in the CD group, we identified statistically significant negative correlation between the abundances of *Peptococcaceae* and IL-1β; between *Fusobacteriales* and *Comamonadaceae* and IL-17A;

between *Fusobacteriales* and TNF-α; and between *Fusobacteriales* and IFN-γ (Fig. 4).

In the group of individuals with UC, we identified statistically significant positive correlation between the abundances of *Cynanobacteria*, *Christensenellaceae*, and *Pseudomonadaceae* and IL-1β; between *Cynanobacteria*, *Bacillales*, and *Verrucomicrobiaceae* and IL-17A; between *Peptococcaceae* and TNF-α; and between *Cynanobacteria*, *Desulfovibrionaceae*, and *Pseudomonadaceae* and IFN-γ. Also in this group, there was statistically significant negative correlation between the abundances of *Streptococcoaceae* and IL-17A and between *Dermabacteraceae* and TNF-α (Fig. 4).

In axSpA we identified statistically significant positive correlation between the abundances of *Rhizobiaceae* and IL-1β; between *Corynebacteriales*, *Dermabacteraceae*, *Microbacteriaceae*, *Deferribacteraceae*, *Cynanobacteria*, *Comamonadaceae*, *Helicobacteraceae*, *Moraxellaceae*, *Rhodobacteraceae*, and *Anaeroplasmataceae* and IL-17A; between *Peptococcaceae* and *Verrucomicrobiaceae* and

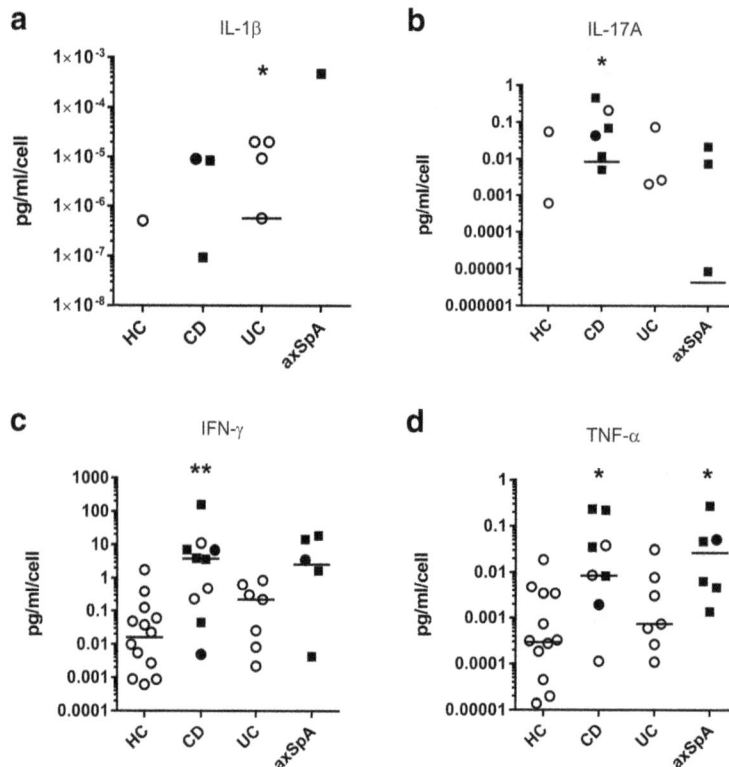

Fig. 2 Cytokines produced by intraepithelial lymphocytes (IELs) are altered in individuals with inflammatory bowel disease (IBD) and axial spondyloarthritis (axSpA). Colonic IELs were mitogen-stimulated overnight and secreted cytokines measured by ELISA. **a** IL-1β, **b** IL-17A, **c** interferon (IFN)-γ, and **d** TNF-α production in pg/ml was normalized to the number of IELs collected from each subject. Each dot represents a case/control analyzed. A solid square indicates subjects on a TNF inhibitor, a solid dot indicates the subject was taking steroids, and an open dot indicates the subject was taking neither. Subjects with undetectable cytokine levels are absent from the graphs due to the logarithmic scale as are means that fall below the axis range. Statistical differences were identified by the Kruskal-Wallis test with Dunn's post-hoc analysis for pairwise differences: *$p < 0.05$ and **$p < 0.01$. HC, healthy controls; CD, Crohn's disease; UC, ulcerative colitis; axSpA, axial spondyloarthritis

TNF-α; and between *Corynebacteriaceae*, *Microbacteriaceae*, *Aerococcaceae*, and *Bradyrhizobiaceae* and IFN-γ. In axSpA, we also identified statistically significant negative correlation between the abundances of *Bacillaceae* and *Leuconostocaceae* and TNF-α (Fig. 4).

Because we identified strong negative correlation between peripheral lymphocyte count and IELs that may suggest mucosal lymphocyte trafficking in the circulation, we queried if this could be driven by specific microbiota. When IEL numbers were compared to the relative abundance of family-level OTUs, we identified only strong negative correlation between IEL number and *Dermatophilaceae*, *Prevotellaceae*, RF16, *Deferribacteraceae*, *Clostridiaceae*, *Anaeroplasmataceae*, and RF9 (Table 2), suggesting that if IELs are trafficking, they may be stimulated by these bacteria.

Discussion

In this study we hypothesized that IEL function would vary by disease type and would be modulated by microbial milieu. Herein, we show for the first time that colonic IELs undergo functional changes in SpA and IBD.

Furthermore, we suggest that changes in the microbiome may drive the functional changes observed in colonic IELs, specifically through interactions affecting cytokine secretion as demonstrated by the unique cytokine-microbiome interactions within each disease.

Our results are in agreement with prior studies that suggested no difference in absolute IEL number in subjects with IBD as compared to healthy controls. However, one of our most interesting findings is that total IEL count is significantly reduced in axSpA. Prior studies document that IELs function to maintain epithelial homeostasis and that IELs promote epithelial barrier function through expressed cytokines, such as IL-6, in response to commensal bacteria [15, 37]. A decrease in IEL count in axSpA would be consistent with the frequently observed barrier dysfunction associated with subclinical colitis in many patients with axSpA [6].

Furthermore, we identified strong, significant, negative correlation between peripheral lymphocyte count and colonic IEL count in patients with axSpA, which may suggest IEL trafficking between blood and colon compartments in this disease, although our data do not

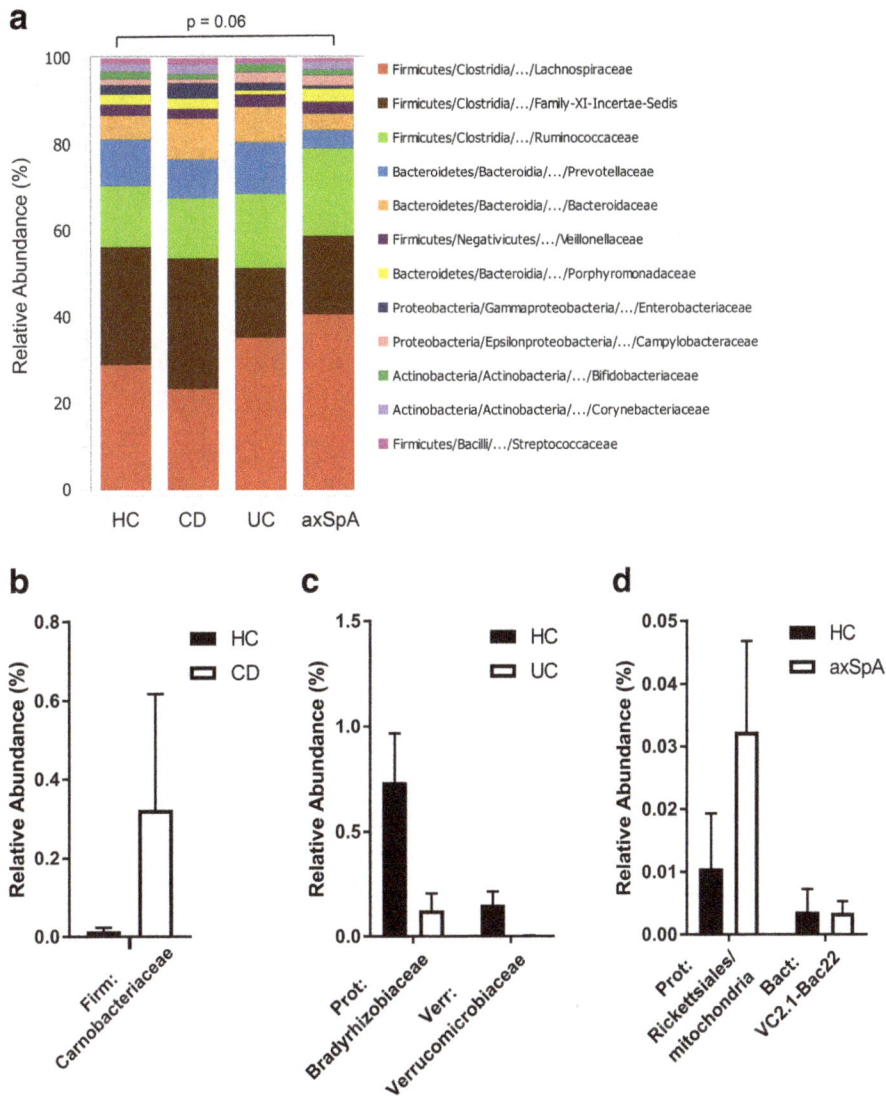

Fig. 3 Microbial community comparisons in individuals with inflammatory bowel disease (IBD) and axial spondyloarthritis (axSpA). Bacterial DNA from fecal swabs from patients (cases) and controls were sequenced for 16S rRNA and analyzed. **a** The percent abundance of the top operational taxonomic unit (OTU) families were compared across subject groups. Differences in the overall composition of microbial communities were determined by permutation-based multiple analysis of variance. **b–d** Pairwise comparisons of OTUs between disease states and controls were performed using the Wilcoxon rank-sum test. The mean relative abundance ± SEM for each OTU that was statistically significant ($p < 0.05$) is shown for Crohn's disease (CD) (**b**), ulcerative colitis (UC) (**c**), and axSpA (**d**). HC, healthy controls

confirm this hypothesis. It has been previously established that in enterogenic SpA, activated T cells originating in inflamed intestinal mucosa develop non-gut-specific adhesion ligands, including synovial ligands, leading to homing of activated T cells from gut into synovium and perpetuating joint inflammation [38, 39]. Unfortunately, our study was not designed to evaluate peripheral blood phenotypes in parallel with mucosal phenotypes. Certainly, additional studies are warranted to validate our findings and support our suggestion that IELs traffic systemically in axSpA.

Because we hypothesized that subjects with axSpA and IBD would exhibit functional changes in IELs, we examined associations between disease type and IEL-produced cytokine quantity and type. Our findings within each disease cohort suggest that IELs may contribute to disease-specific pathology. For example, IELs isolated from colonic tissue secreted significantly increased IL-1β in patients with UC as compared to other cohorts. Since expression of the pro-inflammatory cytokine IL-1β has previously been observed to be increased in mucosal cells from patients with both UC and CD [40], IELs may be an additional local contributor to disease pathogenesis. Colonic IELs secreted significantly increased IL-17A and IFN-γ within the CD cohort

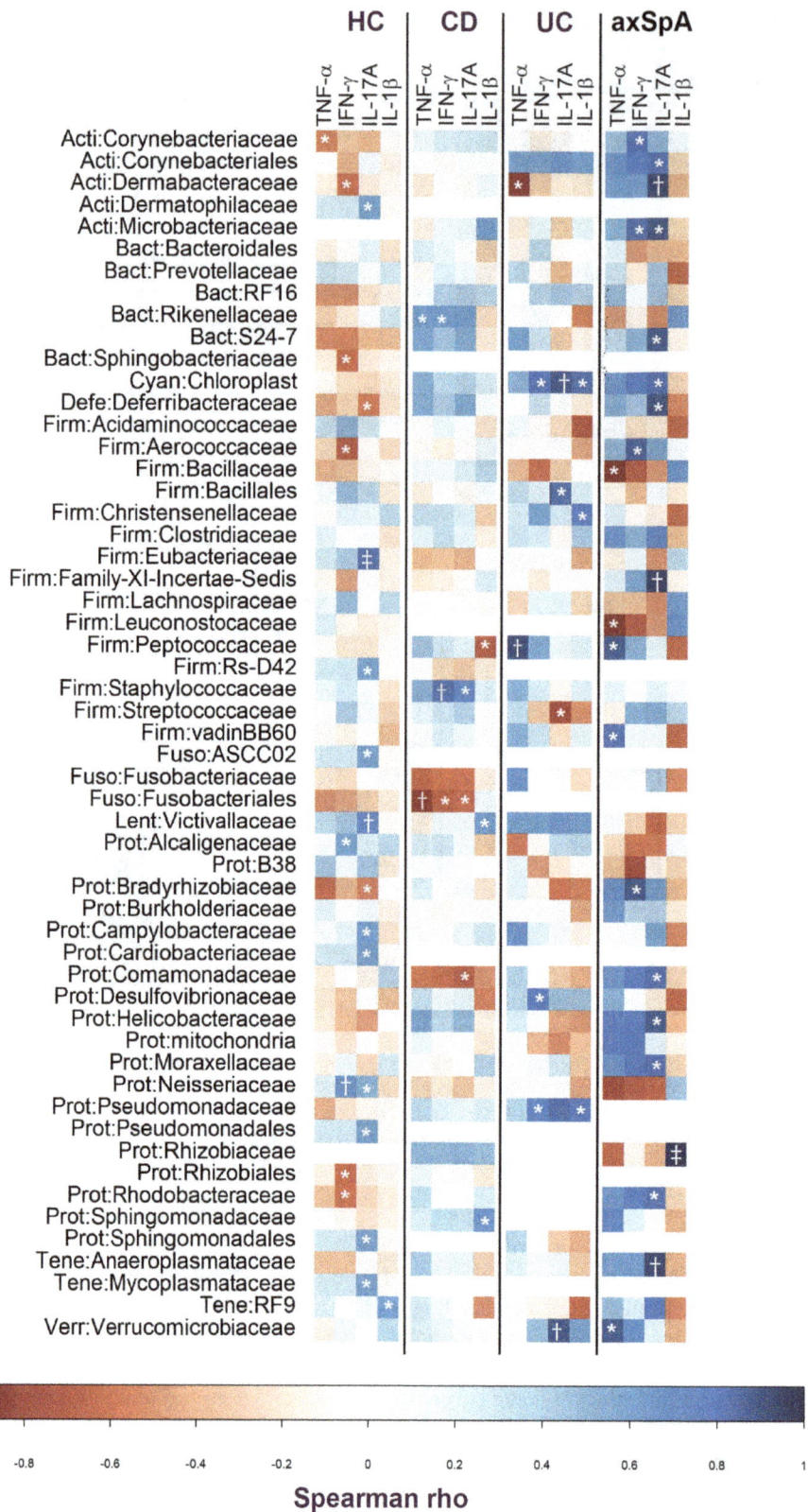

Fig. 4 (See legend on next page.)

(See figure on previous page.)

Fig. 4 There was disease-specific correlation between microbiota and intraepithelial lymphocyte (IEL) production of cytokines. Correlation between the operational taxonomic unit (out) relative abundance and the IEL-produced cytokine value in each case/control group was tested using Spearman's rank test. The data are shown as heatmaps, with the color of each correlation test corresponding to the Spearman rho value: $*p < 0.05$, $^{†}p < 0.01$, and $^{‡}p < 0.001$. HC, healthy controls; CD, Crohn's disease; UC, ulcerative colitis; axSpA, axial spondyloarthritis

compared to other cohorts. Previously published findings corroborate these findings by reporting increased gene expression of IL-17A and IFN-γ in colonic biopsies taken from patients with UC and CD compared to healthy controls [41]. Finally, in patients with CD and axSpA compared to other cohorts, colonic IELs secreted significantly increased TNF-α, which is a well-established pro-inflammatory mediator in both diseases. Thus, while IEL numbers may not be significantly different in individuals with IBD, there are IEL functional changes that may contribute to local inflammation. Because we found no relationship between age, sex, duration of disease, disease activity index, or CRP and IEL abundance or cytokine production, we suggest that alterations in microbiota found in the disease states may influence cytokine production by IELs. Of note, we did find a negative association between smoking and TNFα secretion. This finding is consistent with prior studies as it has previously been shown in rat models that TNFα expression in colonic tissue increases with exposure to cigarette smoke in a dose-dependent fashion [42]. We also noted that TNFi use was associated with increased TNFα production by IELs. TNFα production is likely a reflection of disease activity and TNFi use is presumably a marker of more active disease.

Although not powered for microbiome comparisons, our pilot microbiome sequencing data were consistent with prior studies. Specifically, we noted increased relative abundance of *Ruminococcus* in patients with SpA as compared to healthy controls, which has been previously published [10]. A trend toward decreased number of certain members of the phylum Firmicutes family *Clostridia* was also noted in SpA, as previously published [43, 44].

In the IBD group, certain members of Firmicutes (*Carnobacteriaceae*) were expanded, consistent with prior findings [45].

Our data on correlation between IEL-produced cytokines and the abundance of specific bacterial populations in the setting of IBD and axSpA provides an important link between functional mucosal consequences with changes in gut microbiome. In reviewing the strongest correlation, we note that in patients with CD, strong negative correlation was observed between *Fusobacteriales* and TNF-α. Prior research suggests that phylum Fusobacteria is increased in active CD [46]. Decreased IEL secretion of TNF-α in the setting of increased Fusobacteria and active inflammation could constitute a protective response. In patients with UC, we identified positive correlation between different families within *Firmicutes* (*Chistensenellaceae*) and *Proteobacteria* (*Pseudomonadaceae*) and increased IEL secretion of IL-1β. Prior studies have suggest increased abundance of *Firmicutes* and *Proteobacteria* in active IBD [45]. One mechanism by which these bacteria may be pro-inflammatory in UC is through increased IEL secretion of IL-1β. Finally, in patients with axSpA, we identified both positive and negative correlation between specific species within *Firmicutes* and IEL production of TNF-α. Others have noted increased *Prevotella* species and decreased *Bacteroides* species in axSpA [47]. The new finding that *Firmicutes* species may be linked to pro-inflammatory cytokine secretion is an area for further investigation. Clearly, additional study is required to understand these complicated relationships between IEL-produced cytokines and microbiota.

We acknowledge several limitations to this study: (1) the small number of patients only allows evaluation of changes with large effect sizes; (2) we were not powered to account for confounders, such as medications other than TNFi. TNFi use among 50% of the patients with CD and 83% of patients with axSpA compared to none of the HC and patients with UC is a major limitation to this study as is the use of steroids among three study subjects. Ideally we would have enrolled subjects with new-onset, untreated axSpA and IBD. However, this would have severely limited our enrollment of subjects and the feasibility of this study. Nevertheless, when looking at cytokine production by IELs from those subjects on TNFi or steroids compared to those not on these medications (Figs. 1 and 2), there is no obvious visual difference. This suggests that these medications were

Table 2 Significant correlation between IEL number and OTU in individuals with axSpA

	Spearman's Rho	p value
Bacteroidales: Prevotellaceae	−0.8857	0.0188
Firmicutes: Clostridiaceae	−0.8286	0.0416
Deferribacteres: Deferribacteraceae	−0.9276	0.0077
Tenericutes: Anaeroplasmataceae	−0.8804	0.0206
Actinobacteria: Dermabacteraceae	−0.8804	0.0206
Tenericutes: RF9	−0.9856	0.0003
Bacteroidales: RF16	−0.8452	0.0341
Firmicutes: Eubacteriaceae	0.8697	0.0244

Intraepithelial lymphocyte (IEL) numbers and relative abundance of bacterial operational taxonomic units (OTUs) were compared by Spearman's rank correlation coefficient, which is reported alongside the p value for the most significant results unlikely to have biased our data; (3) while microbiome data was collected via rectal swab instead of directly via mucosal biopsy, prior studies have shown this mainly affects diversity, not OTU abundance [48]; (4) the change in our cytokine expression was small; however, if each pinch biopsy is approximately $4mm^2$ and the average colon is $2m^2$ in surface area then an increase in 1 unit of secretion represents greater than 30,000-fold increase in expression of that cytokine in the colon as a whole. Some subjects displayed high IEL production of certain cytokines; however, subjects producing high levels of one cytokine were not the same for other cytokines. The presence of cytokine secretion was not driven by outliers, as data for TNF-α and IFN-γ graphed on a logarithmic axis demonstrate the full range of values; (5) histologic evidence of disease activity was not assessed when subjects lacked symptoms such as change in bowel function, but all subjects lacked visible evidence of mucosal inflammation; (6) finally, the observational study design did not permit evaluation of causal links between alterations in microbiome and IEL function.

In spite of these limitations, our data provide provocative insights into how the intestinal microbiome interacts with mucosal immune cells to contribute to disease pathogenesis within human subjects. Our findings demonstrate a complex relationship between IEL-produced cytokines and microbial diversity.

Conclusion

The findings of this study indicate differences in IEL function among subjects with axSpA, CD, and UC compared to healthy controls. Our findings demonstrate unique correlation between altered microbiota and IEL function in these distinct populations. We believe the unique interactions between microbiota and IEL function by disease state is relevant to the pathogenesis of disease. Additional research is needed to validate these findings, yet our results give credence to the hypothesis that the gut microbiome is an important mediator in the development of IBD and axSpA.

Abbreviations

ASAS: Assessment of SpondyloArthritis International Society; axSpA: Axial spondyloarthritis; BASDAI: Bath Ankylosing Spondylitis Disease Activity Index; CD: Crohn's disease; CRP: C-reactive protein; ELISA: Enzyme-linked immunosorbent assay; IBD: Inflammatory bowel disease; IELs: Intraepithelial lymphocytes; IFN: Interferon; OTUs: Operational taxonomic units; PBS: Phosphate-buffered saline; SCCAI: Simple Clinical Colitis Activity Index; SpA: Spondyloarthritis; TCR: T cell receptor; TNFi: TNF inhibitor; UC: Ulcerative colitis; WBC: White blood cell

Acknowledgements

The authors would like to thank Lisa Davis, MD, for her participation in ensuring the safety of patients during the study.

Funding

This work was supported by grants from the National Center for Advancing Translational Science (UL1 TR001082 to NO), the National Institute of Arthritis and Musculoskeletal and Skin Diseases (T32 AR007534 to NO and EHR), and the National Institute of Diabetes and Digestive and Kidney Diseases (K08DK107905 to KAK) at the National Institutes of Health. Additional support was provided by the Michelson charitable fund and the UC Denver Gastrointestinal and Liver Innate Immune Program (KAK, DNF, CER, DI). Dr Caplan is supported by VA MERIT IIR 14-083-03.

Authors' contributions

EHR, NO, and KAK designed the study. MEG and BPF performed the endoscopies and obtained study biopsies. EHR, NO, and KAK recruited subjects and performed IEL experiments. WKJ assisted with the IEL experiments. DI, DNF, and CER processed samples and sequenced and analyzed microbiome data. AS and LC assisted with statistical analyses. EHR, NO, AS, LC, and KAK analyzed and interpreted data and wrote the paper. CG and JS assisted with statistical analyses. All authors contributed to reviewing and revising the manuscript and approved the final draft for submission.

Competing interests

The authors declare that they have no competing interests.

Author details

Division of Gastroenterology, Department of Medicine, University of Colorado School of Medicine, Aurora, CO, USA. [2]Division of Rheumatology, Department of Medicine, University of Colorado School of Medicine, Aurora, CO, USA. [3]Division of Infectious Disease, Department of Medicine, University of Colorado School of Medicine, Aurora, CO, USA. [4]Mucosal Inflammation Program, University of Colorado School of Medicine, Aurora, CO, USA. [5]Denver Veterans Affairs Medical Center (Denver VAMC), Denver, CO, USA. [6]Computational Bioscience Program, University of Colorado School of Medicine, Aurora, CO, USA.

References

1. Martindale J, Shukla R, Goodacre J. The impact of ankylosing spondylitis/ axial spondyloarthritis on work productivity. Best Pract Res Clin Rheumatol. 2015;29(3):512–23.
2. Loftus CG, Loftus EV Jr, Harmsen WS, Zinsmeister AR, Tremaine WJ, Melton LJ 3rd, Sandborn WJ. Update on the incidence and prevalence of Crohn's disease and ulcerative colitis in Olmsted County, Minnesota, 1940-2000. Inflamm Bowel Dis. 2007;13(3):254–61.
3. Ranganathan V, Gracey E, Brown MA, Inman RD, Haroon N. Pathogenesis of ankylosing spondylitis - recent advances and future directions. Nat Rev Rheumatol. 2017;13(6):359–67.
4. Turkcapar N, Toruner M, Soykan I, Aydintug OT, Cetinkaya H, Duzgun N, Ozden A, Duman M. The prevalence of extraintestinal manifestations and HLA association in patients with inflammatory bowel disease. Rheumatol Int. 2006;26(7):663–8.
5. Faustini F, Zoli A, Ferraccioli GF. Immunologic and genetic links between spondylarthropathies and inflammatory bowel diseases. Eur Rev Med Pharmacol Sci. 2009;13(Suppl 1):1–9.
6. Jacques P, Elewaut D. Joint expedition: linking gut inflammation to arthritis. Mucosal Immunol. 2008;1(5):364–71.
7. Wright PB, McEntegart A, McCarey D, McInnes IB, Siebert S, Milling SW. Ankylosing spondylitis patients display altered dendritic cell and T cell populations that implicate pathogenic roles for the IL-23 cytokine axis and intestinal inflammation. Rheumatology (Oxford). 2016;55(1):120–32.
8. Catana CS, Berindan Neagoe I, Cozma V, Magdas C, Tabaran F, Dumitrascu DL. Contribution of the IL-17/IL-23 axis to the pathogenesis of inflammatory bowel disease. World J Gastroenterol. 2015;21(19):5823–30.
9. Tito RY, Cypers H, Joossens M, Varkas G, Van Praet L, Glorieus E, Van den Bosch F, De Vos M, Raes J, Elewaut D. Brief report: dialister as a microbial marker of disease activity in spondyloarthritis. Arthritis Rheumatol. 2017;69(1):114–21.

10. Breban M, Tap J, Leboime A, Said-Nahal R, Langella P, Chiocchia G, Furet JP, Sokol H. Faecal microbiota study reveals specific dysbiosis in spondyloarthritis. Ann Rheum Dis. 2017;76(9):1614–22.

11. Costello ME, Ciccia F, Willner D, Warrington N, Robinson PC, Gardiner B, Marshall M, Kenna TJ, Triolo G, Brown MA. Intestinal dysbiosis in ankylosing spondylitis. Arthritis Rheumatol. 2015;67(3):686–91.

12. Frank DN, Robertson CE, Hamm CM, Kpadeh Z, Zhang T, Chen H, Zhu W, Sartor RB, Boedeker EC, Harpaz N, et al. Disease phenotype and genotype are associated with shifts in intestinal-associated microbiota in inflammatory bowel diseases. Inflamm Bowel Dis. 2011;17(1):179–84.

13. Frank DN, St Amand AL, Feldman RA, Boedeker EC, Harpaz N, Pace NR. Molecular-phylogenetic characterization of microbial community imbalances in human inflammatory bowel diseases. Proc Natl Acad Sci U S A. 2007;104(34):13780–5.

14. Gevers D, Kugathasan S, Denson LA, Vazquez-Baeza Y, Van Treuren W, Ren B, Schwager E, Knights D, Song SJ, Yassour M, et al. The treatment-naive microbiome in new-onset Crohn's disease. Cell Host Microbe. 2014;15(3): 382–92.

15. Kuhn KA, Schulz HM, Regner EH, Severs EL, Hendrickson JD, Mehta G, Whitney AK, Ir D, Ohri N, Robertson CE, et al. Bacteroidales recruit IL-6-producing intraepithelial lymphocytes in the colon to promote barrier integrity. Arthritis Rheumatol. 2017;2018. https://doi.org/10.1002/art.40490. [Epub ahead of print].

16. Cheroutre H, Lambolez F, Mucida D. The light and dark sides of intestinal intraepithelial lymphocytes. Nat Rev Immunol. 2011;11(7):445–56.

17. Najarian RM, Hait EJ, Leichtner AM, Glickman JN, Antonioli DA, Goldsmith JD. Clinical significance of colonic intraepithelial lymphocytosis in a pediatric population. Mod Pathol. 2009;22(1):13–20.

18. Torrente F, Barabino A, Bellini T, Murch SH. Intraepithelial lymphocyte eotaxin-2 expression and perineural mast cell degranulation differentiate allergic/eosinophilic colitis from classic IBD. J Pediatr Gastroenterol Nutr. 2014;59(3):300–7.

19. Dalton HR, Dipaolo MC, Sachdev GK, Crotty B, Hoang P, Jewell DP. Human colonic intraepithelial lymphocytes from patients with inflammatory bowel disease fail to down-regulate proliferative responses of primed allogeneic peripheral blood mononuclear cells after rechallenge with antigens. Clin Exp Immunol. 1993;93(1):97–102.

20. Ahn JY, Lee KH, Choi CH, Kim JW, Lee HW, Kim JW, Kim MK, Kwon GY, Han S, Kim SE, et al. Colonic mucosal immune activity in irritable bowel syndrome: comparison with healthy controls and patients with ulcerative colitis. Dig Dis Sci. 2014;59(5):1001–11.

21. Rudwaleit M, van der Heijde D, Landewe R, Listing J, Akkoc N, Brandt J, Braun J, Chou CT, Collantes-Estevez E, Dougados M, et al. The development of assessment of SpondyloArthritis International Society classification criteria for axial spondyloarthritis (part II): validation and final selection. Ann Rheum Dis. 2009;68(6):777–83.

22. Brumbaugh DE, Arruda J, Robbins K, Ir D, Santorico SA, Robertson CE, Frank DN. Mode of delivery determines neonatal pharyngeal bacterial composition and early intestinal colonization. J Pediatr Gastroenterol Nutr. 2016;63(3):320–8.

23. Lemas DJ, Young BE, Baker PR 2nd, Tomczik AC, Soderborg TK, Hernandez TL, de la Houssaye BA, Robertson CE, Rudolph MC, Ir D, et al. Alterations in human milk leptin and insulin are associated with early changes in the infant intestinal microbiome. Am J Clin Nutr. 2016;103(5):1291–300.

24. Markle JG, Frank DN, Mortin-Toth S, Robertson CE, Feazel LM, Rolle-Kampczyk U, von Bergen M, McCoy KD, Macpherson AJ, Danska JS. Sex differences in the gut microbiome drive hormone-dependent regulation of autoimmunity. Science. 2013;339(6123):1084–8.

25. Pandrea I, Xu C, Stock JL, Frank DN, Ma D, Policicchio BB, He T, Kristoff J, Cornell E, Haret-Richter GS, et al. Antibiotic and antiinflammatory therapy transiently reduces inflammation and hypercoagulation in acutely SIV-infected pigtailed macaques. PLoS Pathog. 2016;12(1):e1005384.

26. Frank DN. BARCRAWL and BARTAB: software tools for the design and implementation of barcoded primers for highly multiplexed DNA sequencing. BMC Bioinformatics. 2009;10:362.

27. iGenomes [http://support.illumina.com/sequencing/sequencing_software/igenome.html]. Accessed 8 Dec 2014.

28. Langmead B, Salzberg SL. Fast gapped-read alignment with bowtie 2. Nat Methods. 2012;9(4):357–9.

29. Ewing B, Green P. Base-calling of automated sequencer traces using phred. II. Error probabilities. Genome Res. 1998;8(3):186–94.

30. Ewing B, Hillier L, Wendl MC, Green P. Base-calling of automated sequencer traces using phred. I. Accuracy assessment. Genome Res. 1998;8(3):175–85.

31. Edgar RC, Haas BJ, Clemente JC, Quince C, Knight R. UCHIME improves sensitivity and speed of chimera detection. Bioinformatics. 2011;27(16): 2194–200.

32. Schloss PD, Westcott SL. Assessing and improving methods used in operational taxonomic unit-based approaches for 16S rRNA gene sequence analysis. Appl Environ Microbiol. 2011;77(10):3219–26.

33. Pruesse E, Peplies J, Glockner FO. SINA: accurate high-throughput multiple sequence alignment of ribosomal RNA genes. Bioinformatics. 2012;28(14): 1823–9.

34. Quast C, Pruesse E, Yilmaz P, Gerken J, Schweer T, Yarza P, Peplies J, Glockner FO. The SILVA ribosomal RNA gene database project: improved data processing and web-based tools. Nucleic Acids Res. 2013;41(Database issue):D590–6.

35. Robertson CE, Harris JK, Wagner BD, Granger D, Browne K, Tatem B, Feazel LM, Park K, Pace NR, Frank DN. Explicet: graphical user interface software for metadata-driven management, analysis and visualization of microbiome data. Bioinformatics. 2013;29(23):3100–1.

36. Gorfu G, Rivera-Nieves J, Ley K. Role of beta7 integrins in intestinal lymphocyte homing and retention. Curr Mol Med. 2009;9(7):836–50.

37. Qiu Y, Yang H. Effects of intraepithelial lymphocyte-derived cytokines on intestinal mucosal barrier function. J Interf Cytokine Res. 2013;33(10): 551–62.

38. Fantini MC, Pallone F, Monteleone G. Common immunologic mechanisms in inflammatory bowel disease and spondylarthropathies. World J Gastroenterol. 2009;15(20):2472–8.

39. Kabeerdoss J, Sandhya P, Danda D. Gut inflammation and microbiome in spondyloarthritis. Rheumatol Int. 2016;36(4):457–68.

40. Casini-Raggi V, Kam L, Chong YJ, Fiocchi C, Pizarro TT, Cominelli F. Mucosal imbalance of IL-1 and IL-1 receptor antagonist in inflammatory bowel disease. A novel mechanism of chronic intestinal inflammation. J Immunol. 1995;154(5):2434–40.

41. Olsen T, Rismo R, Cui G, Goll R, Christiansen I, Florholmen J. TH1 and TH17 interactions in untreated inflamed mucosa of inflammatory bowel disease, and their potential to mediate the inflammation. Cytokine. 2011;56(3):633–40.

42. Sun YP, Wang HH, He Q, Cho CH. Effect of passive cigarette smoking on colonic alpha7-nicotinic acetylcholine receptors in TNBS-induced colitis in rats. Digestion. 2007;76(3–4):181–7.

43. Gill T, Asquith M, Rosenbaum JT, Colbert RA. The intestinal microbiome in spondyloarthritis. Curr Opin Rheumatol. 2015;27(4):319–25.

44. Stebbings S, Munro K, Simon MA, Tannock G, Highton J, Harmsen H, Welling G, Seksik P, Dore J, Grame G, et al. Comparison of the faecal microflora of patients with ankylosing spondylitis and controls using molecular methods of analysis. Rheumatology (Oxford). 2002;41(12): 1395–401.

45. Santoru ML, Piras C, Murgia A, Palmas V, Camboni T, Liggi S, Ibba I, Lai MA, Orru S, Loizedda AL, et al. Cross sectional evaluation of the gut-microbiome metabolome axis in an Italian cohort of IBD patients. Sci Rep. 2017;7(1):9523.

46. Forbes JD, Van Domselaar G, Bernstein CN. Microbiome survey of the inflamed and noninflamed gut at different compartments within the gastrointestinal tract of inflammatory bowel disease patients. Inflamm Bowel Dis. 2016;22(4):817–25.

47. Wen C, Zheng Z, Shao T, Liu L, Xie Z, Le Chatelier E, He Z, Zhong W, Fan Y, Zhang L, et al. Quantitative metagenomics reveals unique gut microbiome biomarkers in ankylosing spondylitis. Genome Biol. 2017;18(1):142.

48. Araujo-Perez F, McCoy AN, Okechukwu C, Carroll IM, Smith KM, Jeremiah K, Sandler RS, Asher GN, Keku TO. Differences in microbial signatures between rectal mucosal biopsies and rectal swabs. Gut Microbes. 2012;3(6):530–5.

12

Neuropathic-like knee pain and associated risk factors

Gwen Sascha Fernandes[1,2,3], Ana Marie Valdes[1,2,3,4], David Andrew Walsh[1,2,3,4], Weiya Zhang[1,2,3,4*] and Michael Doherty[1,2,3,4]

Abstract

Background: Neuropathic-like knee pain (NKP) is often reported in individuals with knee pain (KP), but the contribution of specific central and peripheral risk factors to NKP has not been studied previously. The aims of the present study were to determine the prevalence of NKP in a community-derived sample with KP and to identify risk factors associated with NKP.

Methods: A cross-sectional study was undertaken ($n = 9506$) in the East Midlands community among responders (aged 40 + years) to a postal questionnaire. Questions included KP severity (numerical rating scale) and type (neuropathic versus nociceptive) using the modified painDETECT questionnaire, as well as age, body mass index (BMI), significant knee injury, widespread pain, pain catastrophising and fatigue. Multinomial regression analysis was used to determine ORs and 95% CIs. Risk factors were categorised into central and peripheral, and proportional risk contribution (PRC) and 95% CI were estimated using ROC.

Results: KP was reported in 28.2% of responders, of whom 13.65% had NKP (i.e., 3.9% of the total population). Women reported more NKP. After adjustment for age, gender, BMI and pain severity, definite NKP showed associations (aOR, 95% CI) with fibromyalgia (4.07, 2.49–6.66), widespread pain (1.93, 1.46–2.53), nodal osteoarthritis (1.80, 1.28–2.53), injury (1.50, 1.12–2.00), pain catastrophising (5.37, 2.93–9.84) and fatigue (5.37, 3.08–9.35) compared with non-NKP participants. Although only central risk factors contributed to NKP (PRC 8%, 95% CI 2.5–12.5 for central vs. PRC 3%, 95% CI −0.25 to 7.5 for peripheral), both central and peripheral risk factors contributed equally to non-NKP (PRC 10%, 95% CI 5–20 for both).

Conclusions: NKP appears to be driven largely by central risk factors and may require different prevention/treatment strategies.

Keywords: Neuropathic pain, Osteoarthritis, Risk factors, Pain catastrophising, Anxiety, Depression

Background

Knee pain (KP) is a major cause of disability worldwide. In the United Kingdom (UK) approximately 1 in 4 people aged 55 years and over report prevalent KP [1]. KP is often attributed to localised tissue insult that causes nociceptive pain. However, recent data suggest that localised damage to the nervous system and nerve fibres around a joint could result in neuropathic-like knee pain (NKP) that modifies the KP experience [2]. KP can also be modified by central sensitisation following chronic nociceptor stimulation and alterations in central pain transmitting neurons and can result in NKP characteristics [3]. This could be induced by localised insult to the joint, by comorbid conditions or by psychological factors that modify pain physiology and descending pain modulation. However, such modifying factors are rarely studied and are often omitted in clinical assessments of KP [4].

* Correspondence: weiya.zhang@nottingham.ac.uk
[1]Academic Rheumatology, Division of Rheumatology, Orthopedics and Dermatology, Nottingham City Hospital, University of Nottingham, Clinical Sciences Building, Nottingham NG5 1PB, UK
[2]Arthritis Research UK Centre for Sports, Exercise and Osteoarthritis, Queen's Medical Centre, Derby Road, Nottingham NG7 2UH, UK
Full list of author information is available at the end of the article

KP can be broadly categorised into nociceptive (inflammatory or mechanical local mechanisms); neuropathic, involving nerve damage (and potentially involving central mechanisms); and idiopathic pain with no identified cause (presumably driven predominantly by central factors) [5]. Being able to correctly identify different types of KP could have implications for treatment selection and management pathways. KP is the main complaint of knee osteoarthritis (KOA) [6] and is the primary reason patients seek treatment. As Hadler eloquently wrote, 'Knee pain is the malady, not osteoarthritis' [7]. Furthermore, half of those who complain of KP have no definite radiographic evidence of KOA [8], and 20% of people with KOA have persistent severe KP even after total knee replacement [9]. These findings suggest that central factors other than severity of local structural KOA influence KP experience and that identifying and addressing these central factors associated with NKP features, particularly early in the disease, could benefit people with such KP.

NKP associates with characteristic symptoms and pain qualities, including burning pain, tingling or prickling, mechanical and thermal hyperalgesia, allodynia, paroxysmal pain and numbness. Although quantitative sensory testing (QST) is helpful in confirming abnormal pain thresholds, this is impractical for widespread use within a community setting [10]. There are a number of screening tools and questionnaires, such as the SLANNS, painDETECT questionnaire (PDQ) and DN4 (Douleur Neuropathique 4), that use descriptions of pain location, intensity, frequency and pain quality to determine whether pain is likely to be neuropathic or nociceptive [11, 12]. The PDQ was subsequently modified (mPDQ) for use in specific areas of the body, such as the knee, with good face and content validity and good correlation with QST signs of central sensitisation [13, 14]. Hochman et al. [10] reported that one-third of participants with KOA ($n = 259$) described their pain using neuropathic descriptors and were more likely to be younger and female, with higher pain and osteoarthritis (OA) severity as well as longer OA duration, than those who did not use such descriptors. The research suggests the existence of subgroups of participants with shared characteristics that exhibit NKP symptoms. Should that be the case, targeting treatment to the underlying pain mechanism could have the potential to improve pain management and to improve quality of life with individualised treatment interventions. The objectives of this study were to (1) determine the prevalence of NKP in community-derived people with KP and (2) identify risk factors specifically associated with NKP.

Methods
Study design
The Nottingham Knee Pain and Health in the Community (KPIC) study is an ongoing prospective cohort study in the East Midlands region of the UK [15]. The current study used baseline KPIC data to identify people with KP and the proportion of those who reported NKP. A case-control study was conducted with three groups: NKP, non-NKP and no KP. The study was approved by the Nottingham Research Ethics Committee 1 (NREC reference 14/EM/0015) and registered with ClinicalTrials.gov (NCT02098070).

Sample size
Source population
The survey comprised a community-derived sample regardless of whether subjects had experienced KP. A postal questionnaire was developed on the basis of a review of items in previously published questionnaires [16, 17]. Further details on questionnaire logistics and sample size calculations have been published previously [15].

NKP prevalence and risk factors
According to a NKP prevalence in people with KP of 28% (±8%) based on a Canadian community population sample [10], a minimum of 85 participants with KP were required to yield a power of 90% with a 0.05 significance level.

Participants
Inclusion criteria
The inclusion criteria were all men and women aged 40 years and over, located on their general practitioner (GP) register, regardless of KP status.

Exclusion criteria
Exclusion criteria were inability to give informed consent and presence of a terminal illness or severe mental illness. Eligibility was decided by the GPs in each practice. The questionnaire was accompanied by a covering letter from the GP introducing the study and its objectives. Return of a completed questionnaire in a pre-paid envelope to Academic Rheumatology (City Hospital, Nottingham) was taken as implicit consent.

Questionnaire survey
The questionnaire was constructed to capture detailed information about the participants, as well as their medical history and risk factors for KOA [18]. A validated screening question was used to determine presence of current KP: 'Have you ever had knee pain for most days of the past one month?' [19, 20]. Additionally, a body pain manikin [21] was used to locate and define pain in other body regions, allowing definition of widespread pain based on criteria proposed by the American College of Rheumatology which require presence of pain in all four quadrants as well as the axial skeleton [22]. The mPDQ was chosen to identify NKP (PDQ scores ≥ 13 as possible NKP and ≥ 19 as definite NKP) [13]. On the basis of face validity of the questionnaire

content, previous literature [23] and consensus among the authors, the data on risk factors obtained from the questionnaire were divided into three groups: peripheral (related to structural changes in and around the knee joint, such as significant injury and nodal OA [which associates with likelihood of structural KOA]), central (related to pain experience and physiology such as anxiety, depression, fatigue, Pain Catastrophising Scale [PCS] and self-reported GP-diagnosed fibromyalgia) and comorbidities (such as hyperlipidaemia, diabetes and widespread pain as defined using the body pain manikin [15]). Further details on each exposure measured included KP severity, constitutional knee alignment, nodal OA, 2D:4D (index:ring) digit ratio, anxiety, depression, fatigue and pain catastrophising, and high-risk occupations can be found in the published study protocol [15]. Exposures such as 2D:4D digit ratio and nodal OA are recognised risk factors for knee pain and knee OA [1, 13, 15] and were included in order to identify as many possible associations and confounders as possible [10, 13, 14].

Statistical analyses

Categorical variables were reported as frequencies and continuous variables as mean and SD. OR and 95% CI were calculated using multinomial logistic regression for three-group comparisons (NKP, non-NKP and no KP). Each risk factor was adjusted for the same confounding factors (age, body mass index [BMI], gender and pain severity). Statistical significance was defined as $p < 0.05$. There were very few missing data at random (e.g., where BMI was not reported by a participant), so imputation or modelling was not undertaken for occasional missing values. All variables were reported as dichotomous data, with the exception of PCS and fatigue scores. PCS was reported as per official cut-offs in tertiles (< 18 [lowest tertile], 18–24 [middle tertile], ≥24 [highest tertile]). Fatigue data were reported using a Likert-style scale and were categorised as lowest tertile (never), middle tertile (seldom and sometimes) and highest tertile (often and always).

We also used ROC to calculate AUC, from which proportional risk contribution (PRC) of central risk factors, peripheral risk factors and comorbidities was derived. ROC curves were based on the multivariate logistic regression model with definite NKP as an outcome compared with non-NKP. Firstly, we built the full risk model for definite NKP with an ROC curve (ROC1). Secondly, we removed the exposure(s) of interest to examine the contribution of the exposure(s) through the reduction of the ROC curve (i.e., the partial ROC [ROC2]). Thirdly, we calculated the PRC using the following formula:

$$PRC = [ROC1–ROC2]/[ROC1–0.5]$$

The 95% CI of PRC was calculated according to 95% CIs of ROC1 and ROC2. We also calculated ROC curves based

on non-NKP as an outcome compared with no KP to determine the PRC of peripheral and central risk factors and comorbidities. PRCs for each of the groups (central and peripheral risk factors and comorbidities) indicate the contribution of each to the outcome of definite NKP. The ROC curves were generated using STATA software (StataCorp, College Station, TX, USA) with the roctab command and combined graphically [24]. All analysis was conducted using Stata IC version 14 on the Windows 7 operating system, and power calculations were undertaken using Power and Precision version 2.1 software (Biostat, Englewood, NJ, USA).

Results

Of the 40,505 mailed questionnaires, 9506 (23.4%) completed questionnaires were returned which met the inclusion criteria. The characteristics of these participants were compared with those from other national UK cohorts (Appendix). The data showed that the KPIC population is representative of the UK general population in terms of age, percentage of women and BMI (Appendix).

Of the responders, 2681 participants (28.3%) reported KP for most days of the past month. Of these KP participants, 366 (13.65% of those with KP, 3.9% of the total KPIC) had NKP. Proportions of 16.6% of women with KP and 11.6% of men with KP reported definite NKP. Women also reported more NKP in almost every age category than men and peaked 10 years later in the age range of 60–64 years than men in the age range of 50–54 years (Fig. 1).

Comparison of the participants in the four categories (definite NKP, possible NKP, non-NKP and no KP) showed that those with definite NKP were more likely to be younger, female and have greater BMI ($p < 0.01$). They were also more likely to self-report a diagnosis of fibromyalgia, hypertension, hyperlipidaemia and diabetes; report significant knee injury; work in high-risk occupations; present with nodal OA and widespread pain; and have higher scores for anxiety and depression than people without KP ($p < 0.001$). These results are presented in Table 1.

We compared definite NKP participants with no-KP participants to determine which factors were associated with definite neuropathic-like symptoms compared with no KP. Unadjusted and adjusted ORs (for age, BMI, gender and pain severity) for definite NKP compared with no-KP participants were calculated for each risk factor (Table 2). The results of the multinomial regression analysis comparing NKP with no KP showed significant associations, particularly for central factors such as fibromyalgia (aOR 3.19, 95% CI 1.70–5.98), anxiety (aOR 2.48, 95% CI 1.76–3.48), depression (aOR 2.62, 95% CI 1.70–4.04), highest tertile of pain catastrophising (aOR 5.00, 95% CI 2.68–9.36) and highest tertile of fatigue (aOR 5.11, 95% CI 2.86–9.15) (Table 2). The most significant result for peripheral risk factors was significant knee injury and the presence of nodal OA (1.44 [1.04–1.99] and 1.76 [1.19–2.63], respectively).

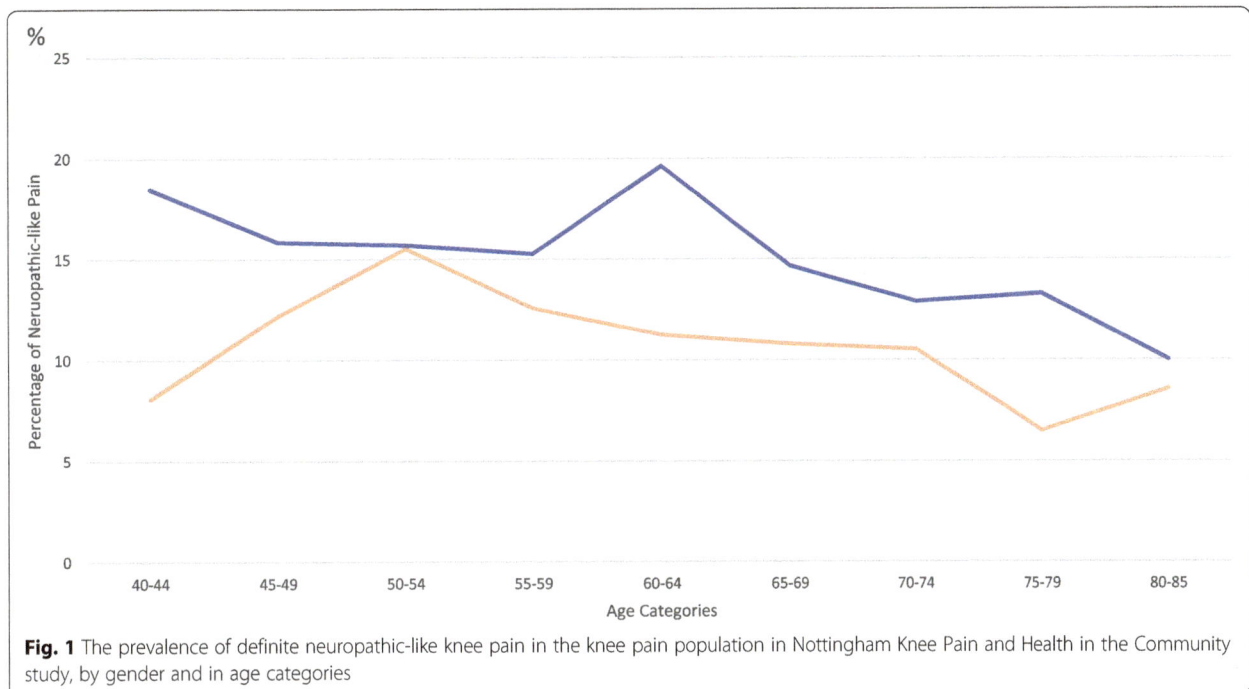

Fig. 1 The prevalence of definite neuropathic-like knee pain in the knee pain population in Nottingham Knee Pain and Health in the Community study, by gender and in age categories

We compared definite NKP participants with non-NKP participants to determine which factors were associated with definite neuropathic-like symptoms compared with non-neuropathic-like knee pain. Unadjusted and adjusted ORs for definite NKP versus non-NKP were also calculated for each risk factor (Table 3). After adjustment for age, BMI, gender and KP severity, definite NKP was significantly associated with two peripheral risk factors (injuries [aOR 1.50, 95% CI 1.12–2.00] and nodal OA [aOR 1.80, 95% CI 1.28–2.53]) and all measured central risk factors (fibromyalgia [aOR 4.07, 95% CI 2.49–6.66], anxiety [aOR 3.17, 95% CI 2.38–4.23], depression [aOR 2.99, 95% CI 2.14–4.19], pain catastrophising [aOR 5.37, 95% CI 2.93–9.84] and fatigue [aOR 5.37, 95% CI 3.08–9.35]). There were also associations with markers of metabolic syndrome, such as diabetes (aOR 1.52, 95% CI 1.04–2.23) and hyperlipidaemia (aOR 1.36, 95% CI 1.01–1.84).

Table 1 Comparison of all characteristics of four groups within the Nottingham Knee Pain and Health in the Community study community

Characteristics	No KP (n = 6822)	Non-NKP (n = 1685)	Possible NKP (n = 462)	Definite NKP (n = 366)	P value
Age, yr, mean (±SD)	62.12 (10.64)	61.94 (10.41)	61.80 (10.32)	61.13 (9.96)	0.03*
Body mass index, kg/m², mean (±SD)	26.61 (4.76)	28.30 (5.42)	29.84 (6.39)	31.49 (7.77)	< 0.001*
Female gender, n (%)	3806 (55.80.09)	956 (56.74)	258 (55.84)	242 (66.12)	0.02*
High-risk occupation, n (%)	2660 (38.99)	783 (46.47)	271 (58.66)	193 (52.73))	< 0.001*
Fibromyalgia, n (%)	101 (1.48)	52 (3.09)	26 (5.63)	57 (15.57)	< 0.001*
Hypertension, n (%)	1890 (27.70)	555 (32.94)	183 (39.61)	146 (39.89)	< 0.001*
High cholesterol, n (%)	1773 (25.99)	495 (29.38)	156 (33.77)	143 (39.07))	< 0.001*
Stroke, n (%)	174 (2.55)	51 (3.02)	14 (3.03)	15 (4.10)	0.05
Diabetes, n (%)	550 (8.06)	172 (10.21)	72 (15.58)	73 (19.95))	< 0.001*
2D:4D digit ratio, n (%)	3256 (47.73)	792 (47.00)	232 (50.22)	142 (38.80)	0.03*
Nodal OA, n (%)	632 (9.62)	234 (14.60)	79 (18.20)	88 (25.36)	< 0.001*
Significant injury, n (%)	972 (14.25)	478 (28.38)	165 (35.71)	130 (35.52)	< 0.001*
Widespread pain, n (%)	1072 (15.71)	537 (31.87)	209 (45.24)	198 (54.10)	< 0.001*
Anxiety, n (%)	754 (11.05)	298 (17.70)	148 (32.03)	191 (52.19)	< 0.001*
Depression, n (%)	266 (3.90)	142 (8.43)	91 (19.70)	133 (36.34))	< 0.001*

Abbreviations: *KP* Knee pain, *NKP* Neuropathic-like knee pain, *OA* Osteoarthritis
* is statistical significance <0.05

Table 2 Regression results of definite neuropathic-like knee pain versus possible neuropathic-like knee pain, non-neuropathic-like knee pain and no knee pain in the whole Nottingham Knee Pain and Health in the Community study population

	No KP	OR (95% CI)					
		Non-NKP		Possible NKP		Definite NKP	
		Crude	Adjusted	Crude	Adjusted	Crude	Adjusted
	(n = 6822)	(n = 1685)		(n = 462)		(n = 366)	
Age	1 (referent)	0.99 (0.99; 1.00)	—	0.99 (0.99;1.00)	—	0.99 (0.98;1.00)	—
Body mass index	1	**1.06 (1.06; 1.08)**	—	1.11 (1.09;1.13)	—	1.15 (1.13;1.17)	—
Gender	1	1.04 (0.93; 1.16)	—	1.03 (0.85; 1.24)	—	1.57 (1.25; 1.96)	—
Pain severity	1	**1.70 (1.64; 1.77)**	—	2.28 (2.15; 2.53)	—	3.44 (3.16; 3.74)	—
Peripheral factors							
High-risk occupation	1	**1.36 (1.22; 1.51)**	0.88 (0.74; 1.05)	2.22 (1.83; 2.69)	**1.38 (1.06; 1.80)**	1.75 (1.41; 2.16)	1.04 (0.77; 1.42)
Significant injury	1	**2.40 (2.12; 2.73)**	0.93 (0.78; 1.12)	3.41 (2.78; 4.18)	1.29 (0.98; 1.69)	3.53 (2.81; 4.44)	**1.44 (1.04; 1.99)**
Nodal OA	1	**1.60 (1.36; 1.89)**	1.01 (0.78; 1.30)	2.09 (1.62; 2.70)	1.34 (0.93; 1.93)	3.19 (2.47; 4.12)	**1.76 (1.19; 2.63)**
2D:4D digit ratio	1	0.99 (0.99; 1.00)	0.99 (0.99; 1.00)	0.99 (0.99; 1.00)	0.99 (0.99; 0.99)	1.00 (0.99; 1.00)	0.99 (0.99; 1.00)
Central factors							
Anxiety	1	**1.73 (1.49; 2.00)**	0.8 (0.63; 1.00)	3.79 (3.08; 4.68)	**1.42 (1.04; 1.94)**	8.78 (7.06; 10.93)	**2.48 (1.76; 3.48)**
Depression	1	**2.27 (1.84; 2.80)**	0.84 (0.60; 1.19)	6.04 (4.66; 7.84)	**1.71 (1.13; 2.59)**	14.06 (11.00; 17.99)	**2.62 (1.70; 4.04)**
Pain Catastrophising Scale							
Lowest tertile	1	—	—				
Middle tertile		**2.00 (1.75; 2.23)**	1.19 (0.97; 1.47)	4.93 (3.35; 7.24)	**2.45 (1.57; 3.82)**	4.04 (2.14; 7.62)	1.60 (0.80; 3.23)
Highest tertile		**2.53 (2.20; 2.91)**	0.87 (0.69; 1.09)	14.98 (10.44; 21.49)	**3.33 (2.16; 5.14)**	40.84 (23.36; 71.42)	**5.00 (2.68; 9.36)**
Fatigue							
Lowest tertile	1	—	—				
Middle tertile		**1.94 (1.70; 2.22)**	1.01 (0.83; 1.24)	2.75 (2.04; 3.69)	1.14 (0.79; 1.65)	6.26 (3.72; 10.55)	**2.38 (1.31; 4.33)**
Highest tertile		**2.80 (2.44; 3.23)**	0.97 (0.77; 1.22)	7.77 (5.86; 10.30)	**1.86 (1.29; 2.68)**	31.20 (19.02; 51.21)	**5.11 (2.86; 9.15)**
Fibromyalgia	1	**2.11 (1.51; 2.97)**	0.79 (0.47; 1.32)	3.97 (2.55; 6.17)	1.27 (0.66; 2.42)	12.28 (8.70; 17.32)	**3.19 (1.70; 5.98)**
Comorbidities							
Hypertension	1	**1.28 (1.14; 1.44)**	1.00 (0.82; 1.21)	1.71 (1.41; 2.07)	1.18 (0.88; 1.57)	1.73 (1.40; 2.15)	1.09 (0.78; 1.53)
Hyperlipidaemia	1	**1.18 (1.05; 1.33)**	1.05 (0.86; 1.28)	1.45 (1.19; 1.77)	1.17 (0.87; 1.56)	1.83 (1.47; 2.27)	**1.44 (1.03; 2.01)**
Stroke	1	1.19 (0.87; 1.64)	1.12 (0.66; 1.89)	1.19 (0.69; 2.07)	1.18 (0.55; 2.50)	1.63 (0.95; 2.80)	1.13 (0.48; 2.68)
Diabetes	1	**1.30 (1.08; 1.55)**	0.91 (0.67; 1.22)	2.10 (1.61; 2.75)	1.20 (0.80; 1.80)	2.84 (2.17; 3.72)	1.38 (0.88; 2.15)
Multiple regional pain	1	**2.50 (2.22;2.83)**	0.97 (0.81; 1.18)	4.43 (3.65; 5.38)	**1.60 (1.23; 2.09)**	6.32 (5.10; 7.84)	**1.90 (1.40; 2.60)**
Pain experience							
ICOAP overall	1	**1.11 (1.10; 1.12)**	**1.08 (1.07; 1.10)**	1.15 (1.14; 1.16)	**1.11 (1.10; 1.13)**	1.19 (1.18; 1.20)	**1.14 (1.13; 1.16)**

Table 2 Regression results of definite neuropathic-like knee pain versus possible neuropathic-like knee pain, non-neuropathic-like knee pain and no knee pain in the whole Nottingham Knee Pain and Health in the Community study population *(Continued)*

	No KP	OR (95% CI)							
		Non-NKP		Possible NKP		Definite NKP			
		Crude	Adjusted	Crude	Adjusted	Crude	Adjusted		
	(n = 6822)	(n = 1685)		(n = 462)		(n = 366)			
ICOAP intermittent	1	**1.09 (1.08; 1.10)**	**1.06 (1.05; 1.07)**	1.13 (1.12; 1.14)	**1.08 (1.07; 1.09)**	1.17 (1.15; 1.18)	**1.10 (1.09; 1.12)**		
ICOAP constant	1	**1.10 (1.09; 1.10)**	**1.07 (1.06; 1.08)**	1.13 (1.13; 1.14)	**1.10 (1.09; 1.11)**	1.18 (1.16; 1.19)	**1.12 (1.11; 1.14)**		

Abbreviations: ICOAP Intermittent and Constant Osteoarthritis Pain measure, *KP* Knee pain, *NKP* Neuropathic-like knee pain, *OA* Osteoarthritis
No KP is no knee pain; non-NKP is non-neuropathic-like knee pain; likely NKP is likely neuropathic pain; and definite NKP is definite neuropathic-like knee pain
The no KP group is the referent group, and hence a '1' represents this in the table
Note: Significant associations are highlighted in bold. For comparison purposes, we only present crude and age-, gender-, body mass index- and pain severity-adjusted OR for each factor

Table 3 Regression results of definite neuropathic-like knee pain versus possible- and non-neuropathic-like knee pain

	Non-NKP	OR (95% CI)			
		Possible NKP		Definite NKP	
		Crude	Adjusted	Crude	Adjusted
	(n = 1685)	(n = 462)		(n = 366)	
Age	1 (Reference)	0.99 (0.99; 1.00)	–	0.99 (0.98; 1.00)	–
Body mass index	1	1.04 (1.02; 1.06)	–	1.08 (1.06; 1.10)	–
Gender	1	0.98 (0.79; 1.21)	–	1.50 (1.18; 1.91)	–
Pain severity	1	1.37 (1.31–1.45)	–	2.08 (1.93; 2.25)	–
Putative factors					
High-risk occupation	1	1.63 (1.33; 2.01)	**1.57 (1.24; 1.99)**	1.29 (1.03–1.61)	1.17 (0.89; 1.54)
Significant injury	1	1.42 (1.14; 1.77)	**1.36 (1.07; 1.73)**	1.47 (1.15; 1.88)	**1.50 (1.12; 2.00)**
2D:4D digit ratio	1	1.00 (0.99; 1.00)	0.99 (0.99; 1.00)	1.00 (0.99; 1.00)	0.99 (0.99; 1.00)
Nodal OA	1	1.30 (0.98; 1.72)	1.34 (0.98; 1.83)	1.99 (1.50; 2.63)	**1.80 (1.28; 2.53)**
Comorbidities					
Hypertension	1	1.34 (1.08; 1.65)	1.18 (0.92; 1.52)	1.35 (1.07; 1.70)	1.09 (0.80; 1.47)
Hyperlipidaemia	1	1.22 (0.98; 1.53)	1.12 (0.86; 1.44)	1.54 (1.22; 1.95)	**1.36 (1.01; 1.84)**
Stroke	1	1.00 (0.55; 1.83)	0.97 (0.52; 1.84)	1.37 (0.76; 2.46)	0.92 (0.44; 1.92)
Diabetes	1	1.62 (1.20; 2.19)	1.32 (0.94; 1.85)	2.19 (1.62; 2.96)	**1.52 (1.04; 2.23)**
Multiple regional pain	1	1.76 (1.43; 2.18)	**1.63 (1.29; 2.05)**	2.52 (2.00; 3.17)	**1.93 (1.46; 2.53)**
Central factors					
Anxiety	1	2.20 (1.74; 2.76)	**1.79 (1.38; 2.32)**	5.08 (3.99; 6.45)	**3.17 (2.38; 4.23)**
Depression	1	2.66 (1.99; 3.55)	**1.96 (1.42; 2.70)**	6.20 (4.71; 8.15)	**2.99 (2.14; 4.19)**
Pain Catastrophising					
Scale					
Lowest tertile	1	Reference			
Middle tertile		2.46 (1.64; 3.67)	**2.03 (1.32; 3.10)**	2.01 (1.05; 3.84)	1.31 (0.66; 2.60)
Highest tertile		5.91 (4.05; 8.62)	**3.63 (2.40; 5.48)**	16.12 (9.12; 28.49)	**5.37 (2.93; 9.84)**
Fatigue					
Lowest tertile	1	Reference			
Middle tertile		1.41 (1.03; 1.93)	1.15 (0.82; 1.62)	3.22 (1.89; 5.48)	**2.45 (1.38; 4.38)**
Highest tertile		2.77 (2.05; 3.75)	**1.91 (1.38; 2.66)**	11.12 (6.69; 18.47)	**5.37 (3.08; 9.35)**
Fibromyalgia	1	1.87 (1.16; 3.03)	1.56 (0.92; 2.66)	5.79 (3.90; 8.61)	**4.07 (2.49; 6.66)**
Treatment					
Opioids	1	1.98 (1.54; 2.54)	**1.46 (1.11; 1.92)**	3.03 (2.35;3.91)	**1.70 (1.26; 2.31)**
NSAIDs	1	1.22 (0.82; 1.81)	1.01 (0.66; 1.56)	2.03 (1.40; 2.95)	**1.75 (1.13; 2.72)**
OTC painkillers	1	1.66 (1.33; 2.07)	**1.39 (1.09; 1.78)**	1.76 (1.38; 2.24)	1.28 (0.96; 1.71)
Aspirin	1	1.31 (0.96; 1.79)	1.12 (0.79; 1.60)	1.66 (1.20; 2.28)	1.40 (0.94; 2.09)
Current statin use	1	0.99 (0.99; 1.00)	0.99 (0.99; 1.00)	0.99 (0.99; 1.00)	**1.00 (0.99; 1.00)**
Statin use ever	1	0.99 (0.99;0.99)	0.99 (0.99; 1.00)	0.99 (0.99; 0.99)	0.99 (0.99; 1.00)
Injection	1	2.04 (1.59; 2.61)	**1.66 (1.27; 2.18)**	3.52 (2.74; 4.52)	**2.39 (1.76; 3.23)**
Pain experience					
ICOAP overall	1	1.04 (1.03; 1.05)	**1.03 (1.02; 1.04)**	1.08 (1.07; 1.09)	**1.05 (1.04; 1.07)**
ICOAP intermittent	1	1.04 (1.03; 1.04)	**1.02 (1.02; 1.03)**	1.07 (1.06; 1.08)	**1.04 (1.04; 1.05)**
ICOAP constant	1	1.04 (1.03; 1.04)	**1.05 (1.04; 1.06)**	1.07 (1.06; 1.08)	**1.05 (1.04; 1.06)**

Abbreviations: ICOAP Intermittent and Constant Osteoarthritis Pain measure, *NKP* Neuropathic-like knee pain, *NSAIDs* Non-steroidal anti-inflammatory drugs, *OA* Osteoarthritis, *OTC* Over the counter
Non-NKP is non-neuropathic-like knee pain; likely NKP is likely neuropathic pain; and definite NKP is definite neuropathic-like knee pain
The non-KP group is the referent group, and hence a '1' represents this in the table
Note: Significant associations are highlighted in bold. For comparison purposes, we only present crude and age-, gender-, BMI- and pain severity-adjusted OR for each factor

The ROC for the full model for definite NKP compared with non-NKP, including central and peripheral risk factors and comorbidities was 0.90 (0.88; 0.92) with the PRC of peripheral, central and comorbidity risk factors as 3%, 8% and 3%, respectively. The ROC for the full model for non-NKP compared with no KP was 0.70 (0.69; 0.72) with the PRC of peripheral, central and comorbidity risk factors as 10%, 10% and 5%, respectively. These ROC graphs are presented in Fig. 2, with further details presented in Table 4.

Discussion

To our knowledge, this is the first community-based study of the prevalence of NKP and associated risk factors. The main findings are as follows: (1) the prevalence of NKP in this sample of people with KP in the Nottingham community is 13.65%; (2) the prevalence of NKP is higher in women and peaks 10 years later than in men; (3) the risk factors associated with definite NKP compared with non-NKP are knee injury; nodal OA; central factors such as depression, anxiety and pain catastrophizing; and comorbidities such as diabetes and hyperlipidaemia; and (4) although contributing factors to NKP are predominantly central, both central and peripheral risk factors contribute equally to non-NKP.

Table 4 ROC and 95% CI for risk factor groups comparing different participants based on neuropathic-like knee pain profile

	ROC	95% CI	PRC (%)	PRC 95% CI
Definite NKP vs. non-NKP				
Full*	0.90	0.88; 0.92	100%	–
Without peripheral	0.89	0.87; 0.91	3%	−2.5; 7.5
Without central	0.87	0.85; 0.89	8%	2.5; 12.5
Without comorbidities	0.89	0.88; 0.91	3%	−2.5; 5
Non-NKP vs. no KP				
Full	0.70	0.69; 0.72	100%	–
Without peripheral	0.68	0.66; 0.69	10%	5; 20
Without central	0.68	0.66; 0.69	10%	5; 20
Without comorbidities	0.69	0.67; 0.70	5%	0; 15

Abbreviations: KP Knee pain, *NKP* Neuropathic-like knee pain, *PRC* Proportional risk contribution
ROC results for the full model including age, gender, body mass index and pain severity
Peripheral = significant injury, nodal osteoarthritis
Central = anxiety, depression, Pain Catastrophising Scale (by highest tertile), fatigue, fibromyalgia
Comorbidities: hyperlipidaemia, diabetes, widespread pain
Pain severity was not included from the second ROC analysis comparing non-NKP with no KP participants

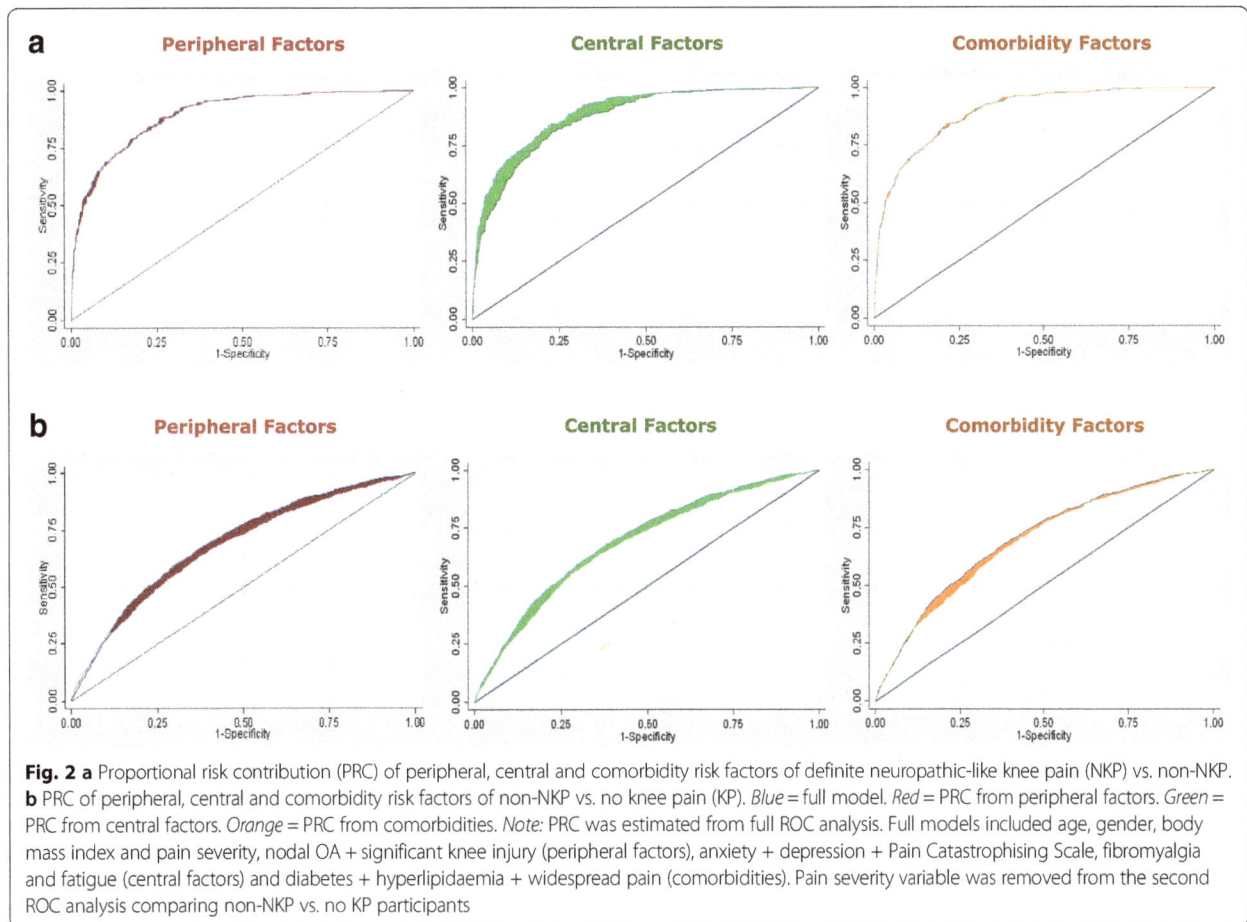

Fig. 2 a Proportional risk contribution (PRC) of peripheral, central and comorbidity risk factors of definite neuropathic-like knee pain (NKP) vs. non-NKP. **b** PRC of peripheral, central and comorbidity risk factors of non-NKP vs. no knee pain (KP). *Blue* = full model. *Red* = PRC from peripheral factors. *Green* = PRC from central factors. *Orange* = PRC from comorbidities. *Note:* PRC was estimated from full ROC analysis. Full models included age, gender, body mass index and pain severity, nodal OA + significant knee injury (peripheral factors), anxiety + depression + Pain Catastrophising Scale, fibromyalgia and fatigue (central factors) and diabetes + hyperlipidaemia + widespread pain (comorbidities). Pain severity variable was removed from the second ROC analysis comparing non-NKP vs. no KP participants

The prevalence of NKP (13.65%) appears higher than in previous questionnaire-based population-wide studies (8.0–8.9%) [25–27]. However, these previous studies defined the prevalence of NKP in the general population, not in a KP population specifically. Conversely, prevalence in our study is also lower than in studies that have reported NKP in symptomatic KOA populations (23%) [28]. This may be because of factors such as different people at risk (KP versus KP plus structural KOA), various definitions of NKP, and sample sizes. In addition to requiring radiographic changes, six of the nine studies in this systematic review used hospital-based samples where more severe cases were included, probably explaining their higher prevalence estimate [29].

Individuals with NKP were more likely to be women and obese (BMI ≥ 30 kg/m^2) than those without NKP. This accords with previous prevalence studies [29, 30] reporting higher overall neuropathic pain prevalence in women of 8–10.2% compared with 6–7.9% in men [25, 31]. The main risk factors associated with NKP are central factors such as depression, anxiety, pain catastrophising and fatigue. This is supported by a composite measure—the PRC—where contribution from the central risk factors to NKP was greater (8%) than that from peripheral risk factors (3%), whereas the contributions from central (10%) and peripheral (10%) risk factors to non-NKP were equal. It is well known that psychological factors such as depression can influence pain perception and behaviour [32]. It is possible that KP, which contributes to functional limitations, fatigue and possible sleep disturbance, may in turn contribute to lower mood, increased anxiety and worse pain and functional scores, resulting in a complex inter-relationship [33, 34].

This study also showed that fibromyalgia and widespread pain were highly associated with NKP in the community when compared with non-NKP and were still significantly associated, but to a lesser extent, when compared with no-KP participants. Fibromyalgia is often considered a predominantly central 'top-down' disorder driven by psychological distress, sleep disturbance and symptoms of anxiety and depression [35], whereas those with neuropathic symptoms have a 'bottom-up' disorder driven by peripheral changes and neurogenic damage [36]. The association reported in this study indicates the overlap between these two conditions that share mechanisms of central sensitisation, but causation cannot be established in a cross-sectional study.

Our study also demonstrated that diabetes associates with NKP compared with non-NKP, but not when compared with the no-KP group. Although we did not differentiate type 1 and type 2 diabetes, it is plausible that the metabolic syndrome underlies the onset and progression of neuropathy and obesity, and its consequences are potential driving adverse factors that propagate altered nerve functioning and injury [37].

There are several clinical implications of this project. Whilst KP has often been treated primarily with frontline analgesic agents, the effect sizes for these drugs are small and do not improve over time [38]. This study supports previous findings [39, 40] that there is a neuropathic component to KP that is predominantly driven by central pain sensitisation processes or, more specifically, central risk factors. Considering that the findings that there is a strong contribution and association of central factors such as depression, anxiety and pain catastrophising to definite NKP, these need to be managed correctly in the KP patient population and early stages of the OA process.

There are several limitations to this study. Firstly, the use of self-reported questionnaires might involve recall bias and possible misclassification of self-reported outcomes. Nevertheless, we used a validated questionnaire and involved patient and public volunteers to help optimize clarity and ease of questionnaire use. Secondly, the low response rate (24%) could have resulted in selection bias because those with KP may be more motivated to participate. However, a comparison of KPIC demographic data was made with other local and national UK community cohorts (Appendix), which demonstrated comparability in terms of age, gender distribution and BMI. Thirdly, whilst the questionnaire covered a spectrum of risk factors associated with KP and NKP, we did not measure smoking status, education level or alcohol consumption at baseline. Similarly, we did not have measures of all potential peripheral risk factors (e.g., radiographic OA scores, synovitis and muscle strength). These have minimised the PRC and do not necessarily reflect the real ratio of central and peripheral risk factor contributions. Further study including more comprehensive measurements of both central and peripheral risk factors is therefore warranted. Furthermore, widespread pain was included as a comorbidity rather than as a central factor because it is widely regarded as such in the literature [41, 42]. However, there are limitations in the understanding of pain physiology, and the groups in our analysis (central, peripheral and comorbidity risk factors) may not be entirely mutually exclusive owing to these overlaps, which is a further caveat to our findings.

Conclusions

In summary, the prevalence of NKP in those with KP in this community sample is approximately 14%. NKP affects more women across all age groups. People with central risk factors such as depression and anxiety and peripheral risk factors such as injury and comorbidities, particularly diabetes, are more likely to have NKP. The results suggest that of the risk factors examined, NKP is predominantly centrally driven, whereas non-NKP is driven equally by both peripheral and central factors. Consideration of NKP characteristics and the balance of central versus peripheral risk factors in individuals with KP could help direct best treatment selection and optimise patient care.

Appendix

Table 5 Comparison of Nottingham Knee Pain and Health in the Community study participants with other population-based cohorts investigation knee pain and knee osteoarthritis in the United Kingdom

Study	Population source, country	Sample size	Age range and mean age (SD)	Female gender, n (percentage)	Body mass index, mean (SD)
Knee Pain in the Community (KPIC)[a]	Community, UK	9506	40–90 and 62.10 yr (10.56)	5262 (55.35%)	27.29 (5.29)
Genetics of Osteoarthritis & Lifestyle Study (GOAL)[b]	Community, UK	3710	40–79 and 66.6 yr (7.9)	1780 (48%)	29.3 (5.3)
English Longitudinal Study of Ageing (ELSA)[c]	Community, UK	12,234	50–100 and 65.1 yr (10.2)	6123 (54.5%)	N/A
Health Survey for England (HSfE) 2010/2011[d]	Community, UK	13,983	16–64 and 40 yr	7834 (56%)	Men: 27.4 (0.11) Women: 27.1 (0.11)

[a] Reference [15]
b Reference [43]
[c] Reference [44]
[d] Reference [45]

Abbreviations
ACR: American College of Rheumatology; aOR: Adjusted odds ratio; BMI: Body mass index; DN4: Douleur Neuropathique 4; GP: General practice; HADS: Hospital and Anxiety Depression Scale; ICOAP: Intermittent and Constant Osteoarthritis Pain measure; KOA: Knee osteoarthritis; KP: Knee pain; mPDQ: Modified painDETECT Questionnaire; NKP: Neuropathic-like knee pain; NREC: Nottingham Research Ethics Committee; OA: Osteoarthritis; PDQ: painDETECT questionnaire; PRC: Proportional risk contribution; QST: Quantitative Sensory Testing; S-LANNS: Self-report version of the Leeds Assessment of Neuropathic Symptoms and Signs

Acknowledgements
We acknowledge the wider KPIC team for their time and contribution to the study set-up and data collection, Helen Richardson, Dr. Aliya Sarmanova, Dr. Michelle Hall, Nadia Frowd, Laura Marshall, Dr. Joanne Stocks, Kehinde Akin-Akinoseye, Dr. Sophie Warner, Dr. Hollie Harvey, Jane Healy, Rose Farrands-Bentley, Ivy Leech, Mandy Broniewski, Fraser Kesteven and Danielle Sinclair.

Funding
This study was supported financially by the Arthritis Research UK Pain Centre (Centre Initiative grant number: 20777) and Arthritis Research UK Centre for Sport, Exercise and Osteoarthritis (Grant reference 20194).

Disclaimer
The opinions, results and conclusions reported in this article are those of the authors and are independent from the funding sources.

Provenance and peer review
Not commissioned; externally peer reviewed.

Authors' contributions
GSF, AV, DW, WZ and MD made substantial contributions to the conception and design of the study. GSF was responsible for the data cleaning and conducted the preliminary analysis and interpretation for the reliability data. All authors have contributed to the work and take public responsibility of the content and guarantee the integrity and accuracy of the work undertaken. All authors have read, provided critical feedback on intellectual content and approved the final manuscript.

Consent for publication
Not applicable.

Competing interests
The authors declare that they have no competing interests.

Author details
[1]Academic Rheumatology, Division of Rheumatology, Orthopedics and Dermatology, Nottingham City Hospital, University of Nottingham, Clinical Sciences Building, Nottingham NG5 1PB, UK. [2]Arthritis Research UK Centre for Sports, Exercise and Osteoarthritis, Queen's Medical Centre, Derby Road, Nottingham NG7 2UH, UK. [3]Arthritis Research UK Pain Centre, University of Nottingham, Nottingham NG5 1PB, UK. [4]NIHR Nottingham Biomedical Research Centre, University of Nottingham, Nottingham NG5 1PB, UK.

References
1. Heidari B. Knee osteoarthritis prevalence, risk factors, pathogenesis and features: part I. Caspian J Int Med. 2011;2(2):205–12.
2. Merskey H, Bogduk N, editors. Classification of chronic pain: descriptions of chronic pain syndromes and definitions of pain terms. 2nd ed. Seattle, WA: IASP Press; 1994. p. 209–14.
3. Kidd BL, Langford RM, Wodehouse T. Arthritis and pain: current approaches in the treatment of arthritic pain. Arthritis Res Ther 2007;9(3):214.
4. Keefe FJ, Lefebvre JC, Egert JR, et al. The relationship of gender to pain, pain behavior, and disability in osteoarthritis patients: the role of catastrophizing. Pain. 2000;87(3):325–34.
5. Thakur M, Dickenson AH, Baron R. Osteoarthritis pain: nociceptive or neuropathic? Nat Rev Rheumatol 2014;10(6):374–80.
6. Courtney CA, O'Hearn MA, Hornby TG. Neuromuscular function in painful knee osteoarthritis. Curr Pain Headache Rep. 2012;16(6):518–24.
7. Hadler NM. Knee pain is the malady—not osteoarthritis. Ann Intern Med. 1992;116(7):598–9.
8. Bedson J, Croft PR. The discordance between clinical and radiographic knee osteoarthritis: a systematic search and summary of the literature. BMC Musculoskelet Disord. 2008;9:116.
9. Beswick AD, Wylde V, Gooberman-Hill R, et al. What proportion of patients report long-term pain after total hip or knee replacement for osteoarthritis? A systematic review of prospective studies in unselected patients. BMJ Open. 2012;2(1):e000435.
10. Hochman JR, Gagliese L, Davis AM, et al. Neuropathic pain symptoms in a community knee OA cohort. Osteoarthritis Cartilage. 2011;19(6):647–54.
11. Freynhagen R, Baron R, Gockel U, et al. painDETECT: a new screening questionnaire to identify neuropathic components in patients with back pain. Curr Med Res Opin. 2006;22(10):1911–20.
12. Bouhassira D. Definition and classification of neuropathic pain [in French]. Presse Med. 2008;37(2 Pt 2):311–4.
13. Hochman JR, Davis AM, Elkayam J, et al. Neuropathic pain symptoms on the modified painDETECT correlate with signs of central sensitization in knee osteoarthritis. Osteoarthritis Cartilage. 2013;21(9):1236–42.
14. Hochman JR, French MR, Bermingham SL, et al. The nerve of osteoarthritis pain. Arthritis Care Res. 2010;62(7):1019–23.
15. Fernandes GS, Sarmanova A, Warner S, et al. Knee Pain and Related Health in the Community Study (KPIC): a cohort study protocol. BMC Musculoskelet Disord. 2017;18(1):404.
16. O'Reilly SC, Muir KR, Doherty M. Screening for pain in knee osteoarthritis: which question? Ann Rheum Dis. 1996;55(12):931–3.
17. Ingham SL, Zhang W, Doherty SA, McWilliams DF, Muir KR, Doherty M. Incident knee pain in the Nottingham community: a 12-year retrospective cohort study. Osteoarthritis Cartilage. 2011;19:847–52.

18. Suri P, Morgenroth DC, Hunter DJ. Epidemiology of osteoarthritis and associated comorbidities. PM R. 2012;4(5 Suppl):S10–9.
19. Thomas KS, et al. Home based exercise programme for knee pain and knee osteoarthritis: randomised controlled trial. BMJ. 2002;325(7367):752.
20. Leyland KM, Gates LS, Nevitt M, et al. Measuring the variation between self-reported osteoarthritis pain assessments [abstract]. Osteoarthritis Cartilage. 2016;24(Suppl 1):S8.
21. Hunt IM, Silman AJ, Benjamin S, McBeth J, Macfarlane GJ. The prevalence and associated features of chronic widespread pain in the community using the 'Manchester' definition of chronic widespread pain. Rheumatology. 1999;38:275–9.
22. Wolfe F, Smythe HA, Yunus MB, et al. The American College of Rheumatology 1990 criteria for the classification of fibromyalgia: report of the Multicenter Criteria Committee. Arthritis Rheum. 1990;33(2):160–72.
23. Silverwood V, Blagojevic-Bucknall M, Jinks C, et al. Current evidence on risk factors for knee osteoarthritis in older adults: a systematic review and meta-analysis. Osteoarthritis Cartilage. 2015;23(4):507–15.
24. Cleves MA. From the help desk: comparing areas under receiver operating characteristic curves from two or moreprobit or logit models. Stata J. 2002; 2(3):301–13.
25. Fayaz A, Croft P, Langford RM, et al. Prevalence of chronic pain in the UK: a systematic review and meta-analysis of population studies. BMJ Open. 2016; 6(6):e010364.
26. Torrance N, Ferguson JA, Afolabi E, et al. Neuropathic pain in the community: more under-treated than refractory? Pain. 2013;(5):154, 690–9.
27. Torrance N, Smith BH, Bennett MI, et al. The epidemiology of chronic pain of predominantly neuropathic origin: results from a general population survey. J Pain. 2006;7(4):281–9.
28. French HP, Smart KM, Doyle F. Prevalence of neuropathic pain in knee or hip osteoarthritis: a systematic review and meta-analysis. Semin Arthritis Rheum. 2017;47(1):1–8.
29. Hall GC, Carroll D, Parry D, et al. Epidemiology and treatment of neuropathic pain: the UK primary care perspective. Pain. 2006;122(1–2):156–62.
30. Fillingim RB, King CD, Ribeiro-Dasilva MC, Rahim-Williams B, Riley JL. Sex, gender, and pain: a review of recent clinical and experimental findings. J Pain. 2009;10(5):447–85.
31. Bouhassira D, Attal N, Alchaar H, et al. Comparison of pain syndromes associated with nervous or somatic lesions and development of a new neuropathic pain diagnostic questionnaire (DN4). Pain. 2005;114(1–2):29–36.
32. Leung L. Pain catastrophizing: an updated review. Indian J Psychol Med. 2012;34(3):204–17.
33. Neogi T. The epidemiology and impact of pain in osteoarthritis. Osteoarthritis Cartilage. 2013;21(9):1145–53.
34. Hawker GA, Mian S, Kendzerska T, et al. Measures of adult pain: Visual Analog Scale for Pain (VAS Pain), Numeric Rating Scale for Pain (NRS Pain), McGill Pain Questionnaire (MPQ), Short-Form McGill Pain Questionnaire (SF-MPQ), Chronic Pain Grade Scale (CPGS), Short Form-36 Bodily Pain Scale (SF-36 BPS), and Measure of Intermittent and Constant Osteoarthritis Pain (ICOAP). Arthritis Care Res. 2011;63(Suppl 11):S240–52.
35. McLean SA, Clauw DJ. Biomedical models of fibromyalgia. Disabil Rehabil. 2005;27(12):659–65.
36. Finnerup NB, Sorensen L, Biering-Sorensen F, et al. Segmental hypersensitivity and spinothalamic function in spinal cord injury pain. Exp Neurol. 2007;207(1):139–49.
37. Wang GS, Tong DM, Chen XD, Yang TH, Zhou YT, Ma XB. Metabolic syndrome is a strong risk factor for minor ischemic stroke and subsequent vascular events. PLoS One. 2016;11(8):e0156243.
38. Zhang W, Nuki G, Moskowitz RW, et al. OARSI recommendations for the management of hip and knee osteoarthritis: part III: changes in evidence following systematic cumulative update of research published through January 2009. Osteoarthritis Cartilage. 2010;18(4):476–99.
39. Dimitroulas T, Duarte RV, Behura A, et al. Neuropathic pain in osteoarthritis: a review of pathophysiological mechanisms and implications for treatment. Semin Arthritis Rheum. 2014;44(2):145–54.
40. Power JD, Perruccio AV, Gandhi R, et al. Neuropathic pain in end-stage hip and knee osteoarthritis: differential associations with patient-reported pain at rest and pain on activity. Osteoarthritis Cartilage. 2018;26(3):363–9.
41. Carlesso LC, Niu J, Segal NA, et al. The effect of widespread pain on knee pain worsening, incident knee osteoarthritis (OA), and incident knee pain: the Multicenter OA (MOST) Study. J Rheumatol. 2017;44(4):493–8.
42. Schiphof D, Kerkhof HJ, Damen J, et al. Factors for pain in patients with different grades of knee osteoarthritis. Arthritis Care Res. 2013;65(5):695–702.
43. McWilliams DF, Muthuri S, Muir KR, et al. Self-reported adult footwear and the risks of lower limb osteoarthritis: the GOAL case control study. BMC Musculoskelet Disord. 2014;15:308.
44. Netuveli G, Wiggins RD, Hildon Z, et al. Quality of life at older ages: evidence from the English Longitudinal Study of Aging (wave 1). J Epidemiol Community Health. 2006;60(4):357–63.
45. Mindell J, Biddulph JP, Hirani V, et al. Cohort profile: the Health Survey for England. Int J Epidemiol. 2012;41(6):1585–93.

13

Recombinant human proteoglycan-4 reduces phagocytosis of urate crystals and downstream nuclear factor kappa B and inflammasome activation and production of cytokines and chemokines in human and murine macrophages

Marwa Qadri[1], Gregory D. Jay[2,3], Ling X. Zhang[2], Wendy Wong[2], Anthony M. Reginato[4], Changqi Sun[4], Tannin A. Schmidt[5] and Khaled A. Elsaid[1*]

Abstract

Background: Gout is an inflammatory arthritis caused by monosodium urate monohydrate (MSU) crystals' joint deposition. MSU phagocytosis by resident macrophages is a key step in gout pathogenesis. MSU phagocytosis triggers nuclear factor kappa B (NFκB) activation and production of cytokines and chemokines. Proteoglycan-4 (PRG4) is a glycoprotein produced by synovial fibroblasts and exerts an anti-inflammatory effect in the joint mediated by its interaction with cell surface receptor CD44. PRG4 also binds and antagonizes TLR2 and TLR4. The objective of this study is to evaluate the efficacy of recombinant human PRG4 (rhPRG4) in suppressing MSU-induced inflammation and mechanical allodynia in vitro and in vivo.

Methods: THP-1 macrophages were incubated with MSU crystals ± rhPRG4 or bovine submaxillary mucin (BSM), and crystal phagocytosis, cytokines and chemokines expression and production were determined. NFκB p65 subunit nuclear translocation, NLRP3 induction, caspase-1 activation and conversion of proIL-1β to mature IL-1β were studied. MSU phagocytosis by $Prg4^{+/+}$ and $Prg4^{-/-}$ peritoneal macrophages was determined in the absence or presence of rhPRG4, BSM, anti-CD44, anti-TLR2, anti-TLR4 and isotype control antibodies. Rhodamine-labeled rhPRG4 was incubated with murine macrophages and receptor colocalization studies were performed. Lewis rats underwent intra-articular injection of MSU crystals followed by intra-articular treatment with PBS or rhPRG4. Weight bearing and SF myeloperoxidase activities were determined.

(Continued on next page)

* Correspondence: elsaid@chapman.edu
Submitted to Arthritis Research and Therapy, November 2017 3rd Revision
Submitted: July 2018.
[1]Department of Biomedical and Pharmaceutical Sciences, Chapman University
School of Pharmacy, Rinker Health Sciences Campus, 9401 Jeronimo Road,
Irvine, CA 92618, USA
Full list of author information is available at the end of the article

(Continued from previous page)

Results: rhPRG4 reduced MSU crystal phagocytosis at 4 h ($p < 0.01$) and IL-1β, TNF-α, IL-8 and MCP-1 expression and production at 6 h ($p < 0.05$). BSM did not alter MSU phagocytosis or IL-1β production in human and murine macrophages. rhPRG4 treatment reduced NFκB nuclear translocation, NLRP3 expression, caspase-1 activation and generation of mature IL-1β ($p < 0.05$). MSU-stimulated IL-1β production was higher in $Prg4^{-/-}$ macrophages compared to $Prg4^{+/+}$ macrophages ($p < 0.001$). rhPRG4, anti-CD44, anti-TLR2 and anti-TLR4 antibody treatments reduced MSU phagocytosis and IL-1β production in murine macrophages ($p < 0.05$). rhPRG4 preferentially colocalized with CD44 on $Prg4^{-/-}$ peritoneal macrophages compared to TLR2 or TLR4 ($p < 0.01$). rhPRG4 normalized weight bearing and reduced SF myeloperoxidase activity compared to PBS in vivo.

Conclusion: rhPRG4 inhibits MSU crystal phagocytosis and exhibits an anti-inflammatory and anti-nociceptive activity in vitro and in vivo. rhPRG4's anti-inflammatory mechanism may be due to targeting CD44 on macrophages.

Keywords: Gout, Proteoglycan-4, Macrophages, Lubricin, Urate, CD44, TLR2, TLR4

Background

Gout is an inflammatory arthritis characterized by deposition of monosodium urate monohydrate (MSU) crystals in synovial joints and periarticular tissues [1, 2]. Gout is characterized by painful episodes of intermittent acute monoarthritis, most often in peripheral joints such as the first metatarsophalangeal and knee joints, in the midst of asymptomatic periods [2, 3]. Tissue MSU crystal deposits initiate inflammation in resident macrophages, mediated in part by pattern recognition receptors of the innate immune system, such as toll-like receptors (TLR2 and TLR4) [4–8]. Other endogenous TLR ligands, such as myeloid-related proteins 8 and 14 and long chain fatty acids may play a role in priming macrophages to the inflammatory effect of MSU crystals [9, 10]. Priming macrophages stimulates nuclear factor kappa B (NFκB) nuclear translocation, proIL-1β expression and induces the expression of NACHT, LRR and PYD-containing protein 3 (NLRP3) inflammasome components: NLRP3 protein, ASC adaptor protein, and caspase-1 [11–13]. NFκB translocation results in inducing the expression and secretion of proinflammatory cytokines, e.g. interleukin-1 beta (IL-1β) and tumor necrosis factor alpha (TNF-α) and chemokines, e.g. interleukin-8 (IL-8) and monocyte chemoattractant protein-1 (MCP-1) [14–17]. Particulate danger signals e.g. MSU crystals are thought to cause lysosomal disruption following their endocytosis by macrophages and thus trigger inflammasome activation and conversion of proIL-1β to IL-1β with downstream enhancement of the inflammatory cascade and inflammatory cell influx to the affected joint [18–22].

Lubricin/Proteoglycan-4 (PRG4) is a mucinous glycoprotein secreted by synovial fibroblasts and superficial zone articular chondrocytes [23–25]. PRG4 is the major lubricating constituent of synovial fluid (SF) and a biological role for PRG4 has been described. The recombinant form of PRG4 exhibits an anti-inflammatory role characterized by its ability to compete with hyaluronan on binding to the CD44 receptor [26]. The downstream effect of engaging CD44 by PRG4 is the inhibition of IL-1β and TNF-α induced NFκB nuclear translocation in synoviocytes from patients with RA and OA [26, 27]. The autocrine anti-inflammatory role of PRG4 on synovial fibroblasts was shown to be mediated by its ability to inhibit the degradation of cytosolic inhibitor kappa B alpha (IκB-α) in a CD44-dependent manner [27]. Related to TLRs, recombinant human PRG4 (rhPRG4) binds to, and regulates agonist-induced activation of TLR2 and TLR4 [28, 29]. Supplementation of OA and RA synovial fluid aspirates with the native form of PRG4 inhibited TLR2 and TLR4 activation by these aspirates [29].

The objective of this study is to evaluate the efficacy of rhPRG4 related to modulation of MSU crystal uptake by human and murine macrophages and subsequent cellular activation and induction of proinflammatory cytokines and chemokines expression and production. Furthermore, we studied the ability of rhPRG4 to reduce inflammation and acute mechanical allodynia in a rat model of intra-articular MSU challenge. We hypothesized that rhPRG4 inhibits MSU crystal phagocytosis by macrophages through the inhibition of TLR receptors or CD44, resulting in a significant reduction in IL-1β, TNF-α, IL-8 and MCP-1 expression and production and an anti-inflammatory and an anti-nociceptive effect in vivo.

Methods

Differentiation of THP-1 monocytes into macrophages and studies of time-dependent MSU phagocytosis and impact of rhPRG4 treatment

THP-1 monocytes (ATCC, USA) were cultured to a density of 1.5×10^6 cells/ml in 75 cm^2 flask in RPMI 1640 medium supplemented with 10% heat-inactivated fetal bovine serum (FBS), 10 mM HEPES, 2 mM glutamine, 100 U/L Penicillin and 100μg/ml streptomycin and maintained at 37 °C. In sterile 12 well plates (Corning, Sigma Aldrich, USA), 500,000 cells in 2 ml RPMI 1640 media were differentiated into macrophages by incubation with phorbol 12-myristate-13-acetate (PMA; Sigma Aldrich) to a final concentration of 5 ng/ml for 48 h [30]. Subsequently, media supernatants were removed and wells were washed with sterile PBS to remove any unattached cells and new RPMI 1640 media was added.

THP-1 macrophages were treated with endotoxin-free MSU crystals (100μg/ml; Invivogen, USA) ± bovine submaxillary mucin (BSM; molecular mass > 1000 KDa) (Sigma Aldrich) (25 μg/ml) or rhPRG4 (molecular mass is approximately 240 KDa) (100 μg/ml) for 2 and 4 h at 37 °C. rhPRG4 is an endotoxin-free full-length product produced by CHO-M cells (Lubris, Framingham, MA, USA) [31]. Subsequently, adherent macrophages were harvested via trypsinization, pelleted and washed with PBS. The phagocytosis of MSU crystals was determined by analyzing change in cell side-scatter using a flow cytometer (BD FACSVerse, BD Biosciences, USA). Two regions of interest were identified. P1 represents the THP-1 macrophage population in the absence of MSU exposure. P2 represents the THP-1 macrophage population with increased side-scatter indicative of MSU internalization. Data are presented as the mean percentage of cells in the P2 region across different time points and different treatments, and were derived from four independent experiments with duplicate wells per group. All flow cytometry experiments were performed using the same acquisition parameters.

Comparative effect of rhPRG4 and BSM on MSU-stimulated production of proinflammatory cytokines and chemokines

THP-1 macrophages (500,000 cells per well) were treated with MSU (100μg/ml) ± rhPRG4 (100μg/ml) or BSM (25μg/ml) for 6 h followed by collection of media supernatants. Media concentrations of IL-1β, TNF-α, IL-8 and MCP-1 were determined using ELISA kits (R&D Systems, USA). Data represent the mean ± S.D. of four independent experiments with duplicate wells per group.

Nuclear p65 NFκB translocation and NLRP3 inflammasome activation following MSU challenge and impact of rhPRG4 treatment

NFκB p65 subunit translocation studies were performed as previously described [32]. THP-1 macrophages (600,000 cells per well) were treated with MSU (100μg/ml) ± rhPRG4 (50 and 100μg/ml) for 1 h followed by cell harvest and nuclear protein extraction. Nuclear levels of p65 subunit were determined using a DNA binding ELISA assay (Abcam) and were normalized to total nuclear protein content using the micro BCA assay and expressed as detectable NFκB p65 levels normalized to untreated controls. Data represent the mean ± S.D. of three independent experiments with duplicate wells per treatment.

THP-1 macrophages (500,000 cells per well) were treated with MSU (100μg/ml) ± rhPRG4 (100 and 200μg/ml) for 12 h. A positive control treatment (H$_2$O$_2$; 5 mM) was also included in the absence or presence of rhPRG4 (200μg/ml). Subsequently, cells were washed twice with ice-cold PBS and lysed on ice in RIPA buffer for 30 min and centrifuged for 5 min (16,000 g at 4 °C). The supernatant was collected and total cellular protein was quantified using BCA protein assay kit (Thermo-Fisher Scientific). Equal amounts of protein (40–50 μg) were loaded and separated by a 12% SDS-PAGE gel. Following blotting, membranes were blocked using 5% non-fat dry milk and probed with primary antibodies overnight at 4 °C. These antibodies included proIL-1β (D3U3E; Cell Signal Technology, USA), cleaved IL-1β (D3A3Z; Cell Signal Technology), NLRP3 (D2P5E; Cell Signal Technology), and capase-1 (MAB6216; R&D Systems). Target proteins were detected using IRDye secondary goat anti-mouse or goat anti-rabbit antibodies (LI-COR Biosciences, USA) and visualized with LI-COR Odyssey Blot Imager (LI-COR Biosciences).

Dose-dependent effect of rhPRG4 treatment on MSU-induced proinflammatory cytokines and chemokines gene expression and production in THP-1 macrophages

THP-1 macrophages (500,000 cells per well) were treated with MSU (100μg/ml) ± rhPRG4 (25, 50, 100 and 200μg/ml) for 6 h. Total RNA was extracted using TRIzol reagent (Thermo Fisher Scientific), and RNA concentrations were determined with a NanoDrop ND-2000 spectrophotometer (NanoDrop Technologies, USA). cDNA was synthesized using Transcriptor First Strand cDNA Synthesis Kit (Roche, USA). Quantitative PCR (qPCR) was performed on Applied Biosystems Step One Plus Real-Time PCR System (Thermo Fisher Scientific) using TaqMan Fast Advanced Master Mix (Life Technologies, USA). Genes of interest included IL-1β (Hs00174097_m1, ThermoFisher Scientific), TNF-α (Hs01113624_g1, ThermoFisher Scientific), IL-8 (Hs00174103_m1, ThermoFisher Scientific) and MCP-1 (Hs00234140_m1, ThermoFisher Scientific). The cycle threshold (Ct) value of target genes was normalized to the Ct value of GAPDH (Hs02758991_g1; Thermo Fisher Scientific) in the same sample, and the relative expression was calculated using the $2^{-\Delta\Delta Ct}$ method [33]. Data are presented as fold target gene expression compared to untreated control. Data represent mean ± S.D. of three independent experiments with duplicate wells per treatment.

THP-1 macrophages (500,000 cells per well) were treated with MSU (100μg/ml) ± rhPRG4 (100 and 200μg/ml) for 24 H. *media* concentrations of IL-1β, TNF-α, IL-8 and MCP-1 were determined using commercially available ELISA kits (R&D Systems). Data represent the mean ± S.D. of three independent experiments with duplicate wells per group.

Isolation of peritoneal macrophages from *Prg4⁺/⁺* and *Prg4⁻/⁻* mice, phagocytosis of MSU crystals by murine macrophages and downstream production of IL-1β and comparative efficacy of rhPRG4, anti-CD44, anti-TLR2 and anti-TLR4 antibody treatments

The phenotype of the *Prg4⁻/⁻* mouse has been previously reported [34], and is characterized by cartilage degeneration and a hyperplastic synovium contributing to joint failure [34]. The *Prg4⁻/⁻* and *Prg4⁺/⁺* mouse colonies are maintained at Rhode Island Hospital. *Prg4⁻/⁻* mouse is also commercially available (stock #025737; The Jackson Laboratory, Maine, USA). Isolation of murine peritoneal macrophages was performed as previously described [35] following IACUC approval at Rhode Island Hospital. A total of 20 *Prg4⁺/⁺* and 20 *Prg4⁻/⁻* mice were euthanized. Subsequently, the abdomen of each mouse was soaked with 70% alcohol and a small incision was made along the midline with scissors. Using blunt dissection, the abdominal skin was retracted to expose the intact peritoneal wall. A 27 G needle attached to a 10 ml syringe filled with sterile cold PBS was inserted through the peritoneal wall at the midline and injected into each mouse, aspirated slowly from the peritoneum, and peritoneal macrophages cells were collected. Subsequently, cells were centrifuged at 10,000 rpm and 4 °C for 10 min. Pelleted cells were re-suspended in RPMI 1640 medium supplemented with 10% FBS and 1% Penicillin/Streptomycin.

Murine peritoneal macrophages were plated onto sterile chamber slides (ThermoFisher Scientific) at a concentration of 1.3×10^6 cells/well. Cells were allowed to adhere by incubation at 37 °C for 24 h. Following incubation, media and non-adherent cells were removed and fresh media was added. Treatments included untreated control cells, MSU (100µg/ml) ± rhPRG4 (100µg/ml), BSM (25µg/ml), anti-CD44 (Abcam; 2µg/ml), anti-TLR2 (Abcam; 2µg/ml), anti-TLR4 (Abcam; 2µg/ml) and isotype control (IC; 2µg/ml) (Abcam) antibodies. Incubations were performed for 4 and 24 h. Subsequently, slides were washed once with PBS and then fixed with 4% formalin for 15 min. Slides were subsequently washed with PBS and cells were permeabilized with 0.1% Triton X100 for 10 min. After washing with PBS for three times, slides were mounted with DAPI mounting medium (Vector Lab, USA) and viewed under a microscope (Nikon E800). The number of intracellular MSU crystals in 8 areas for a total of 900 cells was determined and the total number of MSU crystals was reported. Data represent the mean ± S.D. of four to five independent experiments. Media

supernatants were assayed for IL-1β concentrations using a murine ELISA kit (R&D Systems).

Colocalization of rhPRG4 and CD44, TLR2 and TLR4 receptors in *Prg4⁻/⁻* peritoneal macrophages

Isolation and culture of *Prg4⁻/⁻* peritoneal macrophages was performed as described above. Rhodamine labeling of rhPRG4 was performed using the Pierce NHS-Rhodamine Antibody Labeling Kit (Thermo Fisher Scientific). Rhodamine labeled rhPRG4 (25µg/ml) was incubated with *Prg4⁻/⁻* macrophages for 2 h. Subsequently, media was removed and cells were washed with PBS and fixed using 4% formalin for 15 min at room temperature. Cells were then permeabilized with 0.2% Triton X-100 for 10 min and subsequently blocked with 2% BSA for 30 min. Cells were incubated with CD44 antibody, TLR2 antibody, TLR4 antibody or an isotype control (Abcam) (1:200 dilution) overnight at 4 °C. Cells were then washed with PBS and incubated with Alexa Fluor 488 goat anti-rabbit IgG (Thermo Fisher Scientific) at 1:200 dilution for 1 h at room temperature. After washing with PBS for three times, slides were mounted with DAPI mounting medium (Vector Lab). Confocal images were acquired with a Nikon C1si confocal microscope (Nikon Inc., USA) using diode lasers 402, 488 and 561. Serial optical sections were obtained sequentially with EZ-C1 computer software's frame lambda setting. Z series sections were collected at 0.2 µm with a 60× Plan Apo, 1.4 numerical aperture lens. Six to seven fields were collected per sample for a total minimum number of 100 cells. All colocalization analyses were performed on deconvolved, 3D acquisitions (Elements version 3.2, Nikon Inc.). In each Z stack, cells were outlined and analyzed with Nikon's colocalization macro. Pearson's Correlation Coefficient was used to determine colocalization. A minimum threshold of Pearson's Coefficient > 0.5 was used to indicate positive colocalization. Data is presented as percent of cells positive for rhPRG4 and receptor colocalization and is expressed as mean ± standard deviation of 3 experiments.

Crystal-induced inflammation and mechanical allodynia in the rat and the impact of rhPRG4 treatment

Male Lewis rats ($n = 40$; 10 weeks old) (Charles River, USA) were randomly assigned to three experimental groups; MSU only, MSU + PBS or MSU + rhPRG4. All animals received an intra-articular injection of pyrogen-free MSU suspension (50 µl; 5 mg/ml). Intra-articular injections were performed under gas anesthesia (5% isoflurane). Intra-articular injections were performed in the right knee joints. The skin around the right knee joint was shaved and the injection site was cleansed using a topical iodine-based antiseptic and 70% isopropranolol. At 1 h following MSU injection, animals received PBS (50 µl), rhPRG4 (50 µl; 1 mg/ml) or remained untreated. We have also included 4 animals that received intra-articular PBS (50 µl).

Static weight bearing of the hind limbs of animals at baseline and at 3 and 6 h post-MSU injection ($n = 12$ in the MSU alone group and $n = 14$ in PBS and rhPRG4-treated animals) and at 24 h post-MSU injection ($n = 5$ in MSU alone and $n = 7$ in PBS and rhPRG4-treated animals) was measured using an Incapacitance Meter (Harvard Apparatus, USA). Data are presented as differential weight bearing between the hind right limb and the hind left limb. Animals were euthanized either at 6 h ($n = 7$ in each group) or at 24 h ($n = 5$ in MSU alone and $n = 7$ in PBS and rhPRG4-treated animals) following MSU challenge. Lavaging of the right knee joint was performed by injecting 100 µl of normal saline followed by joint flexion and extension and aspirating ~ 20–30 µl of SF lavage. Animal sera were also collected. Myeloperoxidase (MPO) activity in SF lavage samples was measured using a commercially available kit (Abcam). SF lavage and serum urea concentrations of each animal were determined using a urea assay kit (Abcam) and the fold dilution in SF lavage was calculated [36, 37]. Data are expressed as MPO activity (µU) adjusted to fold urea dilution. SF lavaging was performed for 2 untreated control animals and 4 PBS-injected animals and SF lavage MPO activity was determined as described above. All animal studies were approved by the IACUC committee at MCPHS University.

Statistical analyses

Statistical analyses of gene expression data were performed using ΔCt values (C_t target gene-C_t GAPDH) for each gene of interest in each experimental group and data were graphically presented as fold expression relative to untreated controls using the $2^{-\Delta\Delta Ct}$ method. Continuous variables were initially evaluated whether they satisfy the requirements for parametric statistical tests. Statistical significance comparing two groups or multiple groups with parametric data was assessed by Student's t test or ANOVA followed by post-hoc multiple comparisons using Tukey's post-hoc test. Statistical significance comparing two groups or multiple groups with nonparametric data was assessed by Rank Sum test or ANOVA on the ranks. Analysis of MSU phagocytosis by THP-1 macrophages following 2 and 4-h incubations and impact of rhPRG4 or BSM treatments was performed using 2-way ANOVA. A p value of < 0.05 was considered statistically significant.

Results

rhPRG4 treatment reduced MSU crystal phagocytosis by THP-1 macrophages

Representative MSU phagocytosis flow cytometry scatterplots are presented in Fig. 1. Qualitatively, THP-1 macrophages internalized MSU crystals at 2 and 4 h

with more cells appearing in the P2 region of interest at 4 h compared to 2 h (Fig. 1b and e). rhPRG4 treatment appeared to reduce the number of THP-1 macrophages in the P2 region, especially following incubation for 4 h (Fig. 1f). BSM treatment as a negative control mucin did not appear to modify MSU phagocytosis by THP-1 macrophages (Fig. 1d and g). rhPRG4 or BSM alone did not appear to alter the side scattering of THP-1 macrophages (Fig. 1h and i). The percentage of positive cells in the 2-h MSU group was higher than the percentage of positive cells in the corresponding control group ($p = 0.022$) (Fig. 1j). Similarly, the percentage of positive cells in the 4-h MSU group was higher than the percentage of positive cells in the corresponding control group ($p = 0.0002$). MSU phagocytosis by THP-1 macrophages at 4 h was higher than MSU phagocytosis by THP-1 macrophages at 2 h ($p = 0.003$). rhPRG4 or BSM treatments did not alter MSU phagocytosis by THP-1 macrophages at 2 h ($p = 0.461$; $p = 0.999$) (Fig. 1k). In contrast, rhPRG4 significantly reduced MSU phagocytosis by THP-1 macrophages at 4 h ($p < 0.001$). BSM treatment did not alter MSU phagocytosis by THP-1 macrophages at 4 h ($p = 0.981$), and the percentage of positive cells in the MSU + BSM group was higher than the percentage of positive cells in the MSU + rhPRG4 group ($p = 0.001$). There was no significant difference in percentage of positive cells between rhPRG4-treated or BSM-treated macrophages and untreated controls at 2 or 4 h ($p > 0.999$ for all comparisons).

rhPRG4 treatment reduced MSU stimulated cytokine and chemokine gene expression and production mediated by a reduction in NLRP3 inflammasome activation and NFκB nuclear translocation

Incubation of THP-1 macrophages with MSU crystals resulted in a significant increase in IL-1β, TNF-α, IL-8 and MCP-1 production by the macrophages at 6 h ($p < 0.001$; $p = 0.004$; $p < 0.001$; $p < 0.001$) (Fig. 2a through d). rhPRG4 and BSM treatments did not significantly alter basal cytokine and chemokine production by THP-1 macrophages ($p > 0.05$ for all comparisons). rhPRG4 treatment significantly reduced MSU-induced IL-1β ($p < 0.001$), TNF-α ($p = 0.003$), IL-8 ($p < 0.001$) and MCP-1 ($p = 0.003$) production by THP-1 macrophages at 6 h. In contrast, BSM treatment did not significantly alter MSU-induced cytokines and chemokines production ($p = 0.305$; $p = 0.365$; $p = 0.964$; $p = 0.998$). Media concentrations of IL-1β, IL-8 and MCP-1 were significantly lower in the MSU + rhPRG4 group compared to the MSU + BSM group ($p < 0.001$; $p = 0.002$, $p = 0.003$).

MSU crystals enhanced nuclear NFκB nuclear translocation in THP-1 macrophages compared to untreated control cells (Fig. 2e) ($p < 0.001$). rhPRG4 treatments at 50 and 100 µg/ml significantly reduced MSU stimulated

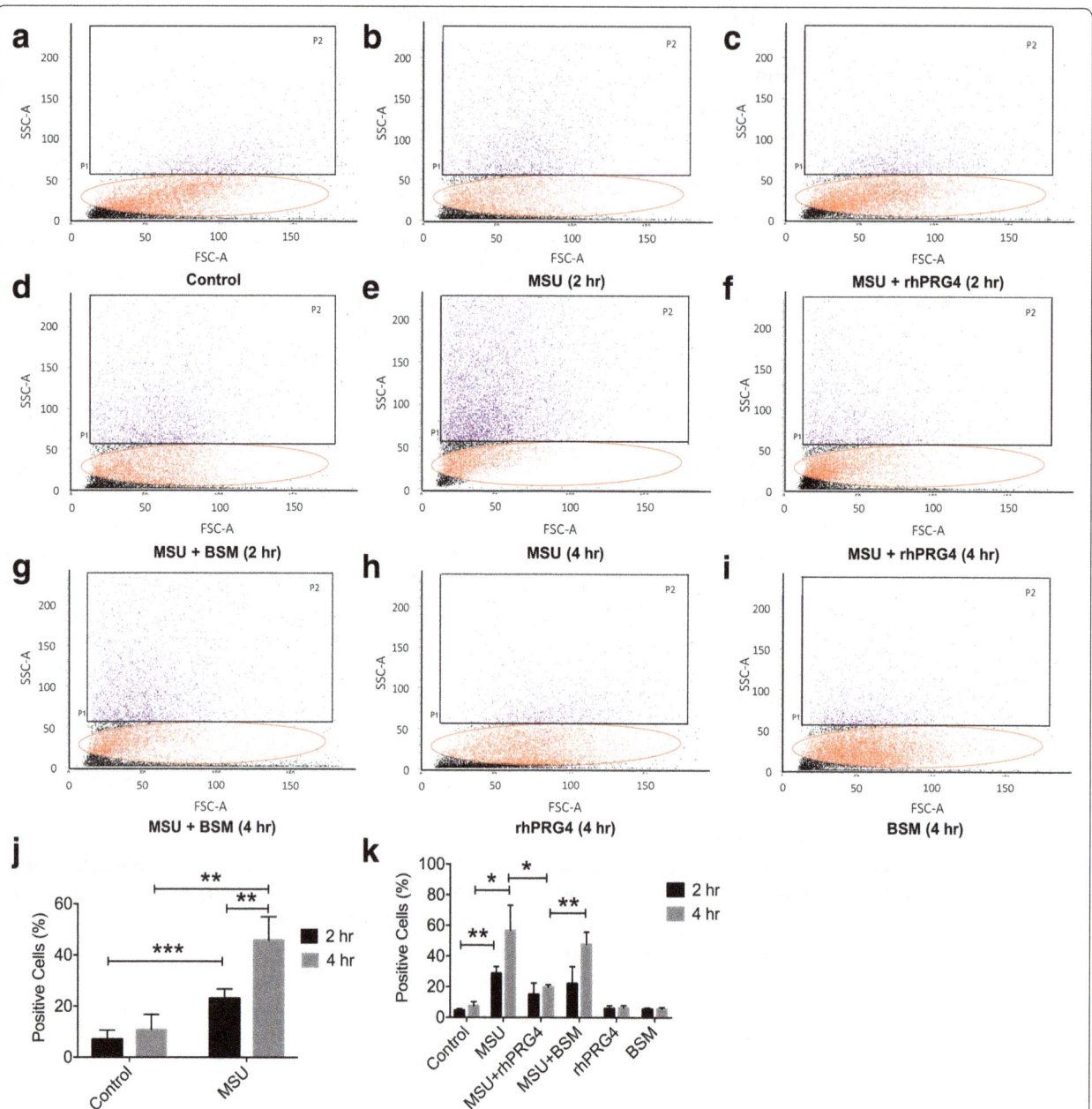

Fig. 1 Time and treatment-dependent phagocytosis of monosodium urate monohydrate (MSU) crystals by differentiated human THP-1 macrophages using flow cytometry and impact of recombinant human proteoglycan-4 (rhPRG4) or bovine submaxillary mucin (BSM) treatments following 2 and 4-h incubations. Quantitative determination of MSU phagocytosis was performed using the percentage of cells in the P2 region of interest. Data represent the mean ± S.D. of four independent experiments. *$p < 0.001$; **$p < 0.01$; ***$p < 0.05$. **a** Representative flow cytometry scatterplot of untreated human THP-1 macrophages. **b** Representative flow cytometry scatterplot of MSU-treated THP-1 macrophages for 2 h. **c** Representative flow cytometry scatterplot of MSU + rhPRG4 (100 µg/ml)-treated THP-1 macrophages for 2 h. **d** Representative flow cytometry scatterplot of MSU + BSM (25 µg/ml)-treated THP-1 macrophages for 2 h. **e** Representative flow cytometry scatterplot of MSU-treated THP-1 macrophages for 4 h. **f** Representative flow cytometry scatterplot of MSU + rhPRG4 (100 µg/ml)-treated THP-1 macrophages for 4 h. **g** Representative flow cytometry scatterplot of MSU + BSM (25 µg/ml)-treated THP-1 macrophages for 4 h. **h** Representative flow cytometry scatterplot of rhPRG4 (100 µg/ml)-treated THP-1 macrophages for 4 h. **i** Representative flow cytometry scatterplot of BSM (25 µg/ml)-treated THP-1 macrophages for 4 h. **j** Phagocytosis of MSU crystals by THP-1 macrophages was higher in following 4-h incubation compared to 2-h incubation. **k** rhPRG4 treatment reduced MSU phagocytosis by THP-1 macrophages at 4 h compared to BSM

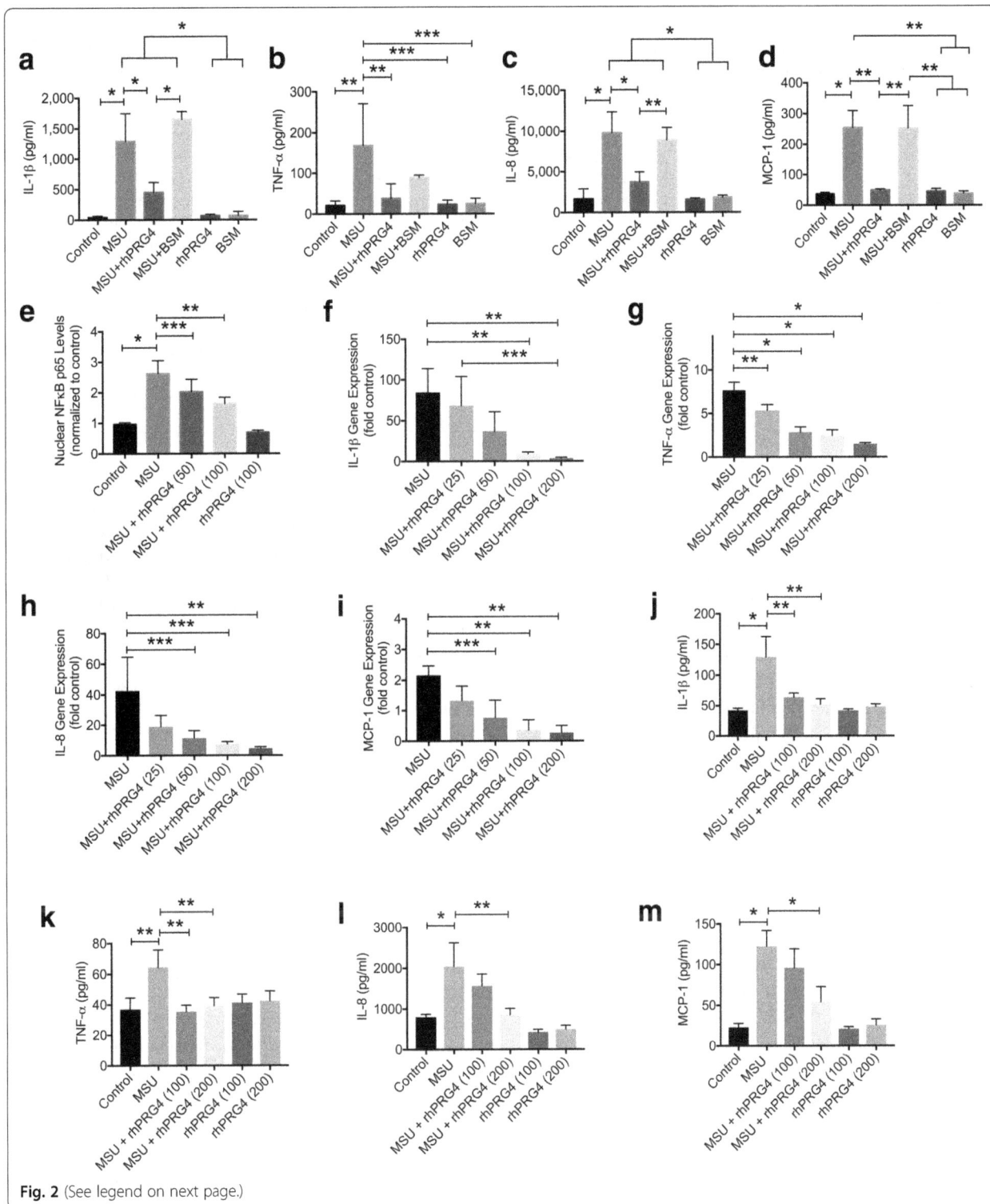

Fig. 2 (See legend on next page.)

(See figure on previous page.)
Fig. 2 Impact of recombinant human proteoglycan-4 (rhPRG4) treatment on monosodium urate monohydrate (MSU) crystal-induced expression and production of proinflammatory cytokines and chemokines and nuclear factor kappa b (NFκB) p65 subunit nuclear translocation in THP-1 macrophages. Cytokines included interleukin-1 beta (IL-1β) and tumor necrosis factor alpha (TNF-α). Chemokines included interleukin-8 (IL-8) and monocyte chemoattractant protein-1 (MCP-1). Gene expression data are presented as fold induction of proinflammatory cytokines and chemokines gene expression compared to control untreated THP-1 macrophages. THP-1 macrophages were treated with MSU crystals (100μg/ml) ± rhPRG4 (100μg/ml) or bovine submaxillary mucin (BSM; 25μg/ml) for 6 h (**a** through **d**). NFκB p65 subunit nuclear translocation in THP-1 macrophages was performed at 1 h following MSU challenge (100μg/ml). Gene expression studies were performed at 6 h (**f** through **i**) and cytokine and chemokine media concentrations were determined at 24 h (**j** through **m**). Data represent the mean ± S.D. of three to four independent experiments with duplicate wells per group. $*p < 0.001$; $**p < 0.01$; $***p < 0.05$. **a** rhPRG4 treatment reduced MSU-stimulated production of IL-1β by THP-1 macrophages. **b** rhPRG4 treatment reduced MSU-stimulated production of TNF-α by THP-1 macrophages. **c** rhPRG4 treatment reduced MSU-stimulated production of IL-8 by THP-1 macrophages. **d** rhPRG4 treatment reduced MSU-stimulated production of MCP-1 by THP-1 macrophages. **e** rhPRG4 treatment reduced MSU-stimulated NFκB p65 subunit nuclear translocation in THP-1 macrophages. **f** rhPRG4 (100 and 200μg/ml) treatment reduced IL-1β gene expression in MSU-stimulated THP-1 macrophages. **g** rhPRG4 (25, 50, 100 and 200μg/ml) treatment reduced TNF-α gene expression in MSU-stimulated THP-1 macrophages. **h** rhPRG4 (50, 100 and 200μg/ml) treatment reduced IL-8 gene expression in MSU-stimulated THP-1 macrophages. **i** rhPRG4 (50, 100 and 200μg/ml) treatment reduced MCP-1 gene expression in MSU-stimulated THP-1 macrophages. **j** rhPRG4 (100 and 200μg/ml) treatment reduced IL-1β production by MSU-stimulated THP-1 macrophages. **k** rhPRG4 (100 and 200μg/ml) treatment reduced TNF-α production by MSU-stimulated THP-1 macrophages. **l** rhPRG4 (200μg/ml) treatment reduced IL-8 production by MSU-stimulated THP-1 macrophages. **m** rhPRG4 (200μg/ml) treatment reduced MCP-1 production by MSU-stimulated THP-1 macrophages

NFκB nuclear translocation in THP-1 macrophages ($p = 0.039$; $p = 0.008$).

MSU crystals induced IL-1β expression compared to untreated macrophages ($p < 0.001$) (Fig. 2f). rhPRG4 (100 and 200μg/ml) treatments reduced IL-1β expression in THP-1 macrophages ($p = 0.002$; $p = 0.001$). Likewise, MSU crystals significantly induced TNF-α expression compared to untreated macrophages ($p < 0.001$) (Fig. 2g). rhPRG4 (25, 50, 100 and 200μg/ml) treatments reduced TNF-α expression compared to MSU alone group ($p = 0.009$; $p < 0.001$; $p < 0.001$; $p < 0.001$). MSU crystals significantly induced chemokines IL-8 and MCP-1 expression compared to untreated macrophages ($p < 0.001$) (Fig. 2h and i). rhPRG4 (50, 100 and 200μg/ml) treatments reduced IL-8 expression compared to MSU alone group ($p = 0.031$; $p = 0.015$; $p = 0.009$). Similarly, rhPRG4 (50, 100 and 200μg/ml) treatments reduced MCP-1 expression compared to MSU alone group ($p = 0.012$; $p = 0.002$; $p = 0.001$).

At 24 h, treatment with MSU crystals resulted in elevated IL-1β media concentrations compared to controls ($p < 0.001$) (Fig. 2j). rhPRG4 (100 and 200μg/ml) treatment reduced MSU-induced IL-1β production by macrophages ($p = 0.003$; $p = 0.001$). MSU crystals significantly increased TNF-α production by THP-1 macrophages ($p = 0.004$) (Fig. 2k). rhPRG4 (100 and 200μg/ml) treatments significantly reduced MSU-induced TNF-α production by macrophages ($p = 0.003$; $p = 0.009$). MSU crystals significantly induced IL-8 and MCP-1 production by macrophages ($p < 0.001$) (Fig. 2l and m). rhPRG4 (200μg/ml) treatment significantly reduced MSU-stimulated IL-8 and MCP-1 production by macrophages ($p = 0.004$; $p < 0.001$). rhPRG4 (100 and 200μg/ml) alone did not alter the basal levels of cytokines and chemokines ($p > 0.05$ for all comparisons).

MSU activated the NLRP3 inflammasome as evidenced by increased cytosolic NLRP3 protein levels in THP-1 macrophages, activated procaspase-1 and increased conversion of proIL-1β to active IL-1β (Fig. 3a). rhPRG4 (100 and 200μg/ml) treatments reduced cytosolic NLRP3 protein levels compared to MSU treatment alone ($p < 0.05$; $p < 0.001$) (Fig. 3b). Similarly, rhPRG4 (100 and 200μg/ml) treatments reduced procaspase-1 activation ($p < 0.001$ for both comparisons; Fig. 3c) and the 200μg/ml treatment level had a lower level of intracellular mature IL-1β ($p < 0.05$; Fig. 3d). rhPRG4 treatment at 200 μg/ml did not alter H_2O_2 induced NLRP3 induction, caspase-1 activation or mature IL-1β generation ($p > 0.05$).

Prg4$^{-/-}$ peritoneal macrophages demonstrated enhanced MSU crystal intracellular localization at 24 h and IL-1β production compared to Prg4$^{+/+}$ peritoneal macrophages

Phagocytosis of MSU crystals by Prg4$^{-/-}$ and Prg4$^{+/+}$ peritoneal macrophages are shown in Figs. 3 and 4. MSU crystals appeared to have been internalized by macrophages from both genotypes as early as 4 h and continued to be detected up to 24 h. At 4 h, there was no significant difference in intracellular MSU crystal count between Prg4$^{-/-}$ and prg4$^{+/+}$ macrophages ($p = 0.739$) (Fig. 4b). In contrast, we have observed a significantly higher number of MSU crystals in Prg4$^{-/-}$ macrophages compared to Prg4$^{+/+}$ macrophages ($p = 0.019$) at 24 h (Fig. 5b). Prg4$^{-/-}$ peritoneal macrophages secreted significantly higher quantities of IL-1β compared to Prg4$^{+/+}$ peritoneal macrophages at 4 h ($p < 0.001$) (Fig. 4c) and 24 h ($p < 0.001$) (Fig. 5c).

Neutralization of CD44, TLR2 and TLR4 receptors reduced MSU crystal phagocytosis and downstream IL-1β production in primary murine peritoneal macrophages similar to rhPRG4

Representative images of DAPI-stained Prg4$^{-/-}$ and Prg4$^{+/+}$ peritoneal macrophages showing the impact of rhPRG4, BSM, anti-CD44, anti-TLR2, anti-TLR4 and IC

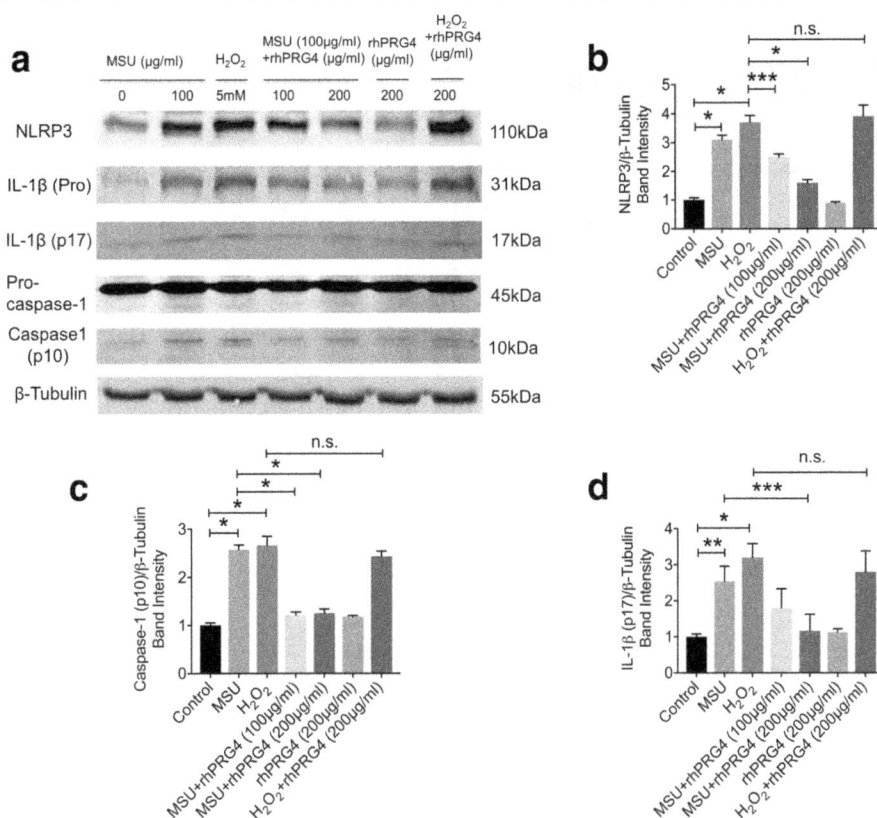

Fig. 3 Impact of recombinant human proteoglycan-4 (rhPRG4) treatment on monosodium urate monohydrate (MSU) crystal-induced NLRP3 inflammasome activation in THP-1 macrophages. THP-1 macrophages were treated with 100µg/ml MSU in the absence or presence of rhPRG4 (100 and 200µg/ml) for 12 h. H_2O_2 (5 mM) was used as a positive control. Data represent the mean ± S.D. of three independent experiments. *$p < 0.001$; **$p < 0.01$; ***$p < 0.05$; n.s.: non-significant. **a** A representative Western Blot of inflammasome components NLRP3 and procaspase-1, pro-IL-1β, active caspase-1 (p10) and active IL-1β (p17). rhPRG4 treatment reduced NLRP3 induction, procaspase-1 activation and conversion of pro IL-1β to active IL-1β (p17) but did not modify H_2O_2 induced inflammasome activation. **b** rhPRG4 (100 and 200µg/ml) treatment reduced NLRP3 protein in MSU-stimulated THP-1 macrophages. **c** rhPRG4 (100 and 200µg/ml) treatment reduced caspase-1 (p10) protein in MSU-stimulated THP-1 macrophages. **d** rhPRG4 (200µg/ml) treatment reduced IL-1β (p17) protein in MSU-stimulated THP-1 macrophages

antibodies treatments at 4 and 24 h are shown in Figs. 4a and 5a. rhPRG4 significantly reduced MSU crystal uptake by peritoneal macrophages from both genotypes at 4 and 24 h ($p < 0.001$ for all comparisons) (Fig. 4b and 5b). In contrast, BSM treatment had no significant effect on MSU phagocytosis ($p > 0.05$ for all comparisons). Neutralization of CD44, TLR2 and TLR4 receptors significantly reduced MSU phagocytosis in $Prg4^{-/-}$ and $Prg4^{+/+}$ peritoneal macrophages at 4 and 24 h incubations ($p < 0.01$ for all comparisons). Treatment with IC did not alter MSU phagocytosis by $Prg4^{-/-}$ and $Prg4^{+/+}$ macrophages at 4 h and crystal phagocytosis by $Prg4^{+/+}$ macrophages at 24 h ($p > 0.05$ for all comparisons). We observed a non-specific effect of antibody treatment on MSU uptake by $Prg4^{-/-}$ peritoneal macrophages at 24 h. MSU phagocytosis in the MSU + IC group was significantly lower than MSU phagocytosis in MSU alone group ($p < 0.05$). The percent positive cells with increased side scattering due to MSU phagocytosis was

significantly reduced with rhPRG4 treatment at 6 h ($p < 0.001$; Fig. 4e).

Media concentrations of IL-1β were significantly lower with rhPRG4, anti-CD44, anti-TLR2 and anti-TLR4 treatments at 4 and 24 h utilizing $Prg4^{-/-}$ peritoneal macrophages ($p < 0.0.5$ for all comparisons) (Fig. 4c and 5c). Likewise, media concentrations of IL-β were significantly lower with rhPRG4, anti-CD44, anti-TLR2 and anti-TLR4 treatments at 24 h utilizing $Prg4^{+/+}$ macrophages. Only rhPRG4 and anti-CD44 treatments significantly reduced IL-1β production in $Prg4^{+/+}$ macrophages at 4 h ($p < 0.01$). Neither anti-TLR2 nor anti-TLR4 significantly reduced IL-1β production in $Prg4^{+/+}$ macrophages at 4 h ($p > 0.05$). We did not detect a non-specific effect by BSM or IC treatments utilizing $Prg4^{+/+}$ peritoneal macrophages at 4 and 24 h or at 4 h utilizing $Prg4^{-/-}$ macrophages. We observed a non-specific effect of antibody treatment on MSU-stimulated IL-1β production in $Prg4^{-/-}$ peritoneal macrophages at 24 h. IL-1β concentrations in

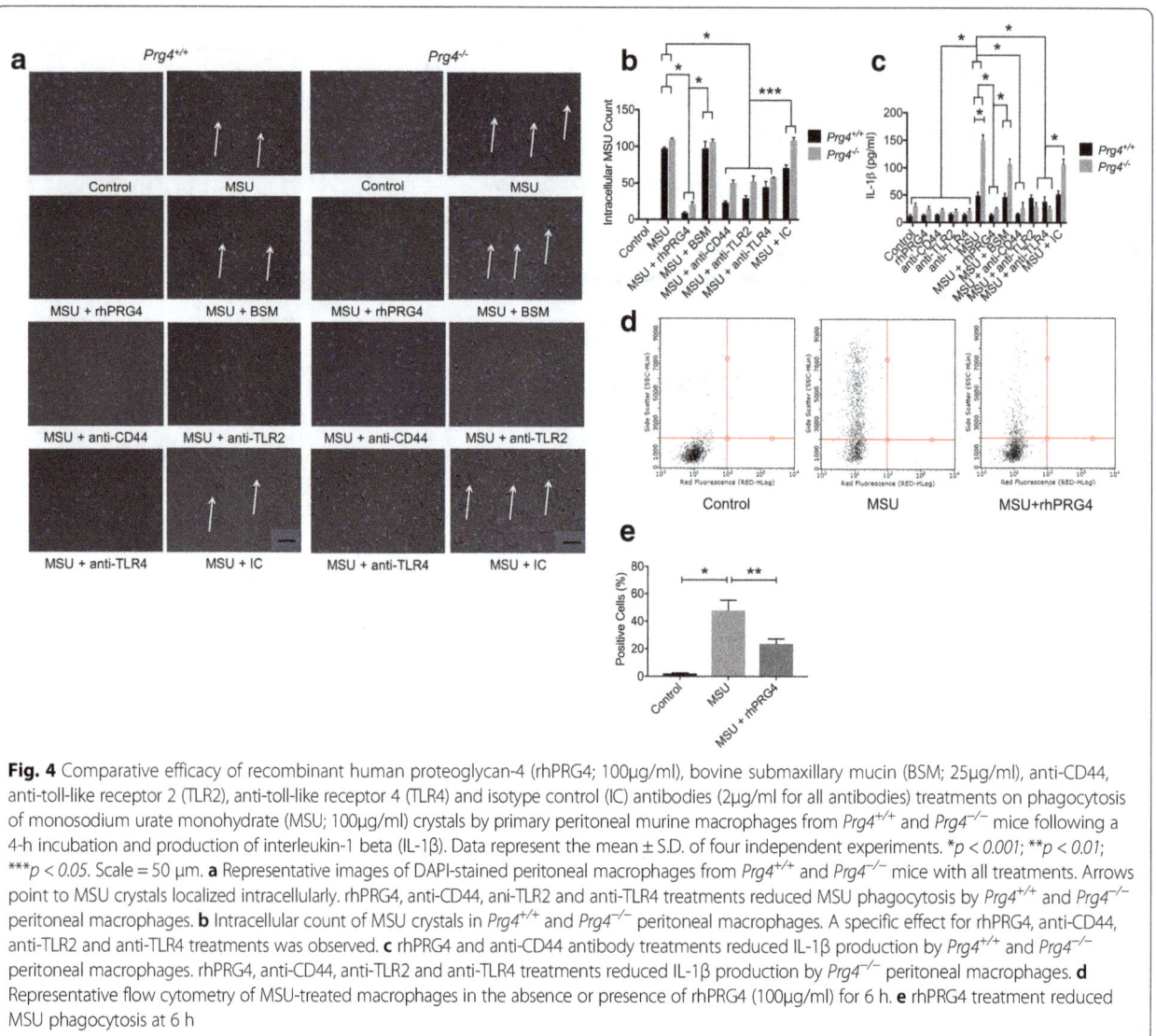

Fig. 4 Comparative efficacy of recombinant human proteoglycan-4 (rhPRG4; 100μg/ml), bovine submaxillary mucin (BSM; 25μg/ml), anti-CD44, anti-toll-like receptor 2 (TLR2), anti-toll-like receptor 4 (TLR4) and isotype control (IC) antibodies (2μg/ml for all antibodies) treatments on phagocytosis of monosodium urate monohydrate (MSU; 100μg/ml) crystals by primary peritoneal murine macrophages from $Prg4^{+/+}$ and $Prg4^{-/-}$ mice following a 4-h incubation and production of interleukin-1 beta (IL-1β). Data represent the mean ± S.D. of four independent experiments. *$p < 0.001$; **$p < 0.01$; ***$p < 0.05$. Scale = 50 μm. **a** Representative images of DAPI-stained peritoneal macrophages from $Prg4^{+/+}$ and $Prg4^{-/-}$ mice with all treatments. Arrows point to MSU crystals localized intracellularly. rhPRG4, anti-CD44, ani-TLR2 and anti-TLR4 treatments reduced MSU phagocytosis by $Prg4^{+/+}$ and $Prg4^{-/-}$ peritoneal macrophages. **b** Intracellular count of MSU crystals in $Prg4^{+/+}$ and $Prg4^{-/-}$ peritoneal macrophages. A specific effect for rhPRG4, anti-CD44, anti-TLR2 and anti-TLR4 treatments was observed. **c** rhPRG4 and anti-CD44 antibody treatments reduced IL-1β production by $Prg4^{+/+}$ and $Prg4^{-/-}$ peritoneal macrophages. rhPRG4, anti-CD44, anti-TLR2 and anti-TLR4 treatments reduced IL-1β production by $Prg4^{-/-}$ peritoneal macrophages. **d** Representative flow cytometry of MSU-treated macrophages in the absence or presence of rhPRG4 (100μg/ml) for 6 h. **e** rhPRG4 treatment reduced MSU phagocytosis at 6 h

the MSU + IC group were significantly lower than corresponding concentrations in the MSU alone group ($p < 0.05$). Antibody-mediated neutralization of the CD44, TLR2 and TLR4 receptors yielded similar efficacy in reducing MSU crystal phagocytosis and IL-1β production similar to rhPRG4 treatment.

rhPRG4 preferentially colocalized with CD44 receptor on $Prg4^{-/-}$ peritoneal macrophages

Representative colocalization images of rhPRG4 and CD44, TLR2 and TLR4 receptors are shown in Fig. 6b, c and d, respectively. We have qualitatively observed more colocalization of rhPRG4 with CD44 compared to TLR2 or TLR4 receptors. Furthermore, internalization of rhPRG4 with CD44 was also observed. The mean percentage of peritoneal macrophages that were positive for rhPRG4 and CD44 colocalization was 55.56% compared to 17.21% for rhPRG4 and TLR2 colocalization and

40.78% for rhPRG4 and TLR4 colocalization. rhPRG4 and CD44 colocalization was significantly higher than rhPRG4 and TLR2 colocalization ($p < 0.001$) and rhPRG4 and TLR4 colocalization ($p < 0.01$) (Fig. 6e). Additionally, rhPRG4 and TLR4 colocalization was significantly higher than rhPRG4 and TLR2 colocalization ($p < 0.01$).

rhPRG4 treatment normalized weight bearing and reduced SF myeloperoxidase activity

Differential weight bearing in the MSU alone group at 3 and 6 h was significantly lower than the differential weight bearing at baseline ($p = 0.007$; $p < 0.001$) (Fig. 7a). Additionally, the differential weight bearing in the MSU alone group at 6 h was significantly lower than corresponding values at 3 h ($p < 0.001$). At 3 h, there was no significant change in differential weight bearing in PBS or rhPRG4-treated animals vs. MSU alone ($p = 0.968$; $p = 0.421$). At 6 h, rhPRG4 treatment normalized weight

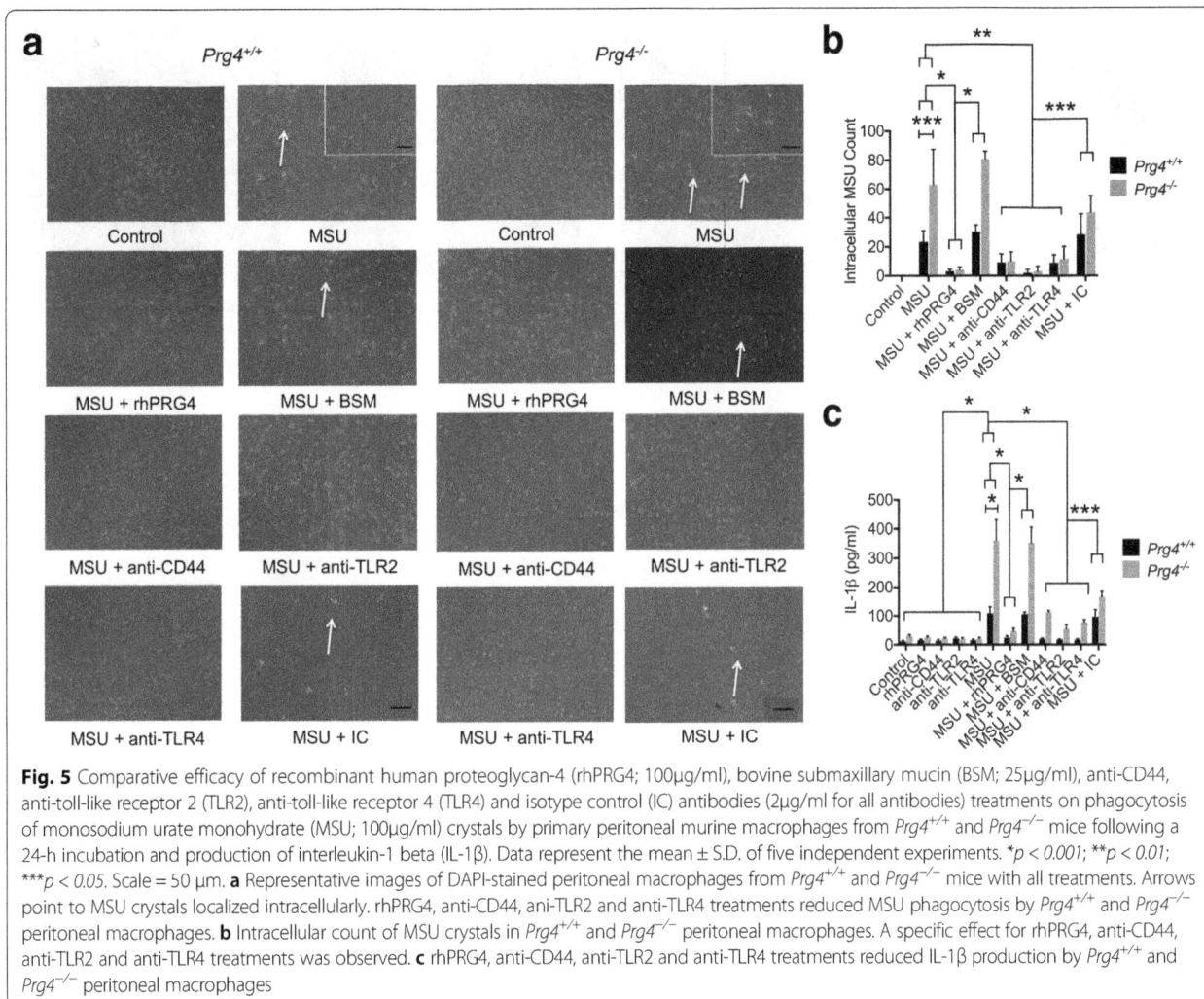

Fig. 5 Comparative efficacy of recombinant human proteoglycan-4 (rhPRG4; 100μg/ml), bovine submaxillary mucin (BSM; 25μg/ml), anti-CD44, anti-toll-like receptor 2 (TLR2), anti-toll-like receptor 4 (TLR4) and isotype control (IC) antibodies (2μg/ml for all antibodies) treatments on phagocytosis of monosodium urate monohydrate (MSU; 100μg/ml) crystals by primary peritoneal murine macrophages from $Prg4^{+/+}$ and $Prg4^{-/-}$ mice following a 24-h incubation and production of interleukin-1 beta (IL-1β). Data represent the mean ± S.D. of five independent experiments. *$p < 0.001$; **$p < 0.01$; ***$p < 0.05$. Scale = 50 μm. **a** Representative images of DAPI-stained peritoneal macrophages from $Prg4^{+/+}$ and $Prg4^{-/-}$ mice with all treatments. Arrows point to MSU crystals localized intracellularly. rhPRG4, anti-CD44, ani-TLR2 and anti-TLR4 treatments reduced MSU phagocytosis by $Prg4^{+/+}$ and $Prg4^{-/-}$ peritoneal macrophages. **b** Intracellular count of MSU crystals in $Prg4^{+/+}$ and $Prg4^{-/-}$ peritoneal macrophages. A specific effect for rhPRG4, anti-CD44, anti-TLR2 and anti-TLR4 treatments was observed. **c** rhPRG4, anti-CD44, anti-TLR2 and anti-TLR4 treatments reduced IL-1β production by $Prg4^{+/+}$ and $Prg4^{-/-}$ peritoneal macrophages

bearing as differential weight bearing values in rhPRG4-treated animals were significantly higher than corresponding values in MSU alone or MSU + PBS groups ($p < 0.001$ for both comparisons). There was no observed effect for PBS treatment compared to MSU alone ($p = 0.2770$). At 24 h, weight bearing in all experimental groups returned to baseline. There was no detectable SF lavage MPO activity in untreated control and PBS-injected animals (Fig. 7b). At 6 h, mean SF lavage MPO activity in rhPRG4 treated animals was significantly lower than corresponding value in PBS-treated and MSU alone animals ($p = 0.018$; $p = 0.007$). There was no significant difference in mean SF lavage MPO activity between MSU alone and MSU + PBS groups at 6 h ($p = 0.894$). At 24 h, there were no significant differences among the different experimental groups ($p > 0.05$ for all comparisons).

Discussion

In this work, we studied the activation of macrophages from human and murine origins by MSU crystals and

evaluated the consequence of rhPRG4 treatment on MSU induced inflammation. MSU crystals were phagocytosed by macrophages in a time-dependent manner resulting in an increase in NFκB p65 subunit nuclear translocation, induction of NLRP3 protein, activation of procaspase-1 enzyme and conversion of proIL-1β to mature IL-1β. The downstream effects included the induction of the expression and production of IL-1β, TNF-α, IL-8 and MCP-1 over a 24-h period. Concentrations of these cytokines and chemokines produced by macrophages subsequent to MSU crystal stimulation were detectable as early as 4 h in murine macrophages and 6 h in human macrophages and remained elevated over a 24-h period. The induction of cytokines and chemokines gene expression and production secondary to MSU stimulation was most pronounced for IL-1β and IL-8. This observation is in agreement with previous reports demonstrating enhanced IL-1β and IL-8 expression and production by macrophages in vitro [22, 38]. PRG4's protein core is 1404 amino acid long with N and C

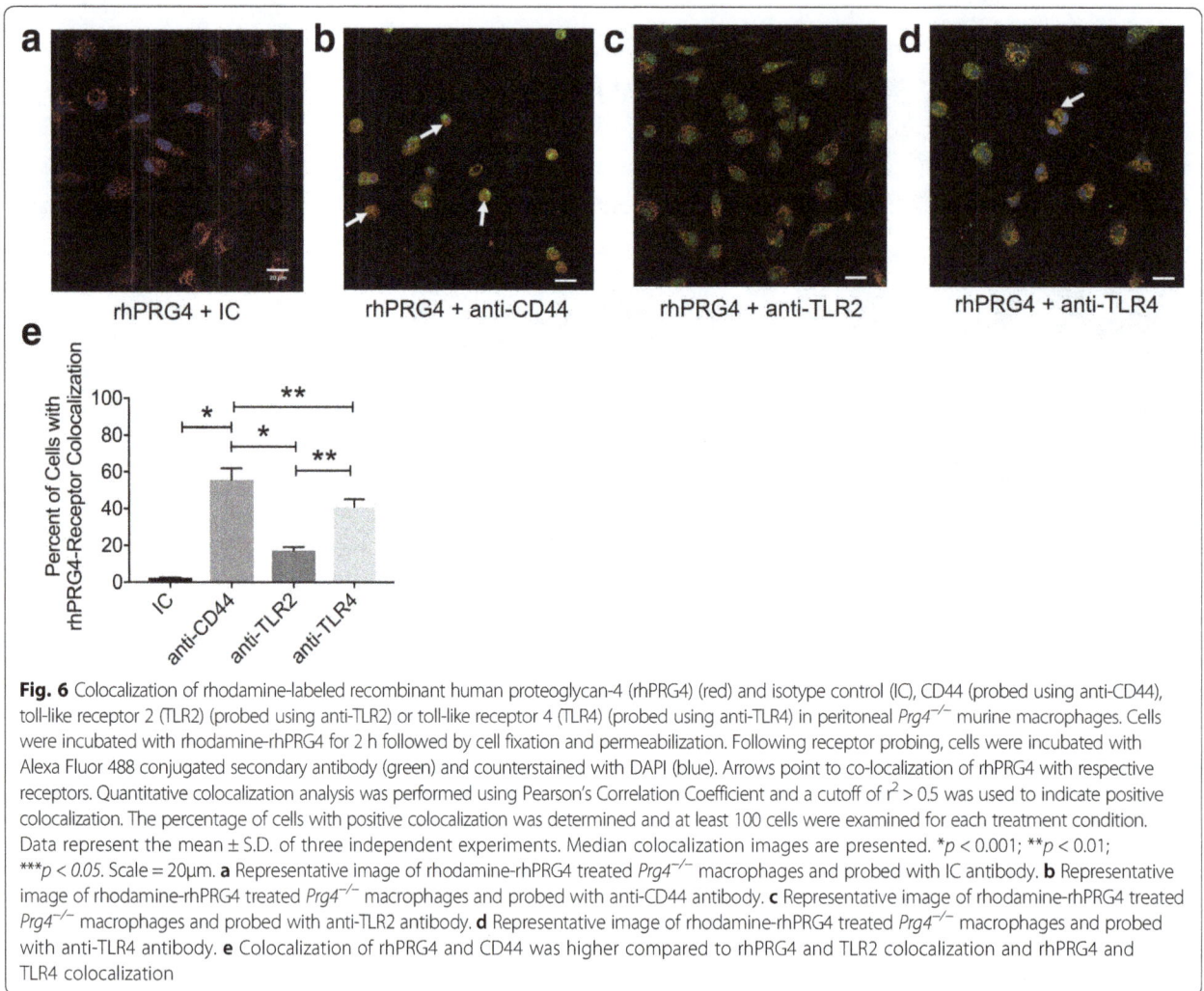

Fig. 6 Colocalization of rhodamine-labeled recombinant human proteoglycan-4 (rhPRG4) (red) and isotype control (IC), CD44 (probed using anti-CD44), toll-like receptor 2 (TLR2) (probed using anti-TLR2) or toll-like receptor 4 (TLR4) (probed using anti-TLR4) in peritoneal $Prg4^{-/-}$ murine macrophages. Cells were incubated with rhodamine-rhPRG4 for 2 h followed by cell fixation and permeabilization. Following receptor probing, cells were incubated with Alexa Fluor 488 conjugated secondary antibody (green) and counterstained with DAPI (blue). Arrows point to co-localization of rhPRG4 with respective receptors. Quantitative colocalization analysis was performed using Pearson's Correlation Coefficient and a cutoff of $r^2 > 0.5$ was used to indicate positive colocalization. The percentage of cells with positive colocalization was determined and at least 100 cells were examined for each treatment condition. Data represent the mean ± S.D. of three independent experiments. Median colocalization images are presented. $*p < 0.001$; $**p < 0.01$; $***p < 0.05$. Scale = 20μm. **a** Representative image of rhodamine-rhPRG4 treated $Prg4^{-/-}$ macrophages and probed with IC antibody. **b** Representative image of rhodamine-rhPRG4 treated $Prg4^{-/-}$ macrophages and probed with anti-CD44 antibody. **c** Representative image of rhodamine-rhPRG4 treated $Prg4^{-/-}$ macrophages and probed with anti-TLR2 antibody. **d** Representative image of rhodamine-rhPRG4 treated $Prg4^{-/-}$ macrophages and probed with anti-TLR4 antibody. **e** Colocalization of rhPRG4 and CD44 was higher compared to rhPRG4 and TLR2 colocalization and rhPRG4 and TLR4 colocalization

termini and a central mucin domain that is heavily glycosylated via O-linked β(1–3) Gal-GalNAc oligosaccharides, and is configured to form a nanofilm that exerts repulsive forces, and provides the basis for its anti-adhesive and lubricating properties [39]. We studied the efficacy of rhPRG4 against submaxillary mucin to evaluate the extent of any non-specific biophysical effect that may have resulted from the mucinous nature of rhPRG4 [40]. Contrary to rhPRG4, submaxillary mucin showed no appreciable effect on MSU phagocytosis or MSU-induced inflammation in both murine and human macrophages. rhPRG4 demonstrated a time-dependent and concentration-dependent inhibition of MSU crystal phagocytosis and NFκB nuclear activation as well as a reduction in NLRP3 inflammasome activation. rhPRG4 dose-dependently reduced MSU-induced gene expression and production of IL-1β, TNF-α, IL-8 and MCP-1. TNF-α and IL-8 gene expression and production were most susceptible to the inhibitory effect of rhPRG4. Overall, rhPRG4 exhibited an anti-inflammatory activity at

physiologically relevant concentrations that have been previously reported in SF aspirates from normal subjects and from patients with OA [41]. The inhibitory effect of rhPRG4 on inflammasome activation was specific for uric acid crystals as rhPRG4 failed to inhibit inflammasome activation due to the generation of reactive oxygen species.

PRG4 plays a homeostatic role in the articular joint with an established role in regulating synovial overgrowth and preserving cartilage integrity [42, 43]. Findings in joints from $Prg4^{-/-}$ mice include synovial hyperplasia, cartilage surface fibrillations and chondrocyte apoptosis [34, 43–45]. These pathological changes are mostly irreversible even with restoration of PRG4 expression [45]. Interestingly, synoviocytes isolated from knee synovial tissues of $Prg4^{-/-}$ mice exhibit a proinflammatory phenotype characterized by upregulation of CD44 receptor and enhanced basal and cytokine induced proliferation compared to synoviocytes isolated from wild type animals [26]. We have isolated peritoneal macrophages from $Prg4^{-/-}$ and $Prg4^{+/+}$ animals and

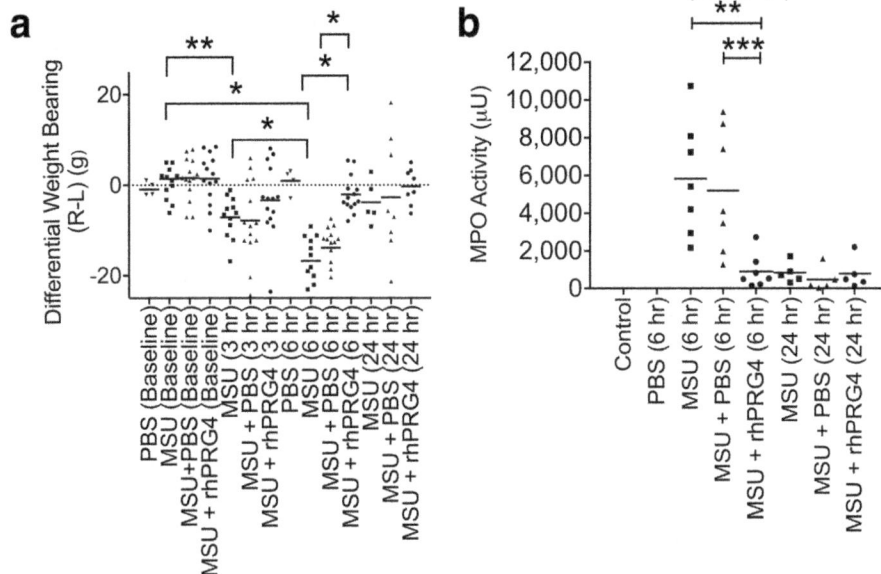

Fig. 7 Impact of recombinant human proteoglycan-4 (rhPRG4) treatment on differential weight bearing (Right hind limb – Left hind limb; R-L) and synovial fluid (SF) lavage myeloperoxidase (MPO) activity following intra-articular administration of monosodium urate monohydrate (MSU) crystals (50μL; 2.5 mg/mL) in the right knee joint of male Lewis rats followed by intra-articular treatments with rhPRG4 (1 mg/mL; 50 μL) or PBS (50 μL) at 1 h following MSU administration, or no treatment. Differential weight bearing was measured at 3 h ($n = 12$ in MSU alone and $n = 14$ in rhPRG4 or PBS treatments), 6 h ($n = 12$ in MSU alone and $n = 14$ in rhPRG4 or PBS treatments) and 24 h ($n = 5$ in MSU alone and $n = 7$ in rhPRG4 or PBS treatments) following MSU administration. SF lavage MPO activities were determined at 6 h ($n = 7$ in each group) and 24 h ($n = 5$ in each group) following MSU administration. Data are presented as a scatterplot with the mean value highlighted. *$p < 0.001$; **$p < 0.01$; ***$p < 0.05$. **a** rhPRG4 treatment decreased MSU-induced differential weight bearing at 6 h compared to PBS treatment or no treatment. **b** rhPRG4 treatment reduced MSU-induced elevation in SF lavage MPO activity at 6 h compared to PBS treatment or no treatment

studied their time-dependent MSU crystal phagocytosis and resultant IL-1β secretion. While we did not observe a marked difference in the extent of MSU internalization by macrophages from *Prg4* null and competent animals at 4 h, MSU crystals have accumulated in the *Prg4*$^{-/-}$ macrophages compared to the wildtype counterparts by 24 h, with approximately 3 times the number of intracellular MSU crystals in *Prg4*$^{-/-}$ macrophages compared to wild-type macrophages. The accumulation of urate crystals inside *Prg4*$^{-/-}$ macrophages may be due to enhanced phagocytosis over time or impaired degradation of intracellular urate crystals in the or a combination of both. The uptake of MSU by *Prg4*$^{-/-}$ and wild type macrophages was reduced by rhPRG4 treatment at 4 h and this effect was sustained over 24 h. We have also observed an enhanced MSU stimulated IL-1β production by *Prg4*$^{-/-}$ macrophages compared to wild type macrophages with approximately 3-fold increase in IL-1β production by knockout macrophages in relation to wild type macrophages after incubation for 4 h and remained up to 24 h. This suggests that *Prg4* null macrophages are primed to the inflammation triggering effect of MSU crystals, which can be rationalized by the low grade inflammatory phenotype of *Prg4*$^{-/-}$ mice [46]. Our combined findings support that PRG4 may have an anti-inflammatory biological role

in regulating the activation of tissue macrophages by danger signals e.g. MSU crystals.

To gain more insight into the molecular target of rhPRG4 that mediates its anti-phagocytic and anti-inflammatory effects, we have conducted comparative efficacy studies of rhPRG4 against antibody-mediated neutralization of CD44, TLR2 and TLR4 receptors using MSU challenged *Prg4*$^{-/-}$ and wildtype macrophages. We have also performed colocalization studies to identify the putative receptor target on the surface of macrophages. Phagocytosis of MSU crystals by human and murine macrophages and downstream IL-1β production were reversed by CD44, TLR2 and TLR4 receptor neutralization. The neutralization of these receptors resulted in a similar anti-inflammatory efficacy to that of rhPRG4. The inhibitory effect of TLR2 and TLR4 neutralizing antibodies supports a role for TLR2 and TLR4 in mediating the initial steps of gout pathogenesis [5]. CD44 is a transmembrane receptor with an important role in inflammation [47]. In addition to regulating cellular migration and adhesion, CD44 receptor has a role in regulating cell signaling pathways owing to its ability to regulate signaling protein assembly [47]. Macrophage CD44 receptor was shown to mediate complement-dependent and independent phagocytosis [48, 49]. In addition to its direct phagocytic role,

CD44 was shown to negatively regulate TLR stimulation [32, 50, 51]. Neutralization of CD44 using a CD44-specific antibody was shown to reduce NFκB nuclear translocation and proinflammatory cytokine expression and production by macrophages in response to TLR2 ligand stimulation [32]. The anti-phagocytic activity of CD44 receptor neutralization, shown in our murine macrophage experiments, provides evidence that CD44 may act as a regulator of MSU induced inflammation in macrophages. The involvement of CD44 is further highlighted by preferential colocalization of rhPRG4 with CD44 compared to TLR2 or TLR4 on the surface of macrophages, likely indicating that the effect of rhPRG4 is based on its CD44 interaction. The involvement of CD44 in mediating rhPRG4's effect is further supported by the higher binding affinity that rhPRG4 exhibit against CD44 compared to either TLR2 or TLR4 [26, 28, 29]. The involvement of CD44 receptor in the function of rhPRG4 cannot definitively rule out other accessory mechanisms. The complexity of the interaction between PRG4 and cell surfaces is highlighted by the unique and multifunctional structure of PRG4. PRG4 was shown to bind to L-selectin in a glycosylation-dependent manner [52, 53]. Additionally, PRG4 amino terminal domains are homologous to somatomedin B domain of vitronectin and the carboxy terminal contains a hemopexin domain and may mediate surface binding of the protein [54].

IL-1β plays a pivotal role in mediating gouty inflammation and IL-1 inhibitors were shown to relieve pain and inflammation in rodent models and in clinical experiences [55–57]. IL-1 inhibitors do not interfere with MSU phagocytosis by macrophages and other cells in the joint and thus do not block the resultant expression and production of proinflammatory cytokines and chemokines. IL-1 inhibitors block the autocrine and paracrine effects of locally produced IL-1β and hence the downstream inflammatory cascade. rhPRG4 works at an earlier point in the gout inflammatory pathway by reducing MSU phagocytosis. The mechanism of action of rhPRG4 results in an indirect IL-1 antagonist effect, via reducing IL-1β production and hence attenuating its role in driving gout pathogenesis. We thus also studied crystal-induced inflammation in vivo in the rat. Intra-articular administration of MSU resulted in a spike in MPO activity at 6 h that gradually resolved by 24 h. MPO is abundantly expressed and released from neutrophils and is a marker of neutrophil tissue infiltration and oxidative stress [58, 59]. Specific to gout, MPO activity in articular joint tissues increased and has been previously correlated with neutrophil influx in a mouse model of crystal-induced inflammation [21]. rhPRG4 treatment reduced joint inflammation following MSU challenge. Hypernociception was evident following MSU challenge and the time course of mechanical allodynia mirrored joint inflammation. This is in accordance with previous reports that demonstrated that synovial tissue COX2 gene expression and associated mechanical allodynia were significantly increased following MSU administration in rat knee or ankle joints [60–62]. This novel in vivo anti-nociceptive and anti-inflammatory efficacy of rhPRG4 builds upon previously reported efficacy of rhPRG4 in pre-clinical PTOA models [63–66] and provides a rationale for further investigation of rhPRG4's efficacy as a treatment for acute gout.

Our study was limited by the brief duration of inflammation that was observed in the rat model, which might have limited our ability to comprehensively characterize the efficacy of rhPRG4 in vivo. Future study will use a higher dose of MSU crystals, which has been recently optimized [67]. Additionally, we have not studied the inflammatory effect of MSU challenge in $Prg4^{+/+}$ and $Prg4^{-/-}$ mice in vivo. In our experiments, we observed a reduction in IL-1β gene expression and secreted IL-1β levels at the 100 μg/ml level following a 6-h incubation period. Alternatively, we detected an inhibitory effect of rhPRG4 on intracellular mature IL-1β at 200 μg/ml following a 12-h incubation period. Collectively, these observations demonstrate the anti-inflammatory potency of rhPRG4.

Conclusion

rhPRG4 inhibited MSU crystal phagocytosis by human and murine macrophages, reduced NFκB p65 subunit nuclear translocation and downstream proinflammatory cytokines and chemokines expression and production in vitro. Neutralization of CD44, TLR2 and TLR4 receptors on murine macrophages yielded similar efficacy to rhPRG4, namely a reduction in MSU phagocytosis and downstream IL-1β production. rhPRG4 demonstrated a higher binding affinity and colocalization with the CD44 receptor compared to TLR2 or TLR4 receptors. These findings suggest that the CD44 receptor may play a role in regulating MSU phagocytosis by macrophages and that rhPRG4's efficacy is partly due to its CD44-based mechanism. Intra-articular administration of rhPRG4 reduced MPO activity and normalized weight bearing in a rat model.

Abbreviations

ANOVA: Analysis of Variance; CD44 receptor: Cluster determinant 44 receptor; Ct: Cycle Threshold; ELISA: Enzyme-linked immunosorbent assay; FBS: Fetal bovine serum; GAPDH: Glyceraldehyde-3-phosphate dehydrogenase; HEPES: (4-(2-hydroxyethyl)-1-piperazineethanesulfonic acid); IκBα: Inhibitor kappa B alpha; IL-1β: Interleukin-1 beta; IL-8: Interleukin-8; MCP-1: Monocyte chemoattractant protein-1; MSU: Monosodium urate monohydrate; NFκB: Nuclear Factor Kappa B; OA: Osteoarthritis; PBS: Phosphate-buffered saline; PRG4: Proteoglycan-4; qPCR: Quantitative PCR; RA: Rheumatoid arthritis; rhPRG4: Recombinant human PRG4; RPMI medium: Roswell Park Memorial Institute medium; S.D.: Standard deviation; TBS-T: Tris-buffered saline Tween 20; TLR2: Toll-like receptor 2; TLR4: Toll-like receptor 4; TNFα: Tumor Necrosis Factor alpha

Funding

This work is supported by R01AR067748 (KE and GJ) and P20GM104937 (AMR).

Authors' contributions

Authors MQ, GJ, LZ, WW, CS and KE carried out the experiments and participated in the analysis of data. Author TS participated in study design and critical interpretation of results. Authors GJ, AR, and KE conceived the study and participated in data analysis and interpretation. All authors have participated in drafting and critical evaluation of the manuscript. All authors have read and approved the final version of the manuscript.

Authors' information

Marwa Qadri, MSc: Ph.D. student, Chapman University School of Pharmacy, Irvine, CA, USA.
Gregory D. Jay, MD, Ph.D.: Professor, Emergency Medicine and Engineering, Brown University, Providence, RI, USA.
Ling Zhang, MD: Senior Research Assistant, Rhode Island Hospital, Providence, RI, USA.
Wendy Wong, MD: Emergency Medicine Resident, Rhode Island Hospital, Providence, RI, USA.
Anthony Reginato, MD, Ph.D.: Associate Professor of Medicine, Brown University, Providence, RI, USA.
Changqi Sun, Ph.D.: Research Assistant, Division of Rheumatology and Department of Dermatology, Rhode Island Hospital, Providence, RI, USA.
Tannin A. Schmidt, Ph.D.: Associate Professor of Biomedical Engineering, University of Connecticut Health Center, Farmington, CT, USA.
Khaled A. Elsaid, Pharm.D, Ph.D.: Associate Professor of Biomedical and Pharmaceutical Sciences, Chapman University, Irvine, CA, USA.

Consent for publication

Not applicable.

Competing interests

Authors MQ, LZ, WW, CS and AR have nothing to disclose.
Author GJ authored patents on rhPRG4 and holds equity in Lubris LLC, MA, USA.
Author TS authored patents on rhPRG4, is a paid consultant for Lubris LLC, MA, USA and holds equity in Lubris LLC, MA, USA.
Author KE authored patents on rhPRG4.
All authors have no non-financial competing interests related to this manuscript.

Author details

[1]Department of Biomedical and Pharmaceutical Sciences, Chapman University School of Pharmacy, Rinker Health Sciences Campus, 9401 Jeronimo Road, Irvine, CA 92618, USA. [2]Department of Emergency Medicine, Rhode Island Hospital, Providence, RI, USA. [3]Department of Biomedical Engineering, Brown University, Providence, RI, USA. [4]Division of Rheumatology and Department of Dermatology, Rhode Island Hospital, Providence, RI, USA. [5]Biomedical Engineering Department, School of Dental Medicine, University of Connecticut Health Center, Farmington, CT, USA.

References

1. Pascual E, Addadi L, Andres M, Sivera F. Mechanisms of crystal formation in gout-a structural approach. Nat Rev Rheumatol. 2015;11:725–30.
2. Bitik B, Akif ÖM. An old disease with new insights: update on diagnosis and treatment of gout. Eur J Rheumatol. 2014;1(2):72–7.
3. Stewart S, Dalbeth N, Vandel A, Rome K. The first metatarsophalangeal joint in gout: a systematic review and meta-analysis. BMC Musculoskeletal Disord. 2016;17:69.
4. Busso N, So A. Mechanisms of inflammation in gout. Arthritis Res Ther. 2010; 12(2):206.
5. Liu-Bryan R, Scott P, Sydalske A, Rose DM, Terkeltaub R. Innate immunity conferred by toll-like receptors 2 and 4 and myeloid differentiation factor 88 expression is pivotal to monosodium urate monohydrate crystal-induced inflammation. Arthritis Rheum. 2005;52(9):2936–46.
6. Scott P, Mia H, Viriyakosol S, Terkeltaub R, Liu-Bryan R. Engagement of CD14 mediates the inflammatory potential of monosodium urate crystals. J Immunol. 2006;177(9):6370–8.
7. Martin WJ, Walton M, Harper J. Resident macrophages initiating and driving inflammation in a monosodium urate monohydrate crystal-induced murine peritoneal model of acute gout. Arthritis Rheum. 2009;60(1):281–9.
8. So AK, Martinon F. Inflammation in gout: mechanisms and therapeutic targets. Nat Rev Rheumatol. 2017;13(11):639–47.
9. Holzinger D, Nippe N, Vogl T, Marketon K, Mysore V, et al. Myeloid-related proteins 8 and 14 contribute to monosodium urate monohydrate crystal-induced inflammation in gout. Arthritis Rheumatol. 2014;66(5):1327–39.
10. Joosten LA, Netea MG, Mylona E, Koenders MI, Malireddi RK, et al. Engagement of fatty acids with toll-like receptor 2 drives interleukin-1β production via the ACS/caspases 1 pathway in monosodium urate monohydrate crystal-induced gouty arthritis. Arthritis Rheum. 2010;62(11):3237–48.
11. Martinon F, Mayor A, Tschopp J. The inflammasomes: guardians of the body. Annu Rev Immunol. 2009;27:229–65.
12. Choi AJ, Ryter SW. Inflammasomes: molecular regulation and implications for metabolic and cognitive diseases. Mol Cells. 2014;37(6):441–8.
13. He Y, Hara H, Nunez G. Mechanism and regulation of NLRP3 inflammasome activation. Trends Biochem Sci. 2016;41(12):1012–21.
14. Chen CJ, Shi Y, Hearn A, Firzgerald K, Golenbock D, et al. MyD88-dependent IL-1 receptor signaling is essential for gouty inflammation stimulated by monosodium urate crystals. J Clin Invest. 2006;116:2262–71.
15. Nishimura A, Akahoshi T, Takahashi M, Takagishi K, Itoman M, et al. Attenuation of monosodium urate crystal-induced arthritis in rabbits by a neutralizing antibody against interleukin-8. J Leukoc Biol. 1997;62:444–9.
16. Pope RM, Tschopp J. The role of interleukin-1 and the inflammasome in Gout. Arthritis Rheum. 2007;56(10):3183–8.
17. Pessler F, Mayer CT, Jung SM, Behrens EM, Dai L, et al. Identification of novel monosodium urate crystal regulated mRNAs by transcript profiling of dissected murine air pouch membranes. Arthritis Res Ther. 2008;10:R64.
18. Castelblanco M, Lugrin J, Ehirchiou D, Nasi S, Ishii I, et al. Hydrogen sulfide inhibits the NLRP3 inflammasome and reduces cytokine production both in vitro and in a mouse model of inflammation. J Biol Chem. 2017; https://doi.org/10.1074/jbc.M117.806869.
19. Ghaemi-Oskouie F, Shi Y. The role of uric acid as an endogenous danger signal in immunity and inflammation. Curr Rheumatol Rep. 2011;13(2):160–6.
20. Martinon F, Petrilli V, Mayor A, Tardivel A, Tschopp J. Gout-associated uric acid crystals activate the NALP3 inflammasome. Nature. 2006;440:237–41.
21. Amaral F, Costa VV, Tavares LD, Sachs D, Coelho FM, et al. NLRP3 inflammasome-mediated neutrophil recruitment and Hypernociception depend on leukotriene B(4) in a murine model of gout. Arthritis Rheum. 2012;64(2):474–84.
22. Pazar B, Ea HK, Narayan S, Kolly L, Bagnoud N, et al. Basic calcium phosphate crystals induce monocyte/macrophage IL-1β secretion through the NLRP3 inflammasome in vitro. J Immunol. 2011;186(4):2495–502.
23. Jay GD, Britt DE, Cha CJ. Lubricin is a product of megakaryocyte stimulating factor gene expression by human synovial fibroblasts. J Rheumatol. 2000; 27(3):594–600.
24. Jay GD, Tantravahi U, Britt DE, Barrach HJ, Cha CJ. Homology of lubricin and superficial zone protein (SZP): products of megakaryocyte stimulating factor (MSF) gene expression by human synovial fibroblasts and articular chondrocytes localized to chromosome 1q25. J Orthop Res. 2001;19(4):677–87.
25. Flannery CR, Hughes CE, Schumacher BL, Tudor D, Aydelotte MB, et al. Articular cartilage superficial zone protein (SZP) is homologous to megakaryocyte stimulating factor precursor and is a multifunctional proteoglycan with potential growth-promoting cytoprotective, and lubricating properties in cartilage metabolism. Biochem Biophys Res Commun. 1999;254(3):535–41.
26. Al-Sharif A, Jamal M, Zhang L, Larson K, Schmidt TA, et al. Lubricin/proteoglycan 4 binding to CD44 receptor: a mechanism of lubricin's suppression of proinflammatory cytokine induced synoviocyte proliferation. Arthritis Rheumatol. 2015;67(6):1503–13.
27. Alquraini A, Jamal M, Zhang L, Schmidt TA, Jay GD, et al. The autocrine role of proteoglycan-4 (PRG4) in modulating osteoarthritic synoviocyte proliferation and expression of matrix degrading enzymes. Arthritis Res Ther. 2017;19:89.
28. Iqbal SM, Leonard C, Regmi SC, De Rantere D, Tailor P, et al. Lubricin/proteoglycan 4 binds to and regulates the activity of toll-like receptors in vitro. Sci Rep. 2016;6:18910.

29. Alquraini A, Garguilo S, D'Souza G, Zhang LX, Schmidt TA, et al. The interaction of lubricin/proteoglycan-4 (PRG4) with toll-like receptors 2 and 4: an anti-inflammatory role of PRG4 in synovial fluid. Arthritis Res Ther. 2015;17:353.

30. Park EK, Jung HS, Yang HI, Yoo MC, Kim C, et al. Optimized THP-1 differentiation is required for the detection of response to weak stimuli. Inflamm Res. 2007;56:45–50.

31. Samson ML, Morrison S, Masala N, Sullivan BD, Sullivan DA, et al. Characterization of full-length recombinant human proteoglycan 4 as an ocular surface boundary lubricant. Exp Eye Res. 2014;127C:14–9.

32. Qadri M, Almadani S, Jay GD, Elsaid KA. Role of CD44 in regulating toll-like receptor 2 (TLR2) activation of human macrophages and downstream expression of proinflammatory cytokines. J Immunol. 2018;200(2):758–67.

33. Livak KJ, Schmittgen TD. Analysis of relative gene expression data using real-time quantitative PCR and the 2(−Delta Delta C(T)) method. Methods. 2001;25:402–8.

34. Rhee DK, Marcelino J, Baker M, Gong Y, Smits P, et al. The secreted glycoprotein lubricin protects cartilage surfaces and inhibits synovial cell overgrowth. J Clin Invest. 2005;115:622–31.

35. Zhang X, Goncalves R, Mosser DM. The isolation and characterization of murine macrophages. Curr Protoc Immunol. 2008;Chapter 14:Unit 14.1.

36. Kraus VB, Huebner JL, Fink C, King JB, Brown S, et al. Urea as a passive transport marker for arthritis biomarker studies. Arthritis Rheum. 2002;46(2):420–7.

37. Elsaid KA, Zhang L, Shaman Z, Patel C, Schmidt TA, et al. The impact of early intra-articular administration of interleukin-1 receptor antagonist on lubricin metabolism and cartilage degeneration in an anterior cruciate ligament transection model. Osteoarthr Cartil. 2015;23:114–21.

38. Orlowsky EW, Stabler TV, Montell E, Verges J, Kraus VB. Monosodium urate crystal induced macrophage inflammation is attenuated by chondroitin sulphate: pre-clinical model for gout prophylaxis? BMC Musculoskelet Disord. 2014;15:318.

39. Zappone B, Ruths M, Greene GW, Jay GD, Israelachvili JN. Adsorption, lubrication, and wear of lubricin on model surfaces: polymer brush-like behavior of a glycoprotein. Biophys J. 2007;92(5):1693–708.

40. Corfield AP. Mucins: a biologically relevant glycan barrier in mucosal protection. Biochem Biophys Acta. 2015;1850(1):236–52.

41. Kosinska MK, Ludwig TE, Liebisch G, Zhang R, Siebert HC, et al. Articular joint lubricants during osteoarthritis and rheumatoid arthritis display altered levels and molecular species. PLoS One. 2015;10:e0125192.

42. Jay GD, Waller KA. The biology of lubricin: near frictionless joint motion. Matrix Biol. 2014;39:17–24.

43. Jay GD, Torres JR, Rhee DK, Helminen HJ, Hytinnen MM, et al. Association between friction and wear in diarthrodial joint lacking lubricin. Arthritis Rheum. 2007;56(11):3662–9.

44. Waller KA, Zhang LX, Elsaid KA, Fleming BC, Warman ML, et al. Role of lubricin and boundary lubrication in the prevention of chondrocyte apoptosis. Proc Natl Acad Sci U S A. 2013;110(15):5852–7.

45. Hill A, Walker KA, Allen JM, Smits P, Zhang LX, et al. Lubricin restoration in a mouse model of congenital deficiency. Arthritis Rheumatol. 2015;67(11):3070–81.

46. Waller KA, Zhang LX, Jay GD. Friction-induced mitochondrial dysregulation contributes to joint deterioration in $Prg4^{-/-}$ mice. Int J Mol Sci. 2017;18(6):1252.

47. Ponta H, Sherman L, Herrlich PA. CD44: from adhesion molecules to signaling regulators. Nat Rev Mol Cell Biol. 2003;4(1):33–45.

48. Fu Q, Wei Z, Xiao P, Chen Y, Liu X. CD44 enhances macrophage phagocytosis and plays a protective role in Streptococcus equi subsp. zooepidemicus infection. Vet Microbiol. 2017;198:121–6.

49. Vachon E, Martin R, Kwok V, Cherepanov V, Chow CW, et al. CD44-mediated phagocytosis induces inside-out activation of complement receptor-3 in murine macrophages. Blood. 2007;110(13):4492–502.

50. Kwana H, Karaki H, Higashi M, Miyazaki M, Hiberg F, et al. CD44 suppresses TLR-mediated inflammation. J Immunol. 2008;180(6):4235–45.

51. Liang J, Jiang D, Griffith J, Yu S, Fan J, et al. CD44 is a negative regulator of acute pulmonary inflammation and lipopolysaccharide-TLR signaling in mouse macrophages. J Immunol. 2007;178(4):2469–75.

52. Estrella RP, Whitelock JM, Packer NH, Karlsson NG. The glycosylation of human synovial lubricin: implication for its role in inflammation. Biochem J. 2010;429(2):359–67.

53. Jin C, Ekwall AK, Bylund J, Björkman L, Estrella RP, et al. Human synovial lubricin expresses sialyl Lewis x determinant and has L-selectin ligand activity. J Biol Chem. 2012;287(43):35922–33.

54. Jones AR, Gleghorn JP, Hughes CE, Fitz LJ, Zollner R, et al. Binding and localization of recombinant lubricin to articular cartilage surfaces. J Orthop Res. 2007;25(3):283–92.

55. Torres R, McDonald L, Croll SD, Reinhardt J, Dore A, et al. Hyperalgesia, synovitis and multiple biomarkers of inflammation are suppressed by interleukin 1 inhibition in a novel animal model of gouty arthritis. Ann Rheum Dis. 2009;68(10):1602–8.

56. Edwards NL, So A. Emerging therapies for gout. Rheum Dis Clin N Am. 2014;40(2):375–87.

57. Ottaviani S, Molto A, Ea HK, Neuveu S, Gill G, et al. Efficacy of Anakinra in gouty arthritis: a retrospective study of 40 cases. Arthritis Res Ther. 2013; 15(5):R123.

58. Pulli B, Ali M, Forghani R, Schob S, Hsieh KC, et al. Measuring myeloperoxidase activity in biological samples. PLoS One. 2013;8(7):e67976.

59. Hampton MB, Kettle AJ, Winterbourn CC. Inside the neutrophil phagosome: oxidants, myeloperoxidase, and bacterial killing. Blood. 1998;92(1):3007–17.

60. Coderre TJ, Wall PD. Ankle joint urate arthritis (AJUA) in rats: an alternative animal model of arthritis to that produced by Freund's adjuvant. Pain. 1987; 28:379–93.

61. Lee HS, Lee CH, Tsai HC, Salter DM. Inhibition of cyclooxygenase 2 expression by diallyl sulfide on join inflammation induced by urate crystal and IL-1β. Osteoarthr Cartil. 2009;17:91–9.

62. Silva CR, Oliveira SM, Hoffmeister C, Funck V, Guerra GP, et al. The role of kinin B1 receptor and the effect of angiotensin I-converting enzyme inhibition on acute gout attacks in rodents. Ann Rheum Dis. 2016;75(1):260–8.

63. Jay GD, Elsaid KA, Kelly KA, Anderson SC, Zhang L, et al. Prevention of cartilage degeneration and gait asymmetry by lubricin tribosupplementation in the rat following anterior cruciate ligament transection. Arthritis Rheum. 2012;64(4):1162–71.

64. Jay GD, Fleming BC, Watkins BA, McHugh KA, Anderson SC, et al. Prevention of cartilage degeneration and restoration of chondroprotection by lubricin tribosupplementation in the rat following anterior cruciate ligament transection. Arthritis Rheum. 2010;62(8):2382–91.

65. Cui Z, Xu C, Li X, Song J, Yu B. Treatment with recombinant lubricin attenuates osteoarthritis by positive feedback loop between articular cartilage and subchondral bone in ovariectomized rats. Bone. 2015;74:37–47.

66. Teeple E, Elsaid KA, Jay GD, Zhang L, Badger GJ, et al. Effects of supplemental intra-articular lubricin and hyaluronic acid on the progression of posttraumatic arthritis in the anterior cruciate ligament-deficient rat knee. Am J Sports Med. 2011;39(1):164–72.

67. Goldberg EL, Asher JL, Malony RD, Shaw AC, Zeiss CJ, et al. β-hydroxybutyrate deactivates neutrophil NLRP3 inflammasome to relieve gout flares. Cell Rep. 2017;18(9):2077–87.

14

Physical activity is related to function and fatigue but not pain in women with fibromyalgia: baseline analyses from the Fibromyalgia Activity Study with TENS (FAST)

Ericka N. Merriwether[1], Laura A. Frey-Law[2,3], Barbara A. Rakel[3], Miriam B. Zimmerman[4], Dana L. Dailey[2], Carol G. T. Vance[2], Meenakshi Golchha[5], Katherine M. Geasland[2], Ruth Chimenti[2], Leslie J. Crofford[5] and Kathleen A. Sluka[2,3,6*]

Abstract

Background: Although exercise is an effective treatment for fibromyalgia, the relationships between lifestyle physical activity and multiple symptomology domains of fibromyalgia are not clear. Thus, the purpose of this study was to comprehensively examine the relationships between lifestyle physical activity with multiple outcome domains in women with fibromyalgia, including pain, fatigue, function, pain-related psychological constructs, and quality of life.

Methods: Women ($N = 171$), aged 20 to 70 years, diagnosed with fibromyalgia, recruited from an ongoing two-site clinical trial were included in this prespecified subgroup analysis of baseline data. Physical activity was assessed using self-report and accelerometry. Symptomology was assessed using questionnaires of perceived physical function, quality of life, fatigue, pain intensity and interference, disease impact, pain catastrophizing, and fear of movement. In addition, quantitative sensory testing of pain sensitivity and performance-based physical function were assessed. Correlation coefficients, regression analyses and between-group differences in symptomology by activity level were assessed, controlling for age and body mass index (BMI).

Results: Lifestyle physical activity was most closely associated with select measures of physical function and fatigue, regardless of age and BMI. Those who performed the lowest levels of lifestyle physical activity had poorer functional outcomes and greater fatigue than those with higher physical activity participation. No relationships between lifestyle physical activity and pain, pain sensitivity, or pain-related psychological constructs were observed.

(Continued on next page)

* Correspondence: kathleen-sluka@uiowa.edu
[2]Department of Physical Therapy and Rehabilitation Science, University of Iowa, Iowa City, IA, USA
[3]College of Nursing, University of Iowa, Iowa City, IA, USA
Full list of author information is available at the end of the article

(Continued from previous page)

Conclusions: Lifestyle physical activity is not equally related to all aspects of fibromyalgia symptomology. Lifestyle physical activity levels have the strongest correlations with function, physical quality of life, and movement fatigue in women with fibromyalgia. No relationships between lifestyle physical activity and pain, pain sensitivity, or psychological constructs were observed. These data suggest that physical activity levels are more likely to affect function and fatigue, but have negligible relationships with pain and pain-related psychological constructs, in women with fibromyalgia.

Keywords: Pain, Fibromyalgia, PROMIS, Function, ActiGraph, Accelerometry, Fatigue, IPAQ

Background

The Centers for Disease Control and Prevention (CDC) recommendations exercise in for healthy adults are at least 150 minutes per week of moderate lifestyle physical activity through daily activities such as walking, stair climbing, or yard work and 2 days per week of strengthening exercises [1]. In the United States, however, the majority of the population does not meet recommended physical activity guidelines [1, 2]. Further, people with chronic pain conditions such as low back pain, osteoarthritis, and fibromyalgia (FM) often show lower levels of physical activity and greater sedentary behaviors than healthy control subjects [3–6], despite exercise being a primary treatment for many pain conditions [7]. Individuals with FM may be particularly at risk for reductions in physical activity due to pain and fatigue that often are initially exacerbated with increased activity [8]. In addition to pain and fatigue, FM is associated with reduced physical function (PF), increased pain sensitivity, reduced pain inhibition, and greater psychological comorbidities such as depression, pain catastrophizing, and fear of movement [9–14]. Thus, the multidimensional symptomology limiting quality of life (QoL) in patients with FM is due to more than just pain alone.

The many benefits of regular physical activity have been widely documented across healthy and patient populations [15]. In particular, reduced pain sensitivity has been observed in healthy adults who regularly perform vigorous daily physical activity, as evidenced by enhanced conditioned pain modulation, a measure of central pain inhibition [16, 17], and reduced temporal summation of pain [17], a measure of pain facilitation. Similarly, reductions in select measures of pain sensitivity were found in a meta-analysis of athletes versus normally active adults [18]. Higher levels of physical activity may also reduce the risk of developing chronic pain, as suggested by large epidemiological studies [19–21]. Last, in patients with chronic pain, significant improvements in pain, function, and disability occur with increased physical activity through prescribed exercise programs [7, 22, 23].

Whereas exercise is an effective treatment for those with chronic pain [7], including adults with FM [22, 23],

there is limited literature examining the relationships between lifestyle physical activity and multidimensional symptomology, with conflicting results. The reported relationships between physical activity and pain outcomes in individuals with FM are variable. For example, some have found no relationship [5], an inverse relationship [6], or a positive relationship between physical activity levels and pain [24]. Also, those reporting moderate to vigorous physical activity (MVPA) levels had more pain than those with only light physical activity, but this varied with the pain scale used [24]. The rationale for these discrepant findings is unclear but may be related to methodological differences in the measurement and analysis of activity levels (e.g., self-report versus accelerometry). Further, these studies did not consider the multidimensional range of FM symptomology.

Hence, the primary purpose of this study was to comprehensively examine a variety of FM symptomology domains: pain, fatigue, PF, pain-related psychological measures, disease impact, and QoL relative to daily lifestyle physical activity (perceived and objectively assessed) in women with FM. Our primary hypothesis was that higher lifestyle physical activity levels would correspond to less pain and fatigue, reduced pain sensitivity, greater PF, lower psychological dysfunction, reduced disease impact, and better QoL. Our secondary aim was to confirm reported relationships between perceived and objectively measured physical activity in this chronic pain population.

Methods
Study design
The current study is a secondary analysis of baseline data from an ongoing clinical trial testing the efficacy of transcutaneous electrical nerve stimulation (TENS) in women with FM (ClinicalTrials.gov identifier NCT01888640; registered on June 28, 2013): the Fibromyalgia Activity Study with TENS (FAST). The FAST study protocol, inclusion/exclusion criteria, and procedures for this phase II, dual-site randomized controlled trial have been described previously [25], but a brief description is provided below. Further, detailed information

on the validity and reliability of the multiple baseline assessments has been published previously [25, 26].

All baseline data were collected at two visits, separated by 7–10 days, in part to minimize participant burden at a single visit. Data were collected using the Research Electronic Data Capture (REDCap) system [25]. At visit 1, participants completed the consent process, were provided an accelerometer to wear on their wrist until visit 2 (*see below* for more details), and completed a demographic survey. At visit 2, participants were asked to complete a battery of instruments to evaluate self-reported pain, fatigue, physical activity, PF, QoL, disease impact, pain catastrophizing, and fear of movement. In addition, quantitative sensory testing to assess pain sensitivity and performance-based assessment of PF were performed during visit 2. Outcome data are described in detail in a paper published on the protocol for the clinical trial, including validity and reliability of the measures [25]. Below we describe those outcomes used in the current study.

Participants

Participants from the FAST clinical trial with complete accelerometry data, recruited through October 2016, were eligible for inclusion in this planned analysis of baseline data (total recruited = 193; $N = 171$ with accelerometry). Women with FM were recruited from the communities surrounding the University of Iowa Hospitals and Clinics and Vanderbilt University Medical Center. Inclusion criteria included women between 20 and 70 years old, native English speakers, diagnosed with FM

based on the 1990 American College of Rheumatology criteria [9], had a prior medical history of cervical or lumbar pain, and had stable medical management of symptoms for at least 4 weeks prior to participation. Exclusion criteria for the FAST study included pain intensity of less than 4 of 10 on the Numeric Rating Scale (NRS), unstable medical or psychiatric diagnoses, prior TENS use in the last 5 years, spinal fusion or other intervention resulting in metal in the spine (cervical, thoracic, or lumbar), pacemaker, or skin sensitivity to adhesives or products with nickel alloys. All participants provided written informed consent as approved by each local institutional review board.

Twenty-two recruited participants were ineligible for this secondary analysis due to missing accelerometry data (e.g., equipment malfunction, < 4 days wear time, or declined). Additional participants had missing data for select items on various survey assessments. Of the 171 women recruited with complete accelerometry data, some individuals had missing responses from their International Physical Activity Questionnaire (IPAQ) or other surveys; thus, total scores were not possible in up to 13 individuals (7.6%). Final sample sizes for each variable (ranging from 158 to 171) are provided in Table 1.

Physical activity measures
Self-reported physical activity
The IPAQ short form was used to measure perceived levels of physical activity over the past 7 days [27]. The IPAQ assesses time spent engaged in vigorous activities,

Table 1 Demographic characteristics and summary statistics ($n = 171$)

	No. of subjects	Mean (SD)	Range
Age (yr)	171	49.3 (11.5)	20–70
BMI (kg/m^2)	171	34.4 (9.1)	19–84
FIQR (0–100)	171	56.1 (17)	17–95
Resting pain (0–10)	171	5.9 (1.5)	3–10
Resting fatigue (0–10)	171	6.4 1.7	1–10
6MWT (ft)	159	1332 (325)	300–2050
5TSTS (s)	156	14.4 (7.0)	6–53
PROMIS PF (T-score)	159	36.8 (4.9)	23.4–53.0
SF-36 PF (T-score)	160	33.1 (7.3)	19.3–55.6
SF-36 PCS (T-score)	160	32.6 (6.5)	17.3–49.5
SF-36 MCS (T-score)	160	39.9 (10.5)	15.8 – 63.6
Pain Catastrophizing Scale (0–52)	160	20.7 (13.1)	0–52
TSK (17–68)	160	36.4 (8.2)	18–58
Time spent in MVPA (min/d)	171	21.9 (23.6)	0.2–153.3
IPAQ (METs*min/wk)	158	2007 (2112)	0–9198

Abbreviations: 5TSTS Five Times Sit to Stand Test, *6MWT* 6-minute walk test, *BMI* Body mass index, *FIQR* Revised Fibromyalgia Impact Questionnaire, *IPAQ* International Physical Activity Questionnaire, *MAF* Multidimensional Assessment of Fatigue, *METs* Metabolic equivalent, *PCS* Physical Component Summary, *PF* Physical function, *PROMIS* Patient-Reported Outcomes Measurement Information System, *SF-36* 36-item Medical Outcomes Study Short Form Health Survey, *TSK* Tampa Scale for Kinesiophobia

moderate-intensity activities, walking, and sitting [27]. The survey data were processed following standardized recommendations (IPAQ guidelines, 2005), including error checking, data cleaning, and truncation at 3 hours for physical activity. Results were summarized as (1) total activity, a continuous variable reported as metabolic equivalents (METs) times minutes throughout the previous week (METs × min/week); and (2) IPAQ-defined activity categories: low, moderate, or high. High is defined as either 3 or more days of vigorous activity totaling at least 1500 METs × min/week or 7 or more days of moderate activity totaling at least 3000 METs × min/week. Moderate activity is defined as 30 or more minutes per day of moderate intensity activity for 5 days. Low activity is defined as not meeting moderate or greater activity categories. The IPAQ short form showed good repeatability (median ρ = 0.73) and good concurrent validity compared with the IPAQ long form (ρ = 0.67) [27]. The short form was chosen for its low subject burden for a clinical trial and is commonly used in clinical populations [28, 29].

Objectively measured physical activity

To objectively measure lifestyle physical activity, participants wore a triaxial accelerometer (ActiGraph GT1M; ActiGraph, LLC, Pensacola, FL, USA) on the nondominant wrist for 7–10 days, 24 hours per day, including showering and sleep. The study assessor provided standard visual and verbal instructions on ActiGraph use. Accelerations were collected at 30 Hz (up to ± 8 g); raw signals were extracted using ActiLife 6 software (ActiGraph, LLC). Flat-line signals prior to and following the 7–10-day period of data collection (i.e., nonwear time) were graphically evaluated and removed prior to further analyses. The raw acceleration signals were processed using a custom MATLAB program (MathWorks, Natick, MA, USA) following previously reported methodology [30]. Briefly, the resultant accelerations (g) across all three axes were determined using the root mean square (Eq. 1), called the vector magnitude. To remove the effects of gravity, 1 g was subtracted from the vector magnitude, referred to as vector magnitude – 1 (VMMO). These VMMO accelerations were averaged over each second and then across each minute, as described by Hildebrand et al. [30].

$$VMMO = \sqrt{x^2 + y^2 + z^2} - 1 \qquad (1)$$

A modified Hildebrand approach was used to estimate activity intensity per minute (i.e., oxygen consumption [VO_2, in ml O_2/kg/min] for each minute throughout the 24-hour period) using a power equation (Eq. 2). The originally reported Hildebrand data, supplemented with new data collected in young and middle-aged healthy men and women, was refit to an exponential (see Eq. 2) equation rather than the linear equation originally

reported by Hildebrand et al. [30]. The linear equation appropriately identified light or higher physical activity [30] but was unable to identify sedentary behaviors owing to the intercept being greater than standard light activity cutoffs [31]. We further validated our updated nonlinear equation with data from another laboratory involving a separate sample of healthy adults, demonstrating equal or better VO_2 estimates for sedentary, light, walking, and vigorous activities compared with three other previously validated approaches [31]. The least accurate VO_2 estimates occurred with moderate-intensity activities that were chosen specifically for isolated arm or leg movements (cycling, typing while walking, throwing), as expected for wrist accelerometry [31].

$$VO_2 = 0.901 * (VMMO \text{ in milli } g's)^{0.534} \qquad (2)$$

Daily minutes of MVPA were calculated as the average number of minutes per 24-hour interval spent in moderate or vigorous activity, operationally defined as VO_2 intensities greater than 11 ml O_2/kg/min [31]. Approximate tertiles of accelerometry average daily MVPA were used to define three physical activity groups in this patient population: very low (0–9 minutes MVPA/day), low (10–21 minutes MVPA/day), and moderate (> 21 minutes MVPA/day). In addition to dividing the cohort into three approximately equal samples, an average of 21 minutes per day equates to 150 minutes per week, which is consistent with CDC physical activity guidelines. However, whereas this meets the CDC guidelines, which do not mention minimum bout durations, it may not meet American College of Sports Medicine guidelines, which indicate MVPA should occur in bouts of 10 or more minutes. No adjustments for bout duration were made. Thus, for both the self-reported and objectively measured assessments of physical activity, both continuous and categorical variables were assessed and analyzed.

Pain and pain sensitivity assessments
Current resting and movement pain intensity

Pain intensity at rest (resting pain) and during movement (movement pain) were assessed using the verbal 0–10 NRS at both baseline visits and averaged. Movement pain was assessed at 5 minutes during the 6-minute walk test (6MWT) and immediately following the Five Times Sit to Stand Test (5TSTS). The 11-point NRS pain scale was anchored with 0 = "no pain" and 10 = "worst pain imaginable."

Overall pain severity and interference

The Brief Pain Inventory (BPI) short form was used to measure overall pain severity and pain interference. This 15-item instrument queries pain intensity (pain severity) and the impact of pain on daily function (pain interference)

[32]. The BPI pain severity scale assesses pain intensity at its "worst," "least," "average," and "right now." Pain severity items are assessed on a 0–10 scale, anchored with 0 = "no pain" and 10 = "pain as bad as you can imagine." Pain interference items assess seven domains of daily activities (general activity, walking, work, mood, enjoyment of life, relations with others, sleep) a 0–10 scale anchored with 0 = "does not interfere" to 10 = "completely interferes" [32, 33].

Deep tissue mechanical pain threshold

Pressure pain threshold (PPT), a measure of deep tissue pain thresholds, was assessed at three sites (cervical, lumbar, anterior lower leg) using a digital pressure algometer at a rate of 40 kPa/second using a 1-cm^2 round tip (Somedic AB, Sösdala, Sweden). These sites included two spine locations, because these are frequently painful regions with FM, and a peripheral site, the lower leg, which is commonly assessed in other research studies including in FM [8]. Participants were instructed to press and release a button when the pressure sensation first transitioned to pain (NRS ~ 1). Following two practice tests on the forearm, four repetitions were performed at each of the cervical and lumbar spine sites (two on each side of the spinous processes) and three repetitions at the lower leg. The mean value at each site was used for analyses. Lower PPTs indicate greater pain sensitivity.

Pain inhibition

Conditioned pain modulation (CPM) is an assessment of descending inhibitory pain processing (the "pain inhibits pain" effect) and was measured using PPTs as the test stimuli before and after cold water immersion as the painful conditioning stimulus [8, 34–36]. PPTs were measured at the lumbar and right lower leg before and immediately after immersion of the participant's left foot in 4 °C water just proximal to the lateral malleolus [8, 34]. An increase in PPT (less pain sensitivity) after the conditioning stimulus (ratio of post-/pre-PPT values > 1) demonstrates presence of descending inhibition, whereas no change or a reduction in PPT (ratio ≤ 1) demonstrates the absence of descending inhibition.

Fatigue assessment
Current resting and movement fatigue intensity

Fatigue intensity at rest (resting fatigue) and during movement (movement fatigue) were assessed using the verbal 0–10 NRS at both baseline visits and averaged. Movement fatigue was assessed at 5 minutes during the 6MWT and immediately following the 5TSTS. The 11-point NRS-Fatigue scale is anchored with 0 = "no fatigue" and 10 = "worst fatigue imaginable" as we previously published [37].

Overall multidimensional fatigue

The Multidimensional Assessment of Fatigue (MAF) survey assesses perception of fatigue across multiple domains and is commonly used in rheumatologic populations [38, 39]. The MAF features 16 items with 4 domains that include distress, severity, timing of fatigue onset, and impact on activities of daily living. Composite scores from each domain comprise the Global Fatigue Index (GFI), with anchors of 0 = "no fatigue" to 50 = "extreme fatigue." Higher scores indicate greater fatigue and fatigue impact.

Physical function assessments
Self-reported physical function

The Patient-Reported Outcomes Measurement Information System–Physical Function 10a static short-form (PROMIS-PF) [26] was used to assess PF. Responses are transformed to standardized T-scores using the PROMIS conversion table, with 50 representing the general population mean and SD of 10. Higher scores indicate better perceived function. The PF subscale from the 36-item Medical Outcomes Study Short Form Health Survey (SF-36) [40] was also assessed as a secondary measure of PF (SF-36 PF) [26]. Participants completed the SF-36 (see below), and the raw response data for the ten items representing PF were converted to a standardized T-score, with higher scores indicating better overall function. We have previously validated this form in FM [26].

Physical endurance

The 6MWT was used to measure physical endurance. The 6MWT measures the distance participants walk on a 100-foot walkway in 6 minutes, with rest periods allowed if necessary [41]. The 6MWT is frequently used in clinical practice and has been used previously to measure physical performance in individuals with FM [8].

Lower extremity strength

The 5TSTS was used as a measure of lower extremity strength [42]. Participants stand up from and sit down in a chair with standard seat height five times as quickly as possible. The time in seconds required to complete the test is recorded.

Pain-related psychological assessments
Pain catastrophizing

Pain catastrophizing was measured using the Pain Catastrophizing Scale. The Pain Catastrophizing Scale is a 13-item instrument that measures the extent to which individuals experience different catastrophic thoughts and feelings related to pain, scored from 0 = "not at all" to 4 = "always" [43]. Scores can range from 0 to 52, with higher scores reflecting greater pain catastrophizing.

Fear of movement

Fear of movement was measured using the Tampa Scale for Kinesiophobia (TSK). The TSK is a 17-item Likert scale instrument that evaluates fear of movement and re-injury associated with a variety of physical activities. TSK total score is the sum of the all items, with scores ranging from 17 to 68. Higher scores indicate greater fear of movement or reinjury [44].

Disease impact and quality-of-life assessments
Disease impact

Disease impact was measured using the Revised Fibromyalgia Impact Questionnaire (FIQR) at both baseline visits. The FIQR contains 21 items divided into 3 domains: (1) "function" (9 items), (2) "overall impact" (2 items), and (3) "symptoms" (10 items) [45]. The total score of the FIQR is the sum of the weighted domain scores and was averaged across both visits. Higher scores indicate greater disease severity and impact.

Quality of life

The SF-36 was used to measure QoL. This 36-item instrument is a common QoL assessment tool [40]. Physical and emotional QoL domains were assessed using the Physical Component Summary (PCS) and the Mental Component Summary scores, respectively, where higher T-scores reflect better QoL.

Statistical analyses

Descriptive statistics were generated for all variables (mean, SD in text and tables; mean, SE in figures). Normality assumptions of the variables were assessed using the Kolmogorov-Smirnoff test. When necessary, natural logarithm transformations were performed to meet normality assumptions, but are reported in original units for clarity. Pearson's correlation coefficients were assessed between measures within each FM outcome domain: pain, pain sensitivity, fatigue, self-reported and performance-based function, psychological traits, and QoL and between the two continuous physical activity variables (accelerometry min of MVPA and IPAQ total METs × min/wk) to characterize relationships between related variables.

To fully characterize the relationships between lifestyle physical activity and the multiple FM symptomology domains, two statistical approaches were used. First, Pearson's correlation coefficients (95% CI) were computed between lifestyle physical activity, both accelerometry and self-reported measures, and the multiple assessments of each symptomology construct. These correlations were assessed with and without adjustment for age and body mass index (BMI) using partial and bivariate correlations, respectively, because obesity (BMI > 30 kg/m^2)

and age (> 60 years) often result in lower levels of lifestyle physical activity [46, 47]. The second approach evaluated for differences in the symptomology variables across categorical levels of physical activity (IPAQ and accelerometry MVPA) using analysis of variance (ANOVA), with and without adjustments for age and BMI. Post hoc group differences were assessed using Tukey's test as needed. All statistical analyses were performed using SAS version 9.4 statistical software (SAS Institute Inc., Cary, NC, USA) or IBM SPSS Statistics version 24.0 software (IBM, Armonk, NY, USA). Significance was set at $p \le 0.05$ for Kolmogorov-Smirnoff tests, demographic comparisons, and necessary post hoc tests. Due to the multiple correlations and ANOVAs evaluating each FM outcome measure, significance was set at $p \le 0.01$ for all tests to minimize the likelihood of type I errors while not overly inflating the likelihood of a type II error.

Results

Demographic characteristics and summary statistics for all physical activity and multidimensional FM symptomology variables are presented in Table 1. Participants had an average (SD) age of 49.4 (11.5) years and BMI of 34.4 (9.1) kg/m^2. Most participants had been diagnosed with FM for less than 10 years (58%) and were white/Caucasian (94%). Physical activity continuous variables (accelerometry and self-report) are presented with original units for clarity in Table 1 but were transformed using a natural logarithm to meet normality assumptions before statistical analyses.

Self-report (IPAQ) and objective (MVPA) assessments of lifestyle physical activity had a moderate positive correlation ($r = 0.32$, $p < 0.001$). Higher levels of MVPA, accelerometry-based MVPA, was associated with younger age ($p < 0.001$) and lower BMI ($p < 0.001$), with age and BMI explaining from 6–12% of the variance in accelerometry physical activity. Using self-report, however, this relationship was weaker for BMI (4% variance explained; $p < 0.02$) and not significant for age. These results are provided in Additional file 1: Table S1.

Correlations between physical activity and FM symptomology

Correlational analyses revealed limited relationships between objective (Table 2) or self-report (Table 3) measures of physical activity and measures representing the multiple symptomology domains of FM, contrary to our initial hypotheses. Greater MVPA (Table 2) was significantly related to higher perceived (PROMIS PF, SF-36 PF) and performance-based (6MWT, 5TSTS) PF, less movement fatigue during the 6MWT, and greater physical QoL (SF-36 PCS) in women with FM. These relationships were maintained for four of the six significant

Table 2 Correlations between objective physical activity and fibromyalgia symptomology assessments

Outcome domain	Outcome variable	No. of subjects	Pearson's correlation (unadjusted)			Partial correlation (BMI and age-adjusted)		
			r	(95% CI)	p Value	r	(95% CI)	p Value
Performance-Based Function	**Endurance (6MWT, ft)**	159	**0.43**	(0.30, 0.55)	**< 0.001**	**0.28**	(0.12, 0.41)	**< 0.001**
	Strength (5TSTS time, s) (ln)	156	**− 0.17**	(− 0.32, − 0.01)	**0.01**	− 0.02	(− 0.18, 0.14)	0.81
Self-reported function	**PROMIS PF**	159	**0.25**	(0.09, 0.39)	**0.002**	0.15	(− 0.01, 0.30)	0.07
	SF-36 PF	160	**0.31**	(0.15, 0.43)	**< 0.001**	**0.20**	(0.06, 0.38)	**0.01**
Pain	Resting pain (0–10)	171	− 0.04	(− 0.19, 0.11)	0.61	0.02	(− 0.14, 0.18)	0.80
	Movement pain (6MWT)	160	− 0.09	(− 0.24, 0.07)	0.28	− 0.01	(− 0.17, 0.14)	0.87
	Movement pain (5TSTS)	159	− 0.04	(− 0.19, 0.12)	0.65	− 0.00	(− 0.16, 0.16)	0.98
	BPI severity	160	0.00	(− 0.16, 0.16)	0.99	0.01	(− 0.14, 0.17)	0.87
	BPI interference	160	− 0.05	(− 0.20, 0.11)	0.52	− 0.02	(− 0.17, 0.14)	0.84
Pain sensitivity	PPT cervical (ln)	159	− 0.10	(− 0.25, 0.06)	0.21	− 0.08	(− 0.24, 0.08)	0.31
	PPT lumbar (ln)	159	− 0.04	(− 0.19, 0.12)	0.65	− 0.03	(− 0.19, 0.13)	0.70
	PPT leg (ln)	159	0.01	(− 0.16, 0.15)	0.92	0.01	(− 0.16, 0.15)	0.88
	CPM lumbar (%)	138	0.14	(− 0.03, 0.30)	0.10	0.14	(− 0.04, 0.30)	0.12
	CPM leg (%)	134	0.07	(− 0.11, 0.23)	0.45	0.11	(− 0.06, 0.28)	0.21
Fatigue	Resting fatigue (0–10)	171	− 0.11	(− 0.25, 0.05)	0.17	− 0.01	(− 0.17, 0.14)	0.86
	Movement fatigue (6MWT)	160	**− 0.20**	(− 0.35, − 0.05)	**0.01**	**− 0.20**	(− 0.35, −0.05)	**0.01**
	Movement fatigue (5TSTS)	160	0.00	(− 0.15, 0.16)	0.96	− 0.02	(− 0.18, 0.14)	0.81
	Multidimensional (MAF)	159	− 0.05	(− 0.21, 0.11)	0.52	− 0.05	(− 0.20, 0.11)	0.58
Psychological constructs	Pain Catastrophizing (Pain Catastrophizing Scale)	160	0.05	(− 0.10, 0.21)	0.52	0.01	(− 0.15, 0.16)	0.93
	Fear of movement (TSK)	160	− 0.01	(− 0.17, 0.14)	0.89	− 0.01	(− 0.17, 0.15)	0.89
Disease impact	FIQR total	171	− 0.12	(− 0.27, 0.03)	0.12	− 0.10	(− 0.25, 0.06)	0.24
Quality of life	**Physical (SF-36 PCS)**	158	**0.27**	(0.11, 0.41)	**0.001**	**0.22**	(0.06, 0.37)	**0.006**
	Emotional (SF-36 MCS)	158	− 0.01	(− 0.17, 0.14)	0.89	− 0.01	(− 0.17, 0.16)	0.99

Abbreviations: MVPA Moderate to vigorous activity, 6MWT 6-minute walk test, 5TSTS Five Times Sit to Stand Test, PF Physical Function T-score for Patient-Reported Outcomes Measurement Information System physical function static short form, SF-36 PCS 36-item Medical Outcomes Study Short Form Health Survey Physical Component Summary, BPI Brief Pain Inventory, PPT Pressure pain threshold, CPM Conditioned pain modulation, MAF Multidimensional Assessment of Fatigue, TSK Tampa Scale for Kinesiophobia, FIQR Revised Fibromyalgia Impact Questionnaire, SF-36 MCS 36-item Medical Outcomes Study Short Form Health Survey Mental Component Score

(ln) The natural logarithm of accelerometry MVPA was used

All significance are bolded

relationships after adjusting for age and BMI. However, MVPA was not related to pain, pain sensitivity, pain-related psychological constructs, disease impact, or emotional QoL (Table 2).

Similar positive correlations were observed for self-reported physical activity with perceived and performance-based PF as well as physical QoL (Table 3). Adjustment for age and BMI resulted in only minor changes to correlation coefficient estimates (Table 3). Similar to objective correlations above, no significant relationships between perceived activity and pain, pain sensitivity, psychological constructs, or disease impact reached significance ($p < 0.01$). However, the relationship between self-reported physical activity and PPTs in the cervical and lumbar spine regions and fear of movement nearly reached significance ($p < 0.05$).

Differences by activity classification

Several demographic characteristics varied between activity group classifications based on MVPA but not self-report assessment (Table 4). Women in the lowest accelerometry MVPA tertile (very low; 0–9 min/d MVPA) were older and had higher BMI than those achieving moderate MVPA levels (moderate; > 21 min/d MVPA). However, no significant differences in age or BMI were noted between any self-report (IPAQ)-based activity classifications (Table 4).

When comparing FM symptomology domains by activity category for MVPA (Fig. 1), there were significant between group differences in function-related indices ($p \leq 0.01$). Post hoc analyses revealed that those achieving the very lowest activity levels (< 9 min/d MVPA) had shorter 6MWT distance, lower self-reported function (PROMIS and SF-36 PF scales, only PROMIS shown Fig. 1,

Table 3 Correlations between self-reported physical activity (International Physical Activity Questionnaire total) and fibromyalgia symptomology assessments

Outcome domain	Outcome variable	No. of subjects	Pearson's correlation (unadjusted)			Partial correlation (BMI and age-adjusted)		
			r	95% CI	p Value	r	95% CI	p Value
Performance-Based Function	**Endurance (6MWT, ft)**	157	**0.30**	(0.12, 0.40)	**< 0.001**	**0.23**	(0.05, 0.30)	**0.005**
	Strength (5TSTS time, s) (ln)	154	− 0.09	(− 0.21, 0.11)	0.26	− 0.02	(− 0.13, 0.18)	0.86
Self-reported function	**PROMIS PF**	157	**0.27**	(0.10, 0.39)	**0.001**	**0.21**	(0.07, 0.34)	**0.009**
	SF-36 PF	157	**0.21**	(0.07, 0.35)	**0.009**	0.15	(− 0.01, 0.32)	0.07
Pain	Resting pain (0–10)	158	0.01	(− 0.15, 0.16)	0.95	− 0.03	(− 0.12, 0.19)	0.73
	Movement pain (6MWT)	158	0.02	(− 0.13, 0.18)	0.77	0.03	(− 0.09, 0.22)	0.70
	Movement pain (5TSTS)	157	− 0.01	(− 0.17, 0.15)	0.88	− 0.02	(− 0.15, 0.17)	0.85
	BPI severity	158	− 0.12	(− 0.24, 0.07)	0.15	− 0.11	(− 0.23, 0.08)	0.17
	BPI interference	158	− 0.15	(− 0.24, 0.04)	0.06	− 0.13	(− 0.22, 0.04)	0.12
Pain sensitivity	PPT cervical (ln)	157	0.15	(− 0.02, 0.29)	0.06	0.17	(0.01, 0.32)	0.04
	PPT lumbar (ln)	157	0.16	(0.02, 0.30)	0.04	0.17	(0.01, 0.32)	0.04
	PPT leg (ln)	157	0.11	(− 0.06, 0.29)	0.18	0.12	(− 0.02, 0.26)	0.13
	CPM lumbar (%)	136	0.06	(− 0.11, 0.23)	0.46	0.05	(− 0.13, 0.21)	0.54
	CPM leg (%)	132	− 0.03	(− 0.22, 0.15)	0.76	− 0.01	(− 0.20, 0.17)	0.94
Fatigue	Resting fatigue (0–10)	158	− 0.08	(− 0.18, 0.03)	0.34	− 0.03	(− 0.18, 0.16)	0.69
	Movement fatigue (6MWT)	158	− 0.08	(− 0.18, 0.03)	0.30	− 0.06	(− 0.16, 0.15)	0.45
	Movement fatigue (5TSTS)	158	− 0.04	(− 0.18, 0.14)	0.47	− 0.04	(− 0.17, 0.14)	0.64
	Multidimensional (MAF)	157	− 0.02	(− 0.18, 0.14)	0.79	− 0.01	(− 0.17, 0.15)	0.99
Psychological constructs	Catastrophizing (Pain Catastrophizing Scale)	158	0.01	(− 0.21, 0.24)	0.94	− 0.02	(− 0.10, 0.22)	0.80
	Fear of movement (TSK)	158	− 0.17	(− 0.31, − 0.02)	0.03	− 0.16	(− 0.29, −0.02)	0.04
Disease impact	FIQR total	158	− 0.02	(− 0.17, 0.14)	0.83	− 0.07	(− 0.15, 0.16)	0.40
Quality of life	**Physical (SF-36 PCS)**	156	**0.22**	(0.06, 0.35)	**0.006**	0.18	(0.02, 0.32)	0.03
	Emotional (SF-36 MCS)	156	− 0.06	(− 0.21, 0.09)	0.48	− 0.05	(− 0.18, 0.08)	0.55

Abbreviations: MVPA Moderate to vigorous activity, *6MWT* 6-minute walk test, *5TSTS* Five Times Sit to Stand Test, *PF* Physical Function T-score for Patient-Reported Outcomes Measurement Information System physical function static short form, *SF-36 PCS* 36-item Medical Outcomes Study Short Form Health Survey Physical Component Summary, *BPI* Brief Pain Inventory, *PPT* Pressure pain threshold, *CPM* Conditioned pain modulation, *MAF* Multidimensional Assessment of Fatigue, *TSK* Tampa Scale for Kinesiophobia, *FIQR* Revised Fibromyalgia Impact Questionnaire, *SF-36 MCS* 36-item Medical Outcomes Study Short Form Health Survey Mental Component Score
(ln) The natural logarithm of accelerometry IPAQ total was used
All significance are bolded

lower movement fatigue during the 6MWT, and lower physical QoL (SF 36 PCS) compared with those with low to moderate minutes of MVPA (10+ min/d MVPA). No differences between accelerometry groups were noted for pain, pain sensitivity, resting or global fatigue, or disease impact. Adjustment of age and BMI did not alter the findings. (*See* Additional file 1: Table S2 for full summary of *p* values.)

Similarly, when comparing across self-report activity categories (Fig. 2), only the perceived function (PROMIS and SF-36 PF), and physical QoL (SF-36 PCS) differed across groups, with or without adjusting for age and BMI. Post hoc tests revealed significant differences between the low and high activity groups, again where higher function and physical QoL were seen only in the

highest self-reported activity group. The only discrepancies between categorical and correlational analyses were the lack of difference in 6MWT distance and associated fatigue ratings across IPAQ categories; yet, a significant correlation between 6MWT and total IPAQ activity was seen (*see* Additional file 1: Table S2 for all *p* values). Correlations between each assessment within each symptomology domain are provided in Additional file 1: Tables S3–S7.

Discussion

The primary finding of this study is that lifestyle physical activity is most closely associated with function, physical QoL, and movement fatigue in women with FM. These

Table 4 Summary statistics (mean, SD) of age and body mass index between activity classifications

	Accelerometry Activity classification				IPAQ Activity classification			
	Very low ($n = 58$)	Low ($n = 56$)	Moderate ($n = 57$)	p Value	Low ($n = 73$)	Moderate ($n = 43$)	High ($n = 42$)	p Value
Age (years)	54.4[a] (10.2)	48.5[b] (10.9)	45.0[b] (11.46)	**< 0.0001**	50.7 (11.2)	49.3 (11.8)	46.6 (12.2)	0.194
BMI (kg/m^2)	37.4[a] (10.1)	35.0[a] (8.7)	30.6[b] (7.0)	**< 0.0001**	35.9 (10.2)	33.3 (7.4)	32.9 (9.3)	0.166

Superscript letters denote which groups differed from one another, where matching superscripts indicate no significant difference
All significance are bolded

findings were consistently observed for self-reported and objectively measured assessments of daily lifestyle physical activity. Accordingly, those with the lowest levels of lifestyle physical activity have worse function, lower physical QoL, and more fatigue with movement. However, contrary to our initial hypotheses, there were no significant associations between lifestyle physical activity and the pain, pain sensitivity, pain-related psychological constructs, resting fatigue, emotional QoL, or disease impact measures.

Our findings are consistent with several previous studies in patient populations but differ somewhat from healthy adults. In one study of patients with FM, there were no observed relationships between peak levels of physical activity or steps per day, and general pain ratings were observed in one study [6]. The al-Andalus study found no association between MVPA and pain using the FIQR pain scale and resting pain ratings, nor with PPTs, a measure of pain sensitivity in those with FM [24, 48]. However, the al-Andalus study researchers observed a significant but weak association between MVPA and pain using the SF-36 pain subscale [24]. It is

not easily explained why this one pain scale but not the others would be related to MVPA. In healthy adults without baseline elevated pain, it is not feasible to study the associations between activity and pain. However, epidemiological data demonstrate a reduced incidence of chronic pain in moderately active individuals compared with sedentary individuals [20, 49]. We also found no relationship between pain sensitivity (PPTs) or pain inhibition (CPM) and daily physical activity in FM, which differs from findings in healthy control subjects, who often exhibit reduced pain sensitivity and/or greater pain inhibition with greater physical activity [17, 50].

People with FM often exhibit altered central nervous system pain processing. These alterations include less descending control of pain inhibition (CPM) and/or greater pressure pain sensitivity, thought to represent a heightened state of central sensitization [21]. Thus, it is possible that central sensitization in a chronic widespread pain condition may be less influenced by physical activity than when in a healthy state. Alternatively, physical activity levels in this specific FM cohort may be subthreshold to influence pain sensitivity.

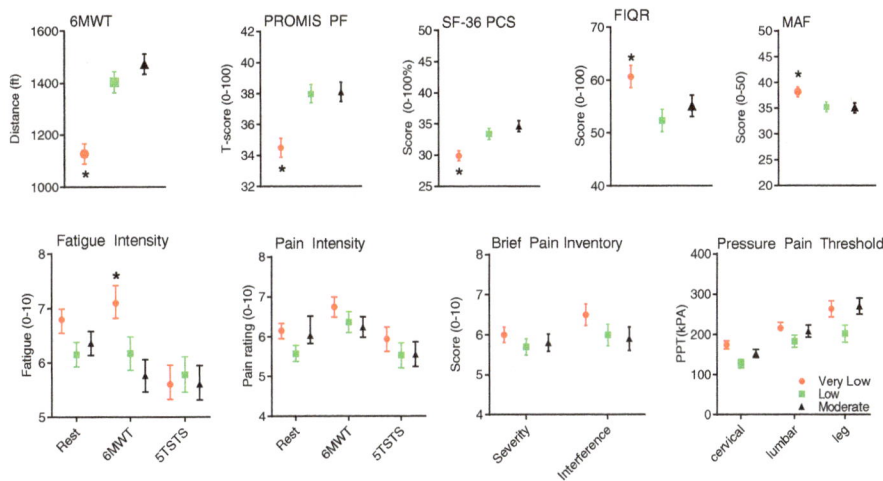

Fig. 1 Mean (SEM) fibromyalgia symptomology by accelerometry activity classification (min/d of moderate to vigorous activity). Select function, fatigue, quality of life, and pain measures are shown. Those with the lowest levels of objectively measured physical activity had the lowest function, highest fatigue with walking, and lowest physical quality of life, but no differences in pain, pain sensitivity or disease impact were noted. * $p < 0.01$. *5TSTS* Five Times Sit to Stand Test, *6MWT* 6-minute walk test, *FIQR* Revised Fibromyalgia Impact Questionnaire, *MAF* Multidimensional Assessment of Fatigue, *PCS* Physical Component Summary, *PF* Physical function, *PROMIS* Patient-Reported Outcomes Measurement Information System, *SF-36* 36-item Medical Outcomes Study Short Form Health Survey

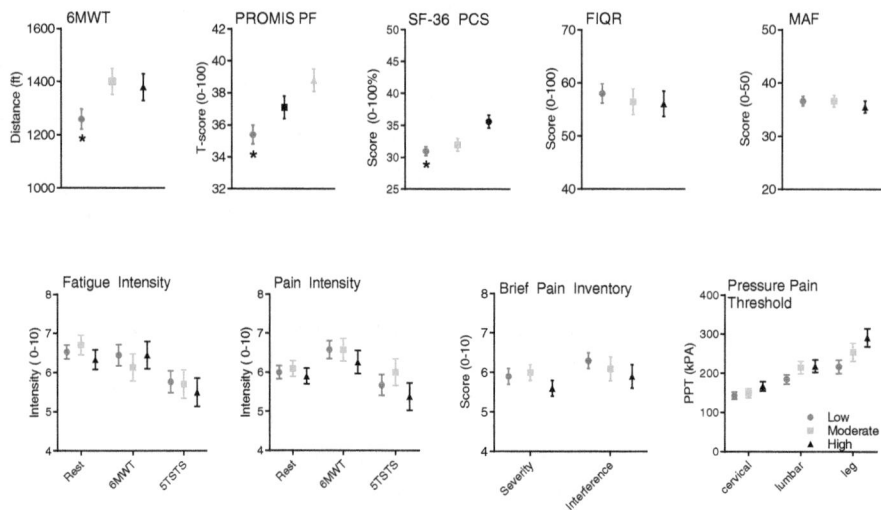

Fig. 2 Mean (SEM) fibromyalgia symptomology by self-reported International Physical Activity Questionnaire short form activity classification. Select function, fatigue, quality of life, and pain measures are shown. Those with the lowest levels of self-reported physical activity had the lowest function and greater fatigue. * *p* < 0.01. *5TSTS* Five Times Sit to Stand Test, *6MWT* 6-minute walk test, *FIQR* Revised Fibromyalgia Impact Questionnaire, *MAF* Multidimensional Assessment of Fatigue, *PCS* Physical Component Summary, *PF* Physical function, *PROMIS* Patient-Reported Outcomes Measurement Information System, *SF-36* 36-item Medical Outcomes Study Short Form Health Survey

In support, a randomized controlled trial designed to increase steps per day in people with FM found reduced pain after 12 weeks compared with an education-only intervention [51]. These differences were lost at 6 and 12 months, when daily steps declined toward preintervention levels, supporting the hypothesis that there is a minimal dose of physical activity needed to modify pain outcomes.

This inconsistency between cross-sectional observations and interventional trials may be a result of underlying pathophysiological pain mechanisms or human behavior. Indeed, we have previously shown in animal studies that acute increases in physical activity can exacerbate pain, whereas regular physical activity over time plays a protective role in reducing or preventing chronic pain [49, 52–55]. Thus, whether activity is routine or recently changed may influence its relationship with pain. Further, individuals may titrate their daily activity levels to their pain so that they are more active when their pain is lower and less active when experiencing greater pain. Prior studies support this premise, where accelerometry-measured physical activity levels were lower when individuals with FM reported higher pain [6], and women with FM are less active than their age-matched control subjects [4, 24]. This inverse relationship, combined with any possible positive relationship between lifestyle physical activity and pain, could partially explain the lack of association between monitored lifestyle activity and pain outcomes. Conversely, lifestyle activity is also dependent on choice, and some choose to be active or inactive regardless of pain levels.

The information in the current study may assist clinicians in discussing the benefits and use of exercise as a pain-relieving and general health promotion strategy with patients. Specifically, it is advisable that health care providers acknowledge that exercise and increasing daily activity are likely to improve function and fatigue but may not reduce pain.

The significant relationships between daily physical activity and function suggest a clear connection between lifestyle daily activity and muscle performance (e.g., strength, endurance) even in the FM patient population. Physical activity guidelines, based largely on reducing cardiovascular disease risk, suggest a minimum of 30 min/d of moderate physical activity [1]. However, whether lower levels of daily physical activity are beneficial for chronic pain patients has not been well defined [56]. The current study shows, for the first time to our knowledge, that just 10 min/d or more of MVPA is associated with better perceived function, 6MWT performance, and physical QoL, regardless of age and BMI. No further benefit in function was observed in those averaging 21+ min/d of MVPA. Indeed, CDC physical activity guidelines and other investigators concur that some physical activity is better than none [1, 57–59]. It remains unclear if further increases in MVPA would result in greater influences on pain, fatigue, or other FM symptom domains, because few in our patient population were vigorously active.

Our results showing an association with lifestyle physical activity and movement fatigue, but not overall perceptions of fatigue, suggest that movement-evoked fatigue is a unique construct that could be modulated by physical activity and exercise. In support of this, prior work shows that individuals with FM with higher MVPA report less fatigue than those with lower MVPA [24], and increasing activity through exercise reduces fatigue in a variety of conditions associated with fatigue, including pain [23, 60, 61]. However, in those with FM, increasing physical activity levels by 50% over 12 weeks had no effect on perceived fatigue measured using the Fatigue Severity Scale [51].

Increasing physical activity and exercise is a first-line nonpharmacological treatment for FM, and systematic reviews show reductions in pain and depression, as well as improved global health and PF [22, 23, 62, 63]. However, systematic reviews report varied effect sizes across FM outcomes and exercise types [62–64]. For example, aerobic exercise produced no to small effect sizes on pain; small effect sizes on fatigue, depression, and global health; and medium effect sizes on PF [63, 64]. This larger effect size of increases in physical activity on function than on the other symptom domains is consistent with our current findings with lifestyle physical activity. Accordingly, we propose that the first expectation for improvement due to increased physical activity in the FM population should be functional gains and improved physical QoL, with secondary potential for improvements in other domains.

Measuring physical activity is inherently challenging, regardless of the method of measurement. Although both objective and subjective methods intend to assess the same construct, lifestyle physical activity, it is well documented that correlations between survey-based and accelerometry-based activity assessment range between $r = 0.14$ and $r = 0.56$ [65]. A major limitation of self-report activity assessments is recall bias, which has led to the belief that accelerometry is a better assessment of lifestyle physical activity. However, there are a number of noted limitations for accelerometry measurements, including the ability to measure only dynamic physical activity, dependence on accelerometer wear placement (e.g., wrist vs. hip), and sensitivity to the analysis used (e.g., step count, activity counts, transformation equations of the raw g signals) [34]. In the current study, both methods resulted in consistent findings with associations between greater physical activity and better function, physical QoL, and movement fatigue, as well as the lack of relationship between physical activity and pain, pain-related psychological constructs, and mental QoL, suggesting the findings are robust. Thus, for this population, either measurement approach is useful, particularly because the relatively low burden of the IPAQ short form makes it a feasible assessment in clinic settings.

The current study has several limitations. First, this is a cross-sectional study and as such we cannot determine causation. Accordingly, better function and QoL may result in greater physical activity levels as opposed to greater physical activity resulting in improved function and QoL. Further, activity over a 7-day period may not be representative of habitual physical activity levels. However, longer durations are not feasible for accelerometry and are likely to involve greater recall bias errors for self-report. Finally, participants in the parent clinical trial, used for these analyses, included only women with NRS pain ratings of at least 4 of 10 and thus may not represent all FM populations, such as those with milder symptoms or men.

Conclusions
Lifestyle physical activity levels have the strongest correlations with function, physical QoL, and movement fatigue in women with FM. These relationships occurred with low levels of moderate physical activity (> 10 min/d), well below most physical activity guidelines. No relationships between lifestyle physical activity and pain, pain sensitivity, or psychological constructs were observed, indicating that some individuals with high pain, pain catastrophizing, or fear remain active, whereas others do not. Clinically, these data support that increasing daily physical activity has the potential to improve function, improve physical QoL, and reduce movement-evoked fatigue in this population.

Abbreviations
5TSTS: Five Times Sit to Stand Test; 6MWT: Six minute walk test; ANOVA: Analysis of variance; BMI: Body mass index; BPI: Brief Pain Inventory; CDC: Centers for Disease Control and Prevention; CPM: Conditioned pain modulation; FAST: Fibromyalgia Activity Study with TENS; FIQR: Revised Fibromyalgia Impact Questionnaire; FM: Fibromyalgia; GFI: Global Fatigue Index; IPAQ: International Physical Activity Questionnaire; MAF: Multidimensional Assessment of Fatigue; MCS: Mental Component Summary; METs: Metabolic equivalent; MVPA: Moderate to vigorous activity; NRS: Numeric Rating Scale; PCS: Physical Component Summary; PF: Physical function; PPT: Pressure pain threshold; PROMIS: Patient-Reported Outcomes Measurement Information System; QoL: Quality of life; REDCap: Research Electronic Data Capture; SF-36: 36-item Medical Outcomes Study Short Form Health Survey; TENS: Transcutaneous electrical nerve stimulation; TSK: Tampa Scale for Kinesiophobia; VMMO: Vector magnitude − 1

Funding
This work was supported by the National Institutes of Health grant numbers UM1 AR06338 and UM1 AR06338-S1. Study data were collected and managed using REDCap electronic data capture tools hosted at the University of Iowa (supported by National Institutes of Health grant number 54TR001013). Data collection was completed at the Institute for Clinical and Translational Science at both the University of Iowa (supported by National Institutes of Health grant number U54TR001356) and Vanderbilt University.

Authors' contributions
ENM AND LAFL were responsible for conception and design, data analysis, manuscript drafting, and writing the final manuscript. BAR and LJC were responsible for manuscript drafting and writing the final manuscript. MBZ was responsible for data analysis, manuscript drafting, and writing the final

manuscript. DLD, CGTV, MG, KMG, and RC were responsible for data collection and writing the final manuscript. KAS was responsible for conception and design, data analysis, manuscript drafting, and writing the final manuscript. All authors read and approved the final manuscript.

Consent for publication
Not applicable.

Competing interests
KAS serves as a consultant for Novartis Consumer Healthcare/GSK Consumer Healthcare, has an active research grant from the American Pain Society/Pfizer, and receives royalties from IASP Press. The remaining authors declare that they have no competing interests.

Author details
[1]Department of Physical Therapy, Steinhardt School of Culture, Education, and Human Development, New York University, New York, NY, USA. [2]Department of Physical Therapy and Rehabilitation Science, University of Iowa, Iowa City, IA, USA. [3]College of Nursing, University of Iowa, Iowa City, IA, USA. [4]College of Public Health, University of Iowa, Iowa City, IA, USA. [5]Department of Medicine/Rheumatology & Immunology, Vanderbilt University, Nashville, TN, USA. [6]Department of Physical Therapy and Rehabilitation Science, 1-242 MEB, University of Iowa Carver College of Medicine, Iowa City, IA 52422-1089, USA.

References
1. Centers for Disease Control and Prevention (CDC). How much physical activity do adults need? Atlanta, GA: CDC; 2016.
2. Hallal PC, Andersen LB, Bull FC, Guthold R, Haskell W, Ekelund U. Global physical activity levels: surveillance progress, pitfalls, and prospects. Lancet. 2012;380(9838):247–57.
3. Heneweer H, Staes F, Aufdemkampe G, van Rijn M, Vanhees L. Physical activity and low back pain: a systematic review of recent literature. Eur Spine J. 2011;20(6):826–45.
4. Segura-Jimenez V, Alvarez-Gallardo IC, Estevez-Lopez F, Soriano-Maldonado A, Delgado-Fernandez M, Ortega FB, Aparicio VA, Carbonell-Baeza A, Mota J, Silva P, et al. Differences in sedentary time and physical activity between female patients with fibromyalgia and healthy controls: the al-Andalus project. Arthritis Rheumatol. 2015;67(11):3047–57.
5. McLoughlin MJ, Colbert LH, Stegner AJ, Cook DB. Are women with fibromyalgia less physically active than healthy women? Med Sci Sports Exerc. 2011;43(5):905–12.
6. Kop WJ, Lyden A, Berlin AA, Ambrose K, Olsen C, Gracely RH, Williams DA, Clauw DJ. Ambulatory monitoring of physical activity and symptoms in fibromyalgia and chronic fatigue syndrome. Arthritis Rheum. 2005;52(1):296–303.
7. Geneen LJ, Moore RA, Clarke C, Martin D, Colvin LA, Smith BH. Physical activity and exercise for chronic pain in adults: an overview of Cochrane reviews. Cochrane Database Syst Rev. 2017;1:CD011279.
8. Dailey DL, Rakel BA, Vance CG, Liebano RE, Amrit AS, Bush HM, Lee KS, Lee JE, Sluka KA. Transcutaneous electrical nerve stimulation reduces pain, fatigue and hyperalgesia while restoring central inhibition in primary fibromyalgia. Pain. 2013;154(11):2554–62.
9. Wolfe F, Smythe HA, Yunus MB, Bennett RM, Bombardier C, Goldenberg DL, Tugwell P, Campbell SM, Abeles M, Clark P, et al. The American College of Rheumatology 1990 criteria for the classification of fibromyalgia: report of the multicenter criteria committee. Arthritis Rheum. 1990;33(2):160–72.
10. Clauw DJ. Fibromyalgia: an overview. Am J Med. 2009;122(12 Suppl):S3–13.
11. Arnold LM, Crofford LJ, Mease PJ, Burgess SM, Palmer SC, Abetz L, Martin SA. Patient perspectives on the impact of fibromyalgia. Patient Educ Couns. 2008;73(1):114–20.
12. Staud R. Treatment of fibromyalgia and its symptoms. Expert Opin Pharmacother. 2007;8(11):1629–42.
13. Staud R, Cannon RC, Mauderli AP, Robinson ME, Price DD, Vierck CJ Jr. Temporal summation of pain from mechanical stimulation of muscle tissue in normal controls and subjects with fibromyalgia syndrome. Pain. 2003; 102(1–2):87–95.
14. Staud R, Robinson ME, Vierck CJ Jr, Price DD. Diffuse noxious inhibitory controls (DNIC) attenuate temporal summation of second pain in normal males but not in normal females or fibromyalgia patients. Pain. 2003; 101(1–2):167–74.
15. Bauman AE. Updating the evidence that physical activity is good for health: an epidemiological review 2000-2003. J Sci Med Sport. 2004;7(1 Suppl):6–19.
16. Geva N, Defrin R. Enhanced pain modulation among triathletes: a possible explanation for their exceptional capabilities. Pain. 2013;154(11):2317–23.
17. Naugle KM, Riley JL 3rd. Self-reported physical activity predicts pain inhibitory and facilitatory function. Med Sci Sports Exerc. 2014;46(3):622–9.
18. Tesarz J, Schuster AK, Hartmann M, Gerhardt A, Eich W. Pain perception in athletes compared to normally active controls: a systematic review with meta-analysis. Pain. 2012;153(6):1253–62.
19. Landmark T, Romundstad P, Borchgrevink PC, Kaasa S, Dale O. Associations between recreational exercise and chronic pain in the general population: evidence from the HUNT 3 study. Pain. 2011;152(10):2241–7.
20. Landmark T, Romundstad PR, Borchgrevink PC, Kaasa S, Dale O. Longitudinal associations between exercise and pain in the general population - the HUNT pain study. PLoS One. 2013;8(6):e65279.
21. Zhang R, Chomistek AK, Dimitrakoff JD, Giovannucci EL, Willett WC, Rosner BA, Wu K. Physical activity and chronic prostatitis/chronic pelvic pain syndrome. Med Sci Sports Exerc. 2015;47(4):757–64.
22. Bidonde J, Busch AJ, Bath B, Milosavljevic S. Exercise for adults with fibromyalgia: an umbrella systematic review with synthesis of best evidence. Curr Rheumatol Rev. 2014;10(1):45–79.
23. Bidonde J, Busch AJ, Schachter CL, Overend TJ, Kim SY, Goes SM, Boden C, Foulds HJ. Aerobic exercise training for adults with fibromyalgia. Cochrane Database Syst Rev. 2017;6:CD012700.
24. Segura-Jiménez V, Borges-Cosic M, Soriano-Maldonado A, Estévez-López F, Álvarez-Gallardo IC, Herrador-Colmenero M, Delgado-Fernández M, Ruiz JR. Association of sedentary time and physical activity with pain, fatigue, and impact of fibromyalgia: the al-Ándalus study. Scand J Med Sci Sports. 2017; 27(1):83–92.
25. Noehren B, Dailey DL, Rakel BA, Vance CG, Zimmerman MB, Crofford LJ, Sluka KA. Effect of transcutaneous electrical nerve stimulation on pain, function, and quality of life in fibromyalgia: a double-blind randomized clinical trial. Phys Ther. 2015;95(1):129–40.
26. Merriwether EN, Rakel BA, Zimmerman MB, Dailey DL, Vance CGT, Darghosian L, Golchha M, Geasland KM, Chimenti R, Crofford LJ, et al. Reliability and construct validity of the Patient-Reported Outcomes Measurement Information System (PROMIS) instruments in women with fibromyalgia. Pain Med. 2017;18(8):1485–95.
27. Craig CL, Marshall AL, Sjostrom M, Bauman AE, Booth ML, Ainsworth BE, Pratt M, Ekelund U, Yngve A, Sallis JF, et al. International Physical Activity Questionnaire: 12-country reliability and validity. Med Sci Sports Exerc. 2003; 35(8):1381–95.
28. Kaleth AS, Ang DC, Chakr R, Tong Y. Validity and reliability of community health activities model program for seniors and short-form International Physical Activity Questionnaire as physical activity assessment tools in patients with fibromyalgia. Disabil Rehabil. 2010;32(5):353–9.
29. Mannerkorpi K. Exercise in fibromyalgia. Curr Opin Rheumatol. 2005;17(2): 190–4.
30. Hildebrand M, Van Hees VT, Hansen BH, Ekelund U. Age group comparability of raw accelerometer output from wrist- and hip-worn monitors. Med Sci Sports Exerc. 2014;46(9):1816–24.
31. Ellingson LD, Hibbing PR, Kim Y, Frey-Law LA, Saint-Maurice PF, Welk GJ. Lab-based validation of different data processing methods for wrist-worn ActiGraph accelerometers in young adults. Physiol Meas. 2017;38(6):1045–60.
32. Cleeland CS, Ryan KM. Pain assessment: global use of the Brief Pain Inventory. Ann Acad Med Singapore. 1994;23(2):129–38.
33. Tan G, Jensen MP, Thornby JI, Shanti BF. Validation of the Brief Pain Inventory for chronic nonmalignant pain. J Pain. 2004;5(2):133–7.
34. Liebano RE, Rakel B, Vance CG, Walsh DM, Sluka KA. An investigation of the development of analgesic tolerance to TENS in humans. Pain. 2011;152(2):335–42.
35. Knudsen L, Drummond PD. Cold-induced limb pain decreases sensitivity to pressure-pain sensations in the ipsilateral forehead. Eur J Pain. 2009;13(10): 1023–9.
36. Tousignant-Laflamme Y, Page S, Goffaux P, Marchand S. An experimental model to measure excitatory and inhibitory pain mechanisms in humans. Brain Res. 2008;1230:73–9.
37. Dailey DL, Keffala VJ, Sluka KA. Cognitive and physical fatigue tasks enhance pain, cognitive fatigue and physical fatigue in people with fibromyalgia. Arthritis Care Res (Hoboken). 2015;67:288–96.
38. Mease PJ, Clauw DJ, Arnold LM, Goldenberg DL, Witter J, Williams DA, Simon LS, Strand CV, Bramson C, Martin S, et al. Fibromyalgia syndrome. J Rheumatol. 2005;32(11):2270–7.

39. Belza BL, Henke CJ, Yelin EH, Epstein WV, Gilliss CL. Correlates of fatigue in older adults with rheumatoid arthritis. Nurs Res. 1993;42(2):93–9.

40. Brazier JE, Harper R, Jones NM, O'Cathain A, Thomas KJ, Usherwood T, Westlake L. Validating the SF-36 health survey questionnaire: new outcome measure for primary care. BMJ. 1992;305(6846):160–4.

41. Steffen TM, Hacker TA, Mollinger L. Age- and gender-related test performance in community-dwelling elderly people: six-minute walk test, Berg Balance Scale, Timed Up & Go Test, and gait speeds. Phys Ther. 2002; 82(2):128–37.

42. Bohannon RW, Bubela DJ, Magasi SR, Wang YC, Gershon RC. Sit-to-Stand Test: performance and determinants across the age-span. Isokinet Exerc Sci. 2010;18(4):235–40.

43. Sullivan MJL, Bishop SR, Pivik J. The Pain Catastrophizing Scale: development and validation. Psychol Assess. 1995;7:524–32.

44. Roelofs J, Goubert L, Peters ML, Vlaeyen JW, Crombez G. The Tampa Scale for Kinesiophobia: further examination of psychometric properties in patients with chronic low back pain and fibromyalgia. Eur J Pain. 2004;8(5): 495–502.

45. Bennett RM, Friend R, Jones KD, Ward R, Han BK, Ross RL. The Revised Fibromyalgia Impact Questionnaire (FIQR): validation and psychometric properties. Arthritis Res Ther. 2009;11(4):R120.

46. Cooper AR, Page A, Fox KR, Misson J. Physical activity patterns in normal, overweight and obese individuals using minute-by-minute accelerometry. Eur J Clin Nutr. 2000;54(12):887–94.

47. Troiano RP, Berrigan D, Dodd KW, Masse LC, Tilert T, McDowell M. Physical activity in the United States measured by accelerometer. Med Sci Sports Exerc. 2008;40(1):181–8.

48. Segura-Jimenez V, Soriano-Maldonado A, Estevez-Lopez F, Alvarez-Gallardo IC, Delgado-Fernandez M, Ruiz JR, Aparicio VA. Independent and joint associations of physical activity and fitness with fibromyalgia symptoms and severity: the al-Andalus project. J Sports Sci. 2017;35(15):1565–74.

49. Gregory NS, Gibson-Corley K, Frey-Law L, Sluka KA. Fatigue-enhanced hyperalgesia in response to muscle insult: induction and development occur in a sex-dependent manner. Pain. 2013;154(12):2668–76.

50. Naugle KM, Ohlman T, Naugle KE, Riley ZA, Keith NR. Physical activity behavior predicts endogenous pain modulation in older adults. Pain. 2017; 158(3):383–90.

51. Fontaine KR, Conn L, Clauw DJ. Effects of lifestyle physical activity on perceived symptoms and physical function in adults with fibromyalgia: results of a randomized trial. Arthritis Res Ther. 2010;12(2):R55.

52. Leung A, Gregory NS, Allen LA, Sluka KA. Regular physical activity prevents chronic pain by altering resident muscle macrophage phenotype and increasing interleukin-10 in mice. Pain. 2016;157(1):70–9.

53. Lima LV, Abner TSS, Sluka KA. Does exercise increase or decrease pain? Central mechanisms underlying these two phenomena. J Physiol. 2017; 595(13):4141–50.

54. Sluka KA, O'Donnell JM, Danielson J, Rasmussen LA. Regular physical activity prevents development of chronic pain and activation of central neurons. J Appl Physiol (1985). 2013;114(6):725–33.

55. Sluka KA, Rasmussen LA. Fatiguing exercise enhances hyperalgesia to muscle inflammation. Pain. 2010;148(2):188–97.

56. Booth J, Moseley GL, Schiltenwolf M, Cashin A, Davies M, Hubscher M. Exercise for chronic musculoskeletal pain: a biopsychosocial approach. Musculoskeletal Care. 2017;15(4):413–21.

57. Pate RR, Pratt M, Blair SN, Haskell WL, Macera CA, Bouchard C, Buchner D, Ettinger W, Heath GW, King AC, et al. Physical activity and public health: a recommendation from the Centers for Disease Control and Prevention and the American College of Sports Medicine. JAMA. 1995;273(5):402–7.

58. Haskell WL, Lee IM, Pate RR, Powell KE, Blair SN, Franklin BA, Macera CA, Heath GW, Thompson PD, Bauman A. Physical activity and public health: updated recommendation for adults from the American College of Sports Medicine and the American Heart Association. Circulation. 2007;116(9): 1081–93.

59. Fontaine KR, Conn L, Clauw DJ. Effects of lifestyle physical activity in adults with fibromyalgia: results at follow-up. J Clin Rheumatol. 2011;17(2):64–8.

60. Larun L, Brurberg KG, Odgaard-Jensen J, Price JR. Exercise therapy for chronic fatigue syndrome. Cochrane Database Syst Rev. 2017;4:CD003200.

61. Kessels E, Husson O, van der Feltz-Cornelis CM. The effect of exercise on cancer-related fatigue in cancer survivors: a systematic review and meta-analysis. Neuropsychiatr Dis Treat. 2018;14:479–94.

62. Busch AJ, Webber SC, Brachaniec M, Bidonde J, Bello-Haas VD, Danyliw AD, Overend TJ, Richards RS, Sawant A, Schachter CL. Exercise therapy for fibromyalgia. Curr Pain Headache Rep. 2011;15(5):358–67.

63. Hauser W, Klose P, Langhorst J, Moradi B, Steinbach M, Schiltenwolf M, Busch A. Efficacy of different types of aerobic exercise in fibromyalgia syndrome: a systematic review and meta-analysis of randomised controlled trials. Arthritis Res Ther. 2010;12(3):R79.

64. Busch AJ, Webber SC, Richards RS, Bidonde J, Schachter CL, Schafer LA, Danyliw A, Sawant A, Dal Bello-Haas V, Rader T, et al. Resistance exercise training for fibromyalgia. Cochrane Database Syst Rev. 2013;12:CD010884.

65. Skender S, Ose J, Chang-Claude J, Paskow M, Bruhmann B, Siegel EM, Steindorf K, Ulrich CM. Accelerometry and physical activity questionnaires - a systematic review. BMC Public Health. 2016;16:515.

15

1,25(OH)$_2$D$_3$ and dexamethasone additively suppress synovial fibroblast activation by CCR6$^+$ T helper memory cells and enhance the effect of tumor necrosis factor alpha blockade

Wendy Dankers[1,2], Claudia González-Leal[1,2], Nadine Davelaar[1,2], Patrick S. Asmawidjaja[1,2], Adriana M. C. Mus[1,2], Johanna M. W. Hazes[1], Edgar M. Colin[3] and Erik Lubberts[1,2,4*] (iD)

Abstract

Background: Despite recent improvements in the treatment of rheumatoid arthritis (RA), an insufficient treatment response and the development of treatment resistance in many patients illustrates the need for new therapeutic strategies. Chronic synovial inflammation could be suppressed by targeting RA synovial fibroblast (RASF) activation by, for example, interleukin (IL)-17A-producing CCR6$^+$ T helper memory (memTh) cells. Here, we modulated this interaction by combining the active vitamin D metabolite 1,25(OH)$_2$D$_3$ with dexamethasone (DEX) and explored the potential therapeutic applications.

Methods: CCR6$^+$ memTh cells from peripheral blood mononuclear cells (PBMCs) of healthy donors or treatment-naive early RA patients were cultured alone or with RASF from established RA patients for 3 days and treated with or without 1,25(OH)$_2$D$_3$, DEX, or etanercept. Treatment effects were assessed using enzyme-linked immunosorbent assay (ELISA) and flow cytometry.

Results: 1,25(OH)$_2$D$_3$, and to lesser extent DEX, reduced production of the pro-inflammatory cytokines IL-17A, IL-22, and interferon (IFN)γ in CCR6$^+$ memTh cells. Tumor necrosis factor (TNF)α was only inhibited by the combination of 1,25(OH)$_2$D$_3$ and DEX. In contrast, DEX was the strongest inhibitor of IL-6, IL-8, and tissue-destructive enzymes in RASF. As a result, 1,25(OH)$_2$D$_3$ and DEX additively inhibited inflammatory mediators in CCR6$^+$ memTh-RASF cocultures. Interestingly, low doses of mainly DEX, but also 1,25(OH)$_2$D$_3$, combined with etanercept better suppressed synovial inflammation in this coculture model compared with etanercept alone.

Conclusion: This study suggests that 1,25(OH)$_2$D$_3$ and DEX additively inhibit synovial inflammation through targeting predominantly CCR6$^+$ memTh cells and RASF, respectively. Furthermore, low doses of DEX and 1,25(OH)$_2$D$_3$ enhance the effect of TNFα blockade in inhibiting RASF activation, thus providing a basis to improve RA treatment.

Keywords: Rheumatoid arthritis, Th17, Vitamin D, Dexamethasone, CCR6

* Correspondence: E.Lubberts@erasmusmc.nl
[1]Department of Rheumatology, Erasmus MC, Rotterdam, the Netherlands
[2]Department of Immunology, Erasmus MC, Rotterdam, the Netherlands
Full list of author information is available at the end of the article

Background

Rheumatoid arthritis (RA) is a chronic inflammatory autoimmune disease characterized by inflamed synovial joints resulting in pain, fatigue, and disability in patients. Although treatment has improved over the last decades, many patients do not reach clinical remission, show progressive joint damage, or become resistant to their treatment [1]. Furthermore, the current therapies include the use of expensive biological disease-modifying antirheumatic drugs (DMARDs) which pose a burden on the healthcare budget. Therefore, there is still a need to find new therapeutic options and to improve currently available treatments.

The main therapeutic goal in RA is to stop the chronic synovial inflammation and thereby prevent the subsequent cartilage and bone damage in the affected joint. Synovial fibroblasts play an important role in this process since they can secrete proinflammatory cytokines that attract and activate immune cells, produce tissue-destructive enzymes, and invade cartilage [2, 3]. How these RA synovial fibroblasts (RASF) are activated is currently unknown, although one of the hypotheses is that they are activated by infiltrating immune cells. Previously we have shown that CCR6$^+$, but not CCR6$^-$, memory T helper (memTh) cells can activate RASF [4].

CCR6$^+$ memTh cells are characterized by interleukin (IL)-17A production and RAR-related orphan C receptor (RORC) expression. This subset contains the classic Th17 cells, but also contains, for example, Th17.1 cells that produce high levels of interferon (IFN)γ [5]. Other evidence that suggests a role for these IL-17A-producing memTh cells is that Th17 cells and IL-17-mediated signaling are required for the development of murine autoimmune arthritis [6, 7]. Furthermore, CCR6$^+$ memTh cells are more activated and more prevalent in the blood of treatment-naive early RA patients and are also found in the synovial fluid of RA patients [4, 8].

Upon interaction with CCR6$^+$ memTh cells, RASF secrete proinflammatory mediators such as IL-6, matrix metalloproteases (MMPs), and prostaglandin E2 (PGE2) via IL-17A and tumor necrosis factor (TNF)α. In turn, these molecules, especially PGE2, further activate the CCR6$^+$ memTh cells to produce more IL-17A, thereby creating a proinflammatory feedback loop that could drive the chronic synovial inflammation [4, 9]. Therefore, inhibiting this proinflammatory loop may be beneficial in the treatment of RA.

We have previously shown that combining the active vitamin D metabolite 1,25(OH)$_2$D$_3$ with TNFα blockade, a commonly used therapy in RA, additively suppresses the proinflammatory loop between CCR6$^+$ memTh and RASF [10]. However, clinical translation of these findings is challenging since high concentrations of 1,25(OH)$_2$D$_3$ were used. Interestingly, the effects of 1,25(OH)$_2$D$_3$ on

Th17-related cytokines, such as IL-17A, TNFα, and IL-22, can be augmented through combination with dexamethasone (DEX) [11]. DEX is a synthetic glucocorticoid (GC) which is clinically used for fast resolution of inflammation and is often combined with vitamin D supplements to prevent the osteoporotic side effects of the drug [12].

Given the immunomodulatory capacities of both DEX and 1,25(OH)$_2$D$_3$, we here investigated whether this combination could suppress CCR6$^+$ memTh cells, RASF, and their interaction. Furthermore, the potential use of these findings for improving current anti-TNFα therapy is explored.

Methods

Subjects

Healthy control peripheral blood mononuclear cells (PBMCs) were obtained from buffycoats (Sanquin, Amsterdam, the Netherlands). For validation of findings in healthy PBMCs, RA PBMCs were isolated from treatment-naive RA patients who were embedded in the tREACH study, which was ethically approved by the METC Rotterdam. Relevant clinical information is summarized in Additional file 1 (Table S1). RASF were grown from synovial explants after joint replacement surgery. All patients signed informed consent.

Cell sorting

PBMCs were isolated from peripheral blood using ficoll-based cell separation and frozen in liquid nitrogen until use. For sorting of CCR6$^+$ memTh cells (CD4$^+$CD45RO$^+$CCR6$^+$CD25$^{low/int}$), PBMCs were stained using antibodies against CD4, CCR6, CD25 (BioLegend, San Diego, CA, USA), and CD45RO (BD Biosciences, San Diego, CA, USA). Before sorting CCR6$^+$ memTh cells, the cells were prepurified using CD4 microbeads via automated magnetic-activated cell sorting (Miltenyi Biotec, Leiden, The Netherlands). Dead cells were excluded using 4′6-diamidino-2-phenylindole dilactate (DAPI) and CCR6$^+$ memTh cells were sorted on a FACSAriaIII sorter (BD Biosciences).

Cell culture

RASF were obtained by culturing small synovial biopsies in a culture flask with Dulbecco's modified Eagle's medium (DMEM; Gibco, Waltham, MA, USA), supplemented with 10% fetal calf serum (FCS; Gibco) and 100 IU/ml penicillin/streptomycin (pen/strep; Lonza, Verviers, Belgium). After RASF were grown out of the synovial biopsies, cells were passaged and used for experiments between passage 3 and 8. For coculture with sorted T cells or stimulation experiments, RASF were plated at a density of 1×10^4 cells/well in a 96-well plate 24 h before the T cells or stimulation medium were added. Where indicated, RASF were stimulated with 2 ng/ml recombinant TNFα and 5 ng/ml recombinant IL-17A (R&D Systems, Minneapolis, MN, USA).

Sorted CCR6$^+$ memTh cells were stimulated with 300 ng/ml soluble anti-CD3 and 400 ng/ml soluble anti-CD28 (Sanquin, Amsterdam, the Netherlands) at a density of 2.5×10^4 cells/ml in Iscove's modified Dulbecco's medium (IMDM; Gibco) supplemented with 10% FCS, 100 IU/ml pen/strep, 2 mM L-glutamine, and 50 μM β-mercaptoethanol (Sigma-Aldrich, St. Louis, MO, USA). Cells were treated with or without 1,25(OH)$_2$D$_3$ (Leo Pharmaceutical Products, Ballerup, Denmark), dexamethasone (Sigma-Aldrich), and etanercept (anti-TNFα, Pfizer, New York, NY, USA) dissolved in 100% ethanol at the indicated concentrations and added for the full duration of the culture simultaneously with the stimulatory compounds. Control conditions contained an equal volume of 100% ethanol which never exceeded 0.1%.

Flow cytometry
Cultured cells were restimulated with 50 ng/ml phorbol 12-myristate 13 acetate (PMA), 500 ng/ml ionomycin (Sigma-Aldrich), and GolgiStop (BD Biosciences) for 4 h. Cells were then stained with Fixable Viability Dye eFluor506 (eBioscience, San Diego, CA, USA), fixated with 2% paraformaldehyde and permeabilized using 0.5% saponine. Intracellular cytokines were stained with monoclonal antibodies against IL-17A, IL-22 (eBioscience), and IFNγ (BioLegend).

Apoptosis was assessed using 7AAD/Annexin V staining, performed according to the manufacturer's instructions (eBioscience). All samples were measured on the FACS-CantoII Flow Cytometer (BD Biosciences).

Enzyme-linked immunosorbent assay (ELISA)
In culture supernatant after 3 days of culture, the concentration of IL-17A, IL-22, IFNγ, TNFα, IL-10, IL-6, IL-8 (Ready-Set-Go, eBioscience), MMP1, MMP3 (DuoSet ELISA, R&D Systems), and PGE2 (Prostaglandin E2 Parameter Assay Kit, R&D Systems) were measured using ELISA. The manufacturers' protocols were followed.

Statistical analysis
Differences between experimental treatment groups were tested using analysis of variance (ANOVA) with Bonferroni post-hoc tests. p values below 0.05 were considered statistically significant. Analyses were performed using Prism software version 6.01 (GraphPad Software, La Jolla, CA, USA).

Results
1,25(OH)$_2$D$_3$-DEX combination treatment suppresses TNFα production from CCR6$^+$ memTh cells
As a first step to examine the potential use of 1,25(OH)$_2$D$_3$ and DEX to inhibit synovial inflammation, CCR6$^+$ memTh cells were sorted from healthy controls and cultured for 3

days with 1,25(OH)$_2$D$_3$, DEX, or both. In line with the previous studies, treatment with 1,25(OH)$_2$D$_3$ reduced the percentage of cells producing IL-17A, IL-22, and IFNγ. On the other hand, treatment with DEX did not affect the percentage of IL-22- or IFNγ-producing cells. The percentage of IL-17A-producing cells was reduced by DEX, but significantly less than by 1,25(OH)$_2$D$_3$. Combining 1,25(OH)$_2$D$_3$ and DEX had a similar effect as 1,25(OH)$_2$D$_3$ single treatment (Fig. 1a, b). Notably, treatment with DEX significantly reduced the amount of IL-17A and IFNγ that was produced during the 3-day culture period (Fig. 1c). Since DEX is known to induce cell death, the treatment effect on apoptosis was investigated. However, the minimal increase in apoptosis on DEX or combination exposure could not explain the difference between flow cytometry and ELISA (Additional file 1: Figure S1). Although no additive effect was observed with 1,25(OH)$_2$D$_3$-DEX combination treatment on IL-17A, IL-22, or IFNγ, TNFα was significantly inhibited by the combined exposure (Fig. 1c). Since 1,25(OH)$_2$D$_3$ can induce an anti-inflammatory phenotype in the CCR6$^+$ memTh cells (Dankers et al., submitted manuscript), the combinatory effects of 1,25(OH)$_2$D$_3$ and DEX on IL-10 were also assessed. However, DEX did not affect IL-10 production when used alone and reduced the induction of IL-10 by 1,25(OH)$_2$D$_3$ when used in combination (Fig. 1c). Overall, these data show that 1,25(OH)$_2$D$_3$ is the strongest modulator of IL-17A, IL-22, IFNγ, and IL-10 production by CCR6$^+$ memTh cells, but the combination of 1,25(OH)$_2$D$_3$ and DEX provides additional value through enhanced TNFα inhibition.

1,25(OH)$_2$D$_3$ and DEX additively suppress the proinflammatory feedback loop between CCR6$^+$ memTh cells and RASF
Since 1,25(OH)$_2$D$_3$ and DEX had additive effects in blocking TNFα and they were both capable of reducing the level of IL-17A that is produced by CCR6$^+$ memTh cells, we hypothesized that the combination treatment would augment inhibition of the proinflammatory loop between CCR6$^+$ memTh cells and RASF when compared with either compound alone. Similar to the effects of 1,25(OH)$_2$D$_3$ and DEX on CCR6$^+$ memTh cell cultures, treatment of the CCR6$^+$ memTh-RASF cocultures significantly reduced IL-17A, IL-22, and IFNγ production, especially with 1,25(OH)$_2$D$_3$. However, the production of TNFα was stimulated upon treatment with DEX, whereas it was still inhibited with the combination treatment. Furthermore, IL-10 was significantly upregulated in response to DEX and the combination of DEX and 1,25(OH)$_2$D$_3$, but not 1,25(OH)$_2$D$_3$ alone (Fig. 2).

Despite the differences in modulation of T cell-derived cytokines by DEX and 1,25(OH)$_2$D$_3$, they equally inhibited the RASF-derived factors IL-6, IL-8, and PGE2. For IL-6 and IL-8 there was also a trend towards additive inhibition

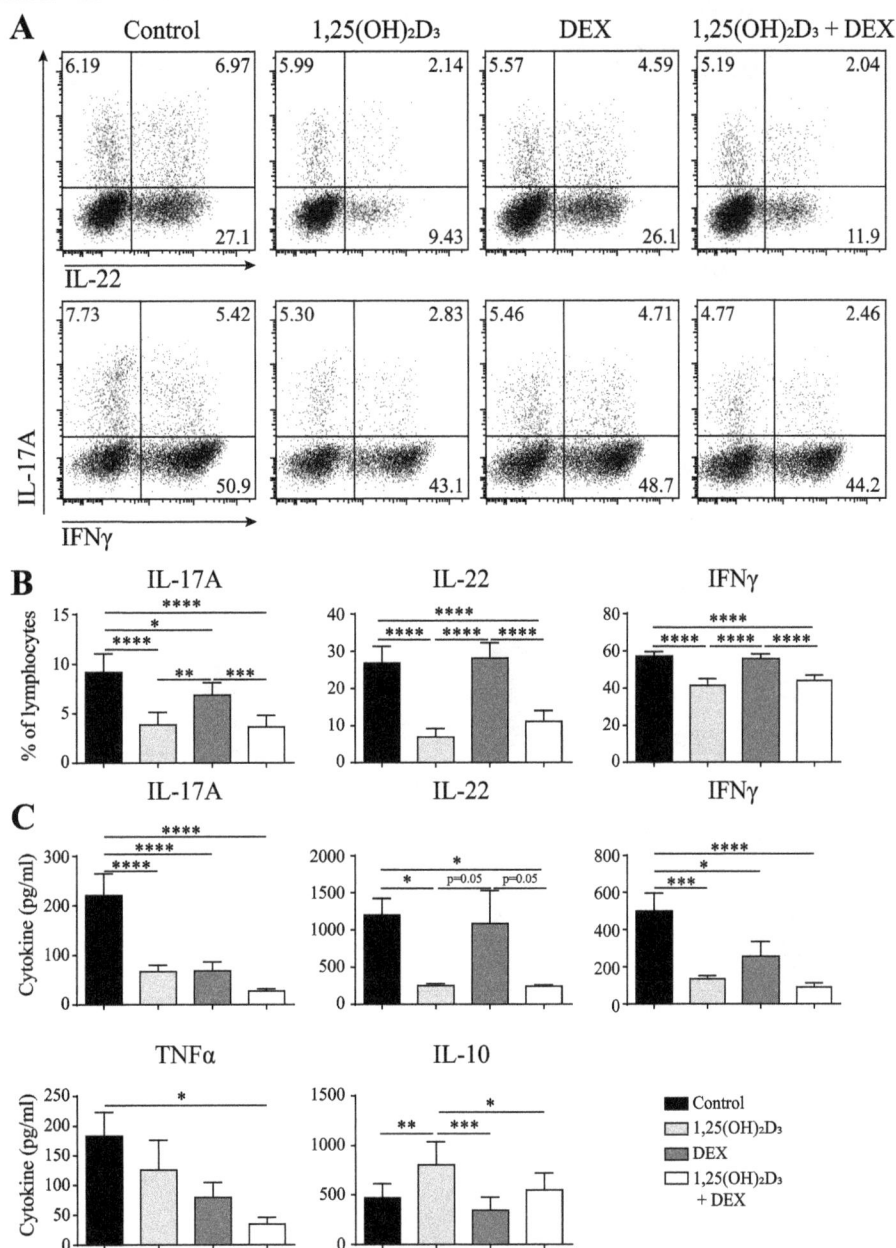

Fig. 1 $1,25(OH)_2D_3$ and DEX additively suppress proinflammatory cytokines secreted by CCR6$^+$ memTh cells. CCR6$^+$ memTh cells were sorted from healthy individuals and cultured for 3 days under stimulation with anti-CD3 and anti-CD28, with or without 100 nM $1,25(OH)_2D_3$ and 1000 nM dexamethasone (DEX). **a** Representative flow cytometry plots of interleukin (IL)-17A-, IL-22-, and interferon (IFN)γ-producing cells. **b** Quantification of flow cytometry as in **a** for six donors. **c** Cytokine production in the culture medium as measured by ELISA. Data show mean ± SEM for $n = 6$–10 healthy individuals, representative of at least three independent experiments. $*p < 0.05$, $**p < 0.01$, $***p < 0.001$, $****p < 0.0001$. TNF tumor necrosis factor

in response to the combination of $1,25(OH)_2D_3$ and DEX. Interestingly, DEX treatment led to a significantly greater inhibition of the tissue-destructive enzymes MMP1 and MMP3 than $1,25(OH)_2D_3$ treatment (Fig. 2). These data suggest that, although no additive effect of $1,25(OH)_2D_3$ and DEX is found on individual cytokines, the two compounds cooperate to reduce the proinflammatory milieu at an inflammatory synovial site by each targeting different

players in the inflammation. Furthermore, the increased production of IL-10 potentially mediates anti-inflammatory effects on other immune cells.

DEX is a stronger inhibitor of proinflammatory factors from RASF than $1,25(OH)_2D_3$

The finding that DEX is an equal inhibitor of IL-6 and IL-8 and stronger inhibitor of MMP1 and MMP3 than

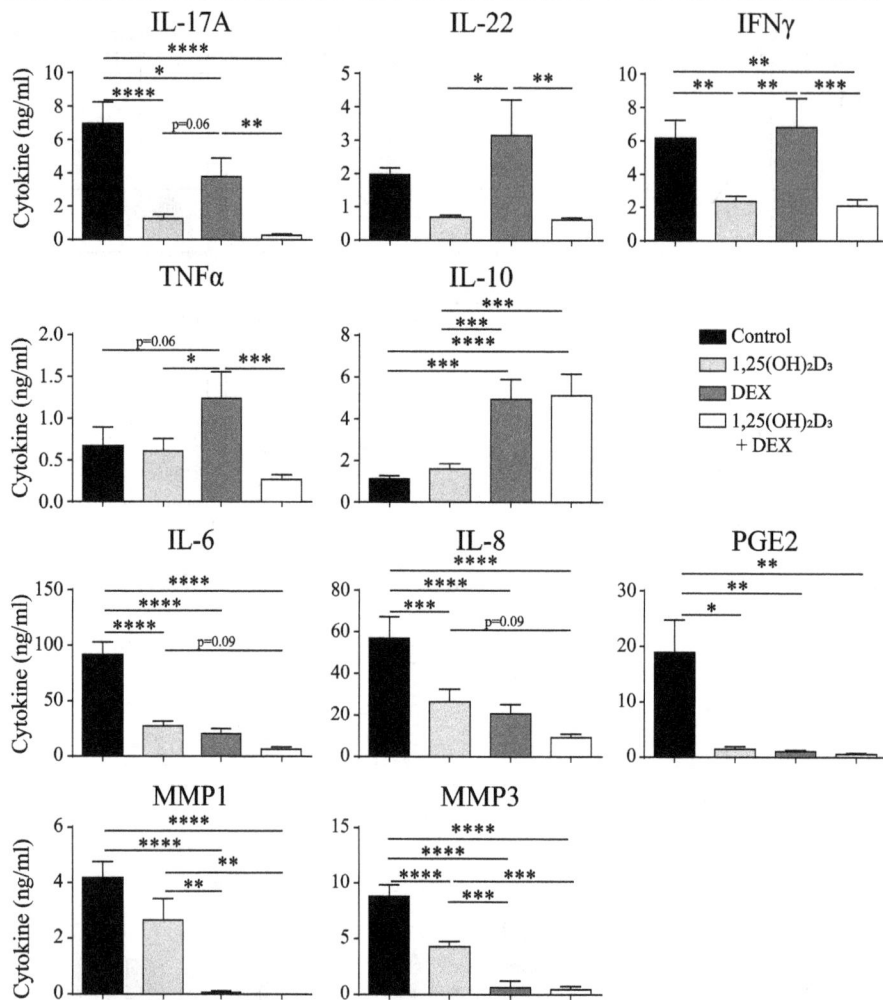

Fig. 2 1,25(OH)$_2$D$_3$ and DEX additively suppress the proinflammatory feedback loop between CCR6$^+$ memTh cells and RASF. CCR6$^+$ memTh sorted from healthy individuals were cultured with RASF for 3 days. The cells were stimulated with anti-CD3 and anti-CD28 and treated with or without 100 nM 1,25(OH)$_2$D$_3$ and 1000 nM dexamethasone (DEX). After 3 days, cytokine production was measured in the culture supernatant using ELISA. Mean ± SEM are given for $n = 10$ healthy donors grown on RASF from two different donors. Data are representative of at least three independent experiments. $*p < 0.05$, $**p < 0.01$, $***p < 0.001$, $****p < 0.0001$. IFN interferon, IL interleukin, MMP matrix metalloprotease, PGE2 prostaglandin E2, TNF tumor necrosis factor

1,25(OH)$_2$D$_3$ while being less efficient in inhibiting T cell-derived cytokines in the CCR6$^+$ memTh-RASF cocultures suggests a direct effect of DEX on RASF. To investigate this, RASF were cultured with or without stimulation of TNFα, IL-17A, or both for 3 days and treated with 1,25(OH)$_2$D$_3$, DEX, or a combination (Fig. 3). Without stimulation, 1,25(OH)$_2$D$_3$ did not significantly affect cytokine production by RASF, whereas DEX reduced the levels of IL-6 and IL-8. Upon stimulation with TNFα, both 1,25(OH)$_2$D$_3$ and DEX inhibited IL-6 and IL-8, whereas MMP1 and MMP3 were only significantly inhibited by DEX or the combination treatment. Similar patterns were observed with stimulation using IL-17A or a combination of IL-17A and TNFα. Together with our previous findings, these data suggest that, although DEX

and 1,25(OH)$_2$D$_3$ can affect both T cells and RASF, DEX acts most strongly on RASF whereas the main effect of 1,25(OH)$_2$D$_3$ is mediated via the T cells.

Low dose of 1,25(OH)$_2$D$_3$ and DEX improves the effects of TNFα blockade in CCR6$^+$ memTh-RASF cocultures

Since 1,25(OH)$_2$D$_3$ and DEX additively inhibit the proinflammatory loop between CCR6$^+$ memTh cells and RASF, we next studied whether the 1,25(OH)$_2$D$_3$-DEX combination can enhance the anti-inflammatory effect of TNFα blockade in this model system. To make these experiments more physiologically relevant, we used a dose-testing experiment to determine whether physiologically relevant dosages of 1,25(OH)$_2$D$_3$ and DEX still affected cytokine production in the CCR6$^+$ memTh-RASF

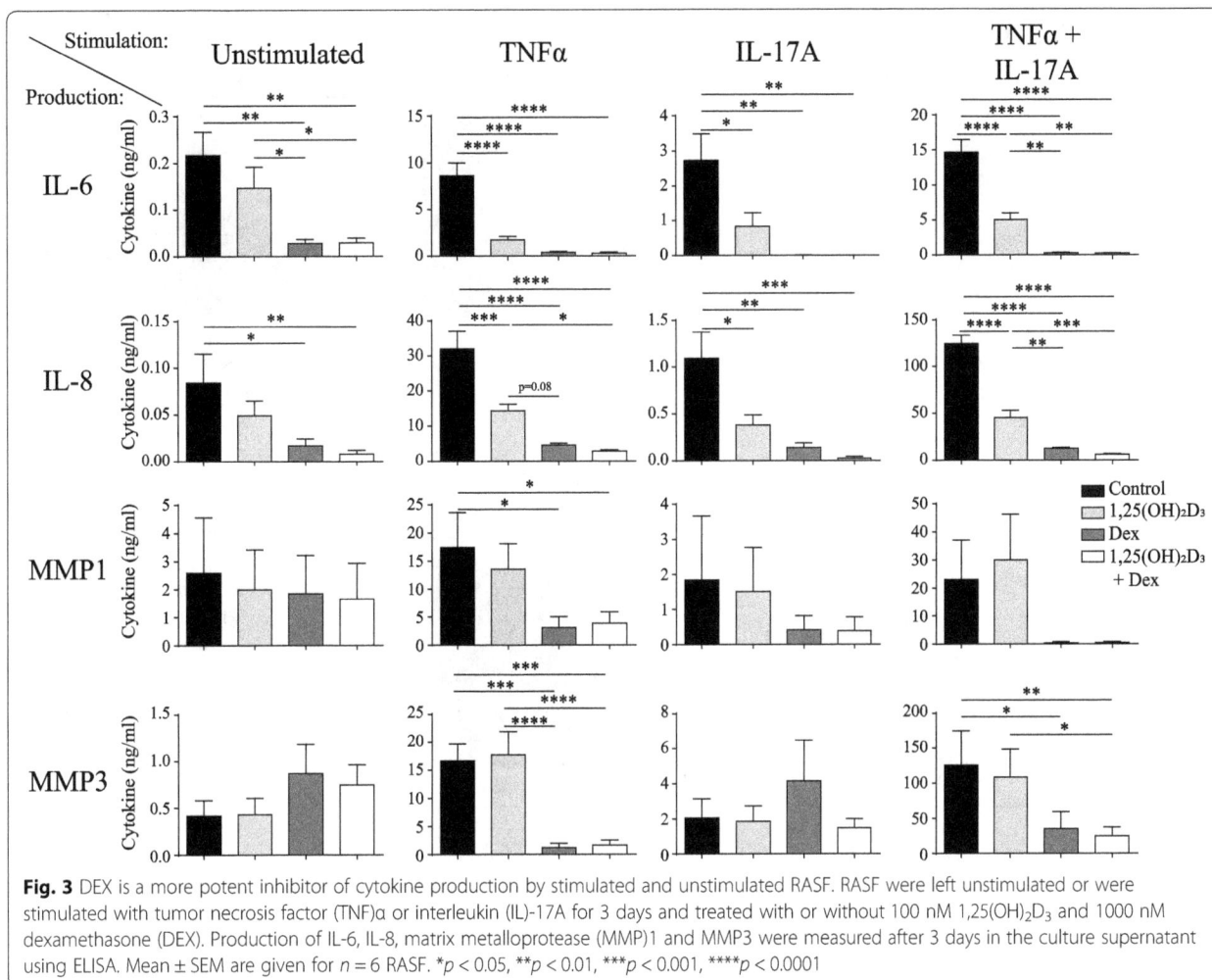

Fig. 3 DEX is a more potent inhibitor of cytokine production by stimulated and unstimulated RASF. RASF were left unstimulated or were stimulated with tumor necrosis factor (TNF)α or interleukin (IL)-17A for 3 days and treated with or without 100 nM $1,25(OH)_2D_3$ and 1000 nM dexamethasone (DEX). Production of IL-6, IL-8, matrix metalloprotease (MMP)1 and MMP3 were measured after 3 days in the culture supernatant using ELISA. Mean ± SEM are given for $n = 6$ RASF. $*p < 0.05$, $**p < 0.01$, $***p < 0.001$, $****p < 0.0001$

coculture system; 10 nM DEX still inhibited IL-6, IL-8, and MMP1 in CCR6[+] memTh-RASF cocultures, but 0.1 nM $1,25(OH)_2D_3$ only slightly affected these proinflammatory factors and did not appear different from the 1 nM dose (Additional file 1: Figure S2). Therefore, the value of adding DEX and $1,25(OH)_2D_3$ to etanercept was assessed using 10 nM DEX and 0.1 or 10 nM $1,25(OH)_2D_3$. CCR6[+] memTh cells were sorted from healthy controls and cultured together with RASF while being exposed to various combinations of $1,25(OH)_2D_3$, DEX, and the TNFα-blocking agent etanercept. Inhibition of IL-17A, IL-6, IL-8, MMP1, and MMP3 is shown as heatmaps in Fig. 4 and further detailed in Additional file 1 (Figure S3).

For IL-17A, etanercept dose-dependently inhibited cytokine expression, but this effect was stronger (darker shades) when the cells were also treated with 10 nM $1,25(OH)_2D_3$. Combining DEX with this dose of $1,25(OH)_2D_3$ further suppresses IL-17A and leaves little added effect for etanercept. IL-6 and IL-8 are more strongly inhibited by etanercept than IL-17A and show a

trend towards a dose response (left column of the heatmap, top to bottom). Adding increasing dosages of $1,25(OH)_2D_3$ augments the effects of etanercept, but the optimal effect is reached when 10 nM DEX, 10 nM $1,25(OH)_2D_3$, and etanercept are combined. Notably, under these conditions there is no significant difference between 0.1 or 10 μg/ml etanercept and cytokine expression is more than 90% reduced. MMP1 and MMP3 show a similar pattern of inhibition as IL-6 and IL-8, except that the effect of DEX is stronger even without additional $1,25(OH)_2D_3$ or etanercept. These data suggest that combining $1,25(OH)_2D_3$ and especially DEX with etanercept has additive effects compared with etanercept alone.

Since the cells from the healthy controls that were used in Fig. 4 and Additional file 1 (Figure S3) may react differently to treatment than the cells from RA patients, the experiment was repeated using sorted CCR6[+] memTh cells from treatment-naive early RA patients cultured with RASF serving as a proof of principle (Fig. 5 and Additional file 1: Figure S4). Due to large variation between patients (Additional file 1: Figure S4), there was

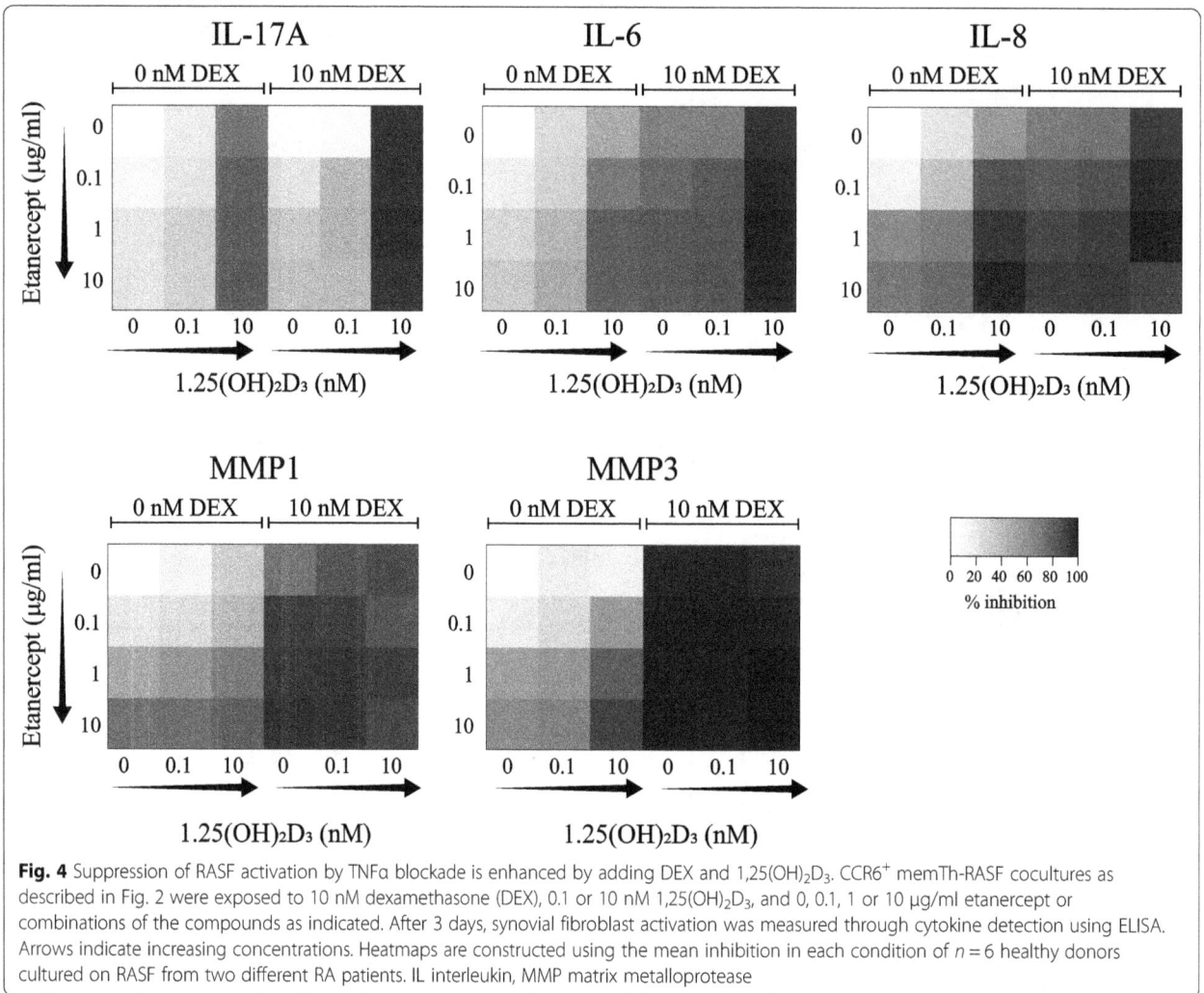

Fig. 4 Suppression of RASF activation by TNFα blockade is enhanced by adding DEX and 1,25(OH)$_2$D$_3$. CCR6$^+$ memTh-RASF cocultures as described in Fig. 2 were exposed to 10 nM dexamethasone (DEX), 0.1 or 10 nM 1,25(OH)$_2$D$_3$, and 0, 0.1, 1 or 10 µg/ml etanercept or combinations of the compounds as indicated. After 3 days, synovial fibroblast activation was measured through cytokine detection using ELISA. Arrows indicate increasing concentrations. Heatmaps are constructed using the mean inhibition in each condition of $n = 6$ healthy donors cultured on RASF from two different RA patients. IL interleukin, MMP matrix metalloprotease

a less clear dose-dependent inhibition of IL-17A in response to etanercept. However, 10 nM 1,25(OH)$_2$D$_3$ still enhanced the effects of etanercept, and IL-17A inhibition was again further increased when 10 nM DEX was added. The inhibition of IL-6 and IL-8 by etanercept was stronger in the CCR6$^+$ memTh cells from RA patients than those from healthy individuals. Similar to the results for the healthy controls, both 1,25(OH)$_2$D$_3$ and DEX enhanced the effects of etanercept. MMP1 and MMP3 were also inhibited by etanercept and their expression was further suppressed by DEX (Fig. 5).

Altogether, the data from Figs. 4 and 5 show that combination with DEX, and to a lesser extent 1,25(OH)$_2$D$_3$, provide a beneficial effect over TNFα blockade alone in a model for synovial inflammation.

Discussion

This study showed that 1,25(OH)$_2$D$_3$ and DEX can additively inhibit synovial inflammation modeled by CCR6$^+$ memTh-RASF cocultures. Furthermore, combining low

doses of DEX and 1,25(OH)$_2$D$_3$ with TNFα blockade demonstrated added value over TNFα blockade alone.

Similar to our previous results in PBMCs and memTh cells [11], 1,25(OH)$_2$D$_3$ was a stronger modulator of IL-17A, IL-22, IFNγ, and IL-10 in CCR6$^+$ memTh cells than DEX. This could be due to the reported resistance of CCR6$^+$ memTh cells to cytokine inhibition and apoptosis induction by GCs [13]. Interestingly, in asthma, GC resistance is increased with decreasing vitamin D serum levels [14]. Since the vitamin D receptor can enhance the activity of the GC receptor at promoter sites, 1,25(OH)$_2$D$_3$ may be able to overcome GC resistance through this mechanism [15]. Notably, in Crohn's disease Th17.1 cells, one of the subpopulations within CCR6$^+$ memTh cells, are the most GC-resistant cells [16]. Since these cells can also be found at the site of inflammation in juvenile idiopathic arthritis [17] and RA (unpublished observations) further research into cell type-specific modulation by GCs may further elucidate its immunosuppressive actions in RA.

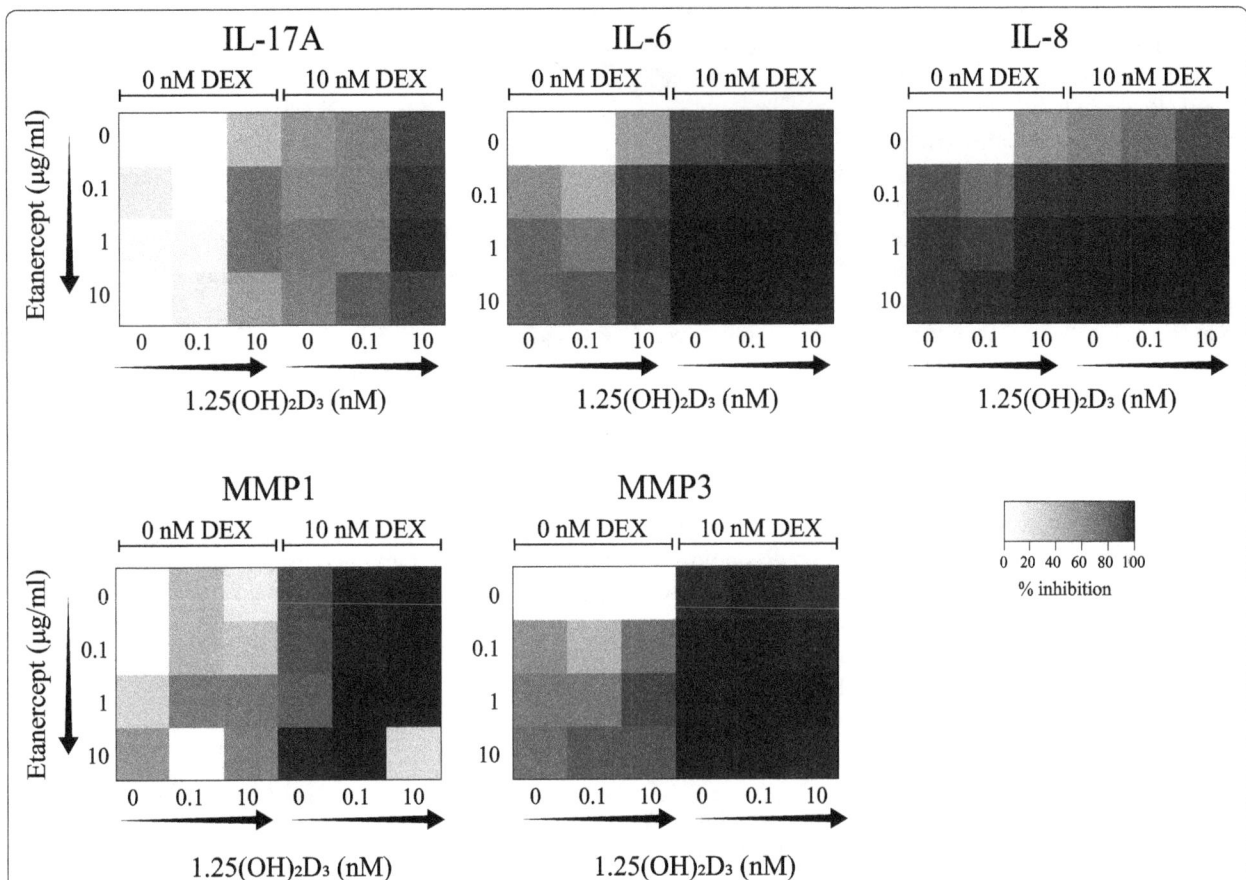

Fig. 5 Additive effects of dexamethasone (DEX) and 1,25(OH)$_2$D$_3$ on the inhibition of RASF activation by TNFα blockade are verified for treatment-naive RA patients. Cocultures were set up as described in Fig. 4 using RASF from established RA patients and allogeneic CCR6$^+$ memTh cells sorted from PBMCs of treatment-naive early RA patients. Cytokine expression was measured using ELISA after 3 days of culture. Arrows indicate increasing concentrations and heatmaps represent the mean inhibition per condition for n = 2–4 treatment-naive early RA patients. IL interleukin, MMP matrix metalloprotease

Independent of the differences in modulation of cytokines derived from CCR6$^+$ memTh cells, either cultured alone or together with RASF, both 1,25(OH)$_2$D$_3$ and DEX inhibited the activation of synovial fibroblasts as demonstrated by decreased IL-6, IL-8, MMP1, MMP3, and PGE2. These data suggest that DEX has strong direct effects on RASF, which was confirmed by RASF-only cultures. Although others have shown that 1,25(OH)$_2$D$_3$ can inhibit MMP1 and MMP3 from RASF under IL-1β stimulation [18], this was not observed in our cultures with stimulation of TNFα and IL-17A. Interestingly, whereas TNFα stimulation of RASF was generally more potent than stimulation with IL-17A, the combination of TNFα and IL-17A induced a higher level of IL-6 and MMP1 and a striking stronger increase in IL-8 and MMP3. It has been previously observed in keratinocytes that IL-8 was more strongly induced by TNFα and IL-17A than IL-6 [19]. Also, another study in RA fibroblast-like synoviocytes suggested a slightly stronger additive effect on IL-8 than IL-6, although they only used

1 ng/ml for both TNFα and IL-17A [20]. Since DEX and 1,25(OH)$_2$D$_3$ inhibit IL-8 and MMP3 both after TNFα single stimulation or TNFα-IL-17A combination, this may be an effective way to suppress even the strong stimulation that is potentially present in the RA joint.

Based on other studies showing that the vitamin D receptor and GC receptor can cooperate to enhance one another's functions [15, 21], we also expected synergistic effects of 1,25(OH)$_2$D$_3$ and DEX in CCR6$^+$ memTh cells or RASF. However, this synergy was not observed, except that TNFα could only be inhibited when 1,25(OH)$_2$D$_3$ and DEX were combined. Instead, the data indicate that 1,25(OH)$_2$D$_3$ and DEX additively suppress inflammation through targeting different inflammatory pathways. 1,25(OH)$_2$D$_3$ indirectly reduces RASF activation through modulation of IL-17A and could reduce activation of other immune cells, such as macrophages, by inhibiting IFNγ [22]. DEX, on the other hand, directly affects the RASF and reduces immune cell activation, immune cell attraction, and tissue destruction through regulation of

IL-6, IL-8, and MMPs, respectively. Finally, $1,25(OH)_2D_3$ and DEX are both capable of inducing the anti-inflammatory cytokine IL-10 in $CCR6^+$ memTh cell monocultures or in coculture with RASF, which could further contribute to inhibiting synovial inflammation.

Because of the strong immunomodulatory effects of $1,25(OH)_2D_3$ and DEX, we postulated that they could be beneficial in the treatment of autoimmune diseases. This study demonstrated that DEX especially could augment the effect of TNFα blockade on RASF activation, even up to the point that no differences could be seen between the lowest and highest dose of anti-TNFα. Adding 0.1 nM $1,25(OH)_2D_3$ did not contribute to this effect, but 10 nM enhanced the effects of DEX and TNFα blockade. The concentration of 0.1 nM (approximately 40 pg/ml) corresponds to the 20–80 pg/ml of $1,25(OH)_2D_3$ that has been found in the synovial fluid of RA patients [23]. However, the synovial fluid is not always a perfect representation of the situation in the synovium. Furthermore, it has been reported that immune cells are capable of converting $25(OH)D_3$ into $1,25(OH)_2D_3$ [24, 25], suggesting that the local concentration of active vitamin D in the inflamed synovium may be higher than 0.1 nM and therefore could contribute to the anti-inflammatory effects of DEX and anti-TNFα.

Although these data indicate that a combination of DEX and TNFα blockade could be beneficial in the treatment of RA, some limitations of this study should be considered. Firstly, the current study has focused on an in-vitro culture model with only T cells and RASF, whereas an inflamed joint also contains other cell types [26]. Although $1,25(OH)_2D_3$ and DEX are both known for their wide range of immunomodulatory properties [12, 27], the exact effects of combining these with TNFα blockade have not been investigated. Furthermore, the data suggest that dose reduction of TNFα blockade could be possible on combination with DEX since there is no dose-dependent effect anymore. It should be noted that the physiological concentration of etanercept in the synovial fluid has not been elaborately studied. One study found the concentration of etanercept in the synovial fluid was around 20 ng/ml in two patients receiving 50 mg etanercept every 2 weeks after 5 weeks, thus in between two dosages [28]. However, one patient who received 50 mg every week had a concentration of 100 ng/ml after 5 weeks, suggesting that the concentration shortly after etanercept injection is in the range of the 0.1 µg/ml that was used in this study [28]. The inhibitory effects of RASF activation by this dose of etanercept have been drastically enhanced by DEX and $1,25(OH)_2D_3$.

A final point to consider is that TNFα blockade has more effects than only suppressing RASF activation [29]. Therefore, it is possible that our in-vitro model overlooks interactions that may arise between the compounds and a more complex environment. To study this, murine models for RA, such as collagen-induced arthritis, could be used as a first validation of our study. After that, a clinical trial should be designed in which a low dose of DEX is combined with TNFα blockade. Due to the perceived immunomodulatory effects of $1,25(OH)_2D_3$, adding vitamin D supplements to this treatment will not only prevent the osteoporotic side effects of DEX, but it may also further enhance the therapeutic effects.

Conclusion

This study suggests an added value of combining $1,25(OH)_2D_3$ with DEX for inhibiting synovial inflammation in RA patients through their distinct cell type-specific modulation properties. Furthermore, the findings in the $CCR6^+$ memTh-RASF functional coculture model provide a rationale for a clinical trial combining low-dose $1,25(OH)_2D_3$ and DEX with TNFα blockade to improve disease management in RA.

Abbreviations
CCR: C-C chemokine receptor; DEX: Dexamethasone; DMARD: Disease-modifying antirheumatic drug; GC: Glucocorticoid; IFN: Interferon; IL: Interleukin; memTh: Memory T helper; MMP: Matrix metalloprotease; PBMC: Peripheral blood mononuclear cell; PGE2: Prostaglandin E2; RA: Rheumatoid arthritis; RASF: Rheumatoid arthritis synovial fibroblasts; RORC: RAR-related orphan receptor C; TNF: Tumor necrosis factor

Acknowledgements
We thank H.J. de Wit and P. van Geel for their extensive help in sorting the cells required for this study.

Funding
This work was supported by research grants from the Dutch Arthritis Foundation (10–1-407 and 15–2-206).

Authors' contributions
WD contributed to study design, performed experiments, analyzed data, and wrote the manuscript. CG-L contributed to study design, performed experiments, analyzed data, and critically revised the manuscript. ND, PSA, and AMCM performed experiments. JMWH provided patient samples, provided input for the study design, and critically revised the manuscript. EMC contributed to the study design and critically revised the manuscript. EL designed and supervised the study and critically revised the manuscript. All authors read and approved the final manuscript.

Consent for publication
Not applicable.

Competing interests
The authors declare that they have no competing interests.

Author details
[1]Department of Rheumatology, Erasmus MC, Rotterdam, the Netherlands. [2]Department of Immunology, Erasmus MC, Rotterdam, the Netherlands. [3]Department of Internal Medicine, Erasmus MC, Rotterdam, the Netherlands. [4]Erasmus MC University Medical Center, Wytemaweg 80, 3015CN Rotterdam, The Netherlands.

References

1. Smolen JS, Aletaha D, McInnes IB. Rheumatoid arthritis. Lancet. 2016;388: 2023–38.
2. Bartok B, Firestein GS. Fibroblast-like synoviocytes: key effector cells in rheumatoid arthritis. Immunol Rev. 2010;233:233–55.
3. Muller-Ladner U, Kriegsmann J, Franklin BN, Matsumoto S, Geiler T, Gay RE, Gay S. Synovial fibroblasts of patients with rheumatoid arthritis attach to and invade normal human cartilage when engrafted into SCID mice. Am J Pathol. 1996;149:1607–15.
4. van Hamburg JP, Asmawidjaja PS, Davelaar N, Mus AM, Colin EM, Hazes JM, Dolhain RJ, Lubberts E. Th17 cells, but not Th1 cells, from patients with early rheumatoid arthritis are potent inducers of matrix metalloproteinases and proinflammatory cytokines upon synovial fibroblast interaction, including autocrine interleukin-17A production. Arthritis Rheum. 2011;63:73–83.
5. Paulissen SM, van Hamburg JP, Dankers W, Lubberts E. The role and modulation of CCR6+ Th17 cell populations in rheumatoid arthritis. Cytokine. 2015;74:43–53.
6. Murphy CA, Langrish CL, Chen Y, Blumenschein W, McClanahan T, Kastelein RA, Sedgwick JD, Cua DJ. Divergent pro- and antiinflammatory roles for IL-23 and IL-12 in joint autoimmune inflammation. J Exp Med. 2003;198:1951–7.
7. Corneth OB, Mus AM, Asmawidjaja PS, Klein Wolterink RG, van Nimwegen M, Brem MD, Hofman Y, Hendriks RW, Lubberts E. Absence of interleukin-17 receptor a signaling prevents autoimmune inflammation of the joint and leads to a Th2-like phenotype in collagen-induced arthritis. Arthritis Rheumatol. 2014;66:340–9.
8. Leipe J, Grunke M, Dechant C, Reindl C, Kerzendorf U, Schulze-Koops H, Skapenko A. Role of Th17 cells in human autoimmune arthritis. Arthritis Rheum. 2010;62:2876–85.
9. Paulissen SM, van Hamburg JP, Davelaar N, Asmawidjaja PS, Hazes JM, Lubberts E. Synovial fibroblasts directly induce Th17 pathogenicity via the cyclooxygenase/prostaglandin E2 pathway, independent of IL-23. J Immunol. 2013;191:1364–72.
10. van Hamburg JP, Asmawidjaja PS, Davelaar N, Mus AM, Cornelissen F, van Leeuwen JP, Hazes JM, Dolhain RJ, Bakx PA, Colin EM, Lubberts E. TNF blockade requires 1,25(OH)2D3 to control human Th17-mediated synovial inflammation. Ann Rheum Dis. 2012;71:606–12.
11. Colin EM, Asmawidjaja PS, van Hamburg JP, Mus AM, van Driel M, Hazes JM, van Leeuwen JP, Lubberts E. 1,25-dihydroxyvitamin D3 modulates Th17 polarization and interleukin-22 expression by memory T cells from patients with early rheumatoid arthritis. Arthritis Rheum. 2010;62:132–42.
12. Cain DW, Cidlowski JA. Immune regulation by glucocorticoids. Nat Rev Immunol. 2017;17:233–47.
13. Banuelos J, Shin S, Cao Y, Bochner BS, Morales-Nebreda L, Budinger GR, Zhou L, Li S, Xin J, Lingen MW, et al. BCL-3 protects human and mouse Th17 cells from glucocorticoid-induced apoptosis. Allergy. 2016;71:640–50.
14. Sutherland ER, Goleva E, Jackson LP, Stevens AD, Leung DY. Vitamin D levels, lung function, and steroid response in adult asthma. Am J Respir Crit Care Med. 2010;181:699–704.
15. Zhang Y, Leung DY, Goleva E. Vitamin D enhances glucocorticoid action in human monocytes: involvement of granulocyte-macrophage colony-stimulating factor and mediator complex subunit 14. J Biol Chem. 2013;288:14544–53.
16. Ramesh R, Kozhaya L, McKevitt K, Djuretic IM, Carlson TJ, Quintero MA, McCauley JL, Abreu MT, Unutmaz D, Sundrud MS. Pro-inflammatory human Th17 cells selectively express P-glycoprotein and are refractory to glucocorticoids. J Exp Med. 2014;211:89–104.
17. Nistala K, Adams S, Cambrook H, Ursu S, Olivito B, de Jager W, Evans JG, Cimaz R, Bajaj-Elliott M, Wedderburn LR. Th17 plasticity in human autoimmune arthritis is driven by the inflammatory environment. Proc Natl Acad Sci U S A. 2010;107:14751–6.
18. Tetlow LC, Woolley DE. The effects of 1 alpha,25-dihydroxyvitamin D(3) on matrix metalloproteinase and prostaglandin E(2) production by cells of the rheumatoid lesion. Arthritis Res. 1999;1:63–70.
19. Chiricozzi A, Guttman-Yassky E, Suarez-Farinas M, Nograles KE, Tian S, Cardinale I, Chimenti S, Krueger JG. Integrative responses to IL-17 and TNF-alpha in human keratinocytes account for key inflammatory pathogenic circuits in psoriasis. J Invest Dermatol. 2011;131:677–87.
20. Fischer JA, Hueber AJ, Wilson S, Galm M, Baum W, Kitson C, Auer J, Lorenz SH, Moelleken J, Bader M, et al. Combined inhibition of tumor necrosis factor alpha and interleukin-17 as a therapeutic opportunity in rheumatoid arthritis: development and characterization of a novel bispecific antibody. Arthritis Rheumatol. 2015;67:51–62.
21. Hidalgo AA, Deeb KK, Pike JW, Johnson CS, Trump DL. Dexamethasone enhances 1alpha,25-dihydroxyvitamin D3 effects by increasing vitamin D receptor transcription. J Biol Chem. 2011;286:36228–37.
22. Schoenborn JR, Wilson CB. Regulation of interferon-γ during innate and adaptive immune responses. In: Advances in immunology. Volume 96. Cambridge: Academic Press; 2007. p. 41–101.
23. Inaba M, Yukioka K, Furumitsu Y, Murano M, Goto H, Nishizawa Y, Morii H. Positive correlation between levels of IL-1 or IL-2 and 1,25(OH)2D/25-OH-D ratio in synovial fluid of patients with rheumatoid arthritis. Life Sci. 1997;61:977–85.
24. Sigmundsdottir H, Pan J, Debes GF, Alt C, Habtezion A, Soler D, Butcher EC. DCs metabolize sunlight-induced vitamin D3 to 'program' T cell attraction to the epidermal chemokine CCL27. Nat Immunol. 2007;8:285–93.
25. Kongsbak M, von Essen MR, Levring TB, Schjerling P, Woetmann A, Odum N, Bonefeld CM, Geisler C. Vitamin D-binding protein controls T cell responses to vitamin D. BMC Immunol. 2014;15:35.
26. Firestein GS, McInnes IB. Immunopathogenesis of rheumatoid arthritis. Immunity. 2017;46:183–96.
27. Dankers W, Colin EM, van Hamburg JP, Lubberts E. Vitamin D in autoimmunity: molecular mechanisms and therapeutic potential. Front Immunol. 2016;7:697.
28. Zhou H. Clinical pharmacokinetics of etanercept: a fully humanized soluble recombinant tumor necrosis factor receptor fusion protein. J Clin Pharmacol. 2005;45:490–7.
29. Farrugia M, Baron B. The role of TNF-alpha in rheumatoid arthritis: a focus on regulatory T cells. J Clin Transl Res. 2016;2:84–90.

16

A comparative clinical study of PF- 06410293, a candidate adalimumab biosimilar, and adalimumab reference product (Humira®) in the treatment of active rheumatoid arthritis

Roy M. Fleischmann[1]*[iD], Rieke Alten[2], Margarita Pileckyte[3], Kasia Lobello[4], Steven Y. Hua[5], Carol Cronenberger[4], Daniel Alvarez[4], Amy E. Bock[6] and K. Lea Sewell[6]

Abstract

Background: This double-blind, randomized, 78-week study evaluated the efficacy, safety, immunogenicity, pharmacokinetics, and pharmacodynamics of PF-06410293, a candidate adalimumab biosimilar, versus adalimumab reference product (Humira®) sourced from the EU (adalimumab-EU) in biologic-naïve patients with active rheumatoid arthritis (RA) despite methotrexate (MTX) (10–25 mg/week). We report results for the first 26 weeks of treatment.

Methods: Patients with active RA ($N = 597$) were randomly assigned (1:1) to PF-06410293 or adalimumab-EU, while continuing with MTX treatment. The primary endpoint was American College of Rheumatology 20% improvement (ACR20) at week 12. Therapeutic equivalence was concluded if the two-sided 95% confidence interval (CI) for the ACR20 difference between the two arms was entirely contained within the symmetric equivalence margin (±14%). Additionally, a two-sided 90% CI was calculated by using an asymmetric equivalence margin (−12%, 15%). Secondary efficacy endpoints to week 26 included ACR20/50/70, change from baseline Disease Activity Score based on high-sensitivity C-reactive protein [DAS28–4(CRP)], European League Against Rheumatism (EULAR) response, DAS28–4(CRP) of less than 2.6, and ACR/EULAR remission. QuantiFERON-TB testing was performed at screening and week 26.

Results: Patients (78.7% of whom were female and whose mean age was 52.5 years) had a mean baseline RA duration of 6.8 years. The mean baseline DAS28–4(CRP) values were 5.9 (PF-06410293) and 6.1 (adalimumab-EU). The observed week-12 ACR20 values were 68.7% (PF-06410293) and 72.7% (adalimumab-EU) in the intention-to-treat population. With non-responder imputation, the treatment difference in week-12 ACR20 was −2.98% and corresponding CIs—95% CI (−10.38%, 4.44%) and 90% CI (−9.25%, 3.28%)—were entirely contained within the equivalence margins (symmetric and asymmetric, respectively). The secondary efficacy endpoints were similar between arms. Over 26 weeks, injection-site reactions occurred in 1.7% versus 2.0%, hypersensitivity events in 4.4% versus 8.4%, pneumonia in 0.7% versus 2.0%, and opportunistic infections in 2.4% versus 1.7% in the PF-06410293 and adalimumab-EU arms, respectively. One death due to myocardial infarction occurred (adalimumab-EU arm). Rates of anti-drug antibody incidence were 44.4% (PF-06410293) and 50.5% (adalimumab-EU).

(Continued on next page)

* Correspondence: rfleischmann@arthdocs.com
[1]Southwestern Medical Center, Metroplex Clinical Research Center, University of Texas, 8144 Walnut Hill Lane, Suite 810, Dallas, TX 75231, USA
Full list of author information is available at the end of the article

(Continued from previous page)

Conclusions: The study results demonstrate that efficacy, safety, and immunogenicity of PF-06410293 and adalimumab-EU were similar during the first 26 weeks of treatment in patients with active RA on background MTX.

Keywords: Rheumatoid arthritis, Adalimumab, Biosimilar, Comparative clinical study

Background

The introduction of biologic disease-modifying anti-rheumatic drugs (bDMARDs) has been a major advance in the treatment of patients with rheumatoid arthritis (RA), providing an important addition to the previously available therapy options [1]. Adalimumab, a recombinant fully human immunoglobulin G1 monoclonal antibody, inhibits the interaction of tumor necrosis factor (TNF) with surface TNF receptors by specifically binding to TNF-α and has been shown to reduce clinical symptoms and inhibit radiographic progression in patients with RA [2–4]. Adalimumab is approved for multiple indications in addition to RA [5, 6].

The US Food and Drug Administration (FDA) defines a biosimilar as "a biopharmaceutical that is highly similar to an already licensed biologic product (the reference product), notwithstanding minor differences in clinically inactive components, and for which there are no clinically meaningful differences in purity, potency, and safety between the two products" [7]. The European Medicines Agency requires that a biosimilar show "similarity to the reference biologic with respect to quality, biologic activity, safety, and efficacy" [8]. Biosimilars may expand patient access to bDMARDs because of potentially lower drug prices as a result of price competition within the product market, resulting in savings for health-care systems and patients [9–11].

PF-06410293 is in development as a candidate adalimumab biosimilar. Peptide mapping data demonstrate that PF-06410293 has a primary amino acid sequence identical to that of adalimumab reference product and is similar in comparative analytical, functional, and binding assessments [12]. Pharmacokinetic (PK) similarity was demonstrated following single-dose administration of PF-06410293 and adalimumab to healthy volunteers (Pfizer unpublished observation) [13]. The current comparative clinical study compared the efficacy, safety, immunogenicity, PK, and pharmacodynamics (PD) of PF-06410293 with adalimumab reference product (Humira®) sourced from the EU (adalimumab-EU) in patients with active RA and an inadequate response to methotrexate (MTX).

Methods
Study population

Patients with active RA and an inadequate response to MTX represent a sensitive and appropriate population for biosimilar comparability trials. Adults (at least 18 years old) with a diagnosis of active RA at least 4 months, based on the 2010 American College of Rheumatology/European League Against Rheumatism (ACR/EULAR) criteria [14], were eligible for inclusion. Active RA was defined as at least six tender and at least six swollen joints (at screening and baseline) with a high-sensitivity C-reactive protein (hs-CRP) of at least 8 mg/L at screening (Additional file 1).

Patients were ineligible if they met any of the following criteria: prior treatment with adalimumab, lymphocyte-depleting therapy, or more than two doses of one biologic therapy; inadequate washout of any second DMARD, pregnancy or breastfeeding, clinically significant laboratory abnormalities, current infection, congestive heart failure (New York Heart Association grade 3/4), untreated or inadequately treated latent or active tuberculosis (TB), malignancy within the previous 5 years, or a positive test for human immunodeficiency virus or hepatitis B or C virus (Additional file 2).

Study design and treatments

This was a multinational, two-arm, double-blind, randomized, comparative clinical study in patients with active RA and was conducted at 173 centers in Australia, Brazil, Bulgaria, Colombia, the Czech Republic, Estonia, Georgia, Germany, Hungary, Japan, Lithuania, Mexico, New Zealand, Peru, Poland, the Republic of Korea, Serbia, South Africa, Spain, Taiwan, Ukraine, the Russian Federation, UK, and the US. Patients were randomly assigned (1:1) on day 1 (stratified by geographic region) to receive either PF-06410293 or adalimumab-EU. There were three 26-week treatment periods and a 16-week follow-up after last dose of study drug (Fig. 1). Prior to dosing at week 26, patients in the adalimumab-EU arm were blindly re-randomized (1:1) to continue on adalimumab-EU or switch to PF-06410293. At week 52, all patients remaining on adalimumab-EU were switched to PF-06410293 for open-label treatment during the third treatment period. Herein, we report data from the first 26 weeks of the study. The number of tender (68) and swollen (66) joints was determined by an independent blinded joint assessor.

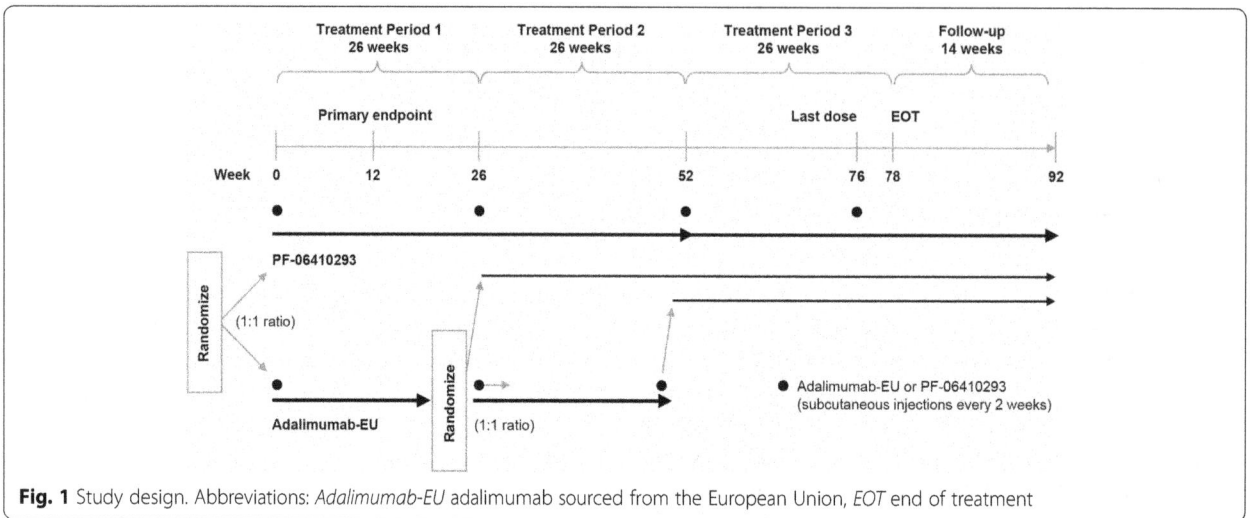

Fig. 1 Study design. Abbreviations: *Adalimumab-EU* adalimumab sourced from the European Union, *EOT* end of treatment

PF-06410293 or adalimumab-EU was administered as a subcutaneous injection (40 mg every other week using a prefilled syringe) in addition to a stable background dose of oral or intramuscular MTX (10–25 mg/week) and oral folic/folinic acid; lower doses of MTX (6 mg/week) were allowed if indicated in local guidance or standards of care. Patients could receive concomitant low-dose oral corticosteroids (≤10 mg prednisone or equivalent per day), one non-steroidal anti-inflammatory drug, and non-opioid or specific opioid analgesics or both. Treatment could be delayed by up to 24 h prior to the next injection for illness or scheduling issues. Dosing could be temporarily held at the discretion of the investigator for an adverse event (AE) and resumed after the AE resolved, unless the patient missed three sequential injections.

Primary study endpoint
The primary efficacy endpoint was the proportion of patients achieving an ACR20 response [15] at week 12. Week 12 is considered the beginning of the plateau of the time-response curve for ACR20 and, as such, is a more sensitive time point for the assessment of rapidity of response in biosimilar comparability trials in RA as suggested by regulatory authorities. Therefore, this trial evaluated the primary endpoint at week 12 rather than week 26, as used in the historical registration trials for adalimumab in patients with RA.

Secondary endpoints and assessments
Secondary efficacy endpoints through week 26 included ACR20 (at time points in addition to week 12), ACR50, ACR70, change from baseline in Disease Activity Score 28 joints: four components based on hs-CRP [DAS28–4(CRP)], EULAR response, DAS28–4(CRP) of less than 2.6, ACR/EULAR remission, and change from baseline in individual ACR components, including Health Assessment Questionnaire

Disability Index (HAQ-DI). The sponsor selected DAS28–4(CRP) rather than DAS28–4(erythrocyte sedimentation rate [ESR]) to determine clinical response, as CRP is performed in a central laboratory. A cutoff of less than 2.6 was used to define DAS28(CRP) "remission" and not more than 3.2 as "low disease activity" rather than the lower numbers that have been shown to best correlate with the DAS28(ESR) formula [16].

Safety endpoints included type, incidence, severity, timing, seriousness, and investigator-determined relatedness of AEs—using the National Cancer Institute Common Terminology Criteria for Adverse Events (Version 4.03)—and laboratory abnormalities (Covance, Indianapolis, IN, USA). Safety evaluations during study treatment included physical examinations, electrocardiograms, and QuantiFERON-TB Gold testing (at screening and week 26).

Prespecified treatment-emergent adverse events (TEAEs) of special interest were injection-site reactions (ISRs), opportunistic infections (defined for this study to include zoster, cytomegalovirus, latent/active TB, atypical mycobacteria, systemic fungal infections and oral thrush, pneumocystis, legionella, salmonellosis, shigellosis, vibrio, and other infections), and anaphylaxis/angioedema/urticaria. Additional prespecified TEAE categories of interest included blood and lymphatic events, cardiovascular events, demyelinating conditions, gastric/hepatic events, hypersensitivity events, infections and infestations, and neoplasms.

Anti-drug antibodies (ADAs) and neutralizing antibodies (NAbs) were tested at baseline and weeks 2, 6, 12, and 26. Serum samples were analyzed by using a tiered approach of laboratory screening, confirmation, and titer determination. Serum samples were analyzed for ADA at QPS, LLC (Newark, DE, USA) by using a single validated electrochemiluminescent immunoassay. ADA-positive samples were then tested for neutralizing activity with a validated cell-based assay using PF-06410293 as the capture agent.

PK serum samples were obtained at baseline and weeks 1, 2, 6, 12, and 26 and evaluated for PF-06410293 or adalimumab-EU concentrations by using a validated, sensitive, and specific enzyme-linked immunosorbent assay with a lower limit of quantification of 250 ng/mL (QPS). The prespecified PD marker was hs-CRP.

Statistical methods

With the assumption of a week-12 ACR20 response rate of 60% for both PF-06410293 and adalimumab-EU, a sample size of 560 patients was determined to provide about 85% power to demonstrate therapeutic equivalence between the treatment arms, and the symmetric margin of ±14% was used for the primary endpoint. This equivalence margin was derived from a meta-analysis of published data from registration studies for adalimumab in patients with RA [2, 3, 17, 18] and was endorsed by both the European Medicines Agency and the Pharmaceuticals and Medical Devices Agency. Exact methods were used to calculate the confidence interval (CI) for the treatment difference in primary efficacy endpoint of week-12 ACR20, using non-responder imputation (NRI) for missing data and for patients with permanent discontinuation of study drug prior to week 12. Therapeutic equivalence was concluded if the two-sided 95% CI for the treatment difference was entirely contained within ±14% margin and additionally if the two-sided 90% CI for the same treatment difference was within the asymmetric margin of –12% to 15% (as requested by the FDA).

The intention-to-treat (ITT) population, defined as all randomly assigned patients, was the primary analysis population. Sensitivity analyses of the primary and secondary endpoints used the per protocol (PP) population, defined as all patients who received study treatment up to week 12, had a week-12 evaluation, and had no major protocol deviations. The DAS28–4(CRP) change from baseline was analyzed by using an analysis of covariance for repeated-measures data approach.

Safety and immunogenicity analyses were performed for the safety population (defined as randomly assigned patients who received any study treatment) on the prespecified TEAEs of special interest and categories of special interest with risk differences (RDs) and 95% CIs by using the asymptotic approach of Miettinen and Nurminen [19]. Transient ADA response after treatment (including the follow-up period) was defined as either a single positive ADA result or two positive sampling time points where the first and last ADA-positive samples (irrespective of any negative samples in between) were separated by less than 16 weeks and the patient's last ADA sampling time result was negative [20]. PK analysis was conducted for all dosed patients who provided at least one post-dose drug concentration measurement and was summarized by treatment and ADA status by using descriptive statistics (mean, standard deviation [SD], median, and minimum and maximum). PD analysis using hs-CRP concentration over time was summarized by descriptive statistics according to treatment.

Results

Patient disposition and demographics

In total, 1231 patients were screened and 597 eligible patients—297 to PF-06410293 and 300 to adalimumab-EU—were randomly assigned to receive study treatment (Additional file 3). Low hs-CRP level was the main reason for screen failure. The safety population included 596 patients, and one adalimumab-EU patient was randomly assigned and not dosed. In both treatment arms, the median duration of study treatment was 24.1 weeks. The first treatment period to week 26 was completed by 286 (96.3%) out of 297 patients in the PF-06410293 arm and 273 (91.0%) out of 300 in the adalimumab-EU arm. Overall, 30 (10.1%) out of 297 patients in the PF-06410293 arm and 46 (15.3%) out of 300 in the adalimumab-EU arm were excluded from the PP population. In most cases, exclusion was due to incomplete study drug dosing up to week 12 for 16 (5.4%) out of 297 patients in the PF-06410293 arm and 34 (11.3%) out of 300 in the adalimumab-EU arm. In the PF-06410293 arm, 29 (9.8%) out of 297 patients, compared with 51 (17.1%) out of 299 in the adalimumab-EU arm, missed one or more doses. This included 18 (6.1%) out of 297 and 34 (11.4%) out of 299 patients who missed one or more doses because of an AE in the PF-06410293 and adalimumab-EU arms, respectively.

Patient demographic and baseline RA characteristics were similar between the treatment arms (Table 1). At baseline, patients had a mean age of 52.5 years, 78.7% were female, and the mean RA duration was 6.8 years. Mean baseline swollen joint counts were 15.4 versus 17.0 and tender joint counts were 24.3 versus 26.7 in the PF-06410293 and adalimumab-EU arms, respectively. Mean baseline DAS28–4(CRP) values were 5.9 (PF-06410293) and 6.1 (adalimumab-EU). Across the two arms, the mean MTX dose was 15.2 mg/week and 55.9% of patients were receiving oral corticosteroids (Table 1).

Efficacy

Primary endpoint

Based on the primary efficacy endpoint of ACR20 response rate at week 12, therapeutic equivalence between PF-06410293 and adalimumab-EU was demonstrated by using both prespecified equivalence margins. With

Table 1 Baseline patient demographic and clinical characteristics (ITT population)

	PF-06410293 $n = 297$	Adalimumab-EU $n = 300$
Demographics[a]		
Gender, n (%)		
Female	241 (81.1)	229 (76.3)
Male	56 (18.9)	71 (23.7)
Age, mean (SD), years	51.5 (13.6)	53.5 (12.9)
Weight, mean (SD), kg	74.7 (17.5)	76.2 (20.8)
Body mass index, mean (SD), kg/m^2	27.5 (6.1)	28.1 (7.3)
Race, n (%)		
White	261 (87.9)	256 (85.3)
Black	6 (2.0)	9 (3.0)
Asian	16 (5.4)	17 (5.7)
Other	14 (4.7)	18 (6.0)
Ethnicity, n (%)		
Hispanic/Latino	25 (8.4)	29 (9.7)
Not Hispanic/Latino	272 (91.6)	271 (90.3)
Clinical characteristics		
RA duration, mean (SD), years	6.8 (7.2)	6.8 (6.9)
Positive RF or anti-CCP antibody or both, n (%)	242 (81.5)	245 (81.7)
Swollen joint count, mean (SD)	15.4 (7.8)	17.0 (9.8)
Tender joint count, mean (SD)	24.3 (12.3)	26.7 (14.8)
hs-CRP, mg/L		
Mean (SD)	21.3 (22.7)	22.8 (25.2)
Median (range)	14.7 (0.2–169)	16.0 (0.2–192)
DAS28–4(CRP), mean (SD)	5.9 (0.9)	6.1 (0.9)
HAQ-DI, mean (SD)	1.5 (0.6)	1.7 (0.6)
Prior use of one biologic drug, n (%)	8 (2.7)	5 (1.7)
Number of prior and current non-biologic DMARDs (in addition to MTX), mean (SD)	1.5 (0.9)	1.5 (0.9)
MTX dose, mean (SD), mg/week	15.2 (4.4)	15.2 (4.5)
Corticosteroid use, n (%)	164 (55.2)	170 (56.7)

Abbreviations: Adalimumab-EU adalimumab sourced from the European Union, *CCP* cyclic citrullinated peptide, *DAS28–4(CRP)* Disease Activity Score-28: four components based on high-sensitivity C-reactive protein, *DMARD* disease-modifying anti-rheumatic drug, *HAQ-DI* Health Assessment Questionnaire Disability Index, *hs-CRP* high-sensitivity C-reactive protein, *ITT* intention-to-treat, *MTX* methotrexate, *n* number of patients in each category, *RA* rheumatoid arthritis, *RF* rheumatoid factor, *SD* standard deviation
[a]Randomization stratified by geographic region (North America and Western Europe; Japan; Republic of Korea and Taiwan; Latin America; rest of world)

observed data in the ITT population, 204 (68.7%) out of 297 patients in the PF-06410293 arm and 218 (72.7%) out of 300 in the adalimumab-EU arm achieved an ACR20 response at week 12, and treatment difference was −3.98%. For the ITT population, response was imputed as non-responder in 19 patients, the treatment difference was −2.98%, based on ACR20 response in 203 (68.4%) out of 297 patients in the PF-06410293 arm and 214 (71.3%) out of 300 in the adalimumab-EU arm, and the 95% CI (−10.38%, 4.44%) was entirely contained within the symmetric margin (Fig. 2a) and 90% CI

(−9.25%, 3.28%) was entirely contained within the asymmetric margin (Fig. 2b).

For the PP population sensitivity analysis, 189 (71.1%) out of 266 patients in the PF-06410293 arm and 191 (75.2%) out of 254 in the adalimumab-EU arm achieved an ACR20 response at week 12. The treatment difference was −4.14%, and the corresponding 95% (−11.79%, 3.61%) and 90% (−10.60%, 2.38%) CIs were entirely contained within the symmetric (±14%) and asymmetric (−12%, 15%) equivalence margins, respectively. Other sensitivity analyses of the primary endpoint, including

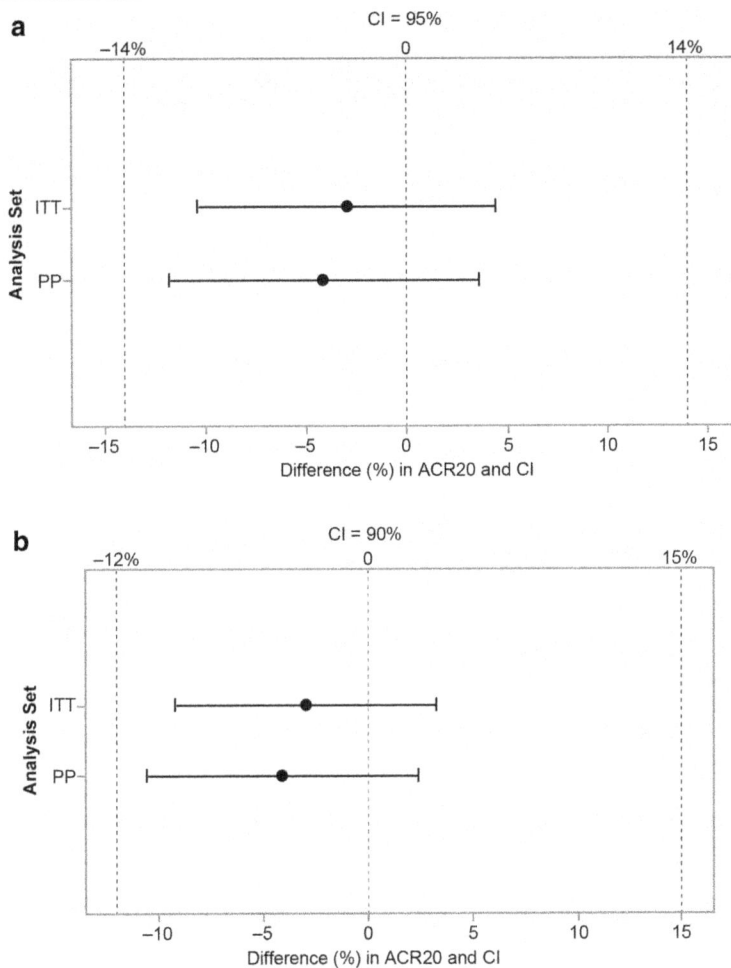

Fig. 2 Primary efficacy endpoint of ACR20 at week 12 (with non-responder imputation). **a** Difference (95% CI) between PF-06410293 and adalimumab-EU using a symmetric equivalence margin. **b** Difference (90% CI) between PF-06410293 and adalimumab-EU using an asymmetric equivalence margin. Abbreviations: *ACR20* American College of Rheumatology 20% improvement, *Adalimumab-EU* adalimumab sourced from the European Union, *CI* confidence interval, *ITT* intention-to-treat, *PP* per protocol

an analysis adjusting for the stratification variable of geographic region and a multiple imputation-based tipping point analysis for missing data, were consistent with the primary result of therapeutic equivalence between PF-06410293 and adalimumab-EU (Additional file 4).

The ACR20 rates at week 12 for subgroups were numerically higher in ADA-negative (70.9% and 77.2%) compared with ADA-positive (63.7% and 65.7%) patients for the PF-06410293 and adalimumab-EU arms, respectively, defined as subjects with a positive ADA test in the first 26 weeks. ACR20 rates for NAb-negative patients were also numerically higher (70.9% and 74.0%) as compared with NAb-positive patients (50.0% and 64.0%) for the PF-06410293 and adalimumab-EU arms, respectively.

Secondary endpoints
The ACR20/50/70 response rates through week 26 were similar between the PF-06410293 and adalimumab-EU

arms (Fig. 3a). Mean changes from baseline in DAS28–4(CRP) were similar between treatment arms at each study visit, and the changes from baseline at week 26 were −2.7 for the PF-06410293 arm and −2.8 for the adalimumab-EU arm (Fig. 3b). At week 26, 162 (54.5%) out of 297 and 147 (49.0%) out of 300 of patients had a good EULAR response in the PF-06410293 and adalimumab-EU arms, respectively (Additional file 5). In the PF-06410293 arm, 87 (29.3%) out of 297 patients achieved DAS28–4(CRP) of less than 2.6 at week 26 compared with 99 (33.0%) out of 300 in the adalimumab-EU arm (Additional file 6). A total of 38 (12.8%) out of 297 patients in the PF-06410293 arm and 44 (14.7%) out of 300 in the adalimumab-EU arm achieved ACR/EULAR remission at week 26, including 26 (8.8%) out of 297 and 27 (9.0%) out of 300 using only the Boolean definition (Additional file 6). At week 26, mean HAQ-DI decreased from baseline by 0.654 in the

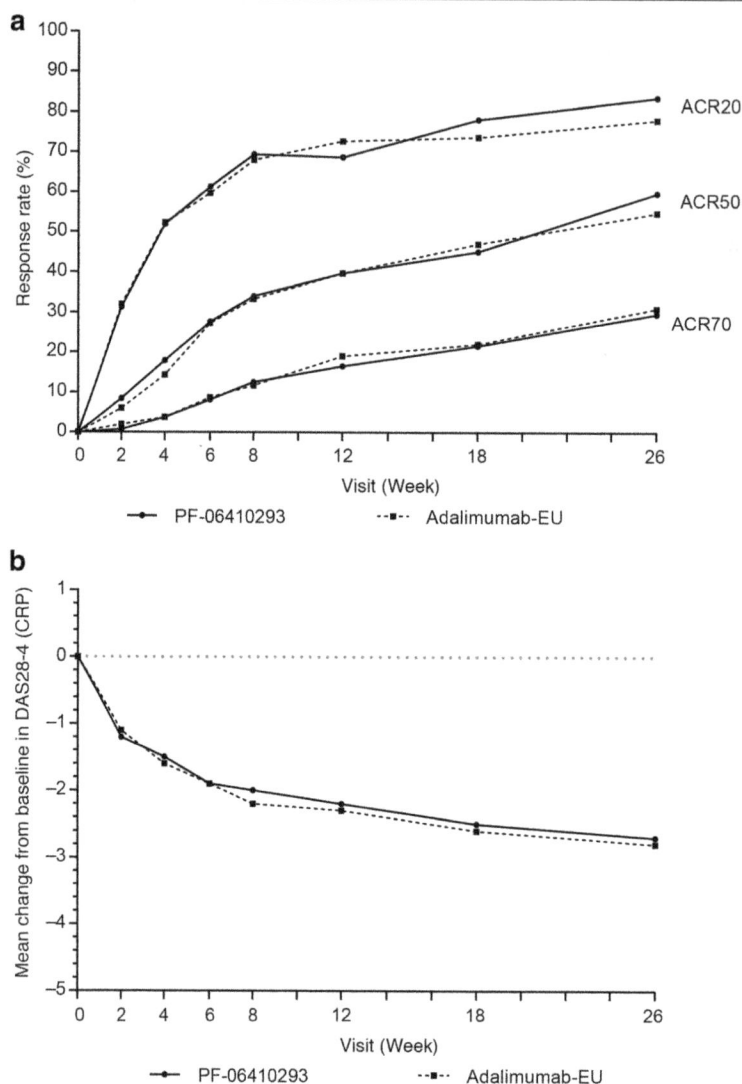

Fig. 3 Secondary efficacy endpoints (intention-to-treat population). **a** ACR20/50/70 response rates by study visit. **b** Mean change from baseline in DAS28–4(CRP) by study visit. Abbreviations: *Adalimumab-EU* adalimumab sourced from the European Union, *ACR20/50/70* American College of Rheumatology 20%/50%/70% improvement, *DAS28–4(CRP)* Disease Activity Score-28: four components based on high-sensitivity C-reactive protein

PF-06410293 arm and by 0.674 in the adalimumab-EU arm (Additional file 7).

Safety

A total of 143 (48.1%) out of 297 patients in the PF-06410293 arm and 143 (47.8%) out of 299 in the adalimumab-EU arm reported one or more TEAEs. The System Organ Classes (SOCs) with the highest proportion of patients with AEs were infections and infestations in 24.9% and 25.1%, musculoskeletal and connective tissue disorders in 10.4% and 8.7%, and investigations in 8.8% and 7.7% for the PF-06410293 and adalimumab-EU patients, respectively. The number of patients who permanently discontinued treatment because of TEAEs was 11 (3.7%) versus 14 (4.7%) and the number of patients who

temporarily discontinued treatment because of TEAEs was 17 (5.7%) versus 29 (9.7%) in the PF-06410293 and adalimumab-EU arms, respectively.

Serious adverse events (SAEs) were reported by 4.0% (PF-06410293) and 4.3% (adalimumab-EU) of patients (Table 2). This included one death due to myocardial infarction in the adalimumab-EU arm. The SOC with the highest proportion of patients with SAEs was infections and infestations, occurring in three patients in each treatment arm.

In total, 5.7% of patients in the PF-06410293 arm and 7.0% in the adalimumab-EU arm reported TEAEs of grade 3 or higher. All-causality grade 4 TEAEs were reported in two patients in the PF-06410293 arm (intentional self-injury, and hemorrhoids with rectal hemorrhage and resulting anemia) and four patients in

Table 2 All-causality treatment-emergent adverse events (safety population)

	PF-06410293 $n = 297$	Adalimumab-EU $n = 299$
Number of AEs	343	379
Patients with events, n (%)		
AEs	143 (48.1)	143 (47.8)
SAEs	12 (4.0)	13 (4.3)
Grade 3 AEs	15 (5.1)	16 (5.4)[a]
Grade 4 AEs	2 (0.7)	4 (1.3)
Grade 5 AEs	0	1 (0.3)
Patients with temporary treatment discontinuation due to AEs, n (%)	17 (5.7)	29 (9.7)
Patients discontinued from treatment due to AEs[c], n (%)	11 (3.7)[b]	14 (4.7)
Patients discontinued from the study due to AEs, n (%)	8 (2.7)	9 (3.0)

AEs were graded in accordance with National Cancer Institute Common Terminology Criteria for Adverse Events version 4.03. Grade 1–5 AEs are defined as mild, moderate, severe, life-threatening AEs, and death related to AE, respectively.
Abbreviations: Adalimumab-EU adalimumab sourced from the European Union, *AE* adverse event, *SAE* serious adverse event
[a]One patient had an AE of neutropenia incorrectly recorded as grade 2; the correct severity was grade 3 (not corrected in this table)
[b]One patient was incorrectly recorded as treatment discontinuation due to an AE; the correct reason was insufficient clinical response (not corrected in this table)
[c]The System Organ Class with the highest proportion of subjects who had AEs leading to permanent treatment discontinuation was infections and infestations (8 [2.7%] subjects on PF-06410293 and 3 [1.0%] subjects on adalimumab-EU)

the adalimumab-EU arm (atrial fibrillation, ileus secondary to colon cancer, gastroenteritis, and papillary thyroid cancer).

The most frequently reported TEAEs occurring in at least 2% of patients in any treatment arm were viral upper respiratory tract infections, increased alanine aminotransferase, hypertension, and headaches (Additional file 8).

Of the TEAEs of special interest, ISRs were reported by five (1.7%) and six (2.0%) patients in the PF-06410293 and adalimumab-EU arms, respectively (Table 3). The primary symptom was redness (three patients in the PF-06410293 arm and two in the adalimumab-EU arm). In addition, one patient in each arm reported pain and swelling. No patients discontinued treatment because of an ISR. For one patient in the PF-06410293 arm and two patients in the adalimumab-EU arm, the ISR occurred on or after the date the patient first tested positive for ADA.

Overall infection rates were similar at 24.9% and 25.1% for the PF-06410293 and adalimumab-EU arms, respectively. Opportunistic infections (predefined in the study as including latent TB) were reported by seven (2.4%) in the PF-06410293 arm and five (1.7%) patients in the adalimumab-EU arm (Table 3). One case of herpes zoster was reported in the PF-06410293 arm and three cases in the adalimumab-EU arm. Five and one cases of seroconversion with a subsequent diagnosis of latent TB (based on specialist consultation following a positive week-26 QuantiFERON-TB Gold test result) were reported in the PF-06410293 and adalimumab-EU arms, respectively. The RD for latent TB (1.35, 95% CI −0.35, 3.59) was not statistically significant. In total, 5.6% of patients in the PF-06410293 arm and 4.9% in the adalimumab-EU arm had a negative QuantiFERON-TB test at screening and a positive test at week 26. There were

Table 3 All-causality treatment-emergent adverse events of special interest with risk difference (safety population)

Event of special interest	PF-06410293 $n = 297$ n (%)	Adalimumab-EU $n = 299$ n (%)	Risk difference (95% CI) (%)
Injection-site reactions	5 (1.7)	6 (2.0)	−0.32 (−2.84, 2.12)
Opportunistic infections	7 (2.4)	5 (1.7)	0.69 (−1.80, 3.32)
Herpes zoster	1 (0.3)	3 (1.0)	−0.67 (−2.61, 0.97)
Latent tuberculosis	5 (1.7)	1 (0.3)	1.35 (−0.35, 3.59)
Confirmed active tuberculosis	0	0	0 (NA)
Oral candidiasis	0	1 (0.3)	−0.33 (−1.87, 0.95)
Pneumocystis jirovecii pneumonia	1 (0.3)	0	0.34 (−0.94, 1.88)
Urticaria, angioedema, anaphylactic reaction[a]	0	2 (0.7)	−0.67 (−2.41, 0.61)

Abbreviations: Adalimumab-EU adalimumab sourced from the European Union, *CI* confidence interval, *NA* not applicable
[a]Only urticaria reported

no cases of active TB in any patient in either treatment arm. One case of oral candidiasis (adalimumab-EU) and one case of *Pneumocystis jirovecii* pneumonia (PF-06410293) were reported. Overall, pneumonia was reported by 0.7% and 2.0% of the PF-06410293 and adalimumab-EU arms, respectively. There were no cases of anaphylaxis or angioedema in either treatment arm; two cases of urticaria were reported in the adalimumab-EU arm.

A total of 39.1% of patients in each arm reported 183 (PF-06410293) and 202 (adalimumab-EU) AEs in one or more prespecified TEAE categories of interest (Table 4). Hypersensitivity TEAEs were reported in 13 (4.4%) out of 297 patients in the PF-06410293 arm compared with 25 (8.4%) out of 299 in the adalimumab-EU arm (RD −3.98, 95% CI −8.15, −0.06). The most frequently reported hypersensitivity TEAEs were cough (5 versus 3), erythema (4 versus 1), and rash (1 versus 3) in the PF-06410293 and adalimumab-EU arms, respectively. Hypersensitivity TEAEs occurring on or after the date a patient first tested positive for ADA included six AEs reported by five patients in the PF-06410293 arm and nine AEs reported by seven patients in the adalimumab-EU arm. Two patients in the PF-06410293 arm reported grade 3 hypersensitivity SAEs, including interstitial lung disease and toxic skin eruption. The rate of blood and lymphatic system events was numerically higher in the PF-06410293 versus adalimumab-EU arms—22 (7.4%) out of 297 versus 14 (4.7%) out of 299—but this was not statistically significant (RD 2.73, 95% CI −1.15, 6.79). The reported malignancies included one (basal cell carcinoma) and two (adenocarcinoma of the colon and papillary thyroid cancer) patients in the PF-06410293 and adalimumab-EU arms, respectively.

Immunogenicity, PK, and PD

Overall, 44.4% and 50.5% of patients in the PF-06410293 and adalimumab-EU treatment arms, respectively, had at least one post-dose sample that tested positive for ADA (Fig. 4; Additional file 9). ADAs were transient in 11.4% of patients in the PF-06410293 arm and in 6.0% in the adalimumab-EU arm. Of the ADA-positive patients, 31.1% in the PF-06410293 and 27.8% in the adalimumab-EU treatment arms tested positive for NAb.

The mean serum drug trough concentrations at week 26 were 8244 and 7190 ng/mL in the PF-06410293 and adalimumab-EU arms, respectively. Mean serum concentrations of both drugs were lower in ADA-positive patients (4683 and 4041 ng/mL) compared with ADA-negative patients (11,090 and 10,460 ng/mL) for the PF-06410293 and adalimumab-EU arms, respectively. The mean hs-CRP concentrations (prespecified PD marker) were decreased at week 26 in both arms (ITT population); the changes from baseline to week 26 were −11.1 (PF-06410293) and −13.6 mg/L (adalimumab-EU).

Discussion

This comparative clinical study was conducted to evaluate the biosimilarity of PF-06410293 and adalimumab-EU. The primary goal of the study was met by demonstrating therapeutic equivalence of PF-06410293 and adalimumab-EU using the symmetric and asymmetric margins for the week-12 ACR20 primary endpoint comparison. Sensitivity analyses of the primary endpoint supported a conclusion of therapeutic equivalence. As expected, ACR20 response rates at week 12 were numerically higher in ADA-negative patients compared with ADA-positive in both treatment arms. Secondary endpoints reported up to week 26, including ACR50, ACR70,

Table 4 Prespecified treatment-emergent adverse event categories of interest with risk difference (safety population)

Category	PF-06410293 n = 297 n (%)	Adalimumab-EU n = 299 n (%)	Risk difference (95% CI) (%)
Blood and lymphatic system events	22 (7.4)	14 (4.7)	2.73 (−1.15, 6.79)
Cardiovascular events	9 (3.0)	16 (5.4)	−2.32 (−5.84, 0.96)
Demyelinating conditions	0	0	0 (NA)
Gastric/hepatic events	11 (3.7)	14 (4.7)	−0.98 (−4.44, 2.39)
Hypersensitivity[a]	13 (4.4)	25 (8.4)	−3.98 (−8.15, −0.06)
Infections and infestations	74 (24.9)	75 (25.1)	−0.17 (−7.13, 6.80)
Neoplasms	5 (1.7)	5 (1.7)	0.01 (−2.38, 2.42)
Other[b]	11 (3.7)	10 (3.3)	0.36 (−2.80, 3.57)

Abbreviations: Adalimumab-EU adalimumab sourced from the European Union, *CI* confidence interval, *MedDRA* Medical Dictionary for Regulatory Activities, *NA* not applicable
[a]Hypersensitivity events identified by Hypersensitivity Standardized MedDRA Query (broad and narrow), Anaphylactic reactions Standardized MedDRA Query (broad and narrow), and High-Level Group Terms Immunology and allergy investigations
[b]Other events identified by High-Level Group Terms Skin Vascular Abnormalities, Central Nervous System Vascular Abnormalities and Medication Errors; Higher Level Terms Connective Tissue Disorders, Vasculitides (not elsewhere classified), Rashes, Eruptions and Exanthems (not elsewhere classified); Lower Level Teams Seizure and Convulsions; and Preferred Terms Lupus-like Syndrome, Headache and Migraine

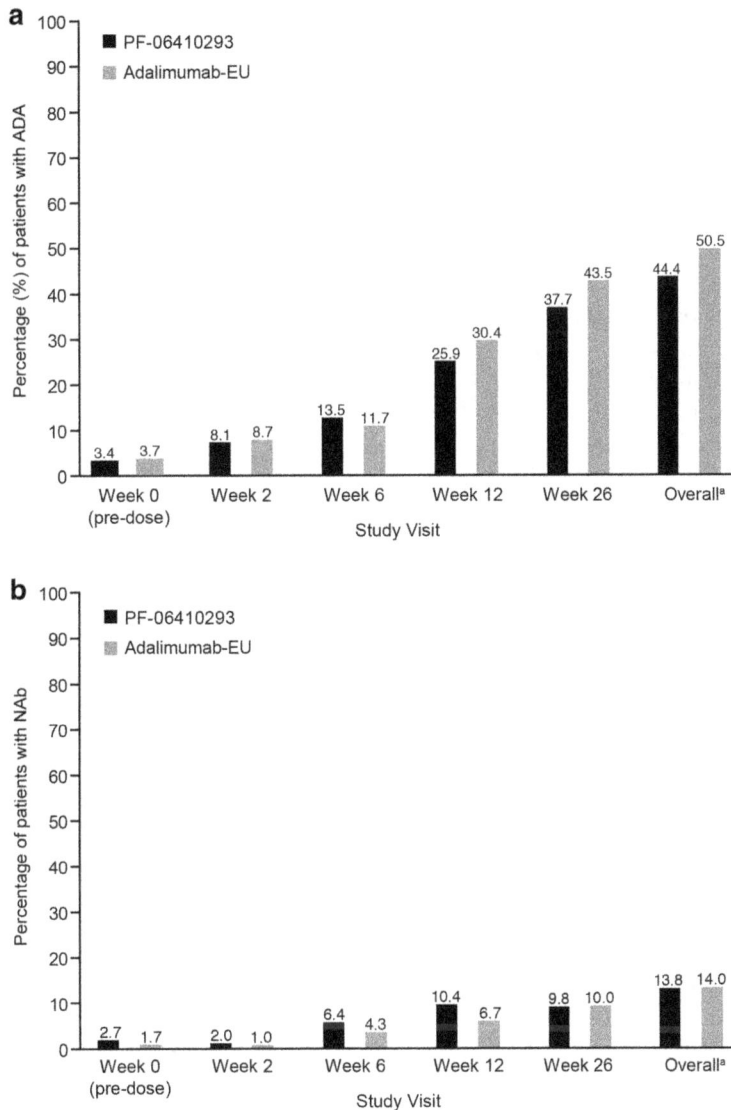

Fig. 4 ADA and NAb incidence by study visit (safety population). **a** ADA incidence. **b** NAb incidence. The percentage of NAb-positive patients is based on the total number of patients in each treatment group. [a]"Overall" includes data from week 2, week 6, week 12, week 26, end-of-treatment/early termination, follow-up, and unplanned visits in treatment period 1. Abbreviations: *ADA* anti-drug antibody, *Adalimumab-EU* adalimumab sourced from the European Union, *NAb* neutralizing antibody

change from baseline in DAS28–4(CRP), EULAR response, DAS28–4(CRP) of less than 2.6, ACR/EULAR remission, and HAQ-DI all supported therapeutic equivalence.

The safety profiles of PF-06410293 and adalimumab-EU to week 26 were comparable, including similar findings with respect to the number of AEs, SAEs, and prespecified TEAEs and TEAE categories of special interest. The only statistically significant safety difference was a lower rate of hypersensitivity events observed in the PF-06410293 arm compared with the adalimumab-EU arm; however, no correction for multiplicity was performed in this study. As might be expected in a single clinical trial, numerical differences were observed between the treatment arms,

including an imbalance in the development of latent TB (more common in the PF-06410293 group) and hypersensitivity events (more common in the adalimumab-EU group). Of note, the diagnosis of latent TB was based on investigator judgment, local practice, and consultation with a pulmonary or infectious disease specialist and after a protocol-mandated QuantiFERON-TB test was performed. The percentage of patients who converted to a QuantiFERON-TB test positive at week 26 was balanced between the treatment arms, suggesting that there was no clinically meaningful difference in the rate of QuantiFERON-TB test conversion between PF-06410293 and adalimumab-EU. The safety profile for both study drugs appears to be consistent with the known safety profile of reference adalimumab-EU.

The immunogenicity profiles observed during the first 26 weeks of treatment were similar for the two treatment arms, and there was a somewhat lower incidence of patients testing positive for ADA in the PF-06410293 arm. Serum drug concentrations were numerically higher in the PF-06410293 arm; however, these differences were not considered clinically meaningful, as the clinical response was similar in the two treatment arms. The hs-CRP response as a PD biomarker supports this lack of clinical significance, as the decrease in hs-CRP was similar for the two arms over the first 26 weeks of treatment. As expected, the serum drug concentrations of PF-06410293 and adalimumab-EU were lower in both treatment arms for ADA-positive compared with ADA-negative patients.

Conclusions

Results from the first 26 weeks of dosing demonstrated no clinically meaningful differences in efficacy, safety, immunogenicity, PK, or PD between PF-06410293 and adalimumab-EU in patients with active RA. Upcoming data from the subsequent 6 months of the trial will provide additional efficacy, safety, and immunogenicity information, including data on patients after a blinded transition from adalimumab-EU to PF-06410293 and those who receive a total of 1 year of treatment with either PF-06410293 or adalimumab-EU.

Abbreviations
ACR: American College of Rheumatology; ACR20: American College of Rheumatology 20% improvement; ADA: Anti-drug antibody; Adalimumab-EU: Adalimumab sourced from the European Union; AE: Adverse event; bDMARD: Biologic disease-modifying anti-rheumatic drug; CI: Confidence interval; DAS28–4(CRP): Disease Activity Score 28 joints: four components based on high-sensitivity C-reactive protein; DMARD: Disease-modifying anti-rheumatic drug; ESR: Erythrocyte sedimentation rate; EULAR: European League Against Rheumatism; FDA: US Food and Drug Administration; HAQ-DI: Health Assessment Questionnaire Disability Index; hs-CRP: High-sensitivity C-reactive protein; ISR: Injection-site reaction; ITT: Intention-to-treat; MTX: Methotrexate; NAb: Neutralizing antibody; PD: Pharmacodynamics; PK: Pharmacokinetics; PP: Per protocol; RA: Rheumatoid arthritis; RD: Risk difference; SAE: Serious adverse event; SOC: System Organ Class; TB: Tuberculosis; TEAE: Treatment-emergent adverse event; TNF: Tumor necrosis factor

Acknowledgments
Medical writing support was provided by Jacqui Oliver and Neel Misra of Engage Scientific Solutions and was funded by Pfizer Inc.

Funding
This study was sponsored by Pfizer Inc.

Authors' contributions
KLS, DA, and AEB made substantial contributions to study conception and design. SYH, CC, KLS, and AEB analyzed the data and SYH provided statistical support. RMF, RA, and MP contributed to the acquisition of data. RMF reviewed for investigator approval all study data in the clinical study report written by KLS. All authors made substantial contributions to the interpretation of data, were involved in drafting the manuscript or revising it critically for important intellectual content or both, and read and approved the final manuscript for submission.

Consent for publication
Not applicable.

Competing interests
RMF has received research grants and consulting fees from Pfizer Inc. and AbbVie. RA has received research grants and honoraria from Pfizer Inc. MP declares that she has no competing interests. SYH was an employee of and held stock holdings or stock options (or both) from Pfizer Inc. at the time of the study. KL, CC, DA, AEB, and KLS are full-time employees of and declare stock holdings or stock options (or both) from Pfizer Inc.

Author details
[1]Southwestern Medical Center, Metroplex Clinical Research Center, University of Texas, 8144 Walnut Hill Lane, Suite 810, Dallas, TX 75231, USA. [2]Schlosspark-Klinik, University Medicine Berlin, Heubnerweg 2, Berlin 14059, Germany. [3]Department of Rheumatology, Hospital of Lithuanian University of Health Sciences, Eiveniu str.2, Kaunas, LT 50161, Lithuania. [4]Pfizer Inc., 500 Arcola Road Collegeville, Collegeville, PA 19426, USA. [5]Pfizer Inc., 10777 Science Center Drive, CB1/2103, San Diego, CA 92121, USA. [6]Pfizer Inc., 300 Technology Square, Cambridge, MA 02139, USA.

References
1. Curtis JR, Singh JA. Use of biologics in rheumatoid arthritis: current and emerging paradigms of care. Clin Ther. 2011;33:679–707. https://doi.org/10.1016/j.clinthera.2011.05.044.
2. Weinblatt ME, Keystone EC, Furst DE, Moreland LW, Weisman MH, Birbara CA, et al. Adalimumab, a fully human anti-tumor necrosis factor alpha monoclonal antibody, for the treatment of rheumatoid arthritis in patients taking concomitant methotrexate: the ARMADA trial. Arthritis Rheum. 2003; 48:35–45. https://doi.org/10.1002/art.10697.
3. Keystone EC, Kavanaugh AF, Sharp JT, Tannenbaum H, Hua Y, Teoh LS, et al. Radiographic, clinical, and functional outcomes of treatment with adalimumab (a human anti-tumor necrosis factor monoclonal antibody) in patients with active rheumatoid arthritis receiving concomitant methotrexate therapy: a randomized, placebo-controlled, 52-week trial. Arthritis Rheum. 2004;50:1400–11. https://doi.org/10.1002/art.20217.
4. Breedveld FC, Weisman MH, Kavanaugh AF, Cohen SB, Pavelka K, van Vollenhoven R, et al. The PREMIER study: a multicenter, randomized, double-blind clinical trial of combination therapy with adalimumab plus methotrexate versus methotrexate alone or adalimumab alone in patients with early, aggressive rheumatoid arthritis who had not had previous methotrexate treatment. Arthritis Rheum. 2006;54:26–37. https://doi.org/10.1002/art.21519.
5. European Medicines Agency. HUMIRA (adalimumab) summary of product characteristics. 2017 (last update: 10 May 2017). http://www.ema.europa.eu/docs/en_GB/document_library/EPAR_-_Product_Information/human/000481/WC500050870.pdf. Accessed 19 Feb. 2018.
6. Abbott Laboratories. HUMIRA (adalimumab) package insert. 2003 (last update: 26 September 2003). https://www.accessdata.fda.gov/drugsatfda_docs/label/2002/adalabb123102LB.htm. Accessed 19 Feb. 2018.
7. US Food and Drug Administration. Scientific considerations in demonstrating biosimilarity to a reference product. Guidance for industry. 2015 (last update: April 2015). https://www.fda.gov/downloads/drugs/guidances/ucm291128.pdf. Accessed 19 Feb. 2018.
8. European Medicines Agency. Guideline on similar biological medicinal products. 2014 (last update: July 2014). http://www.ema.europa.eu/docs/en_GB/document_library/Scientific_guideline/2014/10/WC500176768.pdf. Accessed 19 Feb. 2018.
9. QuintilesIMS. The impact of biosimilar competition in Europe. 2017 (last update: May 2017). http://www.medicinesforeurope.com/wp-content/uploads/2017/05/IMS-Biosimilar-2017_V9.pdf. Accessed 19 Feb. 2018.
10. Mulcahy A, Predmore Z, Soeren M. The cost savings potential of biosimilar drugs in the United States. 2014. https://www.rand.org/content/dam/rand/pubs/perspectives/PE100/PE127/RAND_PE127.pdf. Accessed 19 Feb. 2018.
11. Crespi-Lofton J, Skelton JB. The growing role of biologics and biosimilars in the United States: Perspectives from the APhA Biologics and Biosimilars Stakeholder Conference. J Am Pharm Assoc (2003). 2017;57:e15–27. https://doi.org/10.1016/j.japh.2017.05.014.

12. Derzi D, Ripp S, Ng C, Shoieb A, Finch G, Lorello L, et al. Comparative nonclinical assessments of the potential biosimilar PF-06410293 and adalimumab [abstract no. 276]. In: Society of Toxicology 53rd Annual Meeting and ToxExpo 2014; Phoenix, Arizona; 2014.

13. ClinicalTrials.gov. A study of PF-06410293 (adalimumab-Pfizer) and adalimumab (Humira) In healthy subjects (REFLECTIONS B538–07)) (B538–07). 2014 (last update: 13 April 2015). https://clinicaltrials.gov/ct2/show/NCT02237729. Accessed 19 Feb. 2018.

14. Aletaha D, Neogi T, Silman AJ, Funovits J, Felson DT, Bingham CO 3rd, et al. 2010 rheumatoid arthritis classification criteria: an American College of Rheumatology/European league against rheumatism collaborative initiative. Arthritis Rheum. 2010;62:2569–81. https://doi.org/10.1002/art.27584.

15. Felson DT, Anderson JJ, Boers M, Bombardier C, Furst D, Goldsmith C, et al. American College of Rheumatology. Preliminary definition of improvement in rheumatoid arthritis. Arthritis Rheum. 1995;38:727–35.

16. Fleischmann R, van der Heijde D, Koenig AS, Pedersen R, Szumski A, Marshall L, et al. How much does disease activity score in 28 joints ESR and CRP calculations underestimate disease activity compared with the simplified disease activity index? Ann Rheum Dis. 2015;74:1132–7. https://doi.org/10.1136/annrheumdis-2013-204920.

17. Kim HY, Lee SK, Song YW, Yoo DH, Koh EM, Yoo B, et al. A randomized, double-blind, placebo-controlled, phase III study of the human anti-tumor necrosis factor antibody adalimumab administered as subcutaneous injections in Korean rheumatoid arthritis patients treated with methotrexate. APLAR J Rheumatol. 2007;10:9–16. https://doi.org/10.1111/j.1479-8077.2007.00248.x.

18. Chen DY, Chou SJ, Hsieh TY, Chen YH, Chen HH, Hsieh CW, et al. Randomized, double-blind, placebo-controlled, comparative study of human anti-TNF antibody adalimumab in combination with methotrexate and methotrexate alone in Taiwanese patients with active rheumatoid arthritis. J Formos Med Assoc. 2009;108:310–9. https://doi.org/10.1016/S0929-6646(09)60071-1.

19. Miettinen O, Nurminen M. Comparative analysis of two rates. Stat Med. 1985;4:213–26.

20. Shankar G, Arkin S, Cocea L, Devanarayan V, Kirshner S, Kromminga A, et al. Assessment and reporting of the clinical immunogenicity of therapeutic proteins and peptides-harmonized terminology and tactical recommendations. AAPS J. 2014;16:658–73. https://doi.org/10.1208/s12248-014-9599-2.

17

Increase of circulating memory B cells after glucocorticoid-induced remission identifies patients at risk of IgG4-related disease relapse

Marco Lanzillotta[1,2†], Emanuel Della-Torre[1,2*†], Raffaella Milani[3], Enrica Bozzolo[2], Emanuele Bozzalla-Cassione[1,2], Lucrezia Rovati[1,2], Paolo Giorgio Arcidiacono[4], Stefano Partelli[5], Massimo Falconi[5], Fabio Ciceri[1,6] and Lorenzo Dagna[1,2]

Abstract

Background: Immunoglobulin G4-related disease (IgG4-RD) promptly responds to glucocorticoids but relapses in a considerable fraction of patients. Reliable biomarkers of flare are currently lacking because the pathophysiology of IgG4-RD remains largely elusive. In the present work, we aimed to identify perturbations of B-cell subpopulations that might predict IgG4-RD relapse.

Methods: Thirty patients were treated with glucocorticoids according to international guidelines. Circulating $CD19^+$ and $CD20^+$ cells, naive B cells, memory B cells, plasmablasts, and plasma cells were measured by flow cytometry at baseline and every 6 months for 2 years after the initiation of corticosteroid therapy.

Results: Patients with active untreated IgG4-RD showed significantly reduced $CD19^+$ B cells, $CD20^+$ B cells, and naive B cells compared with healthy subjects ($p < 0.05$), but significantly expanded plasmablasts and plasma cells ($p < 0.01$). After 6 months of corticosteroid treatment, all patients achieved clinical improvement. Naive B cells, plasmablasts, and plasma cells significantly decreased compared with disease onset, whereas memory B cells significantly increased compared with baseline ($p < 0.01$). Increase of memory B cells was observed only in patients who relapsed within 2 years of follow-up, however (HR, 12.24; 2.99 to 50.2; $p = 0.0005$). In these patients, the relapse rates at 12 and 24 months were 30% and 100%, respectively. No abnormalities of other B-cell subpopulations at disease onset or after 6 months of glucocorticoid treatment were found to predict IgG4-RD relapse at 2 years.

Conclusions: Increase of circulating memory B cells after 6 months of glucocorticoid treatment might predict IgG4-RD relapse.

Keywords: IgG4, IgG4-related disease, B cells, Plasmablasts, Corticosteroid, Glucocorticoid, Therapy, Treatment

Background

Immunoglobulin G4-related disease (IgG4-RD) is a systemic fibroinflammatory condition characterized by tumorlike expansive lesions and often by abnormal increase of serum IgG4 concentration [1]. Glucocorticoid treatment leads to remission in the majority of patients, but IgG4-RD relapses within 2 years in up to 50% of cases,

both during tapering and after withdrawal of corticosteroid therapy [2, 3].

Relapses represent a major clinical problem in the long-term management of patients with IgG4-RD, for several reasons. First, flares carry an additional risk of organ damage and life-threatening complications because they might involve the same organs affected at disease onset or different anatomical sites [3]. Second, relapsing patients are at higher risk of steroid-related adverse effects because they are typically treated with higher cumulative doses of glucocorticoids [3, 4]. Also, preventive follow-up and therapeutic strategies cannot be adopted, because we currently lack reliable biomarkers to identify patients who will

* Correspondence: dellatorre.emanuel@hsr.it
†Marco Lanzillotta and Emanuel Della-Torre contributed equally to this work.
[1]Università Vita-Salute San Raffaele, IRCCS-San Raffaele Scientific Institute, Milan, Italy
[2]Unit of Immunology, Rheumatology, Allergy and Rare Diseases (UnIRAR), IRCCS-San Raffaele Scientific Institute, via Olgettina 60, 20132 Milan, Italy
Full list of author information is available at the end of the article

relapse and to predict the timing of flares. Indeed, peripheral blood eosinophilia, elevated serum immunoglobulin E (IgE), and IgG4 at disease onset have traditionally been proposed as predictors of recurrence, but a better understanding of the natural history of IgG4-RD has gradually unveiled the shortcomings of these biomarkers [1, 2, 5, 6]. The majority of patients with IgG4-RD do not in fact show increased eosinophils counts or serum IgE levels at the time of diagnosis, and most of the data regarding the value of IgG4 levels in predicting disease relapse failed to demonstrate any definitive associations in different study cohorts [7, 8]. Reliable predictors of IgG4-RD flare are therefore still missing, and their identification requires a better comprehension of the pathophysiological mechanisms that initiate and sustain disease activity.

Recent observations suggest that the B-cell compartment might be central to IgG4-RD pathogenesis. Indeed, B-cell depletion therapy with rituximab induces prompt clinical responses [9]. Plasmablasts are oligoclonally expanded in patients with active disease [10, 11], disappear with clinical improvement [10, 12], and increase with disease relapse [10, 11]. Given this emerging role of B lymphocytes in the pathogenesis of IgG4-RD, in the present study we aimed to identify alterations of B-cell subsets that might predict IgG4-RD flare after initial response to glucocorticoid treatment.

Methods
Patients, disease activity assessment, and treatment
Thirty patients with active untreated IgG4-RD referred to our tertiary care center between September 2014 and December 2016 were consecutively included in the present prospective monocentric study. IgG4-RD was diagnosed according to the consensus statement on the pathology of IgG4-RD and the comprehensive diagnostic criteria for IgG4-RD [13, 14]. Patients with pancreatic involvement who did not undergo histological confirmation were diagnosed with "definite" IgG4-RD according to the international consensus diagnostic criteria for autoimmune pancreatitis [15]. All patients were treated with oral prednisone at an initial dose of 0.6–1 mg/kg for 1 month. Prednisone was then tapered in accordance with international guidelines and withdrawn whenever possible after 4–6 months [3]. IgG4-RD activity was assessed by means of the immunoglobulin G4-related disease responder index (IgG4-RD RI) [16]. Active disease was defined by an IgG4-RD RI ≥ 3. Complete response vs. disease remission was defined by an IgG4-RD RI < 3 in the presence or absence of concomitant corticosteroid treatment, respectively. A reduction of the IgG4-RD RI but still with a total score ≥ 3 was considered a partial response to treatment. Relapses were defined as increases in the IgG4-RD RI ≥ 2 and/or the need for the reinstitution of treatment. Blood samples for immunological studies were drawn at baseline

and every 6 months for 2 years after the initiation of glucocorticoid treatment. Twenty healthy age- and sex-matched subjects were studied as control subjects. All subjects enrolled provided written informed consent for the analyses performed. The study was conducted according to the Declaration of Helsinki and approved as a descriptive noninterventional study by the ethics committee of the San Raffaele Scientific Institute.

Laboratory and flow cytometric analyses
Laboratory analyses included C-reactive protein (CRP), erythrocyte sedimentation rate (ESR), total serum IgE, total serum immunoglobulin G (IgG), IgG1, IgG2, IgG3, and IgG4 subclasses. Flow cytometry was performed using a Navios cytometer (Beckman Coulter, Brea, CA, USA) on fresh peripheral blood collected in ethylenediaminetetraacetic acid tubes using a lyse-no-wash technique (ammonium chloride) and the following panel of directly conjugated antibodies: CD3-fluorescein isothiocyanate, CD4-ECD, CD8-Pacific Blue, CD19-A700, CD20-allophycocyanin, CD27-phycoerythrin-cyanine 7, CD38-A750, CD45-Krome Orange, CD56-phycoerythrin, CD138-PC5.5 (Beckman Coulter). Naive B cells, memory B cells, plasmablasts, and plasma cells were identified within the $CD19^+$ gate as $CD19^+CD20^+CD27^-CD38^+$ cells, $CD19^+CD20^+CD27^+CD38^-$ cells, $CD19^+CD20^-CD27^+CD38^{+bright}$ cells, and $CD19^+CD20^-CD38^+CD138^+$ cells, respectively. Total B cells were identified both as $CD19^+$ cells ($CD19^+$/side scatter [SSC] within the leukogate) and $CD20^+$ cells ($CD20^+$/SSC within the leukogate).

Statistical analysis
Statistical analysis was performed using Prism software 6.0 (GraphPad Software, La Jolla, CA, USA). Normal distribution of continuous variables was assessed with the D'Agostino and Pearson omnibus normality test. Normally distributed variables were compared using Student's t test. Nonnormally distributed variables were compared using the Mann-Whitney U test. Follow-up nonnormally distributed variables were compared using the Wilcoxon test. Nonparametric correlations were calculated using Spearman's correlation. Linear correlations were measured by Pearson's correlation coefficient. A p value < 0.05 was considered statistically significant. Values are presented as median and IQR, unless specified otherwise. Kaplan-Meier curves were used to assess time to relapse. Times to relapse in subgroups were compared using the log-rank test. The HR was computed using the Mantel-Haenszel approach.

Results
Distribution of B-cell subpopulations in patients with active untreated IgG4-RD
Thirty patients with active untreated IgG4-RD were included in this prospective study. Clinical, serological,

and immunological features of the study cohort are summarized in Table 1. The distribution of B-cell subpopulations in absolute numbers and percentage of CD19$^+$ B lymphocytes is shown in Fig. 1a. At baseline, total lymphocyte count in patients with IgG4-RD was comparable to that of healthy subjects. Flow cytometric analysis revealed a significant CD19$^+$ and CD20$^+$ B-cell lymphopenia in patients with IgG4-RD, both in absolute counts and in percentage of total lymphocytes compared with healthy control subjects ($p < 0.05$). Absolute number of naive B cells—but not the percentage over total

CD19$^+$ lymphocytes—was also significantly reduced in patients with IgG4-RD compared with healthy subjects ($p < 0.01$). The levels of memory B cells were comparable between patients with IgG4-RD and healthy individuals, both in absolute numbers and in percentage of CD19$^+$ B cells. Absolute plasmablast counts and their percentage over total CD19$^+$ B cells were significantly increased in patients with IgG4-RD compared with healthy control subjects ($p < 0.0001$). Circulating plasma cells were detected in 16 (53.3%) patients with IgG4-RD and in none of the healthy individuals.

Table 1 Clinical, serological, and immunological features of the patient cohort at baseline and after treatment with glucocorticoids

	Patients with IgG4-RD before GC ($n = 30$)	Healthy control subjects ($n = 20$)	p Value	Patients with IgG4-RD after GC ($n = 30$)	p Value
Definite IgG4-RD, n (%)	29 (97%)				
Probable IgG4-RD, n (%)	1 (3%)				
Possible IgG4-RD, n (%)	0 (0%)				
Age, yr, median	70 (58–73)	54 (46–65)	0.005		
Male sex, n (%)	23 (77%)	12 (60%)			
ESR (0–20 mm/h)	18 (10–35)				
CRP (< 6 mg/L)	5 (2–6)				
IgG4-RD RI (0–3)	6 (6–9)			2 (1–2.25)	0.0001
Serum IgG4 (< 135 mg/dl)	313 (206–507)			191 (87–230)	0.0001
CD19$^+$ B cells (cells/ml)	162,000 (105,750–217,750)	236,000 (200,000–299,000)	0.0002	163,500 (100,750–233,500)	0.131
CD20$^+$ B cells (cells/ml)	144,500 (93,000–201,700)	224,000 (199,000–279,000)	0.0001	150,500 (85,500–226,250)	0.1
Naive B cells (cells/ml)	15,120 (8895–29,140)	23,810 (17,930–54,020)	0.01	7485 (4195–14,018)	0.0001
Percentage of CD19$^+$ B cells	10.55 (7.94–15.49)	13.02 (7.89–19.39)	0.35	4.78 (3.14–8.33)	0.0001
Memory B cells (cells/ml)	26,475 (13,040–55,450)	37,170 (21,900–57,190)	0.25	41,800 (21,148–69,435)	0.026
Percentage of CD19$^+$ B cells	18.5 (9.26–27.31)	16.60 (9.18–26.34)	0.62	22.89 (11.14–32.50)	0.028
Plasmablasts (cells/ml)	2515 (1023–5550)	340 (170–600)	0.0001	270 (210–1198)	0.0001
Percentage of CD19$^+$ B cells	1.25 (0.6–4.51)	0.19 (0.05–0.29)	0.0001	0.23 (0.1–0.79)	0.0001
Plasma cells (cells/ml)[a]	278 (0–1332)	0 (0–0)	0.0005	55 (0–423)	0.0006
Percentage of CD19$^+$ B cells[a]	0.23 (0–1.27)	0 (0–0)	0.0001	0.07 (0–0.64)	0.0008
Organ involvement, n (%)					
Pancreas	20 (66%)				
Aorta and retroperitoneum	7 (23.3%)				
Lymph nodes	5 (16.6%)				
Biliary tree	5 (16.6%)				
Salivary glands	2 (6.6%)				
Lacrimal glands	2 (6.6%)				
Lung	2 (6.6%)				
Orbit	1 (3.3%)				
Nasal sinuses	1 (3.3%)				
Meninges	1 (3%)				
Kidney	1 (3.3%)				

Abbreviations: *CRP* C-reactive protein, *ESR* Erythrocyte sedimentation rate, *IgG4-RD RI* IgG4-related disease responder index, *GC* Glucocorticoids
Results are expressed as median (IQR), except where indicated otherwise
[a] Results expressed as mean (range)

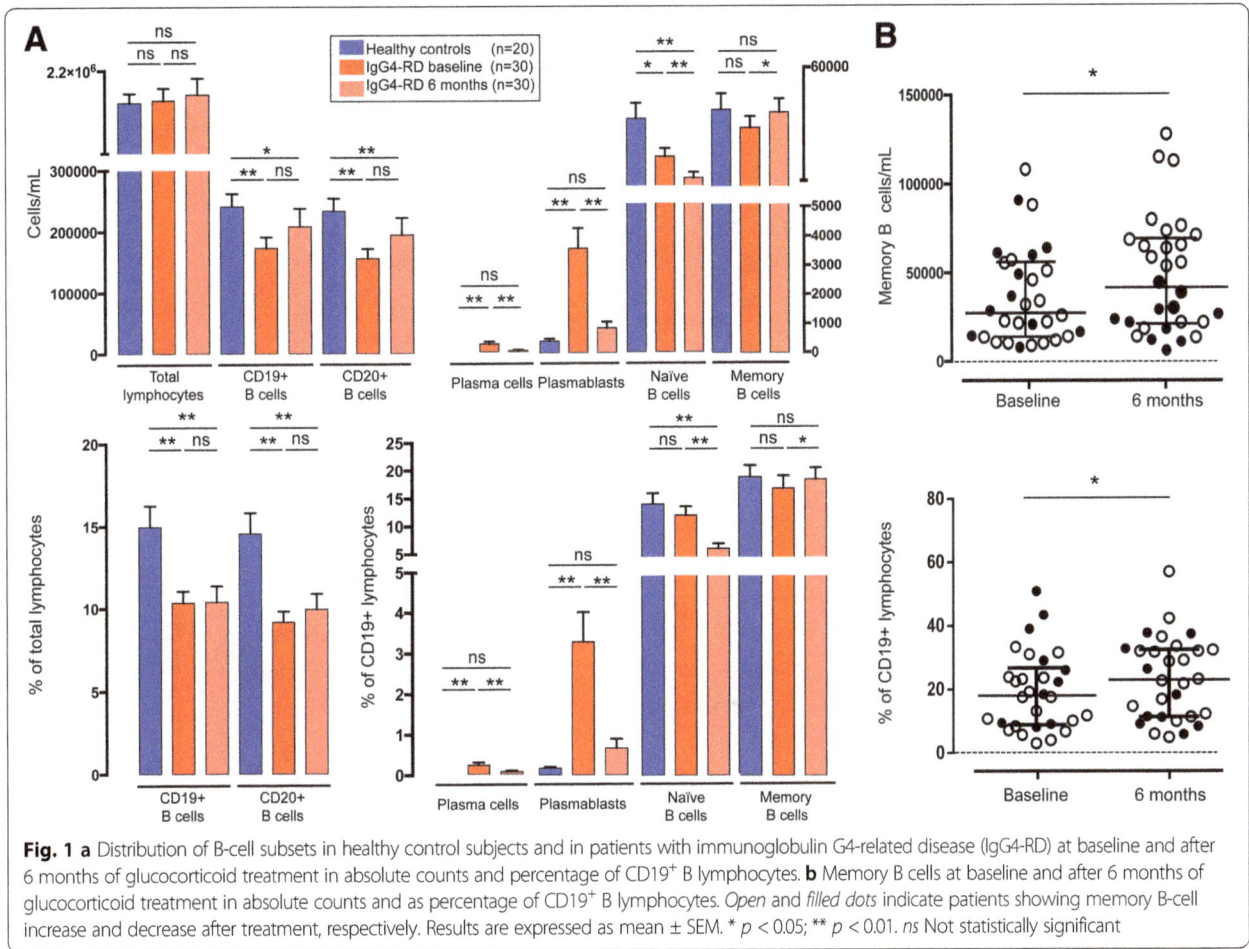

Fig. 1 **a** Distribution of B-cell subsets in healthy control subjects and in patients with immunoglobulin G4-related disease (IgG4-RD) at baseline and after 6 months of glucocorticoid treatment in absolute counts and percentage of CD19$^+$ B lymphocytes. **b** Memory B cells at baseline and after 6 months of glucocorticoid treatment in absolute counts and as percentage of CD19$^+$ B lymphocytes. *Open* and *filled dots* indicate patients showing memory B-cell increase and decrease after treatment, respectively. Results are expressed as mean ± SEM. * $p < 0.05$; ** $p < 0.01$. *ns* Not statistically significant

Effects of glucocorticoids on B-cell subpopulations in patients with IgG4-RD

All patients were treated with glucocorticoids according to international guidelines (*see* the "Methods" section above), and B-cell subpopulations were studied after 6 months of treatment (Table 1) [3]. At that time point, clinical improvement was observed in all patients, with an IgG4-RD RI that decreased from a median baseline value of 6 (IQR, 6–9) to 2 (IQR, 1–2.25) (paired $p < 0.05$). Seven patients achieved partial response, 20 patients achieved complete response, and 3 patients achieved disease remission. The median daily dose of prednisone at the time of follow-up analysis was 5 mg (range, 0–10 mg).

Effects of corticosteroids on B-cell subpopulations are reported in Fig. 1a. Total lymphocytes, CD19$^+$, and CD20$^+$ B-cell counts were not affected by glucocorticoids. Naive B cells, plasmablasts, and plasma cells significantly decreased compared with baseline, both in absolute numbers and as a percentage of total CD19$^+$ B cells (paired $p < 0.01$ for all comparisons). The absolute number of memory B cells and their percentage over CD19$^+$ B lymphocytes significantly increased with disease improvement (paired $p < 0.05$).

Predictors of IgG4-RD relapse at baseline

In order to evaluate differences within the B-cell compartment of relapsing and nonrelapsing patients with IgG4-RD, we further focused our analysis on 15 subjects followed for at least 24 months. Twenty-four months represented a reliable follow-up to identify relapsing and nonrelapsing patients, because most IgG4-RD cases are known to recur within 2 years after initiation of immunosuppressive therapies [2]. The remaining 15 patients of the study cohort were not included in the analysis, because they did not have an adequate follow-up, and we could not classify them as either relapsers or nonrelapsers.

Ten of the fifteen patients followed for 2 years relapsed, on average, 18 months (range, 8–24) after the diagnosis, one on 10 mg of daily prednisone, three on 5 mg, and six off glucocorticoids. The median durations of glucocorticoid treatment in relapsing and nonrelapsing patients were 9 months (range, 6–18) and 7 months (range, 4–13), respectively. Clinical and laboratory features of relapsing and nonrelapsing patients are reported in Table 2. Multiorgan involvement was present in seven of ten relapsing and four of five nonrelapsing patients. The pancreas, the biliary tree, and the aorta were

Table 2 Clinical, serological, and immunological features of relapsing and nonrelapsing patients at baseline and after treatment with glucocorticoids

	Relapsers (n = 10)	Nonrelapsers (n = 5)	p Value
Definite IgG4-RD (%)	9 (90%)	5 (100%)	
Probable IgG4-RD (%)	1 (10%)	0 (0%)	
Possible IgG4-RD (%)	0 (0%)	0 (0%)	
Age, yr, median	69 (60–71)	73 (64–80)	0.13
Male, n (%)	9 (90%)	3 (60%)	
Multiorgan involvement (> 1 organ)	7 (70%)	4 (80%)	
Baseline			
ESR (0–20 mm/h)	10 (9–23)	15 (8–20)	0.59
CRP (< 6 mg/L)	5 (4–6.5)	10 (5–46)	0.06
IgG4-RD RI (0–3)	9 (6–9)	12 (9–12)	0.22
Eosinophils (< 300 cell/µl)	300 (300–500)	200 (150–300)	0.034
Serum IgG4 (< 135 mg/dl)	364 (232–1090)	498 (328–947)	0.5
IgE (mU/ml)	308 (2–1488)	733 (271–1554)	0.11
Prednisone dose (mg/d)	5 (0–5.5)	5 (2.5–5)	0.99
CD19[+] B cells (cells/ml)	138,500 (97,500–172,500)	144,000 (103,000–162,000)	0.66
CD20[+] B cells (cells/ml)	114,000 (86,250–150,000)	128,000 (82,000–140,500)	0.57
Naïve B cells (cells/ml)	14,170 (9518–24,198)	11,170 (2915–38,650)	0.35
Percentage of CD19[+] B cells	11.4 (9.5–13.7)	11.52 (2.33–24.37)	0.09
Memory B cells (cells/ml)	20,450 (10,790–36,070)	48,590 (11,305–62,095)	0.44
Percentage of CD19[+] B cells	15.79 (10.25–23.9)	26.48 (6.9–47.88)	0.67
Plasmablasts (cells/ml)	3280 (985–9868)	5400 (3825–8000)	0.39
Percentage of CD19[+] B cells	3.26 (0.84–7.8)	3.38 (2.06–4.82)	0.76
Plasma cells (cells/ml)[a]	420 (0–1332)	489 (146–1300)	0.86
Percentage of CD19[+] B cells[a]	0.37 (0–1.27)	0.27 (0.1–0.49)	0.95
After 6 mo of treatment			
ESR (0–20 mm/h)	5 (3–21)	9 (8–20)	0.29
CRP (< 6 mg/L)	2 (1–2.25)	2 (1.5–4)	0.47
IgG4-RD RI (0–3)	2.5 (1.75–3.25)	2 (2–2.5)	0.62
Eosinophils (< 300 cell/µl)	200 (100–325)	100 (100–200)	0.37
Serum IgG4 (< 135 mg/dl)	182.5 (107–729)	257 (211–406)	0.42
IgE (mU/ml)	107 (2–299)	425 (384–466)	0.13
Prednisone dose (mg/d)	5 (0–5.62)	5 (2.5–5)	0.99
CD19[+] B cells (cells/ml)	174,500 (93,750–222,250)	128,000 (64,500–157,500)	0.2
CD20[+] B cells (cells/ml)	165,000 (84,750–208,500)	128,000 (52,500–154,000)	0.24
Naïve B cells (cells/ml)	7860 (3988–13,585)	7380 (2950–15,460)	0.8
Percentage of CD19[+] B cells	3.51 (2.57–4.13)	9.27 (4.16–15.73)	0.1
Memory B cells (cells/ml)	60,540 (21,148–75,428)	18,360 (9045–34,650)	0.05
Percentage of CD19[+] B cells	27.46 (19.06–34.9)	24.19 (6.43–37.65)	0.89
Plasmablasts (cells/ml)	355 (138–1263)	1310 (565–3350)	0.07
Percentage of CD19[+] B cells	0.27 (0.07–0.53)	0.88 (0.36–5.3)	0.03
Plasma cells (cells/ml)[a]	56 (0–333)	143 (0–423)	0.22
Percentage of CD19[+] B cells[a]	0.05 (0–0.32)	0.19 (0–0.53)	0.16

Abbreviations: CRP C-reactive protein; *ESR* erythrocyte sedimentation rate; *IgG4-RD RI* IgG4-Related Disease Responder Index
Results are expressed as median (IQR), except where indicated otherwise
[a] Results expressed as mean (range)

affected in five of ten, two of ten, and two of ten relapsing patients and in four of five, one of five, and one of five nonrelapsing patients, respectively. Lymph node involvement was present in two relapsing and two nonrelapsing patients. At baseline, we did not observe any statistically significant difference between the two study groups with respect to the IgG4-RD RI, starting prednisone dose, serum IgE, and IgG4 concentrations ($p > 0.05$ for all comparisons). Eosinophil counts were significantly higher in relapsing patients ($p < 0.05$). In particular, they were elevated in four of ten relapsers (median, 300; range, 200–1800 cell/mm^3) and normal in all nonrelapsers (median, 200; range, 100–300 cell/mm^3) (Table 2). Total CD19$^+$ cells, CD20$^+$ cells, naive B cells, memory B cells, circulating plasmablasts, and plasma cells also did not differ between relapsing and nonrelapsing patients, both in absolute numbers and as a percentage of CD19$^+$ B cells ($p > 0.05$ for all comparisons).

Predictors of IgG4-RD relapse after glucocorticoid treatment

After 6 months of glucocorticoid treatment, all 15 patients experienced clinical improvement, with an IgG4-RD RI that decreased from a median baseline value of 9 (IQR, 6–9) to 2.5 (IQR, 1.75–3.25) in relapsing patients, and from a median baseline value of 12 (IQR, 9–12) to 2 (IQR, 2–2.5) in nonrelapsing patients. In particular, five of ten relapsing patients achieved partial response, three of ten achieved complete response, and two of ten achieved disease remission. One of five nonrelapsing patients achieved partial response, three of five achieved complete response, and one of five achieved disease remission. The median daily dose of prednisone at the time of follow-up was 5 mg, both in relapsing patients (range, 0–10 mg) and in nonrelapsing patients (range, 0–5 mg) ($p = 0.99$). The levels of ESR, CRP, eosinophils, and serum IgE and IgG4 were comparable between the two study groups ($p > 0.05$ for all comparisons).

Total CD19$^+$ cell and CD20$^+$ cell count did not differ between relapsing and nonrelapsing patients ($p > 0.05$). Similarly, the absolute numbers of naive B cells and plasma cells, as well as their percentage over total CD19$^+$ B cells, were comparable between the two study groups ($p > 0.05$ for all comparisons) (Table 2). Conversely, memory B cells and circulating plasmablasts were significantly higher in relapsing and nonrelapsing patients, respectively. Yet, although absolute counts of naive B cells, plasmablasts, and plasma cells uniformly decreased in all patients compared with baseline values, memory B cells decreased only in nonrelapsing patients and increased in all relapsing patients (Fig. 2). A similar trend of the memory B cell/CD19$^+$ B cell ratio—namely, a decrease in nonrelapsing patients and an increase in relapsing patients—was observed in nine of ten relapsing patients and in three of five nonrelapsing patients (Fig. 2).

To further explore the relationship between this opposite behavior of memory B cells in relapsing and nonrelapsing subjects, we performed log-rank survival analysis and confirmed a significantly higher relapse rate among patients with an increase of absolute memory B-cell counts after corticosteroid treatment (HR, 12.24; 2.99 to 50.2; $p = 0.0005$) (Fig. 3a). Relapse rate was also higher in patients showing an increased memory B cell/CD19$^+$ B cell ratio after treatment, but this association did not reach statistical significance (HR, 3.73; 0.91 to 15.24; $p = 0.066$) (Fig. 3b). In particular, the increase of absolute memory B-cell counts after 6 months of therapy was associated with relapse rates of 30% at 12 months and 100% at 24 months. The increase of the memory B cell/CD19$^+$ B cell ratio was associated with relapse rates of 30% at 12 months and 90% at 24 months. Conversely, the relapse rates of patients showing memory B-cell decrease in absolute counts and as a percentage of CD19$^+$ B lymphocytes were 0% and 10%, respectively, at 24 months. A similar opposite trend of memory B cells after corticosteroid treatment was also observed in the remaining 15 patients of the study cohort, but they were not included in the analysis, because their follow-up period was not long enough to identify relapsing and nonrelapsing subjects (Fig. 1b).

Finally, serial measurement of memory B cells and plasmablasts in the ten relapsing patients performed every 6 months until flare showed that disease recurrence was anticipated by a progressive reduction of memory B cells and by a parallel increase of circulating plasmablasts (Fig. 3c). This phenomenon was not observed in nonrelapsing patients, where both memory B cell and plasmablast levels measured every 6 months for 2 years remained comparable to those observed after 6 months of glucocorticoid treatment (or further decreased) (Fig. 3d). Naive B cells did not show any significantly different variation over time between relapsing and nonrelapsing patients (Fig. 3c and d).

Discussion

The identification of reliable biomarkers for predicting disease flare has been identified as a clinical and research priority in the consensus statement on the treatment and management of IgG4-RD [3]. Indeed, although there is unanimous agreement about the strategies to induce IgG4-RD remission, expert opinions still diverge about how to maintain IgG4-RD response through tailored follow-up and preventive interventions [3].

We investigated B-cell subsets in patients with IgG4-RD before and after standardized corticosteroid treatment, seeking potential biomarkers of disease recurrence, and we observed that an increase in memory B-cell counts after glucocorticoid-induced remission predicted relapse at 2 years. This novel finding may provide clinicians with a tool to reliably identify patients at risk of flare, because it

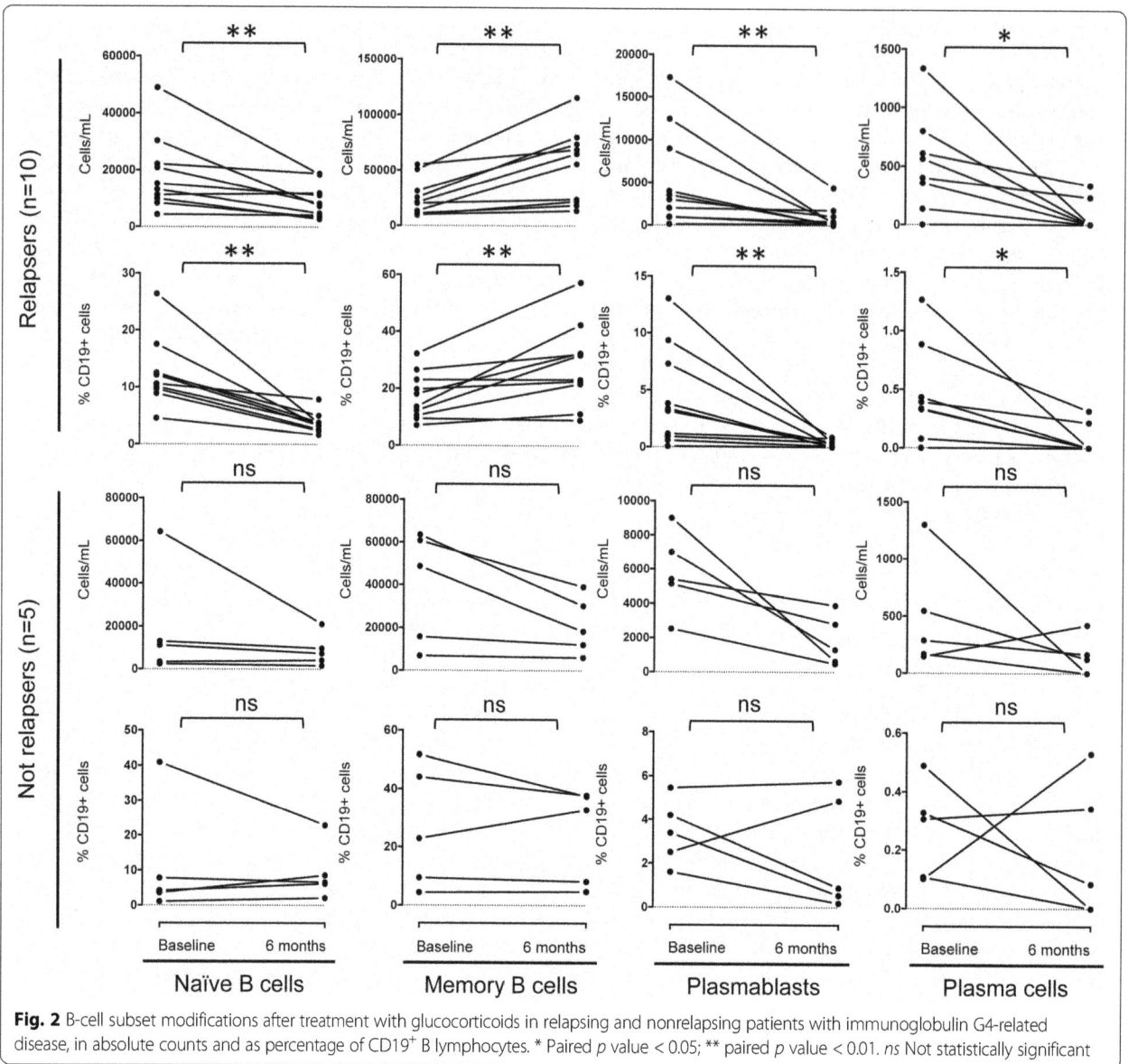

Fig. 2 B-cell subset modifications after treatment with glucocorticoids in relapsing and nonrelapsing patients with immunoglobulin G4-related disease, in absolute counts and as percentage of CD19$^+$ B lymphocytes. * Paired p value < 0.05; ** paired p value < 0.01. ns Not statistically significant

stems from the analysis of B-cell populations that have been causally linked to IgG4-RD [10, 17, 18]. Vice versa, previously reported biomarkers of relapse, such as peripheral blood eosinophilia and serum IgE and IgG4 elevation at baseline, can be considered just bona fide surrogates of disease activity, because their direct involvement in IgG4-RD pathogenesis remains unclear [5, 6]. In addition, relevant shortcomings complicate the use of these biomarkers for preventive follow-up and treatment approaches for the following reasons: (1) cutoff values to identify relapsing and nonrelapsing patients are difficult to establish; (2) the timing of disease relapse remains unpredictable; and (3) as confirmed in the present study, not every patient who ultimately flares shows elevated eosinophils, serum IgE, or IgG4 at disease onset [7, 19]. Conversely, memory B-cell increase after glucocorticoid-

induced remission clearly differentiated patients relapsing within 2 years of follow-up from nonrelapsing patients.

Memory B cells represent a heterogeneous group of antigen-experienced B lymphocytes that exhibit a low proliferation rate in physiological conditions but rapidly expand in response to previously encountered invading organisms. Different lymphocyte subsets with opposing functions are now known to be part of the memory B-cell compartment, and their involvement in human autoimmune diseases has been studied extensively [20]. IgD$^+$CD27$^+$ nonswitched memory B cells with anti-inflammatory properties, for instance, are reduced in systemic lupus erythematosus (SLE) and reconstitute after immunosuppressive treatment [20, 21]. Conversely, proinflammatory IgM$^-$IgD$^-$CD27$^+$ switched and IgD$^-$CD27$^-$ "double-negative" memory B cells are increased in patients

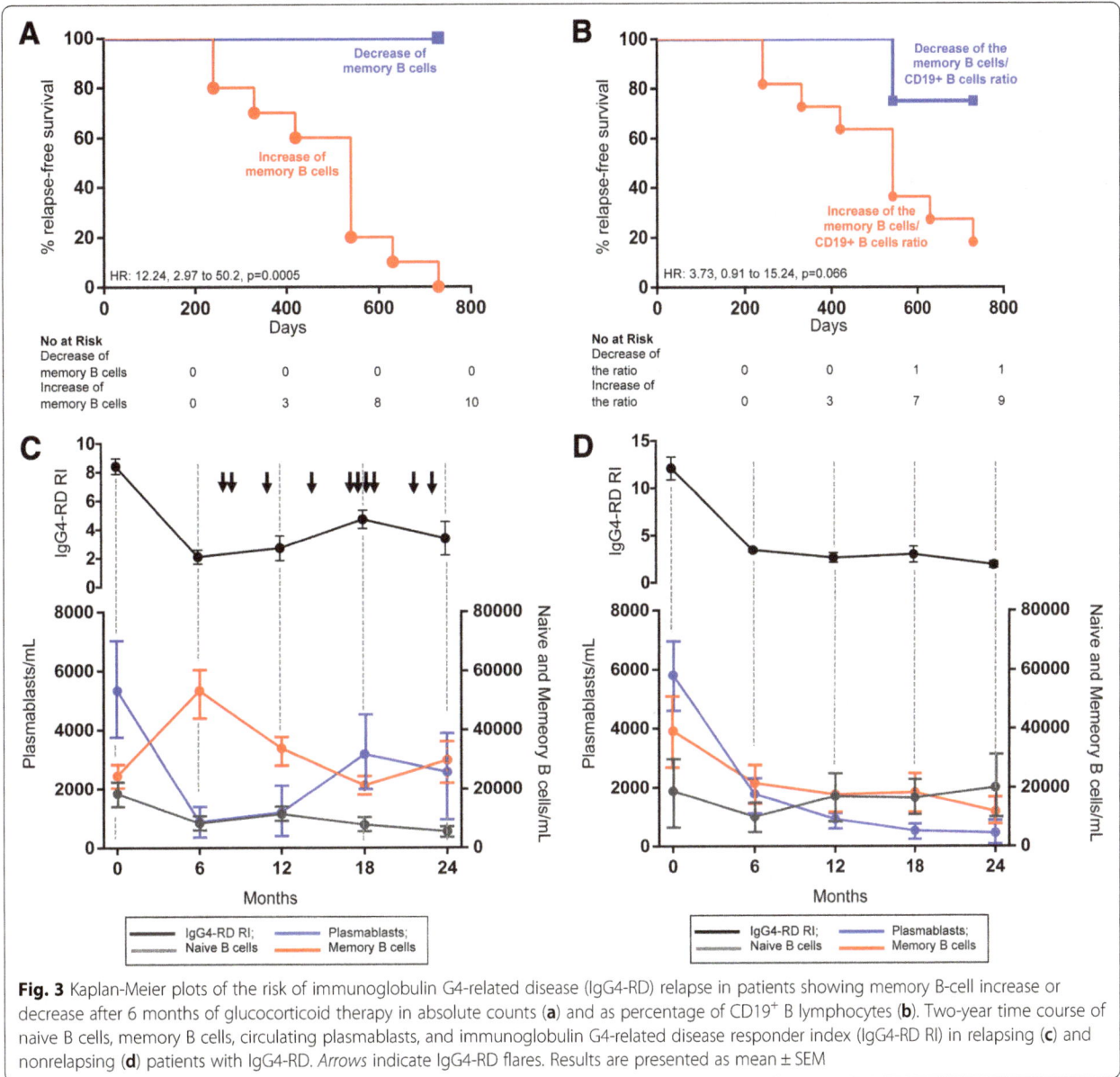

Fig. 3 Kaplan-Meier plots of the risk of immunoglobulin G4-related disease (IgG4-RD) relapse in patients showing memory B-cell increase or decrease after 6 months of glucocorticoid therapy in absolute counts (a) and as percentage of CD19+ B lymphocytes (b). Two-year time course of naive B cells, memory B cells, circulating plasmablasts, and immunoglobulin G4-related disease responder index (IgG4-RD RI) in relapsing (c) and nonrelapsing (d) patients with IgG4-RD. Arrows indicate IgG4-RD flares. Results are presented as mean ± SEM

with SLE and rheumatoid arthritis, and their levels correlate with disease activity [20, 22]. In IgG4-RD, increases of IgG4+ memory B cells and a decrease of IgM+IgD+ memory B cells and of IgG1+ memory B cells were recently described by Heeringa and colleagues, but a clear correlation with IgG4-RD activity was not established [23]. In this sense, although we currently ignore which memory B-cell subset expands following glucocorticoid therapy in relapsing patients with IgG4-RD, our work is the first, to the best of our knowledge, to show an association between memory B cells and IgG4-RD activity. In particular, we hypothesize that an imbalance between anti-inflammatory and proinflammatory memory B-cell subpopulations might be responsible for disease remission and disease recurrence, respectively.

Similarly, although we currently ignore the mechanisms that drive memory B-cell expansion prior to flare, it is reasonable to think that pathogenic B-cell clones within the memory B-cell compartment might bear an increased resistance to immunosuppressive therapy. Indeed, early repopulation of memory B cells after rituximab therapy has already been associated with relapse in autoimmune disorders such as myasthenia gravis, rheumatoid arthritis, and SLE, thus suggesting that the memory B-cell compartment might act as a reservoir for autoreactive clones of antibody-secreting plasmabasts/plasma cells [24–26]. The notion of pathogenic memory B cells driving disease flare is further supported by the gradual reduction of memory B-cell counts and by the concomitant expansion of circulating plasmablasts that we observed in our cohort prior to IgG4-RD relapse.

Our results show significant points of strength but also have some limitations. First, this is the first study, to our knowledge, that correlates the risk of IgG4-RD relapse with cellular biomarkers of IgG4-RD activity. In addition, the present work has been carried out on one of the largest single-center cohorts of patients with IgG4-RD, an aspect that ensured uniform inclusion criteria and treatment [2]. Furthermore, the relapse rate that we observed in our patient population corresponds to that reported in other IgG4-RD cohorts, indicating that a 2-year follow-up period was an adequate time frame for addressing the primary aim of our study [2–28]. Despite a thorough flow cytometric analysis, however, we did not investigate additional B-cell subsets within the naive and memory compartments that might have varied during the disease course. Further molecular and clonal characterization of memory B-cell subtypes at different stages of disease activity, in fact, could have offered a better understanding of their involvement in the pathogenesis of IgG4-RD. We also recognize that a larger study population might have provided more robust results. However, a multicenter study could have generated biases in the cell population analysis and in patient evaluation. Also, half of our cohort did not have a long-enough follow-up period—namely, 2 years—to reliably classify relapsing and nonrelapsing subjects and was therefore excluded from the analysis.

Conclusions

To the best of our knowledge, this is the first study assessing B-lymphocyte subpopulations as biomarkers of relapse in IgG4-RD. Our results suggest that memory B-cell increase after 6 months of standardized glucocorticoid therapy may represent a useful tool for identifying patients at risk of flare, regardless of their organ involvement, clinical presentation, and serological status at disease onset, as well as of the duration of corticosteroid treatment. Careful evaluation of the memory B-cell compartment and of its perturbations might therefore be of value for future mechanistic, interventional, and observational studies on IgG4-RD.

Abbreviations
CRP: C-reactive protein; ESR: Erythrocyte sedimentation rate; IgE: Immunoglobulin E; IgG4-RD RI: Immunoglobulin G4-related disease responder index; IgG4-RD: Immunoglobulin G4-related disease; SLE: Systemic lupus erythematosus

Funding
This work was supported by a "Fondazione Italiana per la Ricerca sull'Artrite (FIRA Onlus) (2014)" award (to EDT) and by a "TRIDEO 2014" award (to EDT) from the "Italian Association for Cancer Research (AIRC)/Cariplo Foundation". EDT received support from the "Collegio Ghislieri" (Pavia, Italy). The funding was employed to cover the cost of the B-cell analysis.

Disclosure
Funding sources do not represent commercial sources but rather private foundations to which the pi applied for grants, fundings, and fellowships. Therefore these fundings do not generate any conflict of interest that the authors must disclose.

Authors' contributions
ML, EDT, LD, and RM conceptualized and designed the study. ML, RM, and EDT acquired the data. ML, RM, EDT, LD, LR, EBC, MF, PGA, EB, SP, and FC analyzed and interpreted the data. All authors were involved in the study design and/or in the collection, analysis, and interpretation of the data; the writing of the manuscript; and the decision to submit the manuscript for publication. All authors are responsible for all content and editorial decisions. All authors read and approved the final manuscript.

Consent for publication
Not applicable.

Competing interests
The authors declare that they have no competing interests.

Author details
[1]Università Vita-Salute San Raffaele, IRCCS-San Raffaele Scientific Institute, Milan, Italy. [2]Unit of Immunology, Rheumatology, Allergy and Rare Diseases (UnIRAR), IRCCS-San Raffaele Scientific Institute, via Olgettina 60, 20132 Milan, Italy. [3]Unit of Immunohematology and Transfusion Medicine, IRCCS-San Raffaele Scientific Institute, Milan, Italy. [4]Pancreato-Biliary Endoscopy and Endosonography Division, IRCCS-San Raffaele Scientific Institute, Milan, Italy. [5]Division of Pancreatic Surgery, Pancreas Translational and Clinical Research Center, IRCCS-San Raffaele Scientific Institute, Milan, Italy. [6]Hematology and Bone Marrow Transplantation Unit, IRCCS-San Raffaele Scientific Institute, Milan, Italy.

References
1. Della-Torre E, Lanzillotta M, Doglioni C. Immunology of IgG4-related disease. Clin Exp Immunol. 2015;181:191–206.
2. Campochiaro C, Ramirez GA, Bozzolo EP, et al. IgG4-related disease in Italy: clinical features and outcomes of a large cohort of patients. Scand J Rheumatol. 2016;45:135–45.
3. Khosroshahi A, Wallace ZS, Crowe JL, et al. International consensus guidance statement on the management and treatment of IgG4-related disease. Arthritis Rheumatol. 2015;67:1688–99.
4. Kamisawa T, Zen Y, Pillai S, Stone JH. IgG4-related disease. Lancet. 2015;385: 1460–71.
5. Culver EL, Sadler R, Bateman AC, et al. Increases in IgE, eosinophils, and mast cells can be used in diagnosis and to predict relapse of IgG4-related disease. Clin Gastroenterol Hepatol. 2017;15:1444–52.
6. Wallace ZS, Mattoo H, Mahajan VS, et al. Predictors of disease relapse in IgG4-related disease following rituximab. Rheumatology (Oxford). 2016;55: 1000–8.
7. Della Torre E, Mattoo H, Mahajan VS, Carruthers M, Pillai S, Stone JH. Prevalence of atopy, eosinophilia, and IgE elevation in IgG4-related disease. Allergy. 2014;69:269–72.
8. Sah RP, Chari ST. Serologic issues in IgG4-related systemic disease and autoimmune pancreatitis. Curr Opin Rheumatol. 2011;23:108–13.
9. Carruthers MN, Topazian MD, Khosroshahi A, et al. Rituximab for IgG4-related disease: a prospective, open-label trial. Ann Rheum Dis. 2015;74:1171–7.
10. Wallace ZS, Mattoo H, Carruthers M, et al. Plasmablasts as a biomarker for IgG4-related disease, independent of serum IgG4 concentrations. Ann Rheum Dis. 2015;74:190–5.
11. Mattoo H, Mahajan VS, Della-Torre E, et al. De novo oligoclonal expansions of circulating plasmablasts in active and relapsing IgG4-related disease. J Allergy Clin Immunol. 2014;134:679–87.
12. Della-Torre E, Feeney E, Deshpande V, et al. B-cell depletion attenuates serological biomarkers of fibrosis and myofibroblast activation in IgG4-related disease. Ann Rheum Dis. 2015;74:2236–43.
13. Deshpande V, Zen Y, Chan JK, et al. Consensus statement on the pathology of IgG4-related disease. Mod Pathol. 2012;25:1181–92.
14. Umehara H, Okazaki K, Masaki Y, et al. Comprehensive diagnostic criteria for IgG4-related disease (IgG4-RD), 2011. Mod Rheumatol. 2012;22:21–30.
15. Shimosegawa T, Chari ST, Frulloni L, et al. International consensus diagnostic criteria for autoimmune pancreatitis: guidelines of the International Association of Pancreatology. Pancreas. 2011;40:352–8.
16. Carruthers MN, Stone JH, Deshpande V, Khosroshahi A. Development of an IgG4-RD responder index. Int J Rheumatol. 2012;2012:259408.

17. Lin W, Zhang P, Chen H, et al. Circulating plasmablasts/plasma cells: a potential biomarker for IgG4-related disease. Arthritis Res Ther. 2017;19:25.
18. Iwata S, Saito K, Hirata S, Tanaka Y. Phenotypic changes of lymphocyte in a patient with IgG4-related disease after corticosteroid therapy. Ann Rheum Dis. 2012;71:2058–9.
19. Khosroshahi A, Stone JH. Treatment approaches to IgG4-related systemic disease. Curr Opin Rheumatol. 2011;23:67–71.
20. Kaminski DA, Wei C, Qian Y, Rosenberg AF, Sanz I. Advances in human B cell phenotypic profiling. Front Immunol. 2012;3:302.
21. Abdulahad WH, Meijer JM, Kroese FG, et al. B cell reconstitution and T helper cell balance after rituximab treatment of active primary Sjögren's syndrome: a double-blind, placebo-controlled study. Arthritis Rheum. 2011; 63:1116–23.
22. Tipton CM, Fucile CF, Darce J, et al. Diversity, cellular origin and autoreactivity of antibody-secreting cell population expansions in acute systemic lupus erythematosus. Nat Immunol. 2015;16:755–65.
23. Heeringa JJ, Karim AF, van Laar JAM, et al. Expansion of blood IgG4+ B, T_H2, and regulatory T cells in patients with IgG4-related disease. J Allergy Clin Immunol. 2018;141:1831–43.
24. Lebrun C, Bourg V, Bresch S, Cohen M, Rosenthal-Allieri MA, Desnuelle C. Therapeutic target of memory B cells depletion helps to tailor administration frequency of rituximab in myasthenia gravis. J Neuroimmunol. 2016;15(298):79–81.
25. Leandro MJ, Cambridge G, Ehrenstein MR, Edwards JC. Reconstitution of peripheral blood B cells after depletion with rituximab in patients with rheumatoid arthritis. Arthritis Rheum. 2006;54:613–20.
26. Vital EM, Dass S, Buch MH, et al. B cell biomarkers of rituximab responses in systemic lupus erythematosus. Arthritis Rheum. 2011;63:3038–47.
27. Sekiguchi H, Horie R, Kanai M, Suzuki R, Yi ES, Ryu JH. IgG4-related disease: retrospective analysis of one hundred sixty-six patients. Arthritis Rheumatol. 2016;68:2290–9.
28. Ebbo M, Daniel L, Pavic M, et al. IgG4-related systemic disease: features and treatment response in a French cohort: results of a multicenter registry. Medicine. 2012;91:49–56.

18

Prognostic profile of systemic sclerosis: analysis of the clinical EUSTAR cohort

Shasha Hu, Yong Hou, Qian Wang, Mengtao Li, Dong Xu[*] and Xiaofeng Zeng[*]

Abstract

Background: Systemic sclerosis is a disease that has significant clinical heterogeneity. This study aims to determine the causes and risk factors of death in a single center European League Against Rheumatism Scleroderma Trials and Research Group (EUSTAR) cohort at the Peking Union Medical College Hospital (PUMCH) in China.

Methods: Patients clinically diagnosed with systemic sclerosis (SSc) between Feb 2009 and Dec 2015 were prospectively recruited from the EUSTAR database and Chinese Rheumatism Data Center (CRDC) of the PUMCH. Baseline and follow-up data were collected. Kaplan-Meier analysis was used to estimate survival, and Cox proportional hazards regression analysis was used to identify factors associated with mortality.

Results: A total of 448 patients were included in the cohort, of whom 56.7% had limited cutaneous systemic sclerosis (lcSSc). The average age at diagnosis was 42.8 ± 12.1 years. The prevalence of interstitial lung disease (ILD) was 382/447 (85.5%). Among 402 patients, 348 of them took glucocorticoid during the disease course; 374 patients received immunosuppressors. Across 2167 patient-years, 40 patients died. Of these, 27 deaths were attributable to SSc, with pulmonary arterial hypertension (PAH) being the leading cause of death. The median survival time was 53 months. Survival rates from disease diagnosis were 97.0%, 94.6%, 91.1% and 87.8% at 1, 3, 5 and 10 years, respectively. Independent prognostic factors for mortality were PAH (HR 6.248, 95% CI 2.855, 13.674) and arrhythmia (HR 4.729, 95% CI 1.588, 14.082). Tripterygium wilfordii Hook F (TwHF) (log-rank test 7.851, p 0.005) and methotrexate (MTX) (log-rank test 7.925, $p = 0.005$) were found in survival analysis to be protective treatments against mortality. Patients who used cyclophosphamide (CTX) during the disease course had poorer prognosis (log-rank test 5.177, $p = 0.023$).

Conclusions: In china, although there is a high prevalence of ILD in patients with SSc (85.5%), most of them have reserved pulmonary function, which means that interstitial lung disease (ILD) is not the most important factor in the death of patients with SSc and also is not a risk factor for poor prognosis. Only ILD with pulmonary dysfunction is associated with poor outcome. The 10-year cumulative rate (87.8%) in patients with SSc in China is slightly lower than the Europe, and pulmonary arterial hypertension (PAH) and arrhythmia at baseline are independent prognostic factors, whereas PAH instead of ILD is the leading cause of death in patients with SSc. Interestingly, the Chinese traditional medicine TwHF, as a protective factor for survival deserves further study.

Keywords: Systemic sclerosis, Prognosis, Cause of death

* Correspondence: xudong74@hotmail.com; xiaofeng.zeng@cstar.org.cn
Department of Rheumatology and Clinical Immunology, Peking Union
Medical College Hospital, Chinese Academy of Medical Sciences & Peking
Union Medical College, Beijing 100730, China

Background

Systemic sclerosis (SSc) is an autoimmune disease of unknown etiology that is characterized by microvasculopathy, immune system disturbances and increased tissue deposition of collagen in the skin and internal organs. The disease course is unpredictable and can remain relatively stable or rapidly progress. Several clinical cohort studies of SSc have been carried out in many countries to determine the clinical features and survival prognosis of patients with SSc [1, 2].

A number of studies suggest that SSc pathogenesis is influenced by multiple factors such as geography and ethnicity, whereas SSc prognosis is closely related to disease subtypes, antibody profile and visceral involvement [3]. Some studies have revealed that the incidence of SSc and diffuse cutaneous SSc (dcSSc) is higher in African-Americans who have worse disease prognosis [4]. A retrospective analysis compared clinical manifestations between Canadian patients of different descent and showed that those of Chinese descent have less severe disease, with less frequent gastrointestinal involvement and less severe vasculopathy than patients of European descent [5]. However, there have been limited clinical and prognostic large-scale clinical analyses of patients with SSc in China. A multicenter study conducted by Jiucun Wang [6], including 419 Chinese patients with SSc in Shanghai, Hebei Province, Sichuan Province and Hunan Province, showed that there are significant differences in the proportion of clinical subsets and frequencies of SSc-related autoantibodies compared to patients of US Caucasian descent. Another study recruited 1479 Taiwan patients based on the health insurance database and showed a lower incidence of SSc in Asian countries than in the USA or Europe [7]. However, neither of these studies had analyzed the clinical characteristics of patients with SSc in China.

Our previous study found that digital ulcers and telangiectasia were common in Chinese patients with SSc, with a prevalence of approximately 30% and 41.7%, respectively, which was similar to those reported abroad [8–11]. The differences in visceral involvement and autoantibody spectrum will determine the prognosis of Chinese patients with SSc. The aim of this study was to determine the prognosis, the cause of death and the risk factors for patients with SSc at a single Chinese center.

Methods

Patients

Patients clinically diagnosed with SSc between Feb 2009 and Dec 2015 were prospectively recruited from the European League Against Rheumatism (EULAR) Scleroderma Trials and Research Group (EUSTAR) and Chinese Rheumatism Data Center (CRDC) database of the Peking Union Medical College Hospital (PUMCH).

Diagnosis of SSc was fulfilled according to the 2013 American College of Rheumatology (ACR)/EULAR criteria. Ethics committee approval was obtained for the EUSTAR and CRDC study and all subjects provided informed written consent.

Data collection

Patients were mainly followed up by outpatient visits at intervals of 6 months to 1 year. Demographic, clinical and laboratory data were collected and entered into a database according to consolidated regulations. Patients whose last follow-up date was more than 1 year from May 2016 were followed up by telephone.

Patients were classified into limited and diffuse cutaneous subsets based on the definition of Leroy et al. [12]. Identification of peripheral vascular involvement included Raynaud's phenomenon (RP), fingertip ulcer, loss of finger pads/pitting scars and telangiectasia. Identification of lung involvement included interstitial lung disease (ILD) and pulmonary arterial hypertension (PAH). ILD was defined as ground glass opacification or fibrosis on high-resolution computed tomography (HRCT). PAH was defined as a mean pulmonary arterial pressure > 25 mmHg at rest, together with pulmonary capillary wedge pressure < 15 mmHg determined by right heart catheterization or pulmonary artery systolic pressure (PASP) > 40 mmHg at rest based on an echocardiogram test. Those who only took echocardiogram test and hadn't taken right heart catheterization once in series and had maximum tricuspid regurgitant velocity (TRV) and pulmonary artery systolic pressure (PASP) of 2.9–3.4 m/s and 37–50 mmHg, respectively, were ruled out as diagnosis of PAH could not be confirmed [13]. Cardiac involvement included arrhythmia, left ventricular dysfunction (LVEF< 50%), decline of left ventricular diastolic function, pericardial effusion and valvular disease that could not otherwise be explained. Gastrointestinal involvement, according to the definition in the EUSTAR database, including esophageal (based on the presence of heartburn, regurgitation or dysphagia symptoms), gastric (based on clinical symptoms of early satiety, flatulence and vomiting) and intestinal involvement (diarrhea or constipation together with pseudo-obstruction secondary to small bowel involvement), in the absence of other explainable causes like treatment, cancer, etc.

Age at disease onset was defined as the age at first non-RP SSc manifestation, and age at disease diagnosis was defined as the age when SSc was diagnosed by a specialist. Length of follow up was defined as the time between the date of SSc diagnosis and last visit or death. Disease duration was defined as the time between the first non-RP SSc manifestation and last visit or death.

Patients who were ≥ 60 years old at the time of disease onset were defined as having late-onset SSc.

Survival status was determined through the end of May 2016 based on database records or telephone tracing of patients for whom no data in the database had been entered for ≥ 12 months. The final status of loss to follow up was defined as having no data entered for ≥ 12 months with a failure to contact the patient on least two attempts. Data on cause of death were collected via medical records for patients who died in the PUMCH or for whom death certification was provided by relatives of patients who died in other hospitals. Deaths attributable to SSc were based on evaluation by three experienced rheumatologists from PUMCH.

Statistical analysis

The data were analyzed using SPSS 19.0 and differences between groups were analyzed by analysis of variance (ANOVA), the Mann-Whitney test or the chi-square (χ^2) test, depending on the distribution of the variables. Bivariate odds ratios with 95% confidence intervals (CI) were calculated. Kaplan-Meier analysis was used to estimate survival from the date of diagnosis, with the Mantel-Haenszel statistic (log-rank test) used to analyze differences in survival. Cox analysis and logistic regression analysis were used to obtain independent risk factors for SSc prognosis.

Results
Clinical and laboratory characteristics

A total of 448 patients with SSc were recruited for this study and 90.4% (405) were female. Limited cutaneous SSc (lcSSc) (254, 56.7%) was more common than diffused cutaneous SSc (dcSSc) (194, 43.3%). Overlap syndrome was present in 36 patients (8%). The mean age at disease onset and diagnosis was 39.0 ± 12.5 (8–75 years) and 42.8 ± 12.1 years, respectively. A significantly greater number of patients experienced disease onset at age< 60 years (427 vs. 21). Across 2167 patient-years, the median disease duration and length of follow up was 7.0 years (0.01, 49.4) and 53.5 months (0.25, 365), respectively. The majority of the cohort was Han Chinese, but 11 ethnic minorities were also included (4 Manchus, 5 Mongolian and 2 Korean). Past history of cardiovascular and respiratory diseases was as follows: 47 patients had a history of hypertension, 9 had previous coronary heart disease, 6 had previous cerebrovascular disease, 1 had rheumatic heart disease and 1 had silicosis.

Raynaud's phenomenon was the most common peripheral vascular involvement in patients with SSc in this cohort (424, 94.6%), 72.3% of whom (315) presented with Raynaud's phenomenon as the first disease manifestation at disease onset. More than half of the patients (271 patients, 60.5%) had different respiratory symptoms,

with shortness of breath after exercise (250, 55.8%) being the most common, followed by cough (106, 23.7%) and dyspnea (38, 8.5%). Most (358 patients, 80.1%) were diagnosed as having SSc-ILD at baseline, whereas 55 had concurrent ILD and PAH.

Pulmonary function test (PFT) had been undertaken in 80.8% of patients (n = 362) at baseline, and the mean ± SD for forced expiratory volume in 1 s (FEV1), total lung capacity (TLC), forced vital capacity (FVC), diffusing capacity for carbon monoxide (DLCO)% on PFT were 82.1 ± 15.4, 7.8 ± 17.5, 81.2 ± 17.0, and 62.2 ± 20.0, respectively. Other organs involved at baseline are shown in Table 1. Elevated erythrocyte sedimentation rate (ESR) occurred in 121 patients (30.9%). C3 and C4 levels at baseline were 1.03 ± 0.25 g/L (in 314 cases) and 0.20 ± 0.09 g/L (in 312 cases), respectively. The average immunoglobulin G (IgG) level was 15 mg/dl (6.5, 52.2). Antinuclear antibodies (ANA) were seen in 97.7% of patients (336/344), whereas the presence of

Table 1 Clinical features at baseline and during follow up

	Total N = 448 Baseline, number (%)	Incident N = 448 Follow up, number
Vascular involvement	430 (96.0)	10
Raynaud phenomenon	424 (94.6)	11
Fingertip ulcer	128 (28.6)	19
Loss of finger pad	137 (30.6)	20
Telangiectasia	153 (34.2)	39
Arthritis	121 (27.0)	66
Muscle involvement	44 (9.8)	11
Pulmonary interstitial disease (ILD)[a]	358/447 (80.1)	24
Pulmonary arterial hypertension (PAH)	67/359 (18.7)	11
Gastrointestinal involvement	274 (61.2)	38
Esophagus	243 (54.2)	40
Gastric	115 (25.7)	20
Intestinal	67 (15.0)	13
Cardiac involvement	177/397 (44.6)	97/411
Arrhythmia	16/396 (4.0)	13/412
LVEF < 50%	1/396 (0.3)	3/411
Left ventricular diastolic dysfunction	69/396 (17.4)	70/411
Pericardial effusion	57/396 (14.4)	53/411
Valvular disease	88/396 (22.2)	70/412
Renal crisis	5 (1.1)	0
Skin Rodnan score	6 (0, 43)	–

LVEF left ventricular ejection fraction
[a]Pulmonary interstitial disease: one patient diagnosed with silicosis at first visit was excluded

anti-ribonucleoprotein (RNP) antibody was less frequent (90/344, 26.2%). Anti Scl-70 and anticentromere antibody (ACA) were present in 46.8% (169/361) and 16.5% (48/291), respectively, of patients, 3 of whom were double positive for anti Scl-70 and ACA.

During follow up (53 months (0.25, 365)), 24 patients developed pulmonary interstitial diseases, and the prevalence of ILD reached 85.5%. PAH was identified in 78/361 patients, accounting for 21.6% of the cohort, and 63 patients had both PAH and ILD. Arrhythmia was present in 29 patients: among those with arrhythmia, only 5 patients experienced palpitations and other symptoms. At baseline, one patient had ovarian cancer and one had thyroid carcinoma, whereas two patients developed tumors during the follow-up period, including one with lung adenocarcinoma and one with leukemia.

Among 402 patients, 348 of them took glucocorticoid during the disease course: 374 patients received immunosuppressors and 43 of them took only immunosuppressors; 11 patients took neither glucocorticoid nor immunosuppressors. Among patients who used immunomodulators during follow up, 250 patients took cyclophosphamide (CTX), 2 took cyclosporin (CsA), 28 took mycophenolate mofetil (MMF), 5 took tacrolimus, 2 took azathioprine (AZA), 9 took leflunomide (LEF), 103 took TwHF, 108 took MTX and 29 took hydroxychloroquine (HCQ); 102 patients used two immunomodulators at the same time and 19 used three immunomodulators at the same time.

Survival analysis

The 448 patients with SSc were followed up for a total of 2167 patient-years. The median survival time for the patient cohort was 53 months (0.25, 365). Survival rates from disease diagnosis were 97.0%, 94.6%, 91.1% and 87.8% at 1, 3, 5 and 10 years, respectively (Fig. 1). The cumulative survival rates at 1, 3, 5 and 10 years in patients with lcSSc were 97.6%, 94.2%, 91.1% and 89.1%, respectively, whereas for patients with dcSSc the rates were 96.3%, 95.1%, 91.2% and 87.0%, respectively.

No significant differences were seen in subgroup survival analysis according to subtypes (log-rank test 0.002, p = 0.968), baseline vascular (log-rank test 2.407, p = 0.121), joint (log-rank test 2.868, p = 0.090), muscular (log-rank test 1.009, p = 0.315), gastrointestinal (GI) involvement (log-rank test 0.027, p = 0.870), gender (log-rank test 0.014, p = 0.907) and age of disease onset (log-rank test 0.249, p = 0.618) (Additional file 1: Figure S2).

The median modified Rodnan skin score (mRSS) was 6 points (0, 43) in this cohort. According to the distribution of skin scores, 87.5% of patients had a skin score < 16 points. Patients with higher skin score (mRSS > 15) had a poorer prognosis (log-rank test 7.977, p = 0.005). However, survival was better in patients who had no respiratory symptoms (Additional file 1: Figure S1) and less pulmonary dysfunction (FVC% < 70%, log-rank test 14.58, p = 0.000, DLCO% < 60%, log-rank test 23.58, p = 0.000) (Fig. 2).

No significant differences were seen in subgroup survival analysis according to use of HCQ (log-rank test

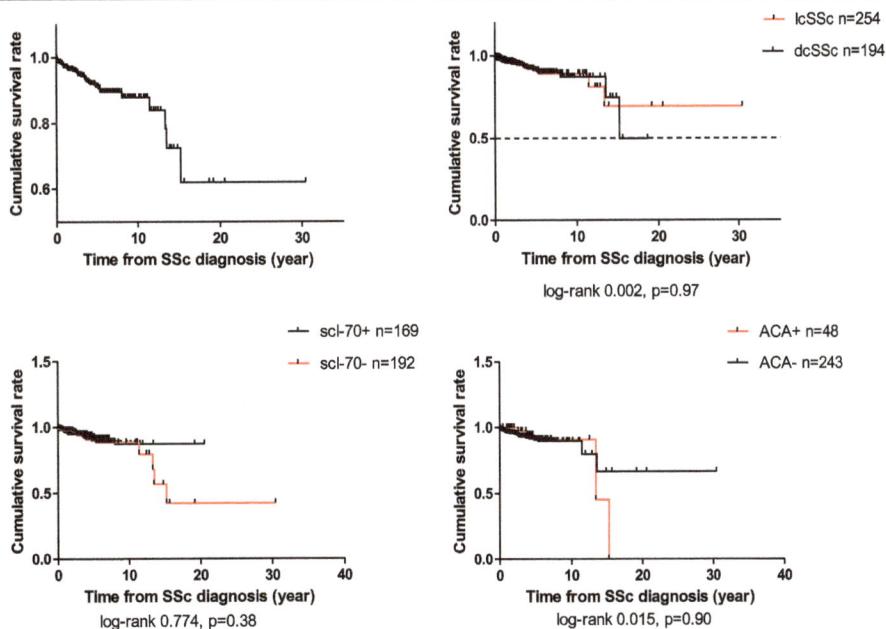

Fig. 1 Survival curve and subgroup study of patients with systemic sclerosis (SSc) in the Peking Union Medical College Hospital (PUMCH) cohort. lcSSc, limited cutaneous SSc; dcSSc, diffuse cutaneous SSc; ACA, anticentromere antibody

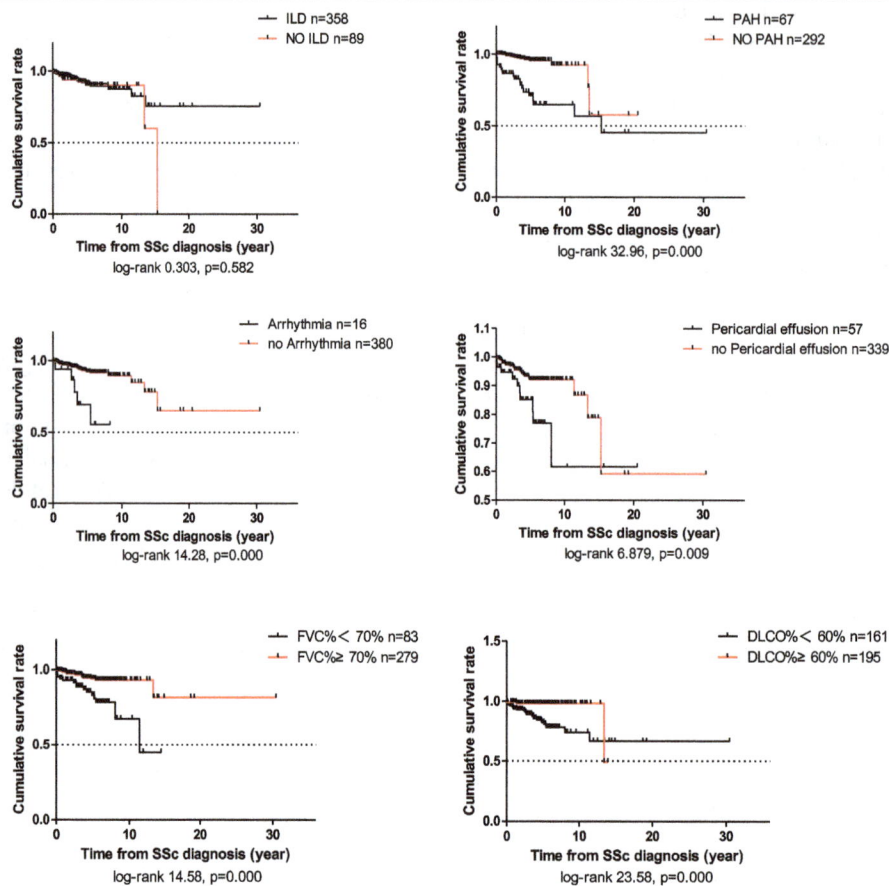

Fig. 2 Survival analysis based on interstitial lung disease (ILD), pulmonary arterial hypertension (PAH), cardiac involvement and pulmonary dysfunction. SSc, systemic sclerosis; FVC, forced vital capacity; DLCO, diffusing capacity for carbon monoxide

1.186, $p = 0.276$) or MMF (log-rank test 0.016, $p = 0.9$). TwHF (log-rank test 7.851, $p = 0.005$) and MTX (log-rank test 7.925, $p = 0.005$) were found to be protective against mortality in survival analysis. Patients who took CTX during the disease course had a poorer prognosis (log-rank test 5.177, $p = 0.023$).

Patients who had PAH (log-rank test 32.96, $p = 0.000$), arrhythmia (log-rank test 14.28, $p = 0.000$) and pericardial effusion (log-rank test 6.879, $p = 0.009$) at baseline had a poorer prognosis than those who did not. However, there was no significant difference between patients with or without ILD at baseline (log-rank test 0.303, $p = 0.582$). Among 288 patients who had both HRCT-confirmed ILD and PFT simultaneously, those who had pulmonary dysfunction (defined as FVC < 70% or DLCO < 60%) had a poorer prognosis (log-rank test 16.266, $p = 0.000$) (Fig. 2).

Among 358 patients who had ILD at baseline, 217 of them had continuous monitoring by HRCT. We qualitatively assess disease progression according to the description in the radiology reports: 64 patients had radiographic evidence of aggravation (median disease duration at baseline was 0 (0, 132) months) during the

disease course, and 153 patients remained stable or improved (median disease duration at baseline was 1 (0, 165) month). A poor prognosis was not confirmed among patients with ILD who had radiographic aggravation (log-rank test 2.629, $p = 0.105$). There were 89 patients who did not have ILD at baseline, and 24 of them developed ILD during the disease course. New onset of ILD was not associated with a poor prognosis (log-rank test 0.111, $p = 0.740$).

Patients with scleroderma renal crisis (SRC) were rare in this cohort. Despite the rarity, patients with SRC at baseline had a poor outcome compared to those patients that did not have SRC (log-rank test 11.36, $p = 0.001$).

Risk factors for prognosis

Univariate survival analysis suggested that SRC, PAH, arrhythmia, pericardial effusion, skin score > 15, FVC% < 70% and DLCO% < 60% on pulmonary function tests (PFT), and respiratory symptoms at baseline were associated with poor prognosis. Further Cox multivariate analysis confirmed that PAH (hazard ratio

(HR) 6.248, 95% CI 2.855, 13.674) and arrhythmia (HR 4.729, 95% CI 1.588, 14.082) at baseline are independent risk factors for poor outcome in patients with SSc.

Cause of death

Among the cohort, 40 patients with SSc died (Table 2): 27 deaths (67.5%) were related to SSc. PAH was the leading cause of death, accounting for 55% of all deaths. The mortality rate in patients who had PAH during the disease course was 28.2% (22/78 patients). Of the 63 patients in this cohort who had both PAH and ILD, 17 died (mortality rate, 27.0%). Among the four patients who died from myocardial infarction and stroke, only one had no history of cardiovascular involvement or hypertension. The two patients who died of lung infection both had SSc-related lung involvement, one had PAH, and the other had ILD. One patient died of bacteremia due to cholecystitis. Two patients who died had tumors and one died of leukemia 5 years after the SSc diagnosis. The other patient was first treated for hemoptysis and within one year of SSc diagnosis this patient died from lung adenocarcinoma that had metastasized to the bone, meninges and liver.

Table 2 Causes of death in the patient cohort

Cause of death	Deaths, N = 40 (%)
All causes of death	40
SSc-related deaths	27 (67.5)
Lungs	23 (57.5)
ILD	1
PAH	22
Heart	1 (2.5)
Arrhythmia	–
Heart failure	1
Renal crisis	3 (7.5)
Non-SSc-related deaths	10 (25.0)
Infection	3 (7.5)
Pulmonary infection	2
Bacteremia	1
Malignant tumor	2 (5.0)
Adenocarcinoma of lung	1
Leukemia	1
CCVd	4 (10.0)
Mi	1
Cerebral apoplexy	3
Digestive tract bleeding	1 (2.5)
Unknown cause of death	3 (7.5)

Results are presented as number (percentage) of patients
ILD interstitial lung disease, *PAH* pulmonary arterial hypertension, *SSc* systemic sclerosis, *CCVd* chronic cerebrovascular disease, *Mi* myocardial infarction

Discussion

Systemic sclerosis is a disease that has significant clinical heterogeneity. Some patients progress rapidly and even die, whereas others remain stable and have limited symptoms such as finger sclerosis and minimal visceral involvement. Therefore, treatment strategies for SSc would benefit from the ability to predict prognosis based on clinical manifestations or laboratory parameters in the early stage of the disease.

Earlier studies reported a 10-year survival rate for SSc that was as low as 50% [14], whereas more recent studies including the EUSTAR registry reported 5-year and 10-year survival rates of 90% and 84%, respectively [15] (Clinical manifestation and survival rates published for different countries since 2008 are listed in (Additional file 2) [16–23]). In recent years, the SSc survival rate has improved. Indeed, Ferri et al. analyzed prognostic cohorts of SSc worldwide at different times and found that the median values of cumulative 10th-year survival rates in patients with SSc increased from 54% to 83.5% [24]. Unfortunately, we could not make comparisons with the EUSTAR study, because no specific organ involvement was mentioned. Compared with two contemporary European studies and one Asian study, the incidence of ILD and PAH in Chinese patients with SSc were much higher than those in Spain, which might partially explain the reduction in 3-year and 5-year survival rates. Compared with the Italian study in 2010, despite a higher incidence rate of PAH in Chinese patients, the 3-year survival rate was similar. The 5-year survival rate in Italy was lower than in China, which might be related to the significant increase in SRC and GI involvement; the latter may result in malnutrition and susceptibility to infection. Although having a high incidence of ILD and PAH, as in China, Thailand had a slightly lower survival rate due to there being a greater proportion of patients with dcSSc in the cohort. Therefore, it can be seen that the characteristics of organ involvement in patients with SSc in different countries determine diverse prognoses.

Survival among patients with dcSSc in our cohort was consistent with that in a Spanish report [2], but was higher than that reported in other studies conducted during the same period [21]. The mortality rate can be underestimated due to the failure to capture data on early death in patients with dcSSc, which could result in overestimation of survival in these patients [25]. Moreover, patients with dcSSc were reported to have worse outcomes [16, 17, 19, 20] relative to patients with lcSSc, due to their predisposition toward internal organ involvement, specifically lung and renal involvement. Our study confirmed that a higher mRSS, which manifests as more extensive skin involvement, was a risk factor for mortality in patients with SSc, but no significant difference in 1, 3, 5 and 10-year survival rates was seen between disease subtypes.

In this study, we found that vital organ involvement such as renal crisis, PAH, cardiac involvement (especially arrhythmia and pericardial effusion), severe skin involvement, presence of respiratory-related symptoms and decreased FVC% and DLCO% on PFT were risk factors for poor prognosis. Multivariate Cox analysis confirmed that PAH and arrhythmia at baseline were independent prognostic factors in this cohort. Arrhythmia can have several origins that are related to primary heart involvement such as cardiac conductive tissue fibrosis and myocardial fibrosis [26, 27], pericardial disease or PAH [28], and was associated with poor outcome [15]. In this study, confirming a diagnosis of arrhythmia during the early disease stage was challenging, as the majority of patients had no clinical symptoms or signs on standard electrocardiogram (ECG) at rest [28].

Although ILD was an independent prognostic factor in a previous study [4], our study did not confirm this, which might be due to the large proportion of patients with ILD and the inclusion of patients with more early or mild interstitial lesions in our study due to the reliance on HRCT imaging features to define ILD. Our study did not confirm a poor prognosis among patients with ILD who had radiographic evidence of aggravation, partially due to individual differences among radiologists in the assessment of images and lack of quantitative assessment. Our findings suggest that ILD with pulmonary dysfunction (FVC $< 70\%$ or DLCO $< 60\%$), rather than the presence of ILD alone, is associated with poor prognosis.

Patients who took CTX during the disease course had poorer prognosis. It was probably because patients requiring CTX were more prone to significant organ involvement and they could have been affected by combined medication and side effects. TwHF, a traditional Chinese herbal medicine, had been widely used in autoimmune diseases, including rheumatoid arthritis (RA), systemic lupus erythematosus (SLE) and SSc etc., mainly due to their anti-inflammatory immunoregulation and favorable cost-benefit ratio. Our previous study showed that TwHF treatment for more than 1 year could improve FVC (0.11 ± 0.25) and FVC% ($3.83 \pm 8.58\%$) ($p < 0.05$) (not published). The protective effect of TwHF on survival in patients with SSc deserves further study.

The median follow-up time of the 40 patients who died was 31.5 months, but the average follow-up time of the survivors was 56 months, indicating that there was no bias associated with a longer observation period among the patients with SSc who died.

A meta-analysis of death in patients with SSc showed that heart and lung involvement had replaced renal crisis as the leading cause of death in patients with SSc [29]. SSc-related deaths, especially lung involvement, were the leading cause of death in patients with SSc in this study, accounting for 67.5% of deaths, which was similar to results for a multinational inception cohort (patients recruited within 4 years of disease onset, 62.1%) [25]. The death rate attributable to lung involvement in patients with SSc increased over time [30]. In the EULAR cohort, 19% of the patients died of ILD, which was higher than that for PAH (14%), but in the study cohort here, only one patient died of ILD, and thus PAH was the leading cause of death, consistent with some other studies [16, 25, 31]. This outcome might also be related to coexisting ILD in 17 out of 22 patients with SSc who died of PAH. To determine the cause of non-sudden cardiac death in patients with both PAH and ILD can be indistinguishable, as the accuracy of the physician's judgment might affect the result and underestimate deaths due to ILD. Only one patient died of cardiac involvement among the SSc related deaths, and this small number was related to the small number cases of patients who had severe cardiac involvement.

With the progress of disease screening and treatment, patients with SSc can have longer life expectancy, and thus long-term complications could become particularly important later in the disease course. Cardiovascular and cerebrovascular disease, infections and tumors were the main causes of non-SSc related deaths in this cohort, as was also seen in a study by Hao et al. [25]. A number of reports confirmed that the incidence of cancer SSc in patients was elevated [32]. The incidence of malignant tumors in patients with SSc is 3–11%, which was 1.5–5 times [33] higher than that for the healthy population. In this cohort, the two patients with malignant tumors during follow up were female, had the lcSSc subtype and were positive for anti scl-70 antibody. Patients with SSc had fewer hematologic malignancies compared with solid tumors, with only a few case reports of hematologic tumor such as multiple myeloma, chronic lymphocytic and myeloid leukemia (CLL and CML), Hodgkin's and non-Hodgkin's lymphoma and hairy cell leukemia [34].

There is no consensus about the incidence of coronary heart and cerebrovascular disease among patients with SSc compared with the general population. A study from the Australian Scleroderma Cohort Study (ASCS) reported that after adjusting for age, sex and traditional risk factors for atherosclerosis, patients with SSc were 3.2 times more likely to have coronary heart disease than the general population [19], whereas studies by Nordin et al. [35] and Hettema et al. [36] concluded that atherosclerosis was not more prevalent in patients with SSc than in controls.

Conclusion

In china, although there is a high prevalence of ILD in patients with SSc (85.5%), most patients have reserved pulmonary function, which means that ILD is not the most important factor in the death of patients with SSc and is also not a risk factor for poor prognosis. Only ILD with pulmonary dysfunction is associated with poor outcome. The 10-year cumulative rate (87.8%) in patients with SSc in China is slightly lower than in Europe, and PAH and arrhythmia at baseline are independent prognostic factors, whereas PAH instead of ILD is the leading cause of death in patients with SSc. Interestingly, the Chinese traditional medicine TwHF deserves further study as a protective factor in survival. This is the first study of prognosis in Chinese patients with SSc, and a study involving multiple centers in China is in progress. The results from this and future studies should help elucidate the influence of various ethnic differences on SSc disease phenotype and prognosis.

Additional files

Additional file 1: Figure S1. Survival analysis based on respiratory symptoms. **Figure S2.** Survival analysis based on organ involvement. (DOCX 550 kb)

Additional file 2: Clinical manifestation and survival rates published by different countries since 2008. (DOCX 19 kb)

Abbreviations

ACA: Anticentromere antibody; ACR: American College of Rheumatology; ANA: Antinuclear antibody; ANOVA: Analysis of variability; ASCS: Australian Scleroderma Cohort Study; CCVd: Chronic cerebrovascular disease; CI: Confidence intervals; CLL: Chronic lymphocytic; CML: Chronic myeloid leukemia; CRDC: Chinese Rheumatism Data Center; CTX: Cyclophosphamide; dcSSc: Diffuse cutaneous systemic sclerosis; DLCO: Diffusing lung capacity for carbon monoxide; ESR: Erythrocyte sedimentation rate; EUSTAR: European League Against Rheumatism Scleroderma Trials and Research Group; FEV1: Forced expiratory volume at 1 min; FVC: Forced vital capacity; GI: Gastrointestinal; HRCT: High-resolution computed tomography; IgG: Immunoglobulin G; ILD: Interstitial lung disease; lcSSc: Limited cutaneous systemic sclerosis; LVEF: Left ventricular ejection fraction; Mi: Myocardial infarction; mRSS: Modified Rodnan skin score; MTX: Methotrexate; PAH: Pulmonary arterial hypertension; PASP: Pulmonary artery systolic pressure; PFT: Pulmonary function test; PUMCH: Peking Union Medical College Hospital; SRC: Scleroderma renal crisis; SSc: Systemic sclerosis; TRV: Tricuspid regurgitant velocity; TwHF: Tripterygium wilfordii Hook F

Acknowledgements

The authors thank Dr Yanhong Wang (PUMC) for data processing.

Funding

This work was supported by the Center for Rare Diseases Research, Chinese Academy of Medical Sciences, Beijing, China (grant number 2016ZX310174–4).

Authors' contributions

All authors participated in design and acquisition of patients' data. SSH analyzed and interpreted the data and drafted the manuscript. DX was a major contributor in revising the manuscript. All authors read and approved the final manuscript.

Consent for publication

Not applicable.

Competing interests

The authors declare that they have no competing interests.

References

1. Al-Dhaher FF, Pope JE, Ouimet JM. Determinants of morbidity and mortality of systemic sclerosis in Canada. Semin Arthritis Rheum. 2010;39(4):269–77.
2. Simeón-Aznar CP, Fonollosa-Plá V, Carles TV, et al. Registry of the Spanish Network for Systemic Sclerosis: survival, prognostic factors, and causes of death. Medicine. 2015;94(43):e1728.
3. Ranque B, Mouthon L. Geoepidemiology of systemic sclerosis. Autoimmun Rev. 2010;9(5):311–8.
4. Nashid M, Khanna PP, Furst DE, et al. Gender and ethnicity differences in patients with diffuse systemic sclerosis–analysis from three large randomized clinical trials. Rheumatology. 2011;50(2):335–42.
5. Low AH, Johnson SR, Lee P. Ethnic influence on disease manifestations and autoantibodies in Chinese-descent patients with systemic sclerosis. J Rheumatol. 2009;36(4):787–93.
6. Wang J, Assassi S, Guo G, et al. Clinical and serological features of systemic sclerosis in a Chinese cohort. Clin Rheumatol. 2013;32(5):617–21.
7. Kuo CF, See LC, Yu KH, et al. Epidemiology and mortality of systemic sclerosis: a nationwide population study in Taiwan. Scand J Rheumatol. 2013;333(5):e401.
8. Xu D, Li MT, Hou Y, et al. Clinical characteristics of systemic sclerosis patients with digital ulcers in China. Clin Exp Rheumatol. 2013;31(2 Suppl 76):46.
9. Sunderkötter C, Herrgott I, Brückner C, et al. Comparison of patients with and without digital ulcers in systemic sclerosis: detection of possible risk factors. Br J Dermatol. 2010;160(4):835–43.
10. Hachulla E, Clerson P, Launay D, et al. Natural history of ischemic digital ulcers in systemic sclerosis: single-center retrospective longitudinal study. J Rheumatol. 2007;34(12):2423.
11. Zhang S, Xu D, Li M, et al. Telangiectasia as a potential clinical marker of microvascular lesions in systemic sclerosis patients from EUSTAR data in China. Clin Exp Rheumatol. 2015;33(4 Suppl 91):S106.
12. LeRoy EC, Medsger TA. Criteria for the classification of early systemic sclerosis. J Rheumatol. 2001;28:1573–6.
13. Gali N, Hoeper MM, Humbert M, et al. Guidelines for the diagnosis and treatment of pulmonary hypertension. Eur Heart J. 2009;30:2493–537.
14. Bennett R, Bluestone R, Holt PJ, Bywaters EG. Survival in scleroderma. Ann Rheum Dis. 1971;30:581–8.
15. Tyndall AJ, Bannert B, Vonk M, Airò P, Cozzi F, Carreira PE, et al. Causes and risk factors for death in systemic sclerosis: a study from the EULAR Scleroderma Trials and Research (EUSTAR) database. Ann Rheum Dis. 2010; 69:1809–15.
16. Joven BE, Almodovar R, Carmona L, et al. Survival, causes of death, and risk factors associated with mortality in Spanish systemic sclerosis patients: results from a single university hospital. Semin Arthritis Rheum. 2010;39(4): 285–93.
17. Vettori S, Cuomo G, Abignano G, et al. Survival and death causes in 251 systemic sclerosis patients from a single Italian center. Reumatismo. 2010; 62(3):202.
18. Walker UA, Tyndall A, Czirják L, et al. Clinical risk assessment of organ manifestations in systemic sclerosis: a report from the EULAR Scleroderma Trials And Research group database. Ann Rheum Dis. 2007;66(6):754–63.
19. Hashimoto A, Tejima S, Tono T, et al. Predictors of survival and causes of death in Japanese patients with systemic sclerosis. J Rheumatol. 2001;38(9): 1931–9.
20. Sampaiobarros PD, Bortoluzzo AB, Marangoni RG, et al. Survival, causes of death, and prognostic factors in systemic sclerosis: analysis of 947 Brazilian patients. J Rheumatol. 2012;39(10):1971–8.
21. Hoffmannvold AM, Molberg Ø, Midtvedt Ø, et al. Survival and causes of death in an unselected and complete cohort of Norwegian patients with systemic sclerosis. J Rheumatol. 2013;40(7):1127–33.
22. Poormoghim H, Andalib E, Jalali A, et al. Survival and causes of death in systemic sclerosis patients: a single center registry report from Iran. Rheumatol Int. 2016;36(7):925–34.
23. Wangkaew S, Prasertwitayakij N, Phrommintikul A, et al. Causes of death, survival and risk factors of mortality in Thai patients with early systemic sclerosis: inception cohort study. Rheumatol Int. 2017;37(12):1–8.

24. Ferri C, Sebastiani M, Monaco AL, et al. Systemic sclerosis evolution of disease pathomorphosis and survival. Our experience on Italian patients' population and review of the literature. Autoimmun Rev. 2014;13(10):1026–34.

25. Hao Y, Hudson M, Baron M, et al. Early mortality in a multinational systemic sclerosis inception cohort. Arthritis Rheumatol. 2017;69(5):1067–77.

26. Chen F, Lu X, Shu X, et al. The predictive value of serum markers for the development of interstitial lung disease in patients with polymyositis and dermatomyositis - a comparative and prospective study. Intern Med J. 2015; 45(6):641–7.

27. Draeger HT, Assassi S, Sharif R, et al. Right bundle branch block: a predictor of mortality in early systemic sclerosis. PLoS One. 2013;8(10):e78808.

28. Vacca A, Meune C, Gordon J, et al. Cardiac arrhythmias and conduction defects in systemic sclerosis. Rheumatology. 2014;53(7):1172–7.

29. Elhai M, Meune C, Avouac J, Kahan A, Allanore Y. Trends in mortality in patients with systemic sclerosis over 40 years: a systematic review and meta-analysis of cohort studies. Rheumatology. 2012;51(6):1017–26.

30. Rubio-Rivas M, Royo, Simeón CP, et al. Mortality and survival in systemic sclerosis. systematic review and meta-analysis. Semin Arthritis Rheum. 2014; 44(2):208–19.

31. Lefèvre G, Dauchet L, Hachulla E, et al. Survival and prognostic factors in systemic sclerosis–associated pulmonary hypertension: a systematic review and meta-analysis. Arthritis Rheum. 2013;65(9):2412–23.

32. Derk CT, Rasheed M, Artlett CM, Jimenez SA. A cohort study of cancer incidence in systemic sclerosis. J Rheumatol. 2006;33(33):1113–6.

33. Szekanecz É, Szamosi S, Horváth Á, et al. Malignancies associated with systemic sclerosis. Autoimmun Rev. 2012;11(12):852–5.

34. Kaşifoğlu T, Korkmaz C, Yaşar Ş, Gülbaş Z. Scleroderma and chronic myeloid leukemia: a sheer coincidence, a consequence of long lasting D-penicillamine therapy or a plausible relationship of both diseases? Rheumatol Int. 2006;27(2):175–7.

35. Nordin A, Jensen-Urstad K, Björnådal L, et al. Ischemic arterial events and atherosclerosis in patients with systemic sclerosis: a population-based case-control study[J]. Arthritis Research & Therapy. 2013;15(4):1–12.

36. Hettema ME, Zhang D, de Leeuw K, Stienstra Y, Smit AJ, Kallenberg CG, et al. Early atherosclerosis in systemic sclerosis and its relation to disease or traditional risk factors. Arthritis Res Ther. 2008;10:R49.

19

CCN family member 2/connective tissue growth factor (CCN2/CTGF) is regulated by Wnt–β-catenin signaling in nucleus pulposus cells

Akihiko Hiyama[1,2]*, Kosuke Morita[1,2], Daisuke Sakai[1,2] and Masahiko Watanabe[1,2]

Abstract

Background: The aims of this study were to investigate the gene expression of CCN family members in rat intervertebral disc (IVD) cells and to examine whether Wnt–β-catenin signaling regulates the expression of CCN family 2 (CCN2)/connective tissue growth factor (CTGF) in rat nucleus pulposus (NP) cells.

Methods: The gene expression of CCN family members were assessed in rat IVD cells using real-time reverse transcription polymerase chain reaction (RT-PCR). The expression pattern of CCN2 was also assessed in rat IVD cells using western blot and immunohistochemical analyses. Gain-of-function and loss-of-function experiments were performed to identify the mechanisms by which Wnt–β-catenin signaling influences the activity of the CCN2 promoter. To further determine if the mitogen-activated protein kinase (MAPK) pathway is required for the Wnt–β-catenin signaling-induced regulation of CCN2 expression in the NP cells, CCN2 expression was analyzed by reporter assay, RT-PCR and western blot analysis.

Results: *CCN2* messenger RNA (mRNA) and protein were expressed in rat IVDs. Expression of *CCN2* was significantly higher than for mRNA of other CCN family members in both rat NP and annulus fibrosus (AF) cells. The relative activity of the CCN2 promoter decreased 24 h after treatment with 6-bromoindirubin-3′-oxime (1.0 μM) (0.773 (95% 0.735, 0.812) $P = 0.0077$) in NP cells. In addition, treatment with the WT–β-catenin vector (500 ng) significantly decreased CCN2 promoter activity (0.688 (95% 0.535, 0.842) $P = 0.0063$), whereas β-catenin small interfering RNA (500 ng) significantly increased CCN2 promoter activity (1.775 (95% 1.435, 2.115) $P < 0.001$). Activation of Wnt–β-catenin signaling decreased the expression of *CCN2* mRNA and protein by NP cells. Regulation of CCN2 by Wnt–β-catenin signaling involved the MAPK pathway in rat NP cells.

Conclusions: This study shows that Wnt–β-catenin signaling regulates the expression of CCN2 through the MAPK pathway in NP cells. Understanding the balance between Wnt–β-catenin signaling and CCN2 is necessary for developing therapeutic alternatives for the treatment of IVD degeneration.

Keywords: Intervertebral disc, Nucleus pulposus cell, Wnt/β-catenin signaling, CCN2/CTGF, MAPK pathway, Intervertebral disc degeneration

* Correspondence: a.hiyama@tokai-u.jp
[1]Department of Orthopaedic Surgery, Surgical Science, Tokai University School of Medicine, 143 Shimokasuya, Isehara, Kanagawa 259-1193, Japan
[2]Research Center for Regenerative Medicine, Tokai University School of Medicine, 143 Shimokasuya, Isehara, Kanagawa 259-1193, Japan

Background

Low back pain (LBP) is often attributed to intervertebral disc (IVD) degeneration, which is also termed degenerative disc disease. The IVD is composed of a soft nucleus pulposus (NP) surrounded by a tough annulus fibrosis (AF). IVD degeneration occurs during aging and is a complex process, and the underlying mechanical and molecular mechanisms remain poorly understood.

CCN family 2 (CCN2)/connective tissue growth factor (CTGF) is a member of the CCN family of secreted multifunctional proteins, which also includes Cyr61/CCN1, NOV/CCN3, WISP1/CCN4, WISP2/CCN5, and WISP3/CCN6 [1–4]. Of the CCN family members, CCN1 appears to possess activity and an expression pattern similar to that of CCN2, whereas CCN3 appears to act antagonistically to CCN2 [5]. The multimodular character of CCN factors allows multiple interactions between them and other growth factors, such as transforming growth factor β (TGF-β), bone morphogenetic protein (BMP), and insulin-like growth factor, and allows networking between growth factors, the extracellular matrix (ECM), and cell surface receptors such as integrins [6].

CCN2 has emerged as a major regulator of chondrogenesis [7]. Previous studies have shown that the addition of exogenous CCN2 to cultured chondrocytes promotes cell proliferation and the synthesis of proteoglycans concomitant with elevated expression of chondrocyte-associated genes [8, 9]. Other in vivo studies have shown that Ccn2-deficient mice die soon after birth as a result of severe skeletal abnormalities associated with impaired chondrocyte proliferation and ECM production [10, 11]. These in vivo findings support the in vitro finding that CCN2 is a promoter of cell proliferation and differentiation during endochondral ossification.

CCN2 protein has also been reported to act within the context of the IVD in vivo and in vitro. For example, CCN2 plays an anabolic role by stimulating matrix production by NP cells [12]. It may be possible to exploit this protein's activity by including it in a regenerative cocktail delivered to IVDs [12–14]. Interestingly, two groups have reported increased levels of CCN2 protein in degenerated and painful human discs [13, 15]. These reports suggested that CCN2 has some influence on the IVD degeneration process.

There is evidence that the expression of some members of the CCN family, namely CCN2 and CCN4, are regulated by the Wnt–β-catenin signaling [16, 17]. However, the relationship between Wnt–β-catenin signaling and CCN2 in the pathogenesis of IVD disease remains unclear. The aims of this study were (1) to investigate the expression of CCN family members messenger RNA (mRNA) in rat IVD cells and (2) to examine whether Wnt–β-catenin signaling regulate the expression of CCN2 in rat NP cells.

Methods

Ethics statement

Animal experiments were performed according to a protocol approved by the Animal Experimentation Committee of the University of Tokai (permit number 131012 and 142055), Tokyo, Japan.

Reagents and plasmids

To determine the β-catenin–T cell factor (TCF)/lymphoid enhancing factor (LEF) transcription activity after treatment with 6-bromoindirubin-3′-oxime (BIO) (number 361550; Calbiochem, San Diego, CA, USA), NP cells were transiently transfected with the TCF/LEF reporter gene Topflash (optimal TCF binding site) (Upstate Biotechnology). CCN2-luc was provided by Dr Xiaolong Yang (Cornell University, Ithaca, NY, USA). The wild-type (WT) β-catenin expression plasmid and the backbone plasmid (pBI-β-catenin) were provided by Dr. Raymond Poon (Hospital for Sick Children, University of Toronto, Toronto, ON, Canada). The β-catenin small interfering RNA (siRNA) (number sc-29209) and control siRNA duplexes were purchased from Santa Cruz Biotechnology (Santa Cruz, California, CA, USA). WT-pcDNA3-T7–extracellular signal-regulated protein kinase (ERK) 1 (#14440) and WT-pcDNA3-HA–ERK2 (#8974) were purchased from the Addgene repository (Cambridge, MA, USA). FLAG-tagged WT-p38α (WT-p38) was provided by Dr Jiahuai Han (Xiamen University, China).

We used the pGL4.74 vector (Promega, WI, USA) containing the Renilla reniformis luciferase gene as an internal transfection control. We used BIO to examine Wnt signaling activity. BIO is a cell-permeable, highly potent, selective, reversible, and ATP-competitive specific inhibitor of glycogen synthase kinase 3α/β activity [18]. The ERK inhibitor (PD98059, #9900) and p38–mitogen-activated protein kinase (MAPK) inhibitor (SB202190, #8158) were obtained from Cell Signaling Technology (Danvers, MA, USA).

Cell isolation and culture

Rat IVD cells were isolated from multiple levels of lumbar discs of 11-week-old Sprague Dawley rats (n = 32). Several samples from the same biological from each of the rats are taken and used as a mass for culturing. Primary rat NP and AF cells were isolated as described [19], and the NP and AF tissues obtained from the same animal were pooled. Isolated cells were maintained in Dulbecco's modified Eagle medium (DMEM) (Invitrogen, Carlsbad, CA, USA) supplemented with 10% fetal bovine serum (FBS) (Invitrogen) and antibiotics at 37 °C in a humidified atmosphere of 5% CO$_2$. Confluent NP and AF cells were harvested and sub-cultured in 10-cm dishes. Low-passage (< 4) cells cultured in monolayers were used for all experiments because cells obtained from the rat IVD tissues exhibited variable morphology until passage 4.

Human NP tissue specimens

We obtained informed consent from patients for the use of their IVD tissues. The participants' written consent was obtained according to the Declaration of Helsinki. Ethical approval was obtained from the Institutional Ethics Review Board of the Tokai University School of Medicine. Human degenerative disc tissues were obtained from seven patients undergoing discectomy or fusion surgery at our hospital. We collected seven disc-samples from seven patients (male/female 4/3). The average age of the patients was 38.1 (16–66) years. The details of the samples are listed in Table 1. The disease state was assessed using Pfirrmann grading [20]. This grading scheme uses T2-weighted magnetic resonance imaging (MRI) and image analysis by three independent observers.

Immediately after surgery, human disc NP tissues were carefully collected from discarded surgical waste and digested in 1% penicillin/streptomycin-supplemented DMEM with 10% FBS and 0.114% collagenase type 2 for 1 h at 37 °C. Isolated cells were grown to ∼ 80% confluence as a monolayer in 1% penicillin/streptomycin-supplemented DMEM with 10% FBS at 37 °C in a humidified atmosphere of 5% CO_2. Human NP cells were then used for real-time PCR analysis to evaluate the gene expression of the CCN family members.

Immunofluorescence staining

Rat NP cells were plated in 96-well flat-bottom plates (3×10^3 cells/well) and incubated for 24 h. The cells were treated with 1.0 μM BIO, fixed with 4% paraformaldehyde, permeabilized with 0.5% Triton X-100 (vol:vol) in phosphate-buffered saline (PBS) for 10 min, blocked with PBS containing 10% FBS, and incubated overnight at 4 °C with antibodies against CCN2 (1:100, Santa Cruz Biotechnology). The cells were washed and incubated with an anti-rabbit Alexa Fluor 488 (green) antibody (Thermo Scientific, IN, USA) at 1:200 and with 10 μM 4′,6-diamidino-2-phenylindole (DAPI) for 1 h at room temperature for nuclear staining. The samples were observed under a fluorescence microscope interfaced with a digital imaging system. Cells treated with normal IgG (Cell Signaling Technology) at equal protein concentrations were used as negative controls.

Immunohistological studies

To gain insight into the expression of CCN2 in the IVD, freshly isolated spines from 11-week-old (mature) ($n = 4$) and 32-week-old (adult) (n = 4) rats were fixed in 4% paraformaldehyde in PBS, decalcified, and embedded in paraffin wax. The IVD tissue specimen was cut into thin sections that can be placed on unstained slides. At least three different IVD tissue specimens were used from the same individual rat. At least 12 different IVD sections per group were immunohistochemically analyzed. Sagittal sections were deparaffinized in xylene, rehydrated through a graded ethanol series, and stained with hematoxylin. Sections were incubated with antibodies to CCN2 (Santa Cruz Biotechnology) in 2% bovine serum albumin (BSA) in PBS at 1:100 overnight at 4 °C. The sections were washed thoroughly and incubated with a biotinylated universal secondary antibody (Vector Laboratories, Burlington, ON, Canada) at 1:20 for 10 min at room temperature. Sections were incubated with a streptavidin–peroxidase complex for 5 min and washed with PBS, and color was developed using 3,3′-diaminobenzidine (Vectastain Universal Quick Kit; Vector Laboratories) and examined under a fluorescence microscope. Non-immune IgG was used as a negative control (Cell Signaling Technology) and mouse ovary was used as positive control. The number of positively immunolabeled cells and the total number of cells per high-power field in each section were determined, and the percentage of positively labeled cells was calculated.

Real-time reverse RT–PCR analysis

Total RNA was extracted from the cells using the TRIzol RNA isolation protocol (Invitrogen). RNA was treated with RNase-free DNAse I. Total RNA (100 ng) was used as the template for the RT-PCR analyses. Complementary DNA (cDNA) was synthesized via the reverse transcription of mRNA, as described previously [21]. Reactions were arranged in triplicate in 96-well plates using 1 μL of cDNA with SYBR Green PCR Master Mix (Applied Biosystems), to which gene-specific forward and reverse PCR primers for BIO were added. The primers were synthesized by Takara Bio Inc. (Tokyo, Japan) or FASMAC Corp. (Tokyo, Japan) and are shown in Table 2. PCR reactions were performed in an Applied Biosystems 7500 Fast system according to the manufacturer's instructions. The expression scores were obtained using the $\Delta\Delta C_t$ calculation method.

Table 1 Information on human disc samples from seven patients

Population of seven patients whose samples were used					
Number	Age	Sex	Diagnosis	IVD level	Grade
1	16	F	Disc herniation	L5/6	4
2	18	F	Disc herniation	L4/5	4
3	26	M	Disc herniation	L4/5	5
4	41	M	Disc herniation	L5/S1	4
5	44	M	Disc herniation	L4/5	4
6	56	F	Disc herniation	L3/4	4
7	66	M	Disc herniation	L1/2	5

M male, *F* female

Table 2 Primers for real-time PCR

Target	NCBI number	Forward primer, 5'- 3'	Reverse primer, 5'- 3'
CCN1 (CYR61)	NM_031327.2	TCACTGAAGAGGCTTCCTGTC	CCAGTTCCGCAGCTCTTG
CCN2 (CTGF)	NM_022266.2	GCTGACCTAGAGGAAAACATTAAGA	CCGGTAGGTCTTCACACTGG
CCN3 (NOV)	NM_030868.2	CGGCCTTGTGAGCAAGAG	TTCTTGGTCCGGAGACACTT
CCN4 (Wisp1)	NM_031716.1	ACATCCGACCACACATCAAG	AAGTTCGTGGCCTCCTCTG
CCN5 (Wisp2)	NM_031590.1	CAGGGCCTGGTTTGTCAG	CCGTCATCCTCATCCAAGA
CCN6 (Wisp3)	NM_001170483.1	CATGGAAGGCAGGGAAGA	CTTTGGGGAGTTGGAAAGTG

The relative quantification of gene expression in the treatment groups versus control (cells isolated freshly before culture) was performed using the comparative threshold cycle method:

$$2^{[(C_{tGAPDH}-C_{tGene})_{treatment}-(C_{tGAPDH}-C_{tGene})_{control}]},$$

where glyceraldehyde 3-phosphate dehydrogenase (GAPDH) was used as the housekeeping control gene. GAPDH is has good feasibility as an endogeneous control for IVD cells [22].

Western blot analysis

Treated rat NP cells were immediately placed on ice and washed with cold PBS. To prepare the total cellular proteins, the cells were lysed with lysis buffer containing 10 mM Tris-HCl (pH 7.6), 50 mM NaCl, 5 mM EDTA, 1% Nonidet P-40, complete protease inhibitor cocktail (Roche, IN, USA), 1 mM NaF, and 1 mM Na_3VO_4. Heat-denatured samples were separated on sodium dodecyl sulfate polyacrylamide gels and electrotransferred onto Immobilon-P polyvinylidene difluoride membranes (Millipore, MA, USA). The membranes were then blocked with blocking buffer (5% BSA and 0.1% NaN_3 in PBS) and subsequently incubated overnight at 4 °C with anti-CCN2 (1:1000, Santa Cruz Biotechnology or Abcam, Cambridge, UK) antibodies diluted in Can Get Signal Immunoreaction Enhancer Solution (Toyobo, Tokyo, Japan). Chemiluminescent signals were visualized with an Immobilon Western Chemiluminescent HRP Substrate (Millipore) and scanned using an Ez-Capture MG imaging system (ATTO, Tokyo, Japan). The western blot data were quantified using Image J pixel analysis (NIH Image software). Western blot data are presented as band intensity normalized to that of the loading control (β-actin). To measure the band intensity, the data shown are representative of at least three independent experiments.

Gene-suppression studies using siRNA

We silenced β-catenin expression in NP cells using siRNA technology. In brief, NP cells were transferred into 24-well plates at a density of 6×10^4 cells/well 1 day before transfection. The next day, cells were treated with β-catenin siRNA or control siRNA duplexes at a final concentration of 100–500 ng/ml using Lipofectamine

2000 (Invitrogen). Cells also received CCN2 promoter constructs and the pGL4.74 plasmid at the time of transfection. At 6 h after transfection, the medium was replaced with complete growth medium, and the cells were allowed to recover for 18 h. Cells were then cultured for 24 h and luciferase activity was measured.

Transfections and Dual-Luciferase™ assay

Rat NP and AF cells were transferred to 24-well plates at 3×10^4 cells/well 1 day before transfection. Cells were cotransfected with 100–500 ng of expression plasmids or the backbone vector together with the reporter plasmids. Lipofectamine 2000 (Invitrogen) was used as the transfection reagent. Reporter activity was measured 48 h after transfection using the Dual-Luciferase™ reporter assay system (Promega) for the sequential measurements of *Firefly* and *Renilla* luciferase activities. The results were normalized to the transfection efficiency and are expressed as the ratio of luciferase to pGL4.74 activity (denoted as "relative activity"). NP and AF cells were transfected with a plasmid encoding green fluorescent protein to check the transfection efficiency, which was 60–70% in NP cells. Luciferase activity and relative ratio were quantified using a Turner Designs Luminometer Model TD-20/20 instrument (Promega).

Statistical analysis

All experiments were performed at least three times or more, and the experiment was replicated at least twice each time. The data are expressed as the mean ± 95% confidence interval (CI). Student's t test and the Mann-Whitney U test were used to compare two groups, and one-way analysis of variance (ANOVA) to compare three or more groups. The positivity of protein and gene expression was analyzed by unpaired Student's t test. One-way ANOVA was used to identify significant differences in transcription levels between the study groups. Statistical analyses were performed using SPSS software (ver. 12.0; SPSS Corp., IL, USA). Significance was set at $P < 0.05$.

Results

Expression of CCN family members in IVD cells

We evaluated the expression of all CCN members in cultured rat IVD cells at the mRNA level using real-time

PCR (Fig. 1a). The mRNA expression of all CCN family members was significantly higher in rat AF than in rat NP cells. In particular, expression of *CCN3* mRNA was more prominent in AF cells than NP cells (9560-fold, $P < 0.001$). In addition, the expression level was significantly higher for *CCN2* mRNA than for mRNA of other CCN family members in both rat NP and rat AF cells (Fig. 1b). Next, we measured the gene expression levels of the CCN family members in the human NP samples. The representative MRI images of discs of different age and different levels of degeneration are shown (Fig. 1c). The gene expression of CCN family members was also confirmed, but the gene expression levels of CCN family members except *CCN1* mRNA and *CCN2* mRNA were equivalent in human NP cells (data not shown). Real-time PCR showed a higher level of the *CCN2* mRNA compared with other CCN family members mRNA in the human NP samples. It is unclear because there were few samples, but it was suggested that expression of *CCN2* mRNA may be lower as age increases (Fig. 1d).We also evaluated the expression of CCN2 protein in cultured rat IVD cells using western blot analysis. Figure 2A shows that both NP and AF cells expressed a prominent 38 kDa CCN2 band. The expression level of

CCN2 protein was higher in AF than in NP cells. The expression of CCN2 protein in IVDs from 11 weeks and 32 weeks rats was immunohistochemically examined. CCN2 was expressed in NP and AF cells in discs from 11-week-old rats. However, there was weak expression of CCN2 protein in IVDs from the 32-week-old rats (Fig. 2B). That is, the percentage of cells in the rat NP that were immunopositive for CCN2 decreased significantly with age (11 weeks, $80.9 \pm 9.1\%$; 32 weeks, $13.7 \pm 5.3\%$; $P < 0.001$).

CCN2/CTGF is regulated by Wnt–β-catenin signaling

To determine whether CCN2 expression is modulated by Wnt–β-catenin signaling in rat NP cells, NP and AF cells were cultured with BIO (0–1.0 μM). We first examined activation of Wnt by BIO stimulation. The results showed that there was an increase in the activity of Topflash upon BIO stimulation (Additional file 1: Figure S1).

The activity of the CCN2 promoter decreased 24 h after BIO treatment (1.0 μM) in both NP cells ($P = 0.0077$) (Fig. 3a) and AF cells ($P = 0.0236$) (Additional file 2: Figure S2). In another experimental approach, we transfected rat NP cells with the WT-β-catenin vector or β-catenin siRNA 24 h before the experiments. Treatment with the

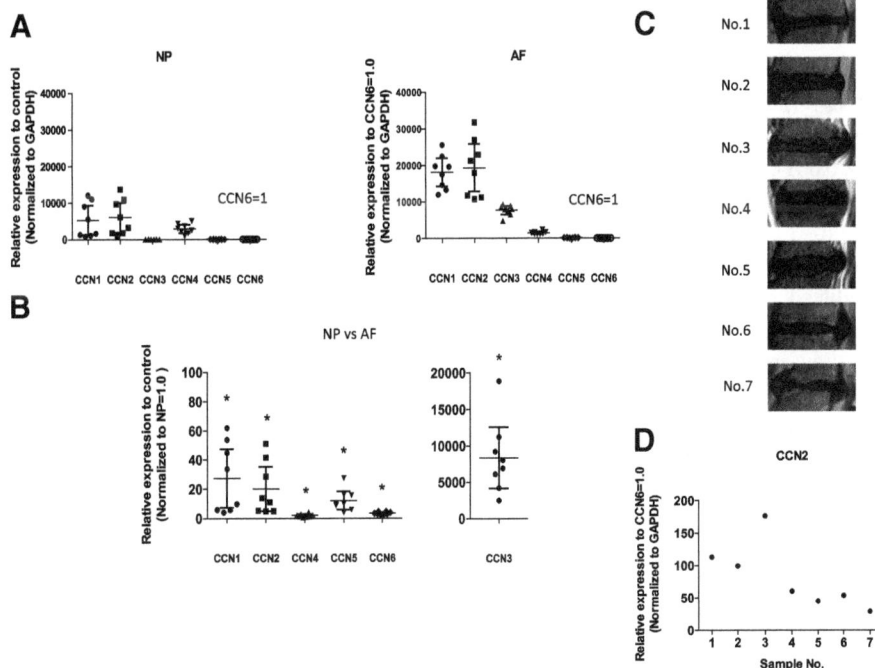

Fig. 1 Expression of CCN family members in rat intravertebral disc (IVD) cells. **a** Real-time RT-PCR analysis of mRNA expression of CCN family members in rat nucleus pulposus (NP) and annulus fibrosus (AF) cells. Results are presented as mean and 95% CI as the fold change relative to the CCN6 (= 1.0) (*n* = 8 for each group) both in NP versus AF cells. **b** Comparison of mRNA expression of CCN family members in NP and AF cells assessed using real-time RT-PCR analysis. Data are the mean and 95% CI (*n* = 8). The unpaired Student's *t* test was used. **c** Lumbar magnetic resonance imaging findings in seven patients. The IVD was low-intensity on T2-weighted images. The IVD was grade 4 in five patients grade 5 in two patients. **d** Real-time RT-PCR analysis of mRNA expression of CCN2 in human NP cells. Glyceraldehyde 3-phosphate dehydrogenase (GAPDH) was used as an endogenous control

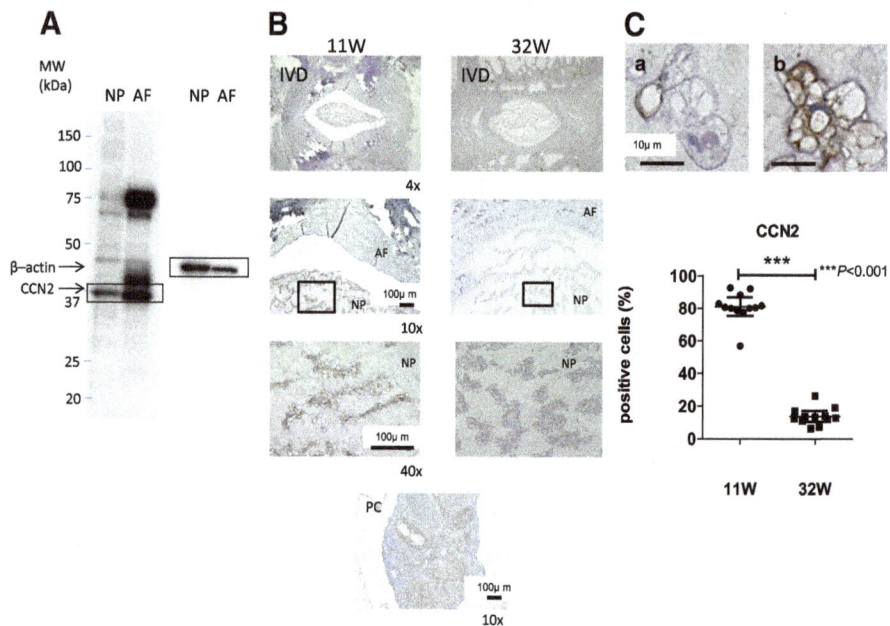

Fig. 2 Expression of CCN2 in rat intravertebral discs (IVDs). **a** Western blot analysis of CCN2 protein in rat nucleus pulposus (NP) and annulus fibrosus (AF) cells. β-actin was used as a loading control. Immunoblots shown are representative of experiments with similar results (n = 8). The unpaired Student's t test was used. **b** Immunohistological staining of CCN2 expression in sagittal sections from 11-week-old (mature) and 32-week-old (adult) rats. Rat kidney was used as positive control (PC). Scale bar = 20–500 μm (× 4–40 original magnification). **c** CCN2 negative (a) and positive (b) cells were immunohistochemically detected in rat NP cells. Cells stained brown are positive cells. The values are the number of CCN2-positive NP cells. The percentage of cells positive for CCN2 in NP cells was calculated from the staining (n = 12). The unpaired Student's t test was used. Scale bar = 10 μm

WT-β-catenin vector significantly decreased CCN2 promoter activity (500 ng) (Fig. 3b) ($P = 0.0063$), whereas β-catenin siRNA significantly increased CCN2 promoter activity (500 ng) ($P < 0.001$) (Fig. 3c). Next, rat NP cells were pretreated with β-catenin siRNA together with a control vector or BIO (0–1.0 μM) 24 h before the experiments. Treatment with β-catenin siRNA significantly attenuated the BIO-induced decrease in CCN2 promoter activity ($P = 0.0419$) (Fig. 3d). These results suggest that Wnt–β-catenin signaling regulates the expression of CCN2 at the transcriptional level.

To confirm the reporter assay data, real-time PCR analysis was performed to analyze the gene expression of CCN family members in both NP and AF cells. As expected, BIO treatment significantly decreased the expression of *CCN1*, *CCN2*, and *CCN5* mRNA at 24 h in NP cells (all $P < 0.001$), while *CCN3* ($P = 0.0037$, $P < 0.01$) and *CCN6* ($P = 0.0037$, $P < 0.01$) mRNA were increased after the BIO treatment (Fig. 4a). Similar results of *CCN1*, *CCN2* and *CCN5* mRNA were obtained with AF cells (Additional file 3: Figure S3). Western blot analysis of cell lysates also indicated that CCN2 protein levels were decreased at 24 h after BIO treatment (Fig. 4b). The expression of the CCN2 protein was further assessed using immunofluorescence microscopy in the BIO-treated NP cells at 24 h after BIO treatment. As shown in (Fig. 4c), CCN2 protein expression was decreased after BIO treatment compared with the untreated control.

Suppression of CCN2 by Wnt–β-catenin signaling through the MAPK pathways in NP cells

To further determine if the MAPK pathway is required for the Wnt–β-catenin signaling-induced regulation of CCN2 expression in the NP cells, we evaluated the activation of the Wnt–β-catenin signaling following treatment with specific inhibitors of ERK1/2 (PD98059) or p38–MAPK (SB202190). NP cells transfected with the CCN2 reporter plasmid together with the pGL4.74 plasmid were treated with specific inhibitors of the MAPK pathway after the BIO (1.0 μM) treatment for 24 h. Figure 5 (a, b) shows that BIO treatment significantly decreased the activity of the CCN2 promoter; this activity was suppressed by the PD98059 (20 μM, $P = 0.017$) and SB202190 (1 μM and 10 μM, $P < 0.001$). To investigate the role of the MAPK pathway in Wnt–β-catenin signaling downregulation of CCN2, we further transfected rat NP cells with WT vector (ERK1, ERK2, and p38) together with BIO, and measured CCN2 promoter activity. The promoter activity of CCN2 was suppressed by BIO treatment, but it was reverse-activated by transfection of WT-ERK1 (Fig. 5c), WT-ERK2 (Fig. 5d) and

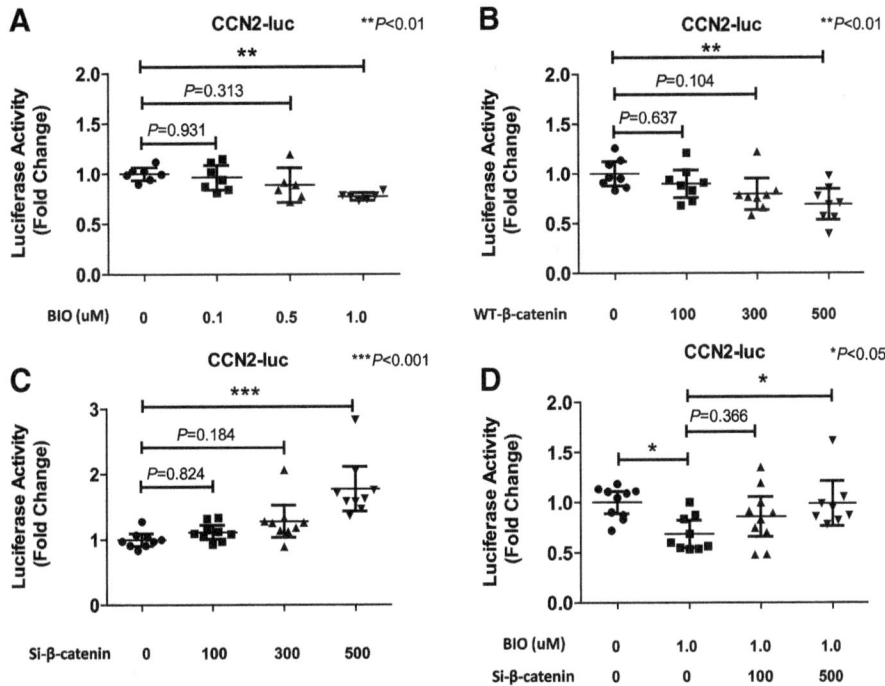

Fig. 3 Effect of Wnt–β-catenin signaling on CCN2 expression in rat nucleus pulposus (NP) cells. **a** Rat NP cells transfected with the CCN2 reporter plasmid together with the pGL4.74 plasmid were treated with different concentrations (0, 0.1, 0.5, 1.0 μM) of 6-bromoindirubin-3′-oxime (BIO) for 24 h. **b**, **c** NP cells were cotransfected with the CCN2 reporter plasmid together with WT-β-catenin (**b**), β-catenin siRNA (si-β-catenin) (**c**), or empty vectors and the pGL4.74 vector. Cells were cultured for 24 h and luciferase (luc) reporter activity was measured. The results were normalized for transfection efficiency and are expressed as the ratio of luciferase relative to pGL4.74 activities (denoted as relative activity). **d** NP cells transfected with the CCN2 reporter plasmid were treated with the β-catenin siRNA (si-β-catenin), which was added during exposure of the cells to 1.0 μM BIO. Results are presented as mean and 95% CI ($n = \geq 8$ for each group). One-way analysis of variance with the Tukey-Kramer post-hoc test was used for all experiments

WT- p38 (Fig. 5e). These results showed that ERK1, ERK2, and p38 abolished the suppression of the transcriptional activity of CCN2 in NP cells treated with BIO. Real-time PCR and western blot analysis also showed that BIO treatment combined with MAPK inhibitors (PD98059 or SB202190) decreased the expression of CCN2 levels further (Fig. 6a) and Fig. 6b).

Densitometric analysis confirms that the MAPK pathway is involved in suppression of CCN2 by Wnt–β-catenin signaling (Fig. 6c). BIO treatment significantly decreased the expression of the *CCN2* mRNA; this activity was not suppressed completely by the JNK inhibitor SP600125 (data not shown). Thus, we did not investigate JNK in this study.

Discussion

The experiments demonstrated for the first time that CCN2 expression in IVD cells is regulated by Wnt–β-catenin signaling. We found that rat IVD cells expressed CCN family members and activation of Wnt–β-catenin signaling reduced activity of the CCN2 promoter, gene, and protein levels in rat NP cells. We have already reported on the involvement of the MAPK pathway in

Wnt–β-catenin signaling [23]. Subsequently, we found that Wnt–β-catenin signaling suppressed CCN2 expression in rat NP cells, and the expression of CCN2 was regulated by Wnt–β-catenin signaling via the MAPK pathway in this study.

CCN2 is a cysteine-rich secretory protein of 36–38 kd containing 349 amino acid residues. It contains a von Willebrand–type C domain that interacts with growth factors such as transforming growth factor (TGF)-β– bone morphogenic proteins (BMPs) and thereby mediates ECM interactions. Erwin et al. found that notochord cells secrete CCN2 and that conditioned medium obtained from these cells upregulates important matrix gene expression, cell proliferation, and proteoglycan production in NP cells [24]. They also suggested that the loss of TGF-β1 and CCN2 is associated with the progression of IVD degeneration [25]. Another group, Oh et al., examined whether CCN2 is regulated by SOX9 in IVD tissues. They not only found that CCN2 expression is regulated directly by the transcription factor SOX9 in chondrocytes, they also detected the SOX9 binding site in NP cells [26]. Although CCN2 is involved in anabolic factors, it is also involved with inflammatory cytokines.

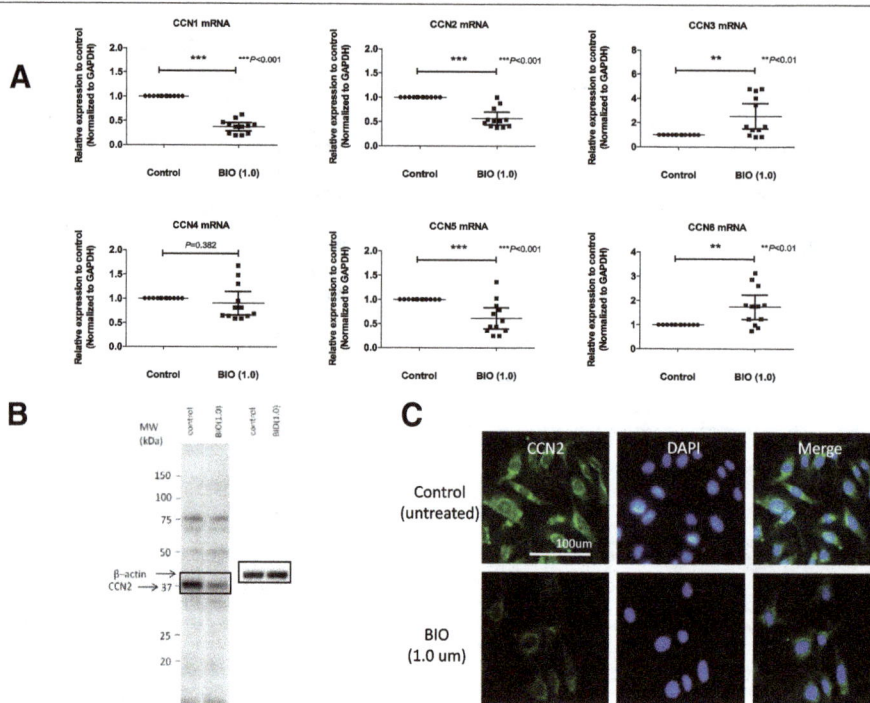

Fig. 4 Effect of Wnt–β-catenin signaling on CCN2 mRNA and protein expression in rat nucleus pulposus (NP) cells. **a** mRNA expression of CCN members (CCN1, CCN2, CCN3, CCN4, CCN5, and CCN6) after exposure of NP cells to 6-bromoindirubin-3'-oxime (BIO) (1.0 μM) for 24 h assessed using real-time PCR. Results are presented as mean and 95% CI ($n = 12$ for each group). Glyceraldehyde 3-phosphate dehydrogenase (GAPDH) was used as an endogenous control. The unpaired Student's t test was used. **b** Western blot analysis of CCN2 protein after treatment of NP cells with BIO (1.0 μM). Western blot analysis showed there was a decrease in the levels of CCN2 protein after BIO treatment. β-actin was used as a loading control. Immunoblots shown are representative of experiments with similar results ($n = 8$). The paired Student's t test was used. **c** Detection of CCN2 protein expression by immunofluorescence microscopy. NP cells were cultured with or without 1.0 μM BIO for 24 h, fixed, and stained with antibody against CCN2. CCN2 protein is decreased with treatment compared with untreated control. Left: cells stained with antibody to CCN2; middle: cells stained with 4',6-diamidino-2-phenylindole (DAPI) to identify healthy nuclei; right: cells stained with antibody to CCN2 and DAPI. Scale bar = 100 μm (× 20 original magnification)

Tran et al. reported that interleukin 1β (IL-1β) and tumor necrosis factor α (TNF-α) suppress CCN2 expression through the nuclear factor-κB signaling pathway in NP cells [12]. These anabolic and catabolic effects suggest that CCN2 may be an important factor in the pathogenesis of IVD disease. Furthermore, from studies using notochord-specific CCN2-null mice, Bedore et al. found that loss of CCN2 in notochord-derived cells resulted in impaired development of IVDs and marked acceleration of age-associated IVD degeneration [27].

Although the involvement of CCN2 in IVD cells has been studied, its regulation remains unknown. Previous studies have demonstrated that Wnt–β-catenin signaling plays a major role in IVD metabolism [19, 28, 29]. Generally, elevated levels of proinflammatory cytokines and other inflammatory mediators, including TNF-α, IL-1β, IL-6, and prostaglandin E_2, are present in degenerating IVDs [30, 31]. We have reported that Wnt–β-catenin signaling regulates TNF-α and that Wnt signaling and TNF-α formed a positive-feedback loop in NP cells [32]. We speculated that blocking the Wnt–β-catenin signaling might protect NP cells against degeneration. However, its relationship with Wnt–β-catenin signaling in the pathogenesis of IVD disease remains unclear. Therefore, the objective of this study was to determine whether CCN2 can be regulated by Wnt–β-catenin signaling.

We first examined the expression and localization of specific CCN family members in rat IVD tissues. The expression of *CCN2* mRNA was significantly higher than that of the mRNA of other CCN family members in both rat NP and AF cells. However, a previous report showed that CCN2 expression is higher in the NP than in the AF and that CCN2 levels are higher in the NP of mature rat discs than in neonatal tissues [13]. This result contrasts with ours because it does not depend on individual differences or age. It may be necessary to perform the same analyses in a larger number of human samples. However, we believe that it is not as important to determine whether CCN2 expression is higher in AF or NP cells as it is to confirm that this expression occurs in both cells.

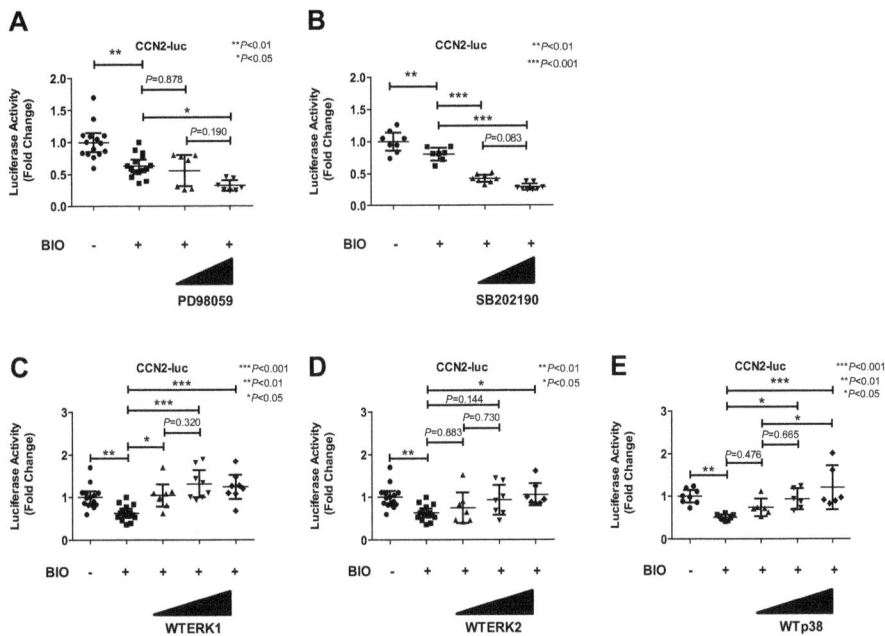

Fig. 5 Wnt–β-catenin signaling suppress CCN2 expression through the mitogen-activated protein kinase (MAPK) pathway in rat nucleus pulposus (NP) cells. **a-b** NP cells transfected with the CCN2 reporter plasmid together with the pGL4.74 plasmid were treated with 6-bromoindirubin-3′-oxime (BIO) (1.0 µM) and the extracellular signal-related protein kinase (ERK) inhibitor (PD98059, 25 or 50 µM) (**a**) or the p38–MAPK inhibitor (SB202190, 1 or 10 µM) (**b**). **c-e** Rat NP cells transfected with the CCN2 reporter plasmid were cotransfected with different concentrations of the wild-type (WT)-ERK1 (**c**), (**d**) WT-ERK2, or (**e**) WT-p38 expression vector together with BIO (1.0 µM). Results are presented as mean and 95% CI ($n = \geq 6$ for each group). One-way analysis of variance with the Tukey-Kramer post-hoc test was used for all experiments

Furthermore, gain-of-function and loss-of-function experiments were performed to identify the mechanism by which Wnt–β-catenin signaling influences the activity of the CCN2 promoter. The results showed that CCN2 promoter activity was regulated by Wnt–β-catenin signaling in NP cells. We speculate that blocking the Wnt–β-catenin signaling might protect NP cells against degeneration by activating CCN2, which stimulates both the proliferation of cells and synthesis of the ECM. We also investigated whether the MAPK pathway is involved in this process. Gain-of-function and loss-of-function experiments were analyzed in the same way. MAPK overexpression increased CCN2 promoter activity, whereas inhibition of the MAPK pathway inhibited its activity. We obtained similar results in gene and protein analysis.

There are several limitations of the present study. First, regulation of the CCN family by Wnt–β-catenin signaling differs between human and rat IVD cells. Animal species and humans differ in many ways in terms of cell populations, anatomy, development, physiology, and mechanical properties of the spine. The central region of the IVD in infant humans is made and maintained by notochordal cells, which disappear during maturation and are replaced by mature chondrocyte-like cells. The disappearance of notochordal cells precedes the onset of IVD degeneration, but whether the disappearance of these cells might be involved in initiating IVD degeneration remains unclear. However, human material is difficult to obtain because of ethical and government regulatory restrictions. Second, as ours is the first report, we conducted the research with simple small animals for analysis. For these reasons, we used normal rat NP cells in several experiments. Third, although we performed cell culture under normoxia, it is well-known that IVD-typical conditions are hypoxic with specific and important effects on cell metabolism. It has been suggested that NP cells are specifically adapted to a hypoxic environment, suggesting that interactions between chemical microenvironment and hypoxia are important questions deserving further study. However, it is very difficult to conclude from all of these study data that low oxygen would be good for the IVD, because there are complex signaling networks involved in IVD degeneration. Finally, we investigated the expression levels of CCN family members in IVD cells and also compared those in the AF and the NP. This showed that the mRNA expression for all CCN family members especially CCN3 was significantly higher in rat AF than in rat NP cells. Thus, we think that further analysis of other CCN family members is necessary, including CCN3.

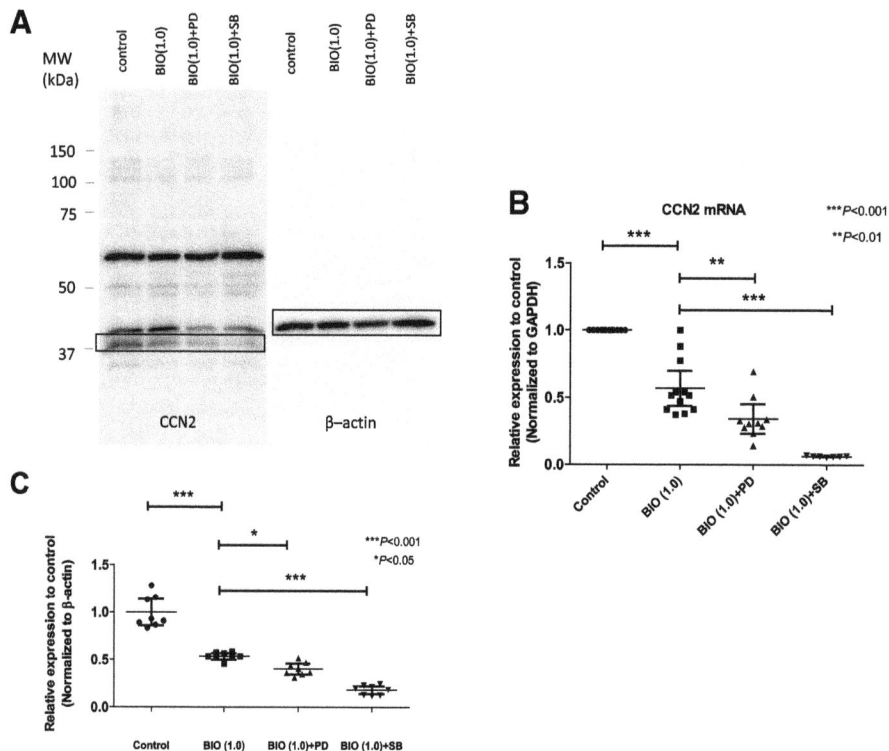

Fig. 6 Regulation of the CCN2 gene and protein by Wnt–β-catenin signaling via the mitogen-activated protein kinase (MAPK) pathway. **a** Western blot analysis of the CCN2 protein in nucleus pulposus (NP) cells after treatment with 6-bromoindirubin-3′-oxime (BIO) with the extracellular signal-related protein kinase (ERK) inhibitor PD98059 (PD) (25 µM) or the p38–MAPK inhibitor SB202190 (SB) (10 µM) in rat NP cells. β-actin was used as a loading control. Data are the mean and 95% CI. One-way analysis of variance with the Tukey-Kramer post-hoc test was used. Immunoblots shown are representative of experiments with similar results ($n = 8$ for each group). **b** Real-time RT-PCR analysis of CCN2 mRNA expression after treatment with BIO with the ERK inhibitor PD98059 (25 µM) or the p38–MAPK inhibitor SB202190 (10 µM) in rat NP cells. Data are the mean and 95% CI expressed as the fold change relative to the control ($n = \geq 7$ for each group). **c** Densitometric analysis as shown (A) confirms that BIO treatment significantly decreased the activity of the CCN2 protein and this activity was suppressed by the MAPK inhibitors treatment. One-way ANOVA with the Tukey-Kramer post-hoc test was used

Conclusion

We found that the expression of CCN2 was regulated by Wnt–β-catenin signaling in IVD cells. That is, activation of Wnt–β-catenin signaling suppressed the expression of CCN2, suggesting the possibility that the MAPK pathway may be involved in this process. However, further studies are needed to investigate whether Wnt–β-catenin signaling has potential as a treatment target for IVD degeneration in vivo.

Abbreviations

AF: Annulus fibrosus; ANOVA: Analysis of variance; BIO: 6-Bromoindirubin-3′-oxime; BMP: Bone morphogenetic proteins; cDNA: Complementary DNA; CTGF: Connective tissue growth factor; ERK: Extracellular signal-regulated protein kinase; FBS: Fetal bovine serum; GAPDH: Glyceraldehyde 3-phosphate dehydrogenase; IL: Interleukin; IVD: Intervertebral disc; LBP: Low back pain; kDa: KiloDalton; MAPK: Mitogen-activated protein kinase; MRI: Magnetic resonance imaging; mRNA: Messenger RNA; PBS: Phosphate-buffered saline; RT-PCR: Reverse transcription polymerase chain reaction; siRNA: Small interfering RNA; TGF-β: Transforming growth factor β; TNF: Tumor necrosis factor; WT: Wild type

Acknowledgements

We greatly appreciate the helpful advice of Dr Tadayuki Sato and the technical assistance of Noboru Kawabe and Masatoshi Ito.

Funding

This study was supported in part by a Grant-in-Aid for Scientific Research (KAKENHI). The study sponsor had no involvement in the study design, collection, analysis, or interpretation of data, writing of the manuscript, or decision to submit the manuscript for publication.

Authors' contributions

AH participated in the design, performed experiments, analyzed data and wrote the paper. KM prepared the isolation of cells and performed experiments and the statistical analysis. DS participated in the design, performed experiments and performed the statistical analysis. MW participated in the design and coordination and helped to draft the manuscript. All authors read and approved the final manuscript.

Ethics approval

All approved animal experiments were performed in accordance with relevant guidelines and regulations of the Ethics Committee at the University of Tokai.

Consent for publication

All authors approved the final version of the manuscript to be published.

Competing interests
The authors declare that they have no competing interests.

References

1. Brigstock DR, Goldschmeding R, Katsube KI, Lam SC, Lau LF, Lyons K, et al. Proposal for a unified CCN nomenclature. Mol Pathol. 2003;56(2):127–8.
2. Jun JI, Lau LF. Taking aim at the extracellular matrix: CCN proteins as emerging therapeutic targets. Nat Rev Drug Discov. 2011;10(12):945–63.
3. Leask A, Abraham DJ. All in the CCN family: essential matricellular signaling modulators emerge from the bunker. J Cell Sci. 2006;119(Pt 23):4803–10.
4. Perbal B. CCN proteins: multifunctional signalling regulators. Lancet (London, England). 2004;363(9402):62–4.
5. Riser BL, Najmabadi F, Perbal B, Rambow JA, Riser ML, Sukowski E, et al. CCN3/CCN2 regulation and the fibrosis of diabetic renal disease. J Cell Comm Signaling. 2010;4(1):39–50.
6. Kubota S, Takigawa M. Role of CCN2/CTGF/Hcs24 in bone growth. Int Rev Cytol. 2007;257:1–41.
7. Takigawa M, Nakanishi T, Kubota S, Nishida T. Role of CTGF/HCS24/ecogenin in skeletal growth control. J Cell Physiol. 2003;194(3):256–66.
8. Nakanishi T, Kimura Y, Tamura T, Ichikawa H, Yamaai Y, Sugimoto T, et al. Cloning of a mRNA preferentially expressed in chondrocytes by differential display-PCR from a human chondrocytic cell line that is identical with connective tissue growth factor (CTGF) mRNA. Biochem Biophys Res Commun. 1997;234(1):206–10.
9. Nishida T, Kubota S, Nakanishi T, Kuboki T, Yosimichi G, Kondo S, et al. CTGF/Hcs24, a hypertrophic chondrocyte-specific gene product, stimulates proliferation and differentiation, but not hypertrophy of cultured articular chondrocytes. J Cell Physiol. 2002;192(1):55–63.
10. Ivkovic S, Yoon BS, Popoff SN, Safadi FF, Libuda DE, Stephenson RC, et al. Connective tissue growth factor coordinates chondrogenesis and angiogenesis during skeletal development. Development (Cambridge, England). 2003;130(12):2779–91.
11. Kawaki H, Kubota S, Suzuki A, Lazar N, Yamada T, Matsumura T, et al. Cooperative regulation of chondrocyte differentiation by CCN2 and CCN3 shown by a comprehensive analysis of the CCN family proteins in cartilage. J Bone Miner Res. 2008;23(11):1751–64.
12. Tran CM, Schoepflin ZR, Markova DZ, Kepler CK, Anderson DG, Shapiro IM, et al. CCN2 suppresses catabolic effects of interleukin-1beta through alpha5beta1 and alphaVbeta3 integrins in nucleus pulposus cells: implications in intervertebral disc degeneration. J Biol Chem. 2014;289(11):7374–87.
13. Tran CM, Markova D, Smith HE, Susarla B, Ponnappan RK, Anderson DG, et al. Regulation of CCN2/connective tissue growth factor expression in the nucleus pulposus of the intervertebral disc: role of Smad and activator protein 1 signaling. Arthritis Rheum. 2010;62(7):1983–92.
14. Tran CM, Shapiro IM, Risbud MV. Molecular regulation of CCN2 in the intervertebral disc: lessons learned from other connective tissues. Matrix Biol. 2013;32(6):298–306.
15. Peng B, Chen J, Kuang Z, Li D, Pang X, Zhang X. Expression and role of connective tissue growth factor in painful disc fibrosis and degeneration. Spine. 2009;34(5):E178–82.
16. Deng YZ, Chen PP, Wang Y, Yin D, Koeffler HP, Li B, et al. Connective tissue growth factor is overexpressed in esophageal squamous cell carcinoma and promotes tumorigenicity through beta-catenin-T-cell factor/Lef signaling. J Biol Chem. 2007;282(50):36571 81.
17. Xu L, Corcoran RB, Welsh JW, Pennica D, Levine AJ. WISP-1 is a Wnt-1- and beta-catenin-responsive oncogene. Genes Dev. 2000;14(5):585–95.
18. Sato N, Meijer L, Skaltsounis L, Greengard P, Brivanlou AH. Maintenance of pluripotency in human and mouse embryonic stem cells through activation of Wnt signaling by a pharmacological GSK-3-specific inhibitor. Nat Med. 2004;10(1):55–63.
19. Hiyama A, Sakai D, Risbud MV, Tanaka M, Arai F, Abe K, et al. Enhancement of intervertebral disc cell senescence by WNT/beta-catenin signaling-induced matrix metalloproteinase expression. Arthritis Rheum. 2010;62(10):3036–47.
20. Pfirrmann CW, Metzdorf A, Zanetti M, Hodler J, Boos N. Magnetic resonance classification of lumbar intervertebral disc degeneration. Spine. 2001;26(17):1873–8.
21. Hiyama A, Mochida J, Iwashina T, Omi H, Watanabe T, Serigano K, et al. Transplantation of mesenchymal stem cells in a canine disc degeneration model. J Orthop Res. 2008;26(5):589–600.
22. Yurube T, Takada T, Hirata H, Kakutani K, Maeno K, Zhang Z, et al. Modified house-keeping gene expression in a rat tail compression loading-induced disc degeneration model. J Orthop Res. 2011;29(8):1284–90.
23. Hiyama A, Sakai D, Tanaka M, Arai F, Nakajima D, Abe K, et al. The relationship between the Wnt/beta-catenin and TGF-beta/BMP signals in the intervertebral disc cell. J Cell Physiol. 2011;226(5):1139–48.
24. Erwin WM, Ashman K, O'Donnel P, Inman RD. Nucleus pulposus notochord cells secrete connective tissue growth factor and up-regulate proteoglycan expression by intervertebral disc chondrocytes. Arthritis Rheum. 2006;54(12):3859–67.
25. Matta A, Karim MZ, Isenman DE, Erwin WM. Molecular therapy for degenerative disc disease: clues from secretome analysis of the notochordal cell-rich nucleus pulposus. Sci Rep. 2017;7:45623.
26. Oh CD, Yasuda H, Zhao W, Henry SP, Zhang Z, Xue M, et al. SOX9 directly Regulates CTGF/CCN2 Transcription in growth plate chondrocytes and in nucleus pulposus cells of intervertebral disc. Sci Rep. 2016;6:29916.
27. Bedore J, Sha W, McCann MR, Liu S, Leask A, Seguin CA. Impaired intervertebral disc development and premature disc degeneration in mice with notochord-specific deletion of CCN2. Arthritis Rheum. 2013;65(10):2634–44.
28. Smolders LA, Meij BP, Riemers FM, Licht R, Wubbolts R, Heuvel D, et al. Canonical Wnt signaling in the notochordal cell is upregulated in early intervertebral disk degeneration. J Orthop Res. 2012;30(6):950–7.
29. Winkler T, Mahoney EJ, Sinner D, Wylie CC, Dahia CL. Wnt signaling activates Shh signaling in early postnatal intervertebral discs, and re-activates Shh signaling in old discs in the mouse. PLoS One. 2014;9(6):e98444.
30. Burke JG, Watson RW, McCormack D, Dowling FE, Walsh MG, Fitzpatrick JM. Spontaneous production of monocyte chemoattractant protein-1 and interleukin-8 by the human lumbar intervertebral disc. Spine. 2002;27(13):1402–7.
31. Le Maitre CL, Hoyland JA, Freemont AJ. Catabolic cytokine expression in degenerate and herniated human intervertebral discs: IL-1beta and TNFalpha expression profile. Arthritis Res Ther. 2007;9(4):R77.
32. Hiyama A, Yokoyama K, Nukaga T, Sakai D, Mochida J. A complex interaction between Wnt signaling and TNF-alpha in nucleus pulposus cells. Arthritis Res Ther. 2013;15(6):R189.

20

Modulation of T-cell responses by anti-tumor necrosis factor treatments in rheumatoid arthritis

Jean-Luc Davignon[1,2*], Benjamin Rauwel[1], Yannick Degboé[1,2,3], Arnaud Constantin[1,2,3], Jean-Fredéric Boyer[1,2], Andrey Kruglov[4,5] and Alain Cantagrel[1,2,3]

Abstract

Tumor necrosis factor (TNF) is a pleiotropic cytokine involved in many aspects of immune regulation. Anti-TNF biological therapy has been considered a breakthrough in the treatment of chronic autoimmune diseases, such as rheumatoid arthritis (RA). In this review, because of the major involvement of T cells in RA pathogenesis, we discuss the effects of anti-TNF biotherapy on T-cell responses in RA patients. We also outline the potential fields for future research in the area of anti-TNF therapy in RA.

This could be useful to better understand the therapeutic efficiency and the side effects that are encountered in RA patients. Better targeting of T cells in RA could help set more specific anti-TNF strategies and develop prediction tools for response.

Keywords: Rheumatoid arthritis, Anti-TNF, Biotherapy, T-cell

Background

The discovery of the role of tumor necrosis factor (TNF) in the pathogenesis of rheumatoid arthritis (RA) has led to anti-TNF biological therapy as a breakthrough in the treatment of chronic autoimmune diseases, such as RA, Crohn's disease, psoriatic arthritis, and spondyloarthritis [1]. Various anti-TNFs are currently used for the treatment of RA, including infliximab (IFX), a chimeric antibody, and two fully human antibodies adalimumab (ADA) and golimumab. Additionally, etanercept (ETA) is a human recombinant dimeric fusion protein consisting of two soluble p75 TNF-RII chains linked to a modified Fc portion of human IgG. Finally, certolizumab pegol (CZP) is a pegylated Fab' fragment of a humanized anti-TNF antibody. Biosimilars of IFX and of ETA are already in use.

TNF is a pleiotropic cytokine involved in many aspects of immune regulation [2]. TNF is first synthesized as a biologically active transmembrane homotrimer (tmTNF), which is further released upon cleavage by tumor necrosis factor-alpha converting enzyme (TACE, also named ADAM17) protease. Soluble TNF binds to the receptors TNF-RI and TNF-RII, while tmTNF binds preferentially to TNF-RII. Anti-TNF biologics can block both soluble and tmTNF [3]. TNF can be produced by multiple cell types such as T and B cells and innate immune cells (dendritic cells, monocytes, neutrophils, mast cells). All these sources may contribute to the development of a pathological state of chronic inflammation, especially in RA. T cells are also targets of TNF either directly, like all cells that express TNF-Rs, or indirectly as a result of antigen presentation or costimulation. The immunomodulatory role of TNF-R2 on T-cell activity has been described in the collagen-induced arthritis (CIA) model of arthritis [4].

In this review, because of the major involvement of T cells in RA pathogenesis, we discuss the effects of anti-TNF biotherapy on T-cell responses in RA patients. This could be of help for the interpretation of the clinical effects (or lack thereof) of anti-TNF treatments, as well as being useful to better understand the side effects which are encountered in RA patients.

* Correspondence: jean-luc.davignon@inserm.fr
[1]Centre de Physiopathologie Toulouse Purpan, INSERM-CNRS-UPS, UMR 1043, CHU Purpan, 1 Place Baylac, 31024 Toulouse Cedex, France
[2]Centre de Rhumatologie, CHU de Toulouse, 31059 Toulouse, France
Full list of author information is available at the end of the article

Role of T cells in RA

Much has been learned from mouse models in the understanding of RA, especially regarding the role of T cells. Collagen-induced, K/BxN, IL-1 RA-KO, and SKG models were shown to depend on T lymphocytes [5]. More specifically, the SKG model, depending on a mutation in ZAP 70 that affects the TcR-ζ chain signaling and T-cell selection, directly implicated the role of T cells in the development of experimental arthritis.

There has been an ongoing debate over the respective importance of macrophages and T cells. The presence of T cells in joints and the expansion of clonotypic T cells, as a result or a cause of inflammation, in the synovium of RA patients has fueled that debate. The role of the HLA-DR shared epitope in the development of RA is a strong indication for the role of T cells [6]. There is a T-cell response to citrullinated T-cell epitopes or PAD peptides [7] in patients who bear the RA susceptibility HLA-DR allele. A direct argument for the role of T lymphocytes in RA has been the successful use of CTLA4-Ig as a biotherapy that blocks the CD28-CD86/CD80 interaction [8]. Thus, the current view is that there is an interplay between pathogenic T cells, macrophages, and cytokines that contributes to the pathogenic imbalance in RA [9] and can be targeted with biologics.

Role of TNF in the development of the immune system

TNF has been shown to be essential in many stages of T-cell development. In the thymus, TNF promotes the apoptosis of triple-negative CD3/CD4/CD8 [10] and double positive CD4/CD8 thymocytes [11], as well as the development of single positive thymocytes [12]. Thus, it is expected that treatment of infants with anti-TNF might alter the development of their T cells. This needs further investigation.

Secondary lymphoid organs (SLO) are crucial for the development of efficient adaptive immune responses. Organized in well-demarcated T-cell zones and B-cell follicles, SLO bring the antigen that is trapped by various subsets of dendritic cells (DCs) in close contact with the immune cells, provide costimulatory signals from DCs, and thereby initiate an appropriate immune response.

TNF-mediated signaling is crucial for the development of some and for structural maintenance of most of the SLO. Distinct cellular sources and molecular forms of TNF contribute to the organization of SLO microarchitecture. TNF from B and T cells cooperates to maintain the structural integrity in lymph nodes, which are indispensable for the generation of efficient local immune responses.

The requirement of TNF signaling for organized lymphoid structures in mice was confirmed by studies in humans. Rheumatoid arthritis patients receiving ETA lack germinal center development in their tonsils [13]. Similar experiments in mice showed that pharmacological inhibition of TNF by ETA leads to inhibition of follicular dendritic cell development and a subsequent decrease in germinal center response, as well as a reduction in the marginal zone [14]. However, the structure of B-cell follicles in the spleen remained unchanged, suggesting that some of the TNF-dependent features of splenic microarchitecture are not inhibited by ETA [14].

Altogether, TNF controls the development and organization of SLO structures and, thereby, influences the development of adaptive immune responses. This could be of importance during the follow-up of RA patients, especially children, treated with anti-TNF.

Role of TNF in T-cell differentiation, activation, and maturation: action of TNF inhibitors

Activation of naive T cells is initiated during their encounter with antigen peptide presented by mature DCs. This activation is dependent on coactivation mediated by the membrane interaction between members of the TNF/TNF-R family other than TNF cytokine on T cells and DCs. As a cytokine, TNF contributes to efficient antigen presentation by inducing DC maturation.

Interaction of T cells with antigen presenting cells leads to differentiation into effector and memory T cells (reviewed in [15]). To understand how anti-TNF treatment may exert an impact on the pathogenicity of T lymphocytes, we first need to overview the role of TNF in the activation of effector, memory, and regulatory T cells.

TNF is reported to negatively regulate the expansion of effector CD4$^+$ and CD8$^+$ T cells during viral infection through apoptosis, thus subsequently limiting the T cell memory compartment [16]. TNF, acting along with interleukin (IL)-33, transforming growth factor (TGF)-β and IL-15, induces resident memory T cells (T$_{RM}$) with CD69 and CD103 expression [15]. These T cells do not recirculate and remain in the lymphoid tissue. Production of TNF by T$_{RM}$ in turn contributes to the maturation of DCs and efficient Ag presentation for recall T-cell activation. Anti-TNF biologics are thus expected to modulate the effector and the memory T-cell response during infections and vaccination (vide infra).

To invade inflamed tissue, T lymphocytes must have the capacity to traffic through endothelial cell junctions. This phenomenon, called diapedesis, has been shown to depend on TNF and interferon (IFN)-γ [17]. Thus, although this has never been tested formally, anti-TNF drugs have the capacity to reduce inflammation by interfering with diapedesis and migration of T cells to the joints.

However, TNF has a contrasting role in T-cell activation [18, 19]. The notion of long-term pathogenic effects of TNF in disease was pioneered by Maini and Feldmann, based on the observation of elevated TNF production in the joints of RA patients. They also reported that chronic exposure of cells to TNF impaired the T cell-specific recall response to tetanus toxoid. This inhibition was later shown to be due to attenuation of TcR signaling. At the molecular level, TNF appeared to inhibit CD3-ζ chain expression via Src-like adaptor protein (SLAP) degradation [20].

Toxicity of IFX for T cells is minimal and the metabolism of T cells is not significantly altered by anti-TNF [21]. However, T-cell subsets were not investigated, and this requires further studies. Regarding in-vitro T-cell activation, impairment of T cells from RA patients can be reversed by anti-TNF and, correspondingly, anti-TNF treatment of RA patients restores in-vitro proliferation in response to soluble antigens [22]. In a model of transmembrane expression of TNF in the Jurkat T-cell line (tm-Jurkat), Mitoma et al. [23] showed that IFX induces JNK activation and IL-10 production, and inhibits proliferation. Reverse signaling is a mechanism of signaling mediated by anti-TNF or TNF-R through binding to tmTNF [3]. Reverse signaling has been suggested to regulate inflammation in macrophages and T cells. However, the molecular mechanisms are not completely understood and demonstration of in-vivo reverse signaling has yet to be demonstrated.

Another possible mechanism of action of anti-TNF on T cells is the regulation of cell death. The action of anti-TNF drugs on cell death was tested using the Jurkat T-cell line transfected with tmTNF [24]. Due to the absence of the Fc fragment, CZP did not induce antibody-dependent cell-mediated cytotoxicity or complement-dependent cytotoxicity, whereas golimumab, IFX, and ADA did. CZP and ETA did not induce apoptosis in tmTNF Jurkat cells [24]. However, those data were obtained with cells overexpressing tmTNF and cannot be extrapolated to physiologic conditions. In tm-Jurkat T-cells, ADCC and CDC, induced by IFX and ADA, were of lower intensity than with ETA, and were not observed with CZP [24].

In patients with active RA, spontaneous apoptosis of CD4+CD25+ cells was evaluated at the start of treatment with IFX and after 3 months of treatment [25]. It was shown that spontaneous in-vitro apoptosis of CD4+CD25+ cells, which was increased in RA patients compared with healthy donors, was reduced after treatment with IFX [25].

Effects of anti-TNF on T-helper cell subset differentiation

There is now a growing literature in RA patients on increased T helper (Th)1 [26–29] and Th17 [26, 27, 29,

30] responses following TNF blockade. Th17 and shifting to nonclassic Th1 have been described as potential components of the pathophysiology of RA, but their overall significance is debated [31].

Hull et al. reported that patients responding to ADA or ETA had an increase in circulating Th17 [30]. Conversely, an increase in Th17 has been reported in patients not responding to TNF inhibitors [27, 32, 33]. Along similar lines, a good response was correlated with low levels of Th17 and was shown to be controlled by regulatory T cells (Tregs) in patients treated with ADA, not in those treated with ETA [34]. Th1 compartments were also reported to be increased in patients not responding to IFX [27] and, conversely, in patients in remission in response to ADA [26].

Furthermore, all the anti-TNF drugs IFX, ADA, CZP, and ETA induce IL-17+CD4+ T cells expressing IL-10 in RA patients [35]. The induction of IL-10 in association with IL-17 by Th17 suggests a modulatory role of those cells, but this needs to be demonstrated.

In conclusion, Th17 and Th1 compartments are increased in response to TNF inhibitors but a definitive answer as to whether they are linked to good or poor responses is needed. This is likely to depend on Th CD4+ T-cell phenotyping techniques, on the biologic administered, and the methodology used.

STAT6, which is associated with the Th2 response, was also induced in T cells from patients treated with ADA [36]. This would suggest a role for ADA in modifying T-cell polarization. Modifications of macrophage polarization induced by anti-TNF (our unpublished data) could also lead to changes in T-cell polarization.

The development of paradoxical psoriasis as a side effect of anti-TNF (ETA, IFX, or ADA) treatment in RA patients has been observed. The mechanism has been shown to involve IFN-α produced by plasmacytoid dendritic cells whose maturation is inhibited by anti-TNF [37] and not to the emergence of Th17 cells during treatment as previously suggested [38]. Recently, a new population of CD4+ T cells, called T peripheral helper (Tph) cells, has been identified in the synovial membrane of RA patients using mass cytometry technology [39]. Tph cells are CD4+ T cells that express high levels of the checkpoint protein PD-1 and, contrary to T-follicular helper cells (Tfh), do not express CXCR5. Tph cells induce the differentiation of plasma cells through IL-21. The inhibition of Tph by anti-TNFs [33] may prevent the differentiation of plasmablasts [39].

Anti-TNF treatments affect Tregs in RA

There are 2 types of CD4CD25 FoxP3-positive Tregs, inducible (iTregs) and natural (nTregs). Inducible Tregs depend on TNF-R2 as exemplified by the observation that TNF-R2 is critical for stabilization and homeostasis of Tregs [40]. TNF has been reported to be either an activator or inhibitor of Tregs depending on the study, as reviewed in [41]. TNF was reported to inhibit both the phosphorylation of FoxP3 and the development of Tregs in correlation with an increase in IL-17- and IFN-γ-producing CD4$^+$ T cells [42]. However, it was shown that Tregs did not lose their suppressive activity in the presence of TNF. Because TNF has costimulatory effects [18], T-effector cells (Teff) may appear resistant to the effect of Tregs [43], and this may have led to previous misinterpretation of the negative role of TNF on Tregs. It was first shown that Tregs from RA patients are present but defective and their function can be restored by IFX treatment. An induced population of iTregs, whose activity is mediated through IL-10 and TGF-β, is restored under the action of IFX, whereas defective nTregs are not [44]. This can be explained by a new mechanism of action with binding of ADA to tmTNF, which is strongly expressed by monocytes

from RA patients. ADA induces higher levels of tmTNF in those monocytes and promotes interaction with TNF-R2-expressing iTregs, which subsequently expand [45]. Such a phenomenon is not observed with ETA. Thus, anti-TNF antibody, but not soluble receptor, induces iTregs through increased expression of tmTNF.

On the T lymphocyte side, the role of soluble versus tmTNF has been explored in several models. T lymphocyte-monocyte contact is important in inflammation. This involves, in part, tmTNF interaction with TNF-R2 on adjacent cells [46]. Blocking tmTNF on T lymphocytes impairs the production of TNF by monocytes [46], and tmTNF expressed by T cells is responsible for the modulation of IL-10 production by monocytes [47].

In T cells, IFX but not ETA induces IL-10 production through reverse signaling, showing disparity in the efficacy of biologics regarding molecular mechanisms [23]

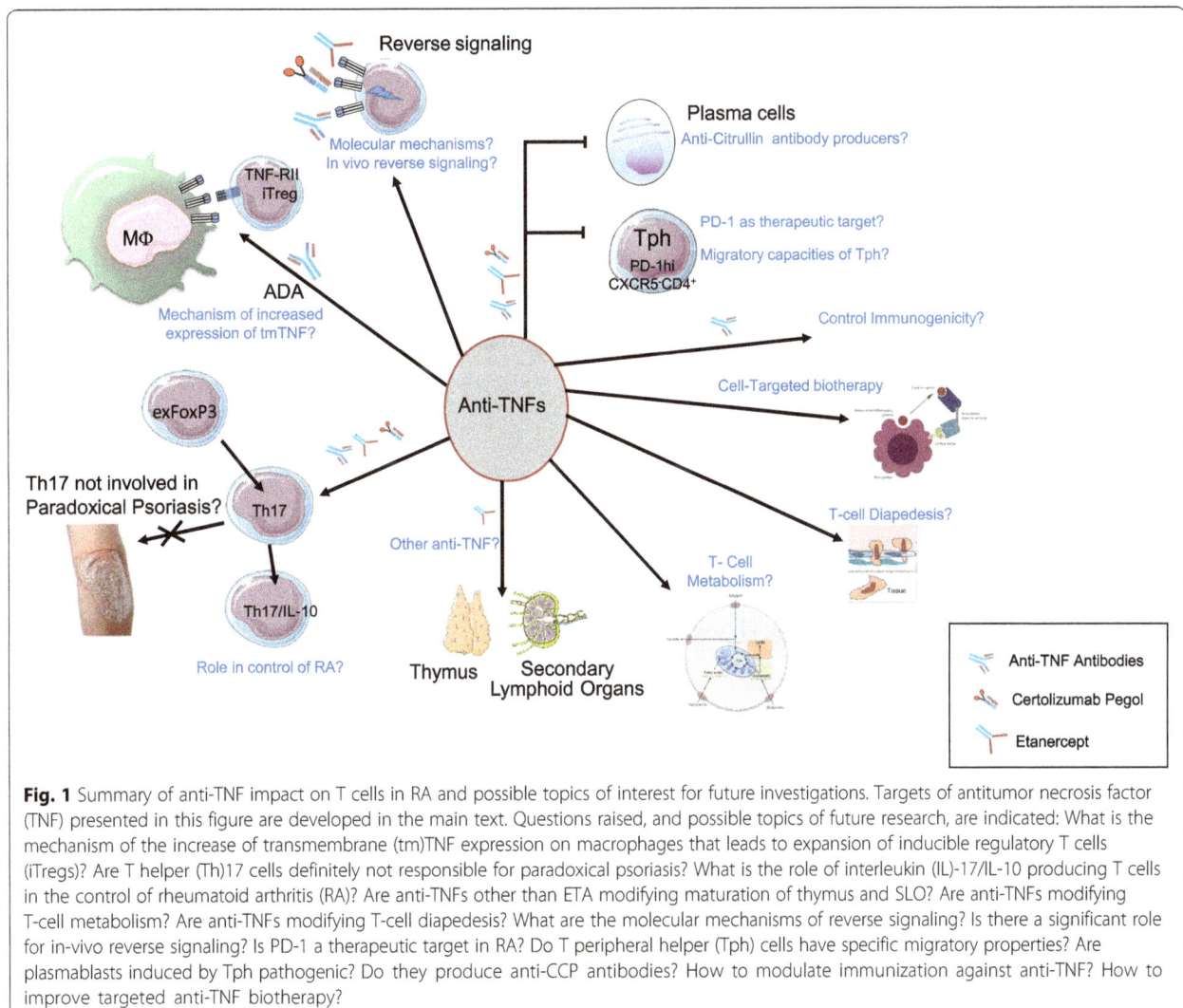

Fig. 1 Summary of anti-TNF impact on T cells in RA and possible topics of interest for future investigations. Targets of antitumor necrosis factor (TNF) presented in this figure are developed in the main text. Questions raised, and possible topics of future research, are indicated: What is the mechanism of the increase of transmembrane (tm)TNF expression on macrophages that leads to expansion of inducible regulatory T cells (iTregs)? Are T helper (Th)17 cells definitely not responsible for paradoxical psoriasis? What is the role of interleukin (IL)-17/IL-10 producing T cells in the control of rheumatoid arthritis (RA)? Are anti-TNFs other than ETA modifying maturation of thymus and SLO? Are anti-TNFs modifying T-cell metabolism? Are anti-TNFs modifying T-cell diapedesis? What are the molecular mechanisms of reverse signaling? Is there a significant role for in-vivo reverse signaling? Is PD-1 a therapeutic target in RA? Do T peripheral helper (Tph) cells have specific migratory properties? Are plasmablasts induced by Tph pathogenic? Do they produce anti-CCP antibodies? How to modulate immunization against anti-TNF? How to improve targeted anti-TNF biotherapy?

Table 1 Summary of specific effects of TNF inhibitors on T cells

	IFX	ADA	CZP	ETA
SLO	–	–	–	Patients lack germinal center development in tonsils [13]
Th1	↗ in nonresponders [27]	↗ in responders [26]	–	↗ in responders [26]
Th17	↗ in nonresponders [27]	↗ in nonresponders [32]	–	↗ in nonresponders [27, 32]
	–	↘ Associated with ultrasound improvement [30]	–	↘ Associated with ultrasound improvement [30]
	–	Good response correlated with low levels of Th17 [34]	-	No correlation of good response with low levels of Th17 [34]
	Induction of IL-17+ IL-10+ CD4+ T cells [35]	Induction of IL-17+ IL-10+ CD4+ T cells [35]	Induction of IL-17+ IL-10+ CD4+ T-cells [35]	Induction of IL-17+ IL-10+ CD4+ T cells [35]
Tph	Decrease in Tph [39]	–	Decrease in Tph [39]	Decrease in Tph [39]
Treg	Restoration of functional Tregs [44]	Expansion of iTregs through tmTNF-Mo/TNF-RII T-cell interaction [45]	–	No expansion of iTregs [45]
T-cell activation	Induction of STAT4 and STAT6 [36]	–	–	–
Reverse signaling	Induction of IL-10 in tm-Jurkat cells [23]	–	–	No induction of IL-10 in tm-Jurkat cells [23]
	Suppression of tm-Jurkat cell proliferation [23]	–	–	No suppression of tm-Jurkat cell proliferation [23]
	JNK activation in tm-Jurkat [23]	–	–	No JNK activation in tm-Jurkat [23]
Metabolism	Not affected [21]	–	–	–
Infections	Tb reactivation [48]	Tb reactivation [48]	Tb reactivation [48]	Lower rate of Tb reactivation than with Abs [48]
	Reduction of Tb-specific CD8+ memory cells [49]	–	–	–
	Inhibition of CD4+ response [50]	Inhibition of CD4+ response [50]	–	Inhibition of CD4+ response less pronounced than with Abs [50]
	Risk of listeria infection [51]	–	–	Lower risk of listeria infection than with sIFX [51]
	CD4+ response to CMV Ags conserved [54]	CD4+ response to CMV Ags conserved [54]	–	CD4+ response to CMV Ags conserved [54]
	Reactivation of HBV chronic infection [55]	Reactivation of HBV chronic infection [55]	–	Possibly less reactivation of HBV chronic infection [55]
Vaccination	Inadvertent vaccination with live vaccines (yellow fever, VZV) suggest they may be safer than expected [62]	Inadvertent vaccination with live vaccines (yellow fever, VZV) suggest they may be safer than expected [62]	Inadvertent vaccination with live vaccines (yellow fever, VZV) suggest they may be safer than expected [62]	Inadvertent vaccination with live vaccines (yellow fever, VZV) suggest they may be safer than expected [62]
	Pneumococcal and influenza vaccine immunogenicity not reduced by anti-TNF [61, 62]	Pneumococcal and influenza vaccine immunogenicity not reduced by anti-TNF [61, 62]	Pneumococcal and influenza vaccine immunogenicity not reduced by anti-TNF [61, 62]	Pneumococcal and influenza vaccine immunogenicity not reduced by anti-TNF [61, 62]
	No specific effect of TNF inhibitors on HBV protective immunity [56]	No specific effect of TNF inhibitors on HBV protective immunity [56]	–	No specific effect of TNF inhibitors on HBV protective immunity [56]
Antidrug antibodies	A proportion of patients develop antidrug antibodies	A proportion of patients develop antidrug antibodies	A proportion of patients develop antidrug antibodies	Fewer patients develop antidrug antibodies which appear to be less neutralizing
Cell death	Induction of ADCC and CDC in tm-Jurkat [24]	Induction of ADCC and CDC in tm-Jurkat [24]	No induction of ADCC and CDC in tm-Jurkat [24]	Lower induction of ADCC or CDC in tm-Jurkat in tm-Jurkat [24]
	Loss of cell viability of tm-Jurkat [24]	Loss of cell viability of tm-Jurkat [24]	No loss of cell viability of tm-Jurkat [24]	No loss of cell viability of tm-Jurkat [24]

Table 1 Summary of specific effects of TNF inhibitors on T cells *(Continued)*

	IFX	ADA	CZP	ETA
Apoptosis	Apoptosis of tm-Jurkat [24]	Apoptosis of tm-Jurkat [24]	No apoptosis of tm-Jurkat [24]	No apoptosis of tm-Jurkat [24]
	Apoptosis of CD3-activated T cells [66]	Apoptosis of CD3-activated T cells [66]	No apoptosis of CD3-activated T cells [66]	Apoptosis of CD3-activated T cells [66]
	Spontaneous in-vitro apoptosis of CD4$^+$CD25$^+$ T cells diminished [25]	–	–	–

Only references in which modifications of Th1/Th17 are correlated with clinical response are listed
tm-TNF Jurkat is a model of Jurkat T cells transfected with a noncleavable form of TNF [23]
Golimumab is not listed because too few data were available on this biologic
– not available, Ab antibody, ADA adalimumab, ADCC antibody-dependent cell-mediated cytotoxicity, Ag antigen, CDC cell-dependent cytotoxicity, CMV cytomegalovirus, CZP certolizumab pegol, ETA etanercept, HBV hepatitis B virus, IFX infliximab, IL interleukin, iTreg inducible regulatory T cell, s soluble, SLO secondary lymphoid organs, Tb tuberculosis, Th T helper, Tph T peripheral helper, tm transmembrane, TNF tumor necrosis factor, Treg regulatory T cell, VZV varicella zoster virus

but suggesting a possible regulatory role for reverse signaling depending on the biologic used.

Consequences of anti-TNF treatments on T-cell control of infections

Reactivation of tuberculosis during anti-TNF therapy by monoclonal antibodies and, to a lesser extent, by ETA has been a major drawback of biotherapies of rheumatic diseases [48]. Production of IFN-γ is, along with TNF, a major element of the T-cell immune response against tuberculosis. Nowadays, recommendations are to test for prior tuberculosis infection before anti-TNF treatments using interferon-gamma release assays (IGRAs) that detect specific T-cell response. Antituberculosis antibiotic prophylaxis has considerably reduced the risks of reactivation.

IFX triggers a reduction in CD8$^+$ terminally differentiated effector memory CD45RA$^+$ T cells (TEMRA cells) with antimicrobial activity against mycobacterium tuberculosis and is responsible for impairing the T-cell defense against microbes [49].

CD4$^+$ T-cell proliferation and IFN-γ production against tuberculosis PPD and CFP-10 antigens were shown to be impaired by a 14-week treatment with anti-TNF in patients with a positive test for prior tuberculosis infection [50]. The inhibition was more pronounced in vitro with antibodies than with ETA.

CD8$^+$-derived TNF is essential for antilisteria activity in mice. Patients treated with IFX are at higher risk for infections with listeria, another intracellular bacteria, than those treated with ETA [51].

Viral infections are controlled at least in part by CD4$^+$ and CD8$^+$ T lymphocytes through their cytotoxic activity and their release of cytokines such as TNF and IFN-γ [52]. Anti-TNF biotherapies have been shown to induce disparate changes in the antivirus immunity which may be due to modifications of SLO and/or direct inhibition of the antiviral effect of TNF. There is no clear evidence for a risk of varicella zoster virus (VZV) and

cytomegalovirus (CMV) reactivation in patients undertaking biotherapies [53] and we have shown that the anti-CMV CD4$^+$ response in RA patients treated with IFX, ADA, or ETA is conserved [54]. However, caution is required with respect to the safety of anti-TNF in patients with those viral infections.

Hepatitis B infections are controlled by T lymphocytes. Depletion of the T-cell response by anti-TNF treatments may explain the resurgence of hepatitis B chronic infections which may occur more frequently with antibodies than with ETA [55]. There is an increased risk of viral reactivation in patients with chronic HBV. Antiviral prophylaxis is required in these patients. It is not known whether the risks with different anti-TNFs are similar or not. Patients with past infection have no particular risk [56].

Recommendations with regard to hepatitis B and C infections in patients treated with anti-TNF have been proposed [57]. Caution is required in patients treated with anti-TNF regarding the follow-up of chronic infection or active infection. In any case, TNF inhibitors can be discontinued as they do not induce irreversible inhibition of TNF production [58].

Consequences of anti-TNF on T-dependent B-cell responses

TNF is involved in T cell-dependent B-cell responses. Resting memory CD45RO$^+$ T cells activated by cytokines, among them TNF, can provide help to B cells for the production of IgM, IgG, and IgA [59]. CD4$^+$ T cells expressing tmTNF provide a costimulatory signal for B cells [60].

Regarding response to vaccines, clinical studies performed with influenza and pneumococcal [61] vaccination reported only modest decreases in antibody titers in patients treated with ADA and safe immunization. Vaccination recommendations for the physician are provided in a recent article [62].

A proportion of RA patients treated with anti-TNF biologics develop antidrug antibodies that can hamper the efficiency of treatments [63]. Due to its structure, ETA has lower immunogenicity than anti-TNF antibodies and anti-ETA antibodies seem to be non-neutralizing [63]. Antigen presenting cells take up anti-TNF antibodies as antigens and present epitopes to CD4$^+$ T cells. Such immunogenicity of anti-TNF antibodies in RA patients suggests that there is no profound decay of T cell-mediated B-cell immunity. Thus, from a functional point of view, only a partial decrease of the B-cell response is observed in RA patients treated with anti-TNF. Although cumbersome, a way of reducing the immunogenicity of anti-TNF antibodies would be to identify T cell epitopes and to modify them accordingly. From a clinical point of view, prescribing anti-TNF with methotrexate, an immunosuppressive drug that reduces the production of Th1 cytokines [64], decreases the risk of antidrug antibodies.

Conclusion

Figure 1 summarizes the consequences of anti-TNF on T-cell homeostasis. Anti-TNF can regulate the T-cell responses in many ways. By inducing iTregs through TNF-RII and restoring T-cell function, these biologics contribute to reducing the autoimmune process. Although apparently contradictory, the induction of iTregs and the restoration of T-cell effector functions suggest that anti-TNF acts on multiple aspects of T-cell homeostasis. Although T cell-dependent B-cell activation is decreased, the risks of immunization resulting in anti-antibodies hampers the efficiency of treatment. In this regard, ETA induces less antidrug antibodies.

Differences between antibodies (IFX and ADA), and monovalent CZP, and ETA were outlined in the present review. They are summarized in Table 1. It appears that ETA and CZP induce less cell death and apoptosis than IFX and ADA. Alteration of the immune response to infections is less pronounced with ETA than with IFX and ADA but control of bacterial and viral infections is decreased by anti-TNF, and assessment of the infection and vaccine status is required. Vaccinations are recommended but not those using attenuated viruses or bacteria.

The mode of action, especially on T cells, of TNF-inhibitors is still not completely understood. For example, reverse signaling induced by TNF inhibitors must be explored in more detail. Future therapeutic strategy for RA should still take TNF inhibitors into account despite the availability of other biologics targeting other cytokines such as IL-6 and the more recent advent of JAKi. The choice of molecule should depend on better knowledge of the mode of action of the various TNF inhibitors. Nonspecific effects of anti-TNF antibodies on the immune system plead for a more targeted action such as bispecific antibodies targeting cells on the one hand and proinflammatory cytokine on the other [65].

Abbreviations
ADA: Adalimumab; CMV: Cytomegalovirus; CZP: Certolizumab pegol; DC: Dendritic cell; ETA: Etanercept; IFX: Infliximab; IFN: Interferon; IL: Interleukin; iTreg: Inducible regulatory T cell; RA: Rheumatoid arthritis; SLO: Secondary lymphoid organs; Th: T helper; TGF: Transforming growth factor; tm: Transmembrane; TNF: Tumor necrosis factor; Tph: T peripheral helper; Treg: Regulatory T cell; T$_{RM}$: Resident memory T cells; VZV: Varicella zoster virus

Acknowledgements
We thank Sergei A. Nedospasov for critical reading of the manuscript.

Funding
This work was supported by CNRS "CoopInter" and a Pfizer "Passerelle" grant.

Authors' contributions
All authors read and approved the final manuscript.

Consent for publication
Not applicable.

Competing interests
The authors declare that they have no competing interests.

Author details
^{1}Centre de Physiopathologie Toulouse Purpan, INSERM-CNRS-UPS, UMR 1043, CHU Purpan, 1 Place Baylac, 31024 Toulouse Cedex, France. ^{2}Centre de Rhumatologie, CHU de Toulouse, 31059 Toulouse, France. ^{3}Faculté de Médecine, Université Paul Sabatier Toulouse III, 31062 Toulouse, France. ^{4}Lomonosov Moscow State University, 119991 Moscow, Russia. ^{5}German Rheumatism Research Center (DRFZ), 10117 Berlin, Germany.

References
1. Feldmann M, Maini RN. Anti-TNF therapy, from rationale to standard of care: what lessons has it taught us? J Immunol. 2010;185:791–4.
2. Kalliolias GD, Ivashkiv LB. TNF biology, pathogenic mechanisms and emerging therapeutic strategies. Nat Rev Rheumatol. 2016;12:49–62.
3. Horiuchi T, Mitoma H, Harashima S, Tsukamoto H, Shimoda T. Transmembrane TNF-alpha: structure, function and interaction with anti-TNF agents. Rheumatology (Oxford). 2010;49:1215–28.
4. McCann FE, Perocheau DP, Ruspi G, Blazek K, Davies ML, Feldmann M, et al. Selective tumor necrosis factor receptor I blockade is antiinflammatory and reveals immunoregulatory role of tumor necrosis factor receptor II in collagen-induced arthritis: immunoregulatory role of TNFRII in CIA. Arthritis Rheumatol. 2014;66:2728–38.
5. Benson RA, McInnes IB, Garside P, Brewer JM. Model answers: rational application of murine models in arthritis research. Eur J Immunol. 2018; 48:32–8.
6. Gourraud P-A, Dieudé P, Boyer J-F, Nogueira L, Cambon-Thomsen A, Mazières B, et al. A new classification of HLA-DRB1 alleles differentiates predisposing and protective alleles for autoantibody production in rheumatoid arthritis. Arthritis Res Ther. 2007;9:R27.
7. Roudier J, Balandraud N, Auger I. HLA-DRB1 polymorphism, anti-citrullinated protein antibodies, and rheumatoid arthritis. J Biol Chem. 2018;293:7038.
8. Kremer JM, Westhovens R, Leon M, Di Giorgio E, Alten R, Steinfeld S, et al. Treatment of rheumatoid arthritis by selective inhibition of T-cell activation with fusion protein CTLA4Ig. N Engl J Med. 2003;349:1907–15.
9. Firestein GS. The T cell cometh: interplay between adaptive immunity and cytokine networks in rheumatoid arthritis. J Clin Invest. 2004;114:471–4.

10. Baseta JG, Stutman O. TNF regulates thymocyte production by apoptosis and proliferation of the triple negative (CD3-CD4-CD8-) subset. J Immunol. 2000;165:5621–30.

11. Guevara Patiño JA, Ivanov VN, Lacy E, Elkon KB, Marino MW, Nikolic-Zugić J. TNF-alpha is the critical mediator of the cyclic AMP-induced apoptosis of CD8+4+ double-positive thymocytes. J Immunol. 2000;164:1689–94.

12. Webb LV, Ley SC, Seddon B. TNF activation of NF-κB is essential for development of single-positive thymocytes. J Exp Med. 2016;213:1399–407.

13. Anolik JH, Ravikumar R, Barnard J, Owen T, Almudevar A, Milner ECB, et al. Cutting edge: anti-tumor necrosis factor therapy in rheumatoid arthritis inhibits memory B lymphocytes via effects on lymphoid germinal centers and follicular dendritic cell networks. J Immunol. 2008;180:688–92.

14. Tumanov AV, Grivennikov SI, Kruglov AA, Shebzukhov YV, Koroleva EP, Piao Y, et al. Cellular source and molecular form of TNF specify its distinct functions in organization of secondary lymphoid organs. Blood. 2010;116:3456–64.

15. Chang JT, Wherry EJ, Goldrath AW. Molecular regulation of effector and memory T cell differentiation. Nat Immunol. 2014;15:1104–15.

16. Suresh M, Singh A, Fischer C. Role of tumor necrosis factor receptors in regulating CD8 T-cell responses during acute lymphocytic choriomeningitis virus infection. J Virol. 2005;79:202–13.

17. Jaczewska J, Abdulreda MH, Yau CY, Schmitt MM, Schubert I, Berggren P-O, et al. TNF-α and IFN-γ promote lymphocyte adhesion to endothelial junctional regions facilitating transendothelial migration. J Leukoc Biol. 2014;95:265–74.

18. Kim EY, Priatel JJ, Teh S-J, Teh H-S. TNF receptor type 2 (p75) functions as a costimulator for antigen-driven T cell responses in vivo. J Immunol. 2006;176:1026–35.

19. Chen X, Oppenheim JJ. Contrasting effects of TNF and anti-TNF on the activation of effector T cells and regulatory T cells in autoimmunity. FEBS Lett. 2011;585:3611–8.

20. Érsek B, Molnár V, Balogh A, Matkó J, Cope AP, Buzás EI, et al. CD3ζ-chain expression of human T lymphocytes is regulated by TNF via Src-like adaptor protein-dependent proteasomal degradation. J Immunol. 2012;189:1602–10.

21. Chimenti MS, Tucci P, Candi E, Perricone R, Melino G, Willis AE. Metabolic profiling of human CD4+ cells following treatment with methotrexate and anti-TNF-α infliximab. Cell Cycle. 2013;12:3025–36.

22. Cope AP, Londei M, Chu NR, Cohen SB, Elliott MJ, Brennan FM, et al. Chronic exposure to tumor necrosis factor (TNF) in vitro impairs the activation of T cells through the T cell receptor/CD3 complex; reversal in vivo by anti-TNF antibodies in patients with rheumatoid arthritis. J Clin Invest. 1994;94:749–60.

23. Mitoma H, Horiuchi T, Hatta N, Tsukamoto H, Harashima S-I, Kikuchi Y, et al. Infliximab induces potent anti-inflammatory responses by outside-to-inside signals through transmembrane TNF-alpha. Gastroenterology. 2005;128:376–92.

24. Ueda N, Tsukamoto H, Mitoma H, Ayano M, Tanaka A, Ohta S, et al. The cytotoxic effects of certolizumab pegol and golimumab mediated by transmembrane tumor necrosis factor α. Inflamm Bowel Dis. 2013;19:1224–31.

25. Toubi E, Kessel A, Mahmudov Z, Hallas K, Rozenbaum M, Rosner I. Increased spontaneous apoptosis of CD4+CD25+ T cells in patients with active rheumatoid arthritis is reduced by infliximab. Ann N Y Acad Sci. 2005;1051:506–14.

26. Aerts NE, De Knop KJ, Leysen J, Ebo DG, Bridts CH, Weyler JJ, et al. Increased IL-17 production by peripheral T helper cells after tumour necrosis factor blockade in rheumatoid arthritis is accompanied by inhibition of migration-associated chemokine receptor expression. Rheumatology (Oxford). 2010;49:2264–72.

27. Talotta R, Berzi A, Atzeni F, Batticciotto A, Clerici M, Sarzi-Puttini P, et al. Paradoxical expansion of Th1 and Th17 lymphocytes in rheumatoid arthritis following infliximab treatment: a possible explanation for a lack of clinical response. J Clin Immunol. 2015;35:550–7.

28. Szalay B, Vásárhelyi B, Cseh A, Tulassay T, Deák M, Kovács L, et al. The impact of conventional DMARD and biological therapies on CD4+ cell subsets in rheumatoid arthritis: a follow-up study. Clin Rheumatol. 2014;33:175–85.

29. Dulic S, Vásárhelyi Z, Sava F, Berta L, Szalay B, Toldi G, et al. T-cell subsets in rheumatoid arthritis patients on long-term anti-TNF or IL-6 receptor blocker therapy. Mediat Inflamm. 2017;2017:6894374.

30. Hull DN, Cooksley H, Chokshi S, Williams RO, Abraham S, Taylor PC. Increase in circulating Th17 cells during anti-TNF therapy is associated with

31. Cosmi L, Liotta F, Maggi E, Romagnani S, Annunziato F. Th17 and non-classic Th1 cells in chronic inflammatory disorders: two sides of the same coin. Int Arch Allergy Immunol. 2014;164:171–7.

32. Chen D-Y, Chen Y-M, Chen H-H, Hsieh C-W, Lin C-C, Lan J-L. Increasing levels of circulating Th17 cells and interleukin-17 in rheumatoid arthritis patients with an inadequate response to anti-TNF-α therapy. Arthritis Res Ther. 2011;13:R126.

33. Alzabin S, Abraham SM, Taher TE, Palfreeman A, Hull D, McNamee K, et al. Incomplete response of inflammatory arthritis to TNFα blockade is associated with the Th17 pathway. Ann Rheum Dis. 2012;71:1741–8.

34. McGovern JL, Nguyen DX, Notley CA, Mauri C, Isenberg DA, Ehrenstein MR. Th17 cells are restrained by Treg cells via the inhibition of interleukin-6 in patients with rheumatoid arthritis responding to anti-tumor necrosis factor antibody therapy. Arthritis Rheum. 2012;64:3129–38.

35. Evans HG, Roostalu U, Walter GJ, Gullick NJ, Frederiksen KS, Roberts CA, et al. TNF-α blockade induces IL-10 expression in human CD4+ T cells. Nat Commun. 2014;5:3199.

36. Aerts NE, Ebo DG, Bridts CH, Stevens WJ, De Clerck LS. T cell signal transducer and activator of transcription (STAT) 4 and 6 are affected by adalimumab therapy in rheumatoid arthritis. Clin Exp Rheumatol. 2010;28:208–14.

37. Conrad C, Di Domizio J, Mylonas A, Belkhodja C, Demaria O, Navarini AA, et al. TNF blockade induces a dysregulated type I interferon response without autoimmunity in paradoxical psoriasis. Nat Commun. 2018;9:25.

38. Wendling D, Prati C. Paradoxical effects of anti-TNF-α agents in inflammatory diseases. Expert Rev Clin Immunol. 2014;10:159–69.

39. Rao DA, Gurish MF, Marshall JL, Slowikowski K, Fonseka CY, Liu Y, et al. Pathologically expanded peripheral T helper cell subset drives B cells in rheumatoid arthritis. Nature. 2017;542:110–4.

40. Chen X, Wu X, Zhou Q, Howard OMZ, Netea MG, Oppenheim JJ. TNFR2 is critical for the stabilization of the CD4+Foxp3+ regulatory T cell phenotype in the inflammatory environment. J Immunol. 2013;190:1076–84.

41. Byng-Maddick R, Ehrenstein MR. The impact of biological therapy on regulatory T cells in rheumatoid arthritis. Rheumatology (Oxford). 2015;54:768–75.

42. Nie H, Zheng Y, Li R, Guo TB, He D, Fang L, et al. Phosphorylation of FOXP3 controls regulatory T cell function and is inhibited by TNF-α in rheumatoid arthritis. Nat Med. 2013;19:322–8.

43. Zaragoza B, Chen X, Oppenheim JJ, Baeyens A, Gregoire S, Chader D, et al. Suppressive activity of human regulatory T cells is maintained in the presence of TNF. Nat Med. 2016;22:16–7.

44. Nadkarni S, Mauri C, Ehrenstein MR. Anti-TNF-alpha therapy induces a distinct regulatory T cell population in patients with rheumatoid arthritis via TGF-beta. J Exp Med. 2007;204:33–9.

45. Nguyen DX, Ehrenstein MR. Anti-TNF drives regulatory T cell expansion by paradoxically promoting membrane TNF-TNF-RII binding in rheumatoid arthritis. J Exp Med. 2016;213:1241–53.

46. Rossol M, Meusch U, Pierer M, Kaltenhäuser S, Häntzschel H, Hauschildt S, et al. Interaction between transmembrane TNF and TNFR1/2 mediates the activation of monocytes by contact with T cells. J Immunol. 2007;179:4239–48.

47. Parry SL, Sebbag M, Feldmann M, Brennan FM. Contact with T cells modulates monocyte IL-10 production: role of T cell membrane TNF-alpha. J Immunol. 1997;158:3673–81.

48. Wallis RS. Infectious complications of tumor necrosis factor blockade. Curr Opin Infect Dis. 2009;22:403–9.

49. Bruns H, Meinken C, Schauenberg P, Härter G, Kern P, Modlin RL, et al. Anti-TNF immunotherapy reduces CD8+ T cell-mediated antimicrobial activity against Mycobacterium tuberculosis in humans. J Clin Invest. 2009;119:1167–77.

50. Hamdi H, Mariette X, Godot V, Weldingh K, Hamid AM, Prejean M-V, et al. Inhibition of anti-tuberculosis T-lymphocyte function with tumour necrosis factor antagonists. Arthritis Res Ther. 2006;8:R114.

51. Slifman NR, Gershon SK, Lee J-H, Edwards ET, Braun MM. Listeria monocytogenes infection as a complication of treatment with tumor necrosis factor alpha-neutralizing agents. Arthritis Rheum. 2003;48:319–24.

52. Kaech SM, Wherry EJ, Ahmed R. Effector and memory T-cell differentiation: implications for vaccine development. Nat Rev Immunol. 2002;2:251–62.

53. Kim SY, Solomon DH. Tumor necrosis factor blockade and the risk of viral infection. Nat Rev Rheumatol. 2010;6:165–74.

54. Davignon J-L, Boyer J-F, Jamard B, Nigon D, Constantin A, Cantagrel A. Maintenance of cytomegalovirus-specific CD4pos T-cell response in rheumatoid arthritis patients receiving anti-tumor necrosis factor treatments. Arthritis Res Ther. 2010;12:R142.

55. Carroll MB, Bond MI. Use of tumor necrosis factor-alpha inhibitors in patients with chronic hepatitis B infection. Semin Arthritis Rheum. 2008;38: 208–17.

56. Nard FD, Todoerti M, Grosso V, Monti S, Breda S, Rossi S, et al. Risk of hepatitis B virus reactivation in rheumatoid arthritis patients undergoing biologic treatment: extending perspective from old to newer drugs. World J Hepatol. 2015;7:344–61.

57. Viganò M, Degasperi E, Aghemo A, Lampertico P, Colombo M. Anti-TNF drugs in patients with hepatitis B or C virus infection: safety and clinical management. Expert Opin Biol Ther. 2012;12:193–207.

58. Balog A, Klausz G, Gál J, Molnár T, Nagy F, Ocsovszky I, et al. Investigation of the prognostic value of TNF-alpha gene polymorphism among patients treated with infliximab, and the effects of infliximab therapy on TNF-alpha production and apoptosis. Pathobiology. 2004;71:274–80.

59. Unutmaz D, Pileri P, Abrignani S. Antigen-independent activation of naive and memory resting T cells by a cytokine combination. J Exp Med. 1994; 180:1159–64.

60. Aversa G, Punnonen J, de Vries JE. The 26-kD transmembrane form of tumor necrosis factor alpha on activated CD4+ T cell clones provides a costimulatory signal for human B cell activation. J Exp Med. 1993;177:1575–85.

61. Kaine JL, Kivitz AJ, Birbara C, Luo AY. Immune responses following administration of influenza and pneumococcal vaccines to patients with rheumatoid arthritis receiving adalimumab. J Rheumatol. 2007;34:272–9.

62. Friedman MA, Winthrop KL. Vaccines and disease-modifying antirheumatic drugs: practical implications for the rheumatologist. Rheum Dis Clin N Am. 2017;43:1–13.

63. van Schouwenburg PA, Rispens T, Wolbink GJ. Immunogenicity of anti-TNF biologic therapies for rheumatoid arthritis. Nat Rev Rheumatol. 2013;9:164–72.

64. Cutolo M, Sulli A, Pizzorni C, Seriolo B, Straub RH. Anti-inflammatory mechanisms of methotrexate in rheumatoid arthritis. Ann Rheum Dis. 2001; 60:729–35.

65. Drutskaya MS, Efimov GA, Kruglov AA, Nedospasov SA. Can we design a better anti-cytokine therapy? J Leukoc Biol. 2017;102:783–90.

66. Nesbitt A, Fossati G, Bergin M, Stephens P, Stephens S, Foulkes R, et al. Mechanism of action of certolizumab pegol (CDP870): in vitro comparison with other anti-tumor necrosis factor alpha agents. Inflamm Bowel Dis. 2007;13:1323–32.

21

Obesity alters the *in vivo* mechanical response and biochemical properties of cartilage as measured by MRI

Amber T Collins[1], Micaela L Kulvaranon[1], Hattie C Cutcliffe[1,2], Gangadhar M Utturkar[1], Wyatt A R Smith[1], Charles E Spritzer[4], Farshid Guilak[5] and Louis E DeFrate[1,2,3*]

Abstract

Background: Obesity is a primary risk factor for the development of knee osteoarthritis (OA). However, there remains a lack of *in vivo* data on the influence of obesity on knee cartilage mechanics and composition. The purpose of this study was to determine the relationship between obesity and tibiofemoral cartilage properties.

Methods: Magnetic resonance images (3T) of cartilage geometry (double-echo steady-state) and T1rho relaxation of the knee were obtained in healthy subjects with a normal (n = 8) or high (n = 7) body mass index (BMI) before and immediately after treadmill walking. Subjects had no history of lower limb injury or surgery. Bone and cartilage surfaces were segmented and three-dimensional models were created to measure cartilage thickness and strain. T1rho relaxation times were measured before exercise in both the tibial and femoral cartilage in order to characterize biochemical composition. Body fat composition was also measured.

Results: Subjects with a high BMI exhibited significantly increased tibiofemoral cartilage strain and T1rho relaxation times (P <0.05). Tibial pre-exercise cartilage thickness was also affected by BMI (P <0.05). Correlational analyses revealed that pre-exercise tibial cartilage thickness decreased with increasing BMI (R^2 = 0.43, P <0.01) and body fat percentage (R^2 = 0.58, P <0.01). Tibial and femoral cartilage strain increased with increasing BMI (R^2 = 0.45, P <0.01; R^2 = 0.51, P <0.01, respectively) and increasing body fat percentage (R^2 = 0.40, P <0.05; R^2 = 0.38, P <0.05, respectively). Additionally, tibial T1rho was positively correlated with BMI (R^2 = 0.39, P <0.05) and body fat percentage (R^2 = 0.47, P <0.01).

Conclusions: Strains and T1rho relaxation times in the tibiofemoral cartilage were increased in high BMI subjects compared with normal BMI subjects. Additionally, pre-exercise tibial cartilage thickness decreased with obesity. Reduced proteoglycan content may be indicative of pre-symptomatic osteoarthritic degeneration, resulting in reduced cartilage thickness and increased deformation of cartilage in response to loading.

Keywords: Obesity, Cartilage, Magnetic resonance imaging (MRI), Proteoglycan, mechanobiology, stress test

Background

Obesity is a major risk factor for osteoarthritis (OA) [1–3] and the incidence of knee OA in obese individuals is four times greater than that in healthy weight controls [4]. Whereas the association between OA and obesity has been established, the mechanisms by which obesity increases the risk for OA are not well understood. Some studies attribute the increased risk of OA with obesity to increased joint loading due to elevated body mass [5, 6]; however, more recently, it has been suggested that a combination of biomechanical and metabolic factors, such as cartilage catabolism due to adipokine-related inflammation, plays an important role in this relationship [7, 8]. Furthermore, the presence of OA in non-weight-bearing joints of obese subjects [9, 10] suggests that factors other than mechanical loading potentially contribute to disease progression.

* Correspondence: lou.defrate@duke.edu
[1]Department of Orthopaedic Surgery, Duke University, Box 3093, Duke University Medical Center, Durham, NC 27710, USA
[2]Department of Biomedical Engineering, Duke University, Campus Box 90281, 101 Science Drive, Durham 27708, NC, USA
Full list of author information is available at the end of the article

Nonetheless, there remains a lack of *in vivo* data describing the effects of obesity on cartilage composition and mechanical function. Although gait analysis studies can provide estimates of the loads experienced by the knee joint [11–13], it is unclear how these estimated loads relate to local *in vivo* cartilage deformation. Cartilage is a biphasic viscoelastic material due to the time-dependent exudation of water that occurs following mechanical loading of the tissue. Owing to the low permeability of the cartilage matrix, recovery of water back into the matrix once unloaded is not immediate [14–17]. Several studies have used magnetic resonance imaging (MRI) to characterize the *in vivo* deformation of cartilage by taking advantage of this time-dependent biomechanical recovery following loading [14–19]. Thus, this technique can be used to assess the effects of obesity on *in vivo* cartilage mechanics.

Previously, Widmyer et al. used MRI to show that increased body mass index (BMI) is associated with increased diurnal cartilage strains in the knee when compared with normal weighted controls; diurnal strain was defined as change in cartilage thickness from morning to evening [18]. However, it is unclear whether these increased cartilage strains associated with obesity are due solely to greater body mass or alterations in cartilage composition or both. Currently, there are limited *in vivo* data quantifying how obesity relates to alterations in cartilage composition and how these changes are related to altered mechanical function. Quantitative MRI techniques, such as T1rho-weighted imaging, have been used to quantify *in vivo* proteoglycan content in cartilage [20–24] and therefore can be used to assess changes in cartilage composition with obesity. The objective of this study was to assess how obesity alters both the *in vivo* mechanical function and composition of cartilage. We hypothesized that obesity is associated with a reduction in proteoglycan content, as evidenced by increased T1rho relaxation times. Additionally, we hypothesized that these alterations in composition result in decreased cartilage stiffness, which will be reflected by increased *in vivo* cartilage strain in response to mechanical loading. Our overall hypothesis is that obese subjects exhibit "pre-OA" changes in both articular cartilage composition and mechanical function that precede the onset of symptomatic OA.

Methods
Subject recruitment
Following approval by the institutional review board of Duke University Medical Center, eight subjects (five males and three females; mean age 30 years, range 23–43; mean height 70 in., range 64–74) with a normal BMI (mean 22.2; range 18–25) and seven subjects (three males and four females; mean age 32, range 22–45;

mean height 66 in., range 63–71) with a high BMI (mean 32.8; range 30–36), who were otherwise healthy, were recruited for participation in this study. The normal BMI and high BMI groups were statistically significantly different with regard to BMI ($P < 0.0001$, t test). However, no statistically significant differences were detected with regard to age ($P = 0.64$, t test), height ($P = 0.08$, t test), or the distribution of males and females between groups ($P = 0.613$, Fisher's exact test). Previous work from our lab investigating cartilage strains in healthy subjects tested eight subjects and found significant changes in cartilage thickness as a result of treadmill walking [15]. Therefore, we aimed to recruit and test a similar number of subjects per group in the present study. All subjects provided informed written consent before beginning the study. Subjects were excluded if they had a history of lower limb injury, surgery, or symptoms related to OA.

Study procedure
In order to minimize the effect of diurnal cartilage loading [14, 18, 19], subjects were tested early in the morning and instructed not to perform any strenuous activities on the day prior to and the morning of testing. Upon arrival, subjects lay supine for 45 min prior to the pre-exercise MRI scan to allow their knee cartilage to relax to its baseline, unloaded state in a room adjacent to the MRI scanner [19]. Following this relaxation period, subjects were transported to the MRI scanner in a wheelchair. Pre-exercise MRI images of each subject's right knee were taken in the sagittal plane using a 3.0 T MRI scanner with an eight-channel knee coil [25] (Trio Tim, Siemens Medical Solutions USA, Malvern, PA, USA). A three-dimensional (3D) double-echo steady-state (DESS) sequence—flip angle: 25°; echo time (TE): 6 ms; repetition time (TR): 17 ms; field of view (FOV): 16 × 16 cm; matrix: 512 × 512 pixels; resolution: 0.3 × 0.3 × 1.0 mm—was used to obtain anatomical images of the bones and articular cartilage, allowing for pre-exercise cartilage thickness measurements. A T1rho-weighted imaging sequence with a 3D fast imaging with steady-state precession (FISP) acquisition—flip angle: 15°; TE: 5.9 ms; TR: 3500 ms; FOV: 14 × 14 cm; matrix: 256 × 256 pixels; resolution: 1.1 × 0.5 × 3.0 mm; B1: 500 Hz; spin lock time (TSL): 5, 10, 40, 80 ms—was collected in order to assess proteoglycan content within the cartilage [14, 15]. Following the pre-exercise MRI scan, subjects were transported by wheelchair to an adjacent room where they walked on a treadmill for 20 min. Walking speed was normalized to the subject's leg length using the Froude number (Fr) ($Fr = v^2/(L \times g)$) [26], which uses leg length (L) as measured from the greater trochanter of the femur to the ground surface, and the gravitational constant ($g = 9.8$ m/s^2) in order to calculate a normalized walking

speed (v). Subjects walked at a Froude number of 0.25, which corresponds to an adult walking at a comfortable pace [26]. Subjects also wore a pedometer to record the number of steps taken during their 20-min walk. Immediately following exercise, subjects were transported back to the MRI scanner for a post-exercise DESS sequence scan which was used to measure post-exercise cartilage thickness. Lastly, each subject's body composition (weight and body fat percentage) was measured immediately following the post-exercise MRI scan by using a bioelectrical impedance scale (InBody230, BioSpace Inc., Cerritos, CA, USA) [27].

Data analysis

The tibial and femoral bony and articular cartilage surfaces were segmented on the DESS images by using solid modeling software (Rhinoceros; Robert McNeel & Associates, Seattle, WA, USA) [14–16]. Segmentations from each DESS MRI slice were compiled to create 3D mesh models of the proximal tibia and distal femur as well as of both the associated articulating surfaces. The pre-exercise and post-exercise models were registered together by using an iterative closest-point algorithm, allowing for site-specific comparisons of cartilage thickness between the pre- and post-exercise scans (Geomagic Studio; Geomagic, 3D Systems, Valencia, CA, USA) [28]. Cartilage thickness maps were generated by calculating the distance from each vertex on the cartilage surface mesh to its nearest vertex on the corresponding bone surface mesh (Fig. 1a). Thickness measurements of both the tibial and femoral cartilage were averaged within uniformly spaced points, each with a radius of 2.5 mm. Eighteen points were placed on the tibial cartilage (9 points on each tibial plateau), and 36 points were placed on the femoral cartilage (18 points on each condyle) (Fig. 1b) [29]. Strain at each of these points was calculated as the difference between the pre- and

post-exercise thickness, divided by the pre-exercise thickness [14]. These strains were averaged to generate mean cartilage strains representing strain across the tibial and femoral cartilage. The methodology used in the present study has been previously validated to measure cartilage thickness in the tibiofemoral joint to within a resolution of 1% [19, 29].

T1rho relaxation time maps were generated from the pre-exercise T1rho MRI images. The tibial and femoral cartilage were manually segmented from the TSL = 5 ms image (Fig. 2). For each voxel within the segmented cartilage regions, T1rho relaxation times were calculated by assessing the exponential decay of the MRI signal intensity with increasing spin lock time (TSL). This was done by fitting the following equation [30]:

$$S(TSL) = S_0 e^{-TSL/T_{1\rho}}.$$

Here, S(TSL) represents signal intensity for a given voxel, S_0 represents initial signal intensity, and TSL represents spin lock time. T1rho relaxation times of all voxels within the segmented region of the tibial cartilage were averaged, as were the relaxation times of all voxels of the femoral cartilage.

T1rho repeatability analysis

The repeatability of this technique was assessed by comparing baseline tibial and femoral cartilage T1rho relaxation times acquired from four male test subjects (mean age 32, range 27–40; mean BMI 22.3, range 18–24) during two separate MRI sessions which occurred within a 2-week period. Subjects were tested at 8 am with a 45-min rest period prior to each testing session. The coefficient of variation of the acquired T1rho relaxation times was determined to be 1.4%.

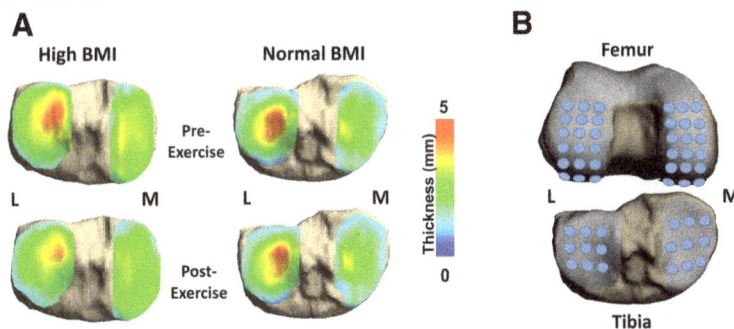

Fig. 1 a Representative tibial cartilage thickness maps from a high body mass index (BMI) subject and a normal BMI subject. The color thickness maps demonstrate greater changes in the high BMI subject compared with the normal BMI subject following the 20-min walking task in both the medial (M) and lateral (L) aspects of the tibial cartilage. **b** Femur and tibia with articular cartilage surfaces demonstrating the grid point sampling locations. The tibial cartilage surfaces were sampled from 18 points, and the femoral cartilage surfaces were sampled from 36 points

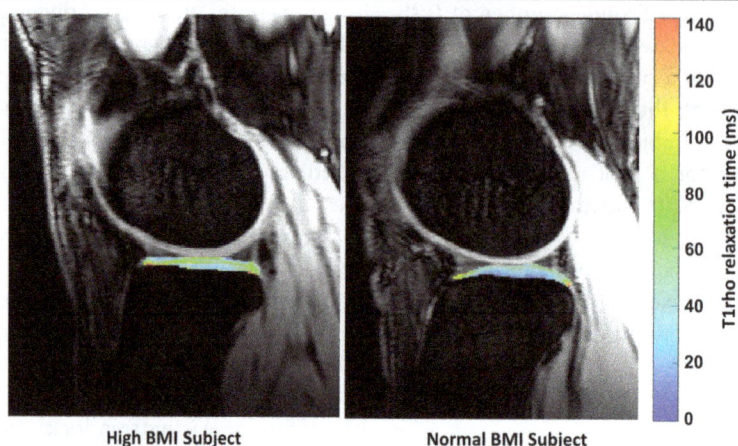

Fig. 2 Color map of tibial cartilage T1rho relaxation times in one representative high body mass index (BMI) subject and one representative normal BMI subject

Statistical analysis

Two-way repeated measures analysis of variance (ANOVA) was performed to determine the influence of BMI (high versus normal) and location (femur versus tibia) on cartilage strain, T1rho relaxation time, and pre-exercise cartilage thickness. Fisher's least significant difference (LSD) test was used for post hoc comparisons in cases where the ANOVA indicated a significant interaction between variables. Additionally, simple linear regressions were performed to analyze relationships between body composition (BMI and body fat percentage) and tibial and femoral cartilage properties (cartilage thickness, strain, and T1rho relaxation time). Statistical significance was defined as a P value of less than 0.05.

Results

Overall, high BMI subjects had significantly decreased resting tibial cartilage thickness ($P <0.05$, Fig. 3a) compared with normal BMI subjects. Additionally, high BMI subjects had increased compressive tibiofemoral cartilage strains compared with normal BMI subjects ($P <0.01$, Fig. 3b). Finally, high BMI subjects had elevated tibiofemoral T1rho relaxation times compared with normal BMI subjects ($P = 0.03$, Fig. 3c), and femoral T1rho relaxation times were greater than tibial T1rho relaxation times ($P <0.01$).

As expected, BMI was significantly correlated with body fat percentage ($P <0.05$, $R^2 = 0.79$). Additionally, tibial pre-exercise cartilage thickness was negatively correlated with BMI ($P <0.01$, $R^2 = 0.43$, Fig. 4a), with 12% thinner cartilage in high BMI subjects compared with normal BMI subjects. Pre-exercise tibial cartilage thickness was also negatively correlated with body fat percentage ($P <0.01$, $R^2 = 0.58$, Fig. 4b). Tibial cartilage strain was positively correlated with BMI ($P <0.01$, $R^2 = 0.45$, Fig. 5a), with a nearly fourfold increase in high BMI subjects compared with normal BMI subjects. Tibial strain was also positively correlated with body fat percentage ($P <0.05$, $R^2 = 0.40$, Fig. 5b).

Femoral pre-exercise cartilage thickness was not significantly correlated to either BMI ($P = 0.79$, $R^2 = 0.006$) or body fat percentage ($P = 0.71$, $R^2 = 0.011$). However, femoral cartilage strain was positively correlated with BMI ($P <0.01$, $R^2 = 0.51$, Fig. 5c), again with a nearly

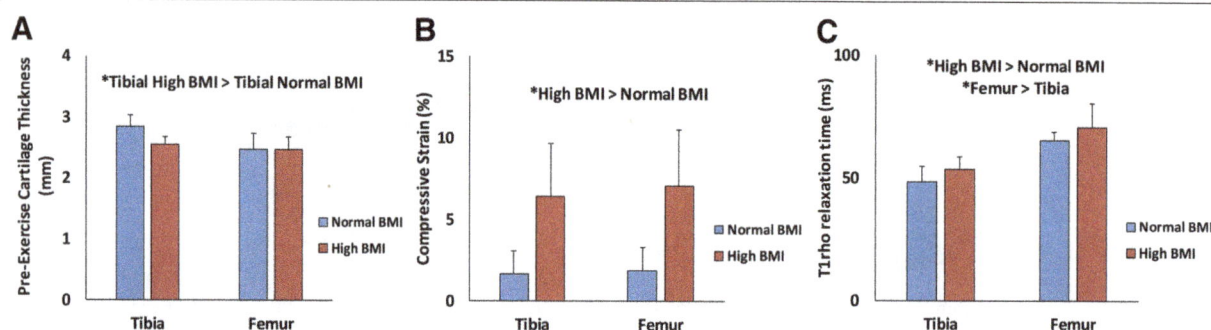

Fig. 3 a Pre-exercise cartilage thickness **b** Cartilage compressive strain and **c** T1rho relaxation time. Data are presented as mean ± standard deviation. Asterisk indicates a significant effect. Abbreviation: *BMI* body mass index

fourfold increase in high BMI subjects compared with normal BMI subjects. Additionally, femoral strain was also positively correlated with body fat percentage ($P < 0.05$, $R^2 = 0.38$, Fig. 5d).

Pre-exercise tibial T1rho relaxation times were significantly correlated with BMI ($P < 0.05$, $R^2 = 0.39$, Fig. 6a), and high BMI subjects had 13% greater T1rho relaxation times compared with normal BMI subjects. Likewise, pre-exercise tibial T1rho was significantly correlated with body fat percentage ($P < 0.01$, $R^2 = 0.47$, Fig. 6b). However, pre-exercise femoral T1rho relaxation times were not correlated with BMI ($P = 0.31$, $R^2 = 0.08$) or body fat percentage ($P = 0.6$, $R^2 = 0.08$, Fig. 6c, d).

Discussion

Obesity is a major risk factor for the development of knee OA; however, the relative contribution of biochemical and biomechanical factors to the obesity–OA relationship is unclear. In order to better understand the mechanisms by which obesity leads to OA, this study aimed to quantify both biomechanical and biochemical changes in tibiofemoral articular cartilage that occur with high BMI and increased body fat percentage. Specifically, this study explored the influence of obesity on changes in both *in vivo* cartilage strain in response to an acute, dynamic loading task (20-min treadmill walk) as well as baseline cartilage proteoglycan content using T1rho relaxation imaging. Our study found that obese subjects, who had no history of joint injury or surgery and no symptoms of knee OA, exhibited lower pre-exercise tibial cartilage thickness as well as greater

tibiofemoral cartilage compressive strain following loading. Additionally, we found that high BMI subjects exhibited increased tibiofemoral T1rho relaxation times, which may be indicative of decreased proteoglycan content within the cartilage [22, 31, 32].

Increased tibial and femoral *in vivo* cartilage strains demonstrated with increased BMI are consistent with previous work from our lab which investigated diurnal changes in cartilage thickness [18]. Widmyer et al. found that over the course of normal daily activities, subjects with a high BMI (25–31) had significantly higher compressive strains in the tibial cartilage compared with those with a normal BMI (18.5–24.9) [18]. Whereas Widmyer et al. compared cartilage thickness in the morning and evening to obtain measures of diurnal strain, the current study demonstrated similar changes in tibial and femoral cartilage thickness between BMI groups as a result of a controlled and shorter duration loading activity. Specifically, this study investigated cartilage strains in response to treadmill walking for 20 min at a speed normalized to each subject's lower limb length by using the Froude number (Fr) [26]. Controlling for walking speed across subjects by using the Froude number was important in this study as previous work has shown that given the option of self-selected walking speed, obese individuals walk slower than lean individuals, thus possibly influencing ground reaction forces and subsequent loads experienced by the knee joint [33].

Gait analysis studies have been previously used to approximate joint reaction forces in response to obesity [34–36]. For example, Harding et al. demonstrated that

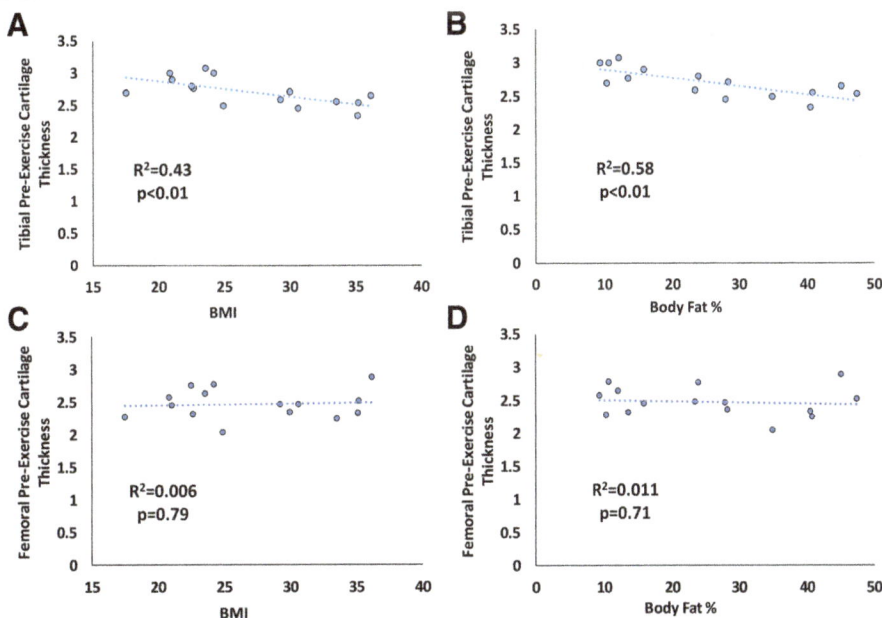

Fig. 4 a, b Tibial cartilage pre-exercise thickness was significantly correlated with body mass index (BMI) (*P* <0.01) and body fat percentage (*P* <0.01). **c, d** Femoral cartilage pre-exercise thickness was not significantly correlated with BMI (*P* = 0.79) or body fat percentage (*P* = 0.71)

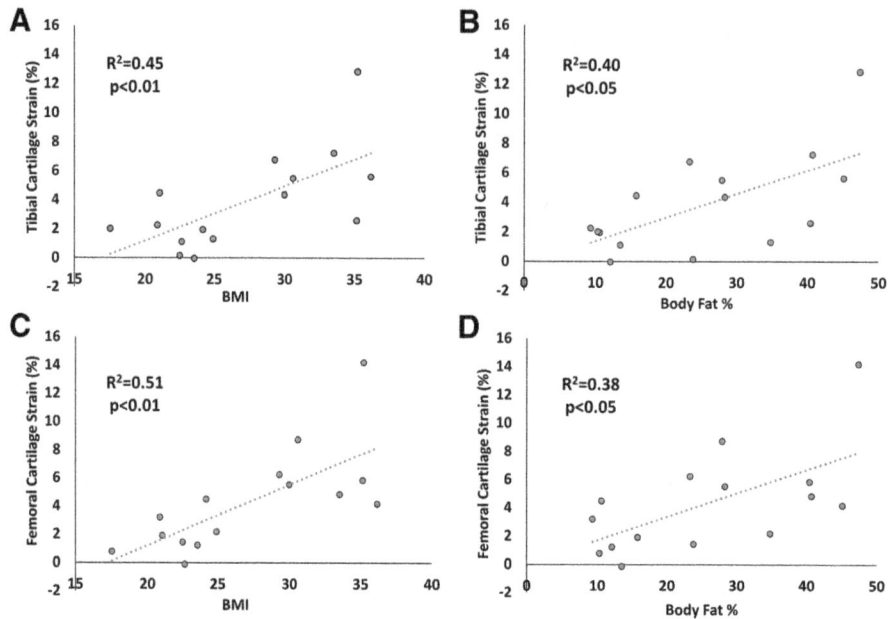

Fig. 5 a, b Tibial cartilage compressive strain was significantly correlated with body mass index (BMI) (*P* <0.01) and body fat percentage (*P* <0.05). **c, d** Femoral cartilage strain was also significantly correlated with BMI (*P* <0.01) and body fat percentage (*P* <0.05)

high BMI is associated with higher absolute tibiofemoral compressive forces by using a sagittal plane contact force model [34]. In a separate weight loss study, DeVita et al. demonstrated that weight loss of approximately 34% of initial body weight reduced maximum compressive forces in the knee as measured through gait analysis techniques, but these changes were later attenuated by gait adaptations following weight loss [35]. Additionally, Liukkonen et al. showed that weight loss induced by bariatric surgery altered knee kinetics and kinematics during gait [36]. In general, such gait analysis studies provide a wealth of information regarding knee joint

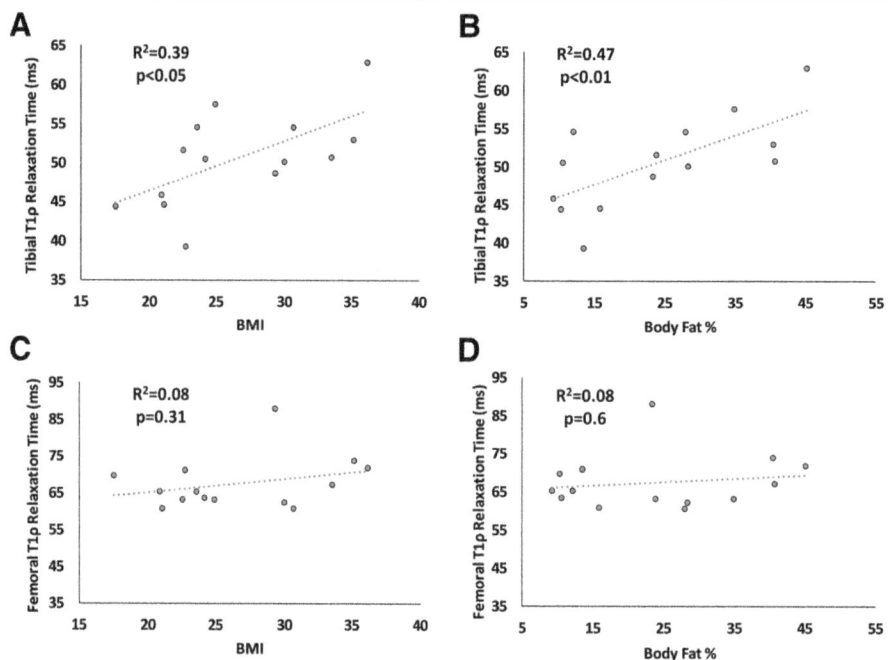

Fig. 6 a, b Tibial T1rho relaxation time was significantly correlated with body mass index (BMI) (*P* <0.05) and body fat percentage (*P* <0.01). **c, d** Femoral T1rho relaxation time was not significantly correlated with BMI (*P* = 0.31) or body fat percentage (*P* = 0.6)

loading in various populations. The present study further suggests that, in addition to potentially altering joint loading, obesity may be associated with presymptomatic alterations in the mechanical response and composition of cartilage.

In addition to changes in the mechanical function of the cartilage, we observed alterations in cartilage biochemical composition occurring with obesity. Specifically, we observed decreased proteoglycan content in the tibiofemoral cartilage of high BMI subjects as measured using T1rho imaging. Consistent with these findings, one previous study used delayed gadolinium-enhanced magnetic resonance imaging of cartilage (dGEMRIC) to estimate proteoglycan content in the articular cartilage of subjects before and after a weight loss program [37]. They concluded that weight loss was associated with protective effects on proteoglycan content and cartilage thickness [37]. Changes in cartilage composition have important implications for the mechanical behavior of cartilage and thus the development of OA [22, 31]. Specifically, decreased proteoglycan content has been shown to be related to decreased aggregate modulus, or stiffness, of cartilage resulting in increased deformation in response to load [31, 38]. Structural modifications to cartilage components such as proteoglycan loss may directly affect the ability of cartilage to withstand and transfer load. To this point, one study found that, in a diet-induced mouse model, high fat gain was associated with cartilage proteoglycan loss and reduced the aggregate modulus of cartilage in high fat–fed mice [39]. These results demonstrate that a high-fat diet may alter the material properties of cartilage by reducing proteoglycan content and decreasing tissue stiffness, potentially leading to increased deformation due to mechanical loading as observed in the present study. Importantly, chondrocyte metabolism is closely related to its mechanical environment [40], and several studies have shown that hyperphysiologic magnitudes of cartilage loading can lead to decreased synthesis of extracellular matrix components, increased production of pro-inflammatory cytokines, and potentially cell death [41–44]. Thus, altered mechanical properties related to changes in biochemical composition can change the mechanical environment experienced by chondrocytes, thus changing their metabolic activity and potentially contributing to a progressive cycle of degeneration [45]. Further support for this hypothesis is provided by evidence of decreased pre-exercise tibial cartilage thickness observed in obese subjects in this study, which may be indicative of cartilage degeneration.

The exact mechanism of obesity-related OA is unclear but may be the result of alterations in both the local mechanical loading and inflammatory environments. Specifically, it is possible that local mechanical factors, such as increased joint loading, exacerbate the effects of inflammatory cytokines (either systemic or localized),

thus furthering the cycle of cartilage degeneration. Additionally, obesity is considered a systemic inflammatory disease which has been shown to induce OA in non-weight-bearing joints such as the wrist and hand [10, 46]. Recent studies suggest that metabolic factors occurring with obesity alter the activity of inflammatory cytokines that are associated with OA [47, 48]. Specifically, increased pro-inflammatory biomarkers—tumor necrosis factor alpha (TNF-α), interleukin-1 beta (IL-1β), and IL-6—have been observed in obese children with no comorbidities [47] as well as in obese patients with OA [49]. However, diet and exercise can reduce these cytokine levels [49, 50]. Such increased inflammatory cytokine activity can induce chondrocyte catabolism, resulting in degenerative changes such as decreased proteoglycan content [51, 52]. Similarly, the increased tibial T1rho relaxation time (corresponding to decreased proteoglycan content) with both increasing BMI and body fat percentage observed in the present study may be due to increased activity of inflammatory cytokines [51, 52]. The stronger correlation of tibial T1rho relaxation time with body fat percentage than with BMI demonstrated in this study may be suggestive of adipose-related inflammation playing a greater role than mechanical loading in the obesity–cartilage degeneration relationship. Future studies may further investigate the relative contributions of body mass and body fat percentage on cartilage deformation and composition.

In this study, measures of cartilage strain may have been underestimated because of inadequate recovery of the cartilage prior to the pre-exercise MRI scan or because of partial recovery prior to the post-exercise MRI scan. Although subjects were asked to refrain from strenuous activity 24 h prior to and the morning of testing, and a 45-min period of supine resting time was included to allow cartilage thickness to reach its baseline unloaded state, it is possible that the cartilage was not fully recovered prior to pre-exercise imaging. Additionally, the period between completion of the walking activity and the post-exercise MRI scan was less than 4 min. Previous work has demonstrated that cartilage volume recovers to about 50% of its original volume after 45 min of being unloaded [53]. Therefore, it is possible that some cartilage recovery occurred during this time; however, there was no difference between groups either in the study tasks completed or in the time between the completion of the walking activity and the post-exercise MRI scan. Nonetheless, cartilage recovery occurring within this 4-min period may result in underestimations of cartilage strain.

Conclusions

The present study demonstrates a significant relationship between body composition and the biomechanical and biochemical properties of cartilage. We found that a short treadmill walking task resulted in greater tibiofemoral cartilage strains in subjects with a high BMI as compared with subjects with a normal BMI. Additionally, we found that tibiofemoral T1rho relaxation times increased in high BMI subjects, indicative of a decrease in cartilage proteoglycan concentration. Taken together with our previous work [18], these data indicate that the changes in cartilage strain observed here may be the result of alterations in both biomechanics (that is, increased joint load) and cartilage composition (loss of proteoglycan) leading to changes in mechanical properties. Importantly, decreases in proteoglycan content and cartilage thickness in obese subjects may be indicative of a "pre-osteoarthritic" state of cartilage. Characterizing the effects of BMI and body fat percentage on *in vivo* cartilage properties is a critical first step in understanding the mechanisms by which obesity alters the mechanical and biochemical properties of cartilage, thus contributing to the initiation and progression of knee OA.

Abbreviations
3D: Three-dimensional; ANOVA : Analysis of variance; BMI: Body mass index; DESS: Double-echo steady-state; FOV: Field of view; Fr: Froude number; IL: Interleukin; MRI: Magnetic resonance imaging; OA: Osteoarthritis; TE: Echo time; TNF: Tumor necrosis factor alpha; TR: Repetition time; TSL: Spin lock time

Acknowledgments
The authors would like to thank Jean Shaffer at the Duke University Center for Advanced Magnetic Resonance Development (Durham, NC, USA) for technical assistance.

Funding
This study was supported by the National Institutes of Health, specifically the National Institute of Arthritis and Musculoskeletal and Skin Diseases and the National Institute on Aging (AR066477, AR065527, AR50245, and AG46927).

Authors' contributions
AC contributed to this article through study design, collection of all data, analysis and interpretation of data, and the writing of the article. MK, HC, and WS contributed to this article through data analysis and editing of the article. GU and CS contributed to this article through analysis and interpretation of data and editing of the article. FG and LD contributed to this article through the conception and design of the study, analysis and interpretation of data, and the writing of the article. All authors contributed to this work, agree with its contents, and have provided their final approval for submission.

Consent for publication
Not applicable.

Competing interests
The authors declare that they have no competing interests.

Author details
[1]Department of Orthopaedic Surgery, Duke University, Box 3093, Duke University Medical Center, Durham, NC 27710, USA. [2]Department of Biomedical Engineering, Duke University, Campus Box 90281, 101 Science Drive, Durham 27708, NC, USA. [3]Department of Mechanical Engineering and Materials Science, Duke University, Campus Box 90300, Hudson Hall, Durham 27708, NC, USA. [4]Department of Radiology, Duke University, Box 3808, Duke University Medical Center, Durham 27710, NC, USA. [5]Department of Orthopaedic Surgery, Washington University and Shriners Hospitals for Children, Campus Box 8233, Couch Research Building, Room 3121, St. Louis 63110, MO, USA.

References
1. Felson DT. Relation of obesity and of vocational and avocational risk factors to osteoarthritis. J Rheumatol. 2005;32:1133–5. http://www.ncbi.nlm.nih.gov/pubmed/15977343.
2. Runhaar J, Koes BW, Clockaerts S, Bierma-Zeinstra SM. A systematic review on changed biomechanics of lower extremities in obese individuals: a possible role in development of osteoarthritis. Obes Rev. 2011;12:1071–82. https://doi.org/10.1111/j.1467-789X.2011.00916.x.
3. Felson DT. Weight and osteoarthritis. J Rheumatol Suppl. 1995;43:7–9. http://www.ncbi.nlm.nih.gov/pubmed/7752143.
4. Murphy L, Schwartz TA, Helmick CG, Renner JB, Tudor G, Koch G, et al. Lifetime risk of symptomatic knee osteoarthritis. Arthritis Rheum. 2008;59: 1207–13. https://doi.org/10.1002/art.24021.
5. Powell A, Teichtahl AJ, Wluka AE, Cicuttini FM. Obesity: a preventable risk factor for large joint osteoarthritis which may act through biomechanical factors. Br J Sports Med. 2005;39:4–5. https://doi.org/10.1136/bjsm.2004.011841.
6. Felson DT. Does excess weight cause osteoarthritis and, if so, why? Ann Rheum Dis. 1996;55:668–70. http://www.ncbi.nlm.nih.gov/pubmed/8882146.
7. Griffin TM, Guilak F. Why is obesity associated with osteoarthritis? Insights from mouse models of obesity. Biorheology. 2008;45:387–98. http://www.ncbi.nlm.nih.gov/pubmed/18836239.
8. Aspden RM. Obesity punches above its weight in osteoarthritis. Nat Rev Rheumatol. 2011;7:65–8. https://doi.org/10.1038/nrrheum.2010.123.
9. Grotle M, Hagen KB, Natvig B, Dahl FA, Kvien TK. Obesity and osteoarthritis in knee, hip and/or hand: an epidemiological study in the general population with 10 years follow-up. BMC Musculoskelet Disord. 2008;9:132. https://doi.org/10.1186/1471-2474-9-132.
10. Oliveria SA, Felson DT, Cirillo PA, Reed JI, Walker AM. Body weight, body mass index, and incident symptomatic osteoarthritis of the hand, hip, and knee. Epidemiology. 1999;10:161–6. https://www.ncbi.nlm.nih.gov/pubmed/10069252.
11. Hurwitz D, Sumner D, Andriacchi T, Sugar D. Dynamic knee loads during gait predict proximal tibial bone distribution. J Biomech. 1998;31:423–30.
12. Landry SC, McKean KA, Hubley-Kozey CL, Stanish WD, Deluzio KJ. Knee biomechanics of moderate OA patients measured during gait at a self-selected and fast walking speed. J Biomech. 2007;40:1754–61. http://www.ncbi.nlm.nih.gov/entrez/query.fcgi?cmd=Retrieve&db=PubMed&dopt=Citation&list_uids=17084845.
13. Fregly BJ, D'Lima DD, Colwell CW Jr. Effective gait patterns for offloading the medial compartment of the knee. J Orthop Res. 2009;27:1016–21. https://doi.org/10.1002/jor.20843.
14. Cher WL, Utturkar GM, Spritzer CE, Nunley JA, DeFrate LE, Collins AT. An analysis of changes in in vivo cartilage thickness of the healthy ankle following dynamic activity. J Biomech. 2016;49:3026–30. https://doi.org/10.1016/j.jbiomech.2016.05.030.
15. Lad NK, Liu B, Ganapathy PK, Utturkar GM, Sutter EG, Moorman CT 3rd, et al. Effect of normal gait on in vivo tibiofemoral cartilage strains. J Biomech. 2016;49:2870–6. https://doi.org/10.1016/j.jbiomech.2016.06.025.
16. Liu B, Lad NK, Collins AT, Ganapathy PK, Utturkar GM, McNulty AL, et al. In vivo tibial cartilage strains in regions of cartilage-to-cartilage contact and cartilage-to-meniscus contact in response to walking. Am J Sports Med. 2017;45:2817–23. https://doi.org/10.1177/0363546517712506.
17. Eckstein F, Lemberger B, Gratzke C, Hudelmaier M, Glaser C, Englmeier KH, et al. In vivo cartilage deformation after different types of activity and its dependence on physical training status. Ann Rheum Dis. 2005;64:291–5. https://doi.org/10.1136/ard.2004.022400.
18. Widmyer MR, Utturkar GM, Leddy HA, Coleman JL, Spritzer CE, Moorman CT 3rd, et al. High body mass index is associated with increased diurnal strains in the articular cartilage of the knee. Arthritis Rheum. 2013;65:2615–22. https://doi.org/10.1002/art.38062.
19. Coleman JL, Widmyer MR, Leddy HA, Utturkar GM, Spritzer CE, Moorman CT 3rd, et al. Diurnal variations in articular cartilage thickness and strain in the human knee. J Biomech. 2013;46:541–7. https://doi.org/10.1016/j.jbiomech.2012.09.013.

20. Tsushima H, Okazaki K, Takayama Y, Hatakenaka M, Honda H, Izawa T, et al. Evaluation of cartilage degradation in arthritis using T1rho magnetic resonance imaging mapping. Rheumatol Int. 2012;32:2867–75. https://doi.org/10.1007/s00296-011-2140-3.

21. Li X, Benjamin Ma C, Link TM, Castillo DD, Blumenkrantz G, Lozano J, et al. In vivo T(1rho) and T(2) mapping of articular cartilage in osteoarthritis of the knee using 3 T MRI. Osteoarthritis Cartilage. 2007;15:789–97. https://doi.org/10.1016/j.joca.2007.01.011.

22. Keenan KE, Besier TF, Pauly JM, Han E, Rosenberg J, Smith RL, et al. Prediction of glycosaminoglycan content in human cartilage by age, T1rho and T2 MRI. Osteoarthritis Cartilage. 2011;19:171–9. https://doi.org/10.1016/j.joca.2010.11.009.

23. Li X, Pai A, Blumenkrantz G, Carballido-Gamio J, Link T, Ma B, et al. Spatial distribution and relationship of T1rho and T2 relaxation times in knee cartilage with osteoarthritis. Magn Reson Med. 2009;61:1310–8. https://doi.org/10.1002/mrm.21877.

24. Souza RB, Kumar D, Calixto N, Singh J, Schooler J, Subburaj K, et al. Response of knee cartilage T1rho and T2 relaxation times to in vivo mechanical loading in individuals with and without knee osteoarthritis. Osteoarthritis Cartilage. 2014;22:1367–76. https://doi.org/10.1016/j.joca.2014.04.017.

25. Taylor KA, Cutcliffe HC, Queen RM, Utturkar GM, Spritzer CE, Garrett WE, et al. In vivo measurement of ACL length and relative strain during walking. J Biomech. 2013;46:478–83. https://doi.org/10.1016/j.jbiomech.2012.10.031.

26. Alexander RM, Jayes AS. A dynamic similarity hypothesis for the gaits of quadrupedal mammals. J Zool. 1983;201:135–52 <Go to ISI>://WOS: A1983RH79100010.

27. von Hurst PR, Walsh DCI, Conlon CA, Ingram M, Kruger R, Stonehouse W. Validity and reliability of bioelectrical impedance analysis to estimate body fat percentage against air displacement plethysmography and dual-energy X-ray absorptiometry. Nutr Diet. 2016;73:197–204. https://doi.org/10.1111/1747-0080.12172.

28. Okafor EC, Utturkar GM, Widmyer MR, Abebe ES, Collins AT, Taylor DC, et al. The effects of femoral graft placement on cartilage thickness after anterior cruciate ligament reconstruction. J Biomech. 2014;47:96–101. https://doi.org/10.1016/j.jbiomech.2013.10.003.

29. Van de Velde SK, Bingham JT, Hosseini A, Kozanek M, DeFrate LE, Gill TJ, et al. Increased tibiofemoral cartilage contact deformation in patients with anterior cruciate ligament deficiency. Arthritis Rheum. 2009;60:3693–702. https://doi.org/10.1002/art.24965.

30. Borthakur A, Wheaton A, Charagundla SR, Shapiro EM, Regatte RR, Akella SV, et al. Three-dimensional T1rho-weighted MRI at 1.5 Tesla. Journal of magnetic resonance imaging. JMRI. 2003;17:730–6. https://doi.org/10.1002/jmri.10296.

31. Hatcher CC, Collins AT, Kim SY, Michel LC, Mostertz WC 3rd, Ziemian SN, et al. Relationship between T1rho magnetic resonance imaging, synovial fluid biomarkers, and the biochemical and biomechanical properties of cartilage. J Biomech. 2017;55:18–26. https://doi.org/10.1016/j.jbiomech.2017.02.001.

32. Wheaton AJ, Dodge GR, Borthakur A, Kneeland JB, Schumacher HR, Reddy R. Detection of changes in articular cartilage proteoglycan by T(1rho) magnetic resonance imaging. J Orthop Res. 2004;23:102–8. https://doi.org/10.1016/j.orthres.2004.06.015.

33. DeVita P, Hortobagyi T. Obesity is not associated with increased knee joint torque and power during level walking. J Biomech. 2003;36:1355–62. https://www.ncbi.nlm.nih.gov/pubmed/12893044.

34. Harding GT, Dunbar MJ, Hubley-Kozey CL, Stanish WD, Astephen Wilson JL. Obesity is associated with higher absolute tibiofemoral contact and muscle forces during gait with and without knee osteoarthritis. Clin Biomech (Bristol, Avon). 2016;31:79–86. https://doi.org/10.1016/j.clinbiomech.2015.09.010.

35. DeVita P, Rider P, Hortobagyi T. Reductions in knee joint forces with weight loss are attenuated by gait adaptations in class III obesity. Gait Posture. 2016;45:25–30. https://doi.org/10.1016/j.gaitpost.2015.12.040.

36. Liukkonen MK, Mononen ME, Vartiainen P, Kaukinen P, Bragge T, Suomalainen JS, et al. Evaluation of the effect of bariatric surgery-induced weight loss on knee gait and cartilage degeneration. J Biomech Eng. 2018;140(4). https://doi.org/10.1115/1.4038330.

37. Anandacoomarasamy A, Leibman S, Smith G, Caterson I, Giuffre B, Fransen M, et al. Weight loss in obese people has structure-modifying effects on medial but not on lateral knee articular cartilage. Ann Rheum Dis. 2012;71:26–32. https://doi.org/10.1136/ard.2010.144725.

38. Setton LA, Elliott DM, Mow VC. Altered mechanics of cartilage with osteoarthritis: human osteoarthritis and an experimental model of joint degeneration. Osteoarthritis Cartilage. 1999;7:2–14. https://doi.org/10.1053/joca.1998.0170.

39. Griffin TM, Fermor B, Huebner JL, Kraus VB, Rodriguiz RM, Wetsel WC, et al. Diet-induced obesity differentially regulates behavioral, biomechanical, and molecular risk factors for osteoarthritis in mice. Arthritis Res Ther. 2010;12:R130. https://doi.org/10.1186/ar3068.

40. Sanchez-Adams J, Leddy HA, McNulty AL, O'Conor CJ, Guilak F. The mechanobiology of articular cartilage bearing the burden of osteoarthritis. Curr Rheumatol Rep. 2014;16:451. https://doi.org/10.1007/s11926-014-0451-6.

41. Coleman MC, Ramakrishnan PS, Brouillette MJ, Martin JA. Injurious loading of articular cartilage compromises chondrocyte respiratory function. Arthritis Rheumatol. 2016;68:662–71. https://doi.org/10.1002/art.39460.

42. Lee W, Leddy HA, Chen Y, Lee SH, Zelenski NA, McNulty AL, et al. Synergy between Piezo1 and Piezo2 channels confers high-strain mechanosensitivity to articular cartilage. Proc Natl Acad Sci U S A. 2014;111:E5114–22. https://doi.org/10.1073/pnas.1414298111.

43. Mohanraj B, Meloni GR, Mauck RL, Dodge GR. A high-throughput model of post-traumatic osteoarthritis using engineered cartilage tissue analogs. Osteoarthritis Cartilage. 2014;22:1282–90. https://doi.org/10.1016/j.joca.2014.06.032.

44. Honda K, Ohno S, Tanimoto K, Ijuin C, Tanaka N, Doi T, et al. The effects of high magnitude cyclic tensile load on cartilage matrix metabolism in cultured chondrocytes. Eur J Cell Biol. 2000;79:601–9. https://doi.org/10.1078/0171-9335-00089.

45. Guilak F. Biomechanical factors in osteoarthritis. Best Pract Res Clin Rheumatol. 2011;25:815–23. https://doi.org/10.1016/j.berh.2011.11.013.

46. Carman WJ, Sowers M, Hawthorne VM, Weissfeld LA. Obesity as a risk factor for osteoarthritis of the hand and wrist: a prospective study. Am J Epidemiol. 1994;139:119–29. https://www.ncbi.nlm.nih.gov/pubmed/8296779.

47. Aygun AD, Gungor S, Ustundag B, Gurgoze MK, Sen Y. Proinflammatory cytokines and leptin are increased in serum of prepubertal obese children. Mediat Inflamm. 2005;2005:180–3. https://doi.org/10.1155/MI.2005.180.

48. Wellen KE, Hotamisligil GS. Inflammation, stress, and diabetes. J Clin Invest. 2005;115:1111–9. https://doi.org/10.1172/JCI25102.

49. Messier SP, Mihalko SL, Legault C, Miller GD, Nicklas BJ, DeVita P, et al. Effects of intensive diet and exercise on knee joint loads, inflammation, and clinical outcomes among overweight and obese adults with knee osteoarthritis: the IDEA randomized clinical trial. JAMA. 2013;310:1263–73. https://doi.org/10.1001/jama.2013.277669.

50. Huebner JL, Landerman LR, Somers TJ, Keefe FJ, Guilak F, Blumenthal JA, et al. Exploratory secondary analyses of a cognitive-behavioral intervention for knee osteoarthritis demonstrate reduction in biomarkers of adipocyte inflammation. Osteoarthritis Cartilage. 2016;24:1528–34. https://doi.org/10.1016/j.joca.2016.04.002.

51. McNulty AL, Miller MR, O'Connor SK, Guilak F. The effects of adipokines on cartilage and meniscus catabolism. Connect Tissue Res. 2011;52:523–33. https://doi.org/10.3109/03008207.2011.597902.

52. Hui W, Litherland GJ, Elias MS, Kitson GI, Cawston TE, Rowan AD, et al. Leptin produced by joint white adipose tissue induces cartilage degradation via upregulation and activation of matrix metalloproteinases. Ann Rheum Dis. 2012;71:455–62. https://doi.org/10.1136/annrheumdis-2011-200372.

53. Eckstein F, Tieschky M, Faber S, Englmeier KH, Reiser M. Functional analysis of articular cartilage deformation, recovery, and fluid flow following dynamic exercise in vivo. Anat Embryol. 1999;200:419–24. http://www.ncbi.nlm.nih.gov/pubmed/10460479.

22

From association to mechanism in complex disease genetics: the role of the 3D genome

Yao Fu[1], Kandice L Tessneer[1], Chuang Li[2] and Patrick M Gaffney[1]* (iD)

Abstract

Genome-wide association studies (GWAS) and fine mapping studies in autoimmune diseases have identified thousands of genetic variants, the majority of which are located in non-protein-coding enhancer regions. Enhancers function within the context of the three-dimensional (3D) genome to form long-range DNA looping events with target gene promoters that spatially and temporally regulate gene expression. Investigating the functional significance of GWAS variants in the context of the 3D genome is essential for mechanistic understanding of these variants and how they influence disease pathology by altering DNA looping between enhancers and the target gene promoters they regulate. In this review, we discuss the functional complexity of the 3D genome and the technological approaches used to characterize DNA looping events. We then highlight examples from the literature that illustrate how functional mapping of the 3D genome can assist in defining mechanisms that influence pathogenic gene expression. We conclude by highlighting future advances necessary to fully integrate 3D genome analyses into the functional workup of GWAS variants in the continuing effort to improve the health of patients with autoimmune diseases.

Keywords: Autoimmune disease, 3D genome, Chromatin conformation, Complex genetic disease, DNA looping, Functional genomics, GWAS, Enhancer, Promoter

Background

Genome-wide association studies (GWAS) have significantly advanced the identification of variants associated with complex genetic diseases, including autoimmune diseases [1, 2]. GWAS leverages the phenomenon of linkage disequilibrium—the tendency for common variants to be inherited in correlated haplotype blocks—to identify statistical associations between genetic diseases and haplotypes of single nucleotide polymorphisms (SNPs) [3]. Statistical associations, while powerful for locus discovery, cannot distinguish risk-driving variants within a haplotype block that are responsible for the genetic association from non-risk neutral variants. Large-scale GWAS have shown that the vast majority (~ 80–90%) of GWAS variants are located in regions of

genomic DNA that do not code for protein sequences [4, 5]. These variants are thought to exert their influence on disease risk by modulating gene expression, which can vary based on cell type and cell state. Compared to genetic variants in protein coding sequences for which the impact of an amino acid change on protein function can be reasonably predicted, the function of non-coding DNA variants must be empirically determined through experimentation, hindering translation of GWAS data into clinically meaningful information.

To demystify the function of non-coding DNA in chromatin regulation and gene expression, several large-scale collaborative efforts (Encyclopedia of DNA Elements (ENCODE) Project, National Institutes of Health (NIH) Roadmap Epigenomics Mapping Consortium, and International Human Epigenome Consortium (IHEC)) have successfully mapped the locations of regulatory sequences that bind over 400 transcription factors and histone post-translational modifications that mark enhancers, promoters, repressors, and insulator regions

* Correspondence: gaffneyp@omrf.org
[1]Division of Genomics and Data Sciences, Arthritis and Clinical Immunology Research Program, Oklahoma Medical Research Foundation, 825 Northeast 13th Street, Oklahoma City, OK 73104, USA
Full list of author information is available at the end of the article

in a large variety of cell lines and primary cells [6–8]. Collectively, these studies provided a detailed "parts list" of non-coding DNA elements, suggesting that over 80% of what was once referred to as "junk DNA" may have a role in gene regulation [6]. With this "parts list" and their precise genomic locations, it is now possible to develop and test functional hypotheses about how variants associated with complex genetic diseases potentially alter the function of enhancers to influence the expression of target genes.

Enhancer elements are short DNA sequences (~ 50–1500 bp) that bind transcription factors leading to the expression of a gene [9]. It is estimated that the human genome has nearly one million enhancer sequences scattered throughout all 23 pairs of chromosomes, a number that far exceeds the estimated 20,000 genes in the human genome [9, 10]. Moreover, approximately 60% of autoimmune disease GWAS variants reside in enhancer elements, suggesting that much of autoimmune disease risk is concentrated on modulating gene expression [5]. Enhancers influence gene expression by delivering their payload of transcription factors to the gene promoter most often located on the same chromosome, but at varying distances, through a process of DNA looping

[11]. The mechanisms that govern DNA looping and the technologies to measure them are a burgeoning area of research and have been the subject of many detailed reviews [11–15]. Knowledge of DNA looping mechanisms is important because it reveals how specific enhancer–promoter interactions occur and are modulated in response to specific cellular contexts. Traditionally, it has been naively assumed that the gene promoter closest to an enhancer is the target promoter that is regulated by that enhancer (Fig. 1a); however, we now know that enhancers likely engage multiple distant promoters within an enhancer's "regulatory network"—defined as all physical interactions between a given enhancer and gene promoters in the region (Fig. 1b) [16, 17]. Furthermore, formation of enhancer regulatory networks is likely cell type-specific and influenced significantly by autoimmune disease-associated SNPs enriched in the enhancer region [17].

In this review, we discuss the functional complexity of the 3D genome, contrast the various aspects of how the 3D genome is measured, and provide specific examples of how knowledge of the 3D genome has helped decipher GWAS results. We conclude by highlighting future advancements needed to generalize 3D genome

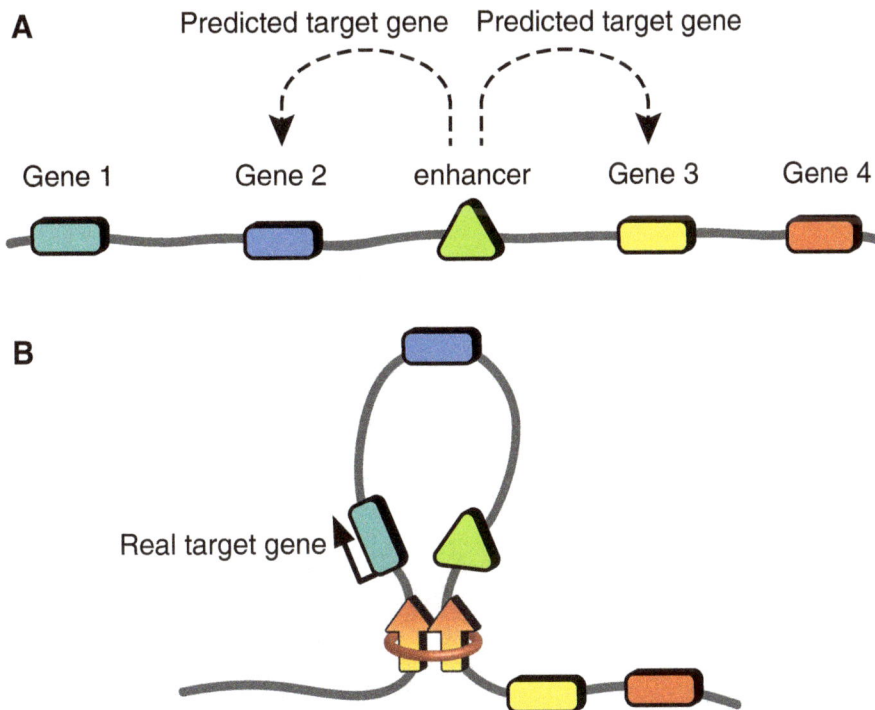

Fig. 1 Predicting enhancer–promoter interactions using linear proximity versus 3D proximity. **a** Traditional modeling of enhancer function in the context of a linear genome where an enhancer (*green triangle*) is predicted to modulate the function of the promoter in closest linear proximity (gene 2 (*blue rectangle*) or gene 3 (*yellow rectangle*)). **b** Modeling in the context of the 3D genome where an enhancer (*green triangle*) often regulates distant gene expression through long-range DNA looping to the gene promoter (gene 1 (*green rectangle*)). Due to spatial proximity, the enhancer "skips" gene 2 (*blue rectangle*). Enhancer function is restricted within the insulated loop structure formed by a CTCF-CTCF (*arrows*)–cohesion (*red ring*) complex, and therefore cannot activate gene 3 (*yellow rectangle*) or gene 4 (*red rectangle*) despite close linear proximity

data into the routine analysis of GWAS-associated risk variants.

Main Text
Functional complexity of the 3D genome
The human genome is organized into complex layers of intricate folds and loops that allow for proper gene expression regulation while fitting roughly three meters of histone-wrapped DNA into an interphase nucleus averaging 6 μm in diameter [11, 14, 15]. Each of the 23 homologous chromosomes are organized into specific regions of the nucleus, called chromosome territories, that restrict interactions between different chromosomes (Fig. 2a) [18, 19]. Each chromosome undergoes additional organization into active "A" and inactive "B" compartments [20–23]. B compartments contain densely packed regions of DNA, called heterochromatin, that are enriched with histone marks of inactivity [20]. A compartments of DNA are typically areas of open chromatin. A/B compartments are further organized to create thousands of megabase-sized sub-regions, called topologically associating domains (TADs), that promote chromatin interactions within the TAD and restrict interactions outside the TAD (Fig. 2a) [18, 20–24]. TAD boundaries are enriched with CCCTC-binding factors (CTCF) and cohesin proteins which facilitate loop formation through a process of loop extrusion (Fig. 2b) [13, 25, 26]. During loop extrusion, cohesin binds to and facilitates the "sliding" of DNA through the cohesin ring structure. The

"sliding" on one side of the small loop tends to stop when a CTCF-bound sequence encounters the cohesin. The other side of the loop continues to "slide" and "grow" until another CTCF-bound sequence with convergent orientation reaches the cohesin. The two CTCF proteins homodimerize and create a stabilizing complex with cohesin [25]. The unknotted loop of DNA "extruding" from the newly established CTCF-CTCF–cohesin complex forms the TAD [25]. TADs are largely evolutionarily conserved and maintained during cellular differentiation and embryonic development [18, 27, 28]. In contrast, CTCF-CTCF–cohesion bound regions known as "insulated neighborhoods" organize dynamic enhancer–promoter interactions during cellular differentiation or in response to stimuli (Fig. 2a) [14, 15, 29, 30]. Typically, more than one dynamic insulated neighborhood is nested within a larger evolutionarily conserved TAD.

Characterizing the complex layers of organization that occur within the 3D genome and the regulatory mechanisms that dictate them have provided a framework from which current explorations of gene expression regulation are often based. Approximately 90% of identified enhancer–promoter loops occur within the CTCF-CTCF–cohesin boundaries of TADs and insulated neighborhoods [31]. As reported in several types of cancer, disrupting these boundaries can alter gene expression by relieving restrictions and allowing new loops to form between what was once an insulated enhancer and genes outside of the original loop [32]. What's more, enhancer–promoter loops

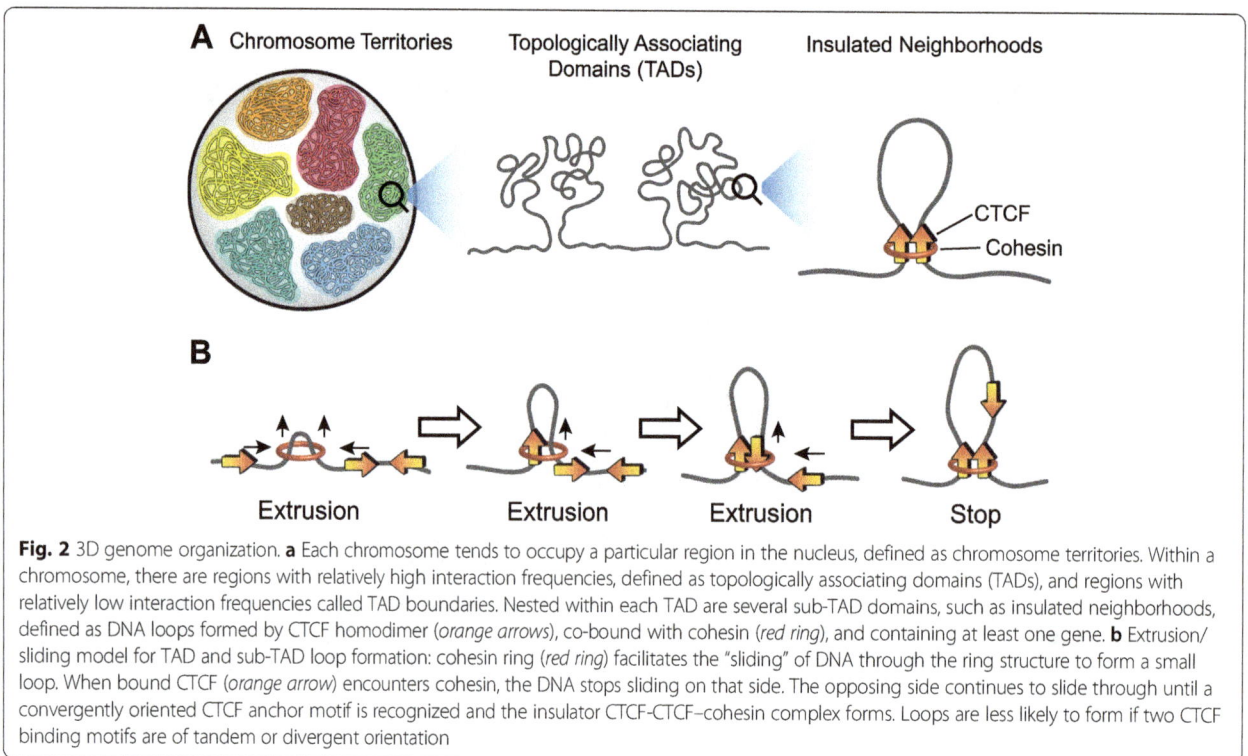

Fig. 2 3D genome organization. **a** Each chromosome tends to occupy a particular region in the nucleus, defined as chromosome territories. Within a chromosome, there are regions with relatively high interaction frequencies, defined as topologically associating domains (TADs), and regions with relatively low interaction frequencies called TAD boundaries. Nested within each TAD are several sub-TAD domains, such as insulated neighborhoods, defined as DNA loops formed by CTCF homodimer (*orange arrows*), co-bound with cohesin (*red ring*), and containing at least one gene. **b** Extrusion/sliding model for TAD and sub-TAD loop formation: cohesin ring (*red ring*) facilitates the "sliding" of DNA through the ring structure to form a small loop. When bound CTCF (*orange arrow*) encounters cohesin, the DNA stops sliding on that side. The opposing side continues to slide through until a convergently oriented CTCF anchor motif is recognized and the insulator CTCF-CTCF–cohesin complex forms. Loops are less likely to form if two CTCF binding motifs are of tandem or divergent orientation

function not in isolation, but as regulatory networks where one enhancer has the potential to influence multiple genes and one gene can be influenced by multiple enhancers [16]. Given that a large majority of GWAS variants are located within enhancers that likely modulate distant, as well as neighboring, gene function, establishing detailed maps of enhancer–promoter loops and regulatory networks have the potential to more accurately predict the functional mechanisms influenced by causal GWAS variants and provide translational insights into how such alterations influence disease pathogenesis [5].

Investigating the 3D genome

The majority of techniques used to investigate the 3D genome are derivatives of the original chromatin conformation capture (3C) method, which uses a process called proximity ligation to capture interactions between two sequences of DNA that are in 3D proximity but are separated by linear distance (Fig. 3) [33, 34]. To capture a long-distance interaction, cells are first crosslinked, or fixed, to preserve interactions between the two regions of DNA and associated proteins, and then the entire genome is digested into small pieces using restriction enzymes. Because crosslinking keeps the interacting regions of DNA and associated proteins in close proximity after digestion, the remaining regions of DNA can be enzymatically ligated together to make a chimeric strand of DNA that, once de-crosslinked, can be used in downstream 3D chromatin applications. Building upon this basic methodologic framework, variations have been developed to facilitate both targeted and genome-wide 3D chromatin exploration.

Targeted hypothesis-driven methodologies are used to analyze looping events for one or more selected targets (Table 1). Original 3C uses a unique set of primers and quantitative PCR to measure the frequency of interactions captured by proximity ligation [35]. Despite low throughput, 3C remains one of the most commonly used methods because it is cost-effective, easily adaptable to PCR-capable laboratories, quantitative, and the unique primers define a specific region of interest, thus providing relatively high resolution of the interacting regions (~ 250 bp to 4 kb) [34, 35]. Typically, 3C is used to

confirm suspected looping events and quantitatively measure changes in looping patterns caused by allelic variation in enhancer SNPs. For example, 3C was used to solve the long-time mystery of how paternal imprinting at the insulin-like growth factor 2 (IGF2) and H19 gene loci alters expression of the non-coding RNA, H19 [36]. 3C revealed an enhancer region that forms either an enhancer–promoter loop with the H19 gene promoter on the maternal allele or with the IGF2 gene promoter on the paternal allele. Further functional analyses revealed that a control region upstream of H19 is methylated on the imprinted paternal allele which blocks looping to the H19 promoter, thus silencing H19 expression and activating IGF2 expression [37, 38]. More recently, 3C has been used to demonstrate how SNPs in loop boundaries and anchors can significantly alter gene expression. In isocitrate dehydrogenase (IDH) mutant gliomas, 3C revealed that a gain-of-function mutation caused hypermethylation at the CTCF binding site defining an insulated neighborhood containing the oncogene, platelet-derived growth factor receptor alpha (PDGFRA) [39]. Hypermethylation disrupted formation of the insulated neighborhood, allowing a constitutive enhancer outside of the loop to promote oncogenic expression of PDGFRA [39].

Innovative modifications to traditional 3C, including methodologies such as 4C, 5C, and Capture-C (Table 1), have coupled 3C with microarray or high-throughput next generation sequencing (NGS) technologies to improve throughput with only minor reductions in resolution, but at the expense of quantitative capabilities [40–42]. Improved throughput has allowed for larger-scale targeted studies, like the Promoter Capture-C study by Hughes et al. that comparatively mapped the interactions between 6000 promoters and their regulatory elements in mouse embryonic stem cells and mature erythroid cells [42]. This study not only demonstrated the complexity of enhancer–promoter networks and that the promoter of a specific gene can be regulated by interactions with multiple regulatory elements, but also provided strong evidence that disease-associated risk variants are enriched in gene regulatory elements such as enhancers. Currently, most targeted methodologies still require over 100 million cells to

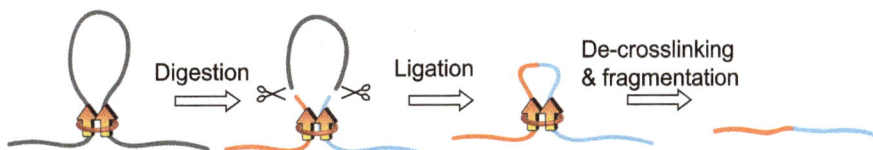

Fig. 3 Proximity ligation. Chromatin are crosslinked to preserve interactions between proximal regions of DNA and associated proteins. Crosslinked chromatin are digested using restriction enzymes (*scissors*) to create two short DNA fragments complexed with associated proteins. "Sticky ends" of the two DNA fragments originally in close 3D proximity are then ligated using DNA ligase to create a chimeric strand of DNA. After de-crosslinking, the chimeric DNA can be used in downstream applications to identify and characterize loop formation

Table 1 Advantages and disadvantages of current 3D genome technologies

Technique		Assay name/description	Target size	Assay platform	Cell input	Advantages	Disadvantages	References
Targeted								
3C		Chromosome conformation capture	One target	Quantitative PCR	> 100 M	• Quantitative measurement of long-range interactions between two targeted loci • No sequencing required	• Low throughput • Large amount of input cells	[34, 35]
4C		Circular chromosome conformation capture or chromosome conformation capture-on-chip	Multiple targets	Microarray	> 100 M	• Identification of multiple DNA regions that interact with a target locus • Modified protocol: 4C-seq	• Relatively low throughput • Large amount of input cells	[40, 63]
5C		Chromosome conformation carbon copy	Multiple targets	Microarray or sequencing	> 100 M	• Multiplexed conformation capture • Higher efficiency and lower background compared to 3C	• Not all sites are compatible to 5C primer design • 5C cannot detect contacts larger than a few megabases	[41]
Capture-C		3C with specific oligonucleotides capture	Multiple targets	Sequencing	10-20 M	• Unbiased capture of all regions interacting with a specific target sequence • Reduced background signal compared to Hi-C • More informative contacts • Modified protocol: Capture Hi-C	• Interaction detection depends on the design of the target "bait"	[42]
Genome-wide								
Non-protein-mediated	Hi-C	Chromosome conformation capture by high-throughput sequencing	All interactions	Sequencing	20-25 M	• High throughput • Improved efficiency • First genome-wide assay • Modified protocol: in situ Hi-C; single cell Hi-C	• High background due to random ligations • Requires deep sequencing • Relatively low resolution	[21, 44–48]
Protein-mediated	ChIA-PET	Chromatin interaction analysis by paired-end tag sequencing	All interactions	Sequencing	> 100 M	• Identify specific protein-mediated DNA loop structures • Reduced background noise in sequencing data	• Long processing time (> 6 days) • Requires high efficiency ChIP-grade antibodies	[49]
	HiChIP/ PLAC-seq	In situ Hi-C with protein-centric ChIP/proximity ligation-assisted ChIP-seq	All interactions	Sequencing	1-10 M	• Faster protocol (2 days) • Higher efficiency than ChIA-PET • Less sequencing	• Requires high efficiency ChIP-grade antibodies	[50–52]

get chromatin quantities necessary to obtain meaningful results, thus restricting use to immortalized cell lines [15]. Given the cell type- and context-specific nature of chromatin dynamics, restricted use of 3C-based technologies to immortalized cell lines has hindered functional characterization of GWAS variants in more relevant primary cell models.

To capture 3D chromatin interactions on a genome-wide scale, proximity ligation was coupled with NGS to create an innovative method called Hi-C (Table 1) [21]. Following proximity ligation, chimeric strands are sequenced and aligned to a reference genome to identify where the two interacting regions were originally located within the linear DNA sequence, thereby identifying the anchor points where chromatin organizing proteins form a DNA loop. Early investigations using Hi-C revealed, for the first-time, chromatin substructures, i.e., TADs, within the context of previously characterized chromosome territories [18]. Subsequent advances in Hi-C methodology have improved resolution from > 100 kb in 2012 to ~ 5–10 kb in 2017, allowing for the generation of 3D genome maps that are now widely used to predict enhancer–promotor interactions occurring within a population of cells at a fixed time [28, 43–45]. Javierre et al. used promoter capture Hi-C (PCHi-C) to map the interacting regions of 31,253 promoters in 17 human primary blood cell types [46]. Not only did this study successfully use primary human cells to perform PCHi-C, but also successfully demonstrated that active enhancers significantly and quantitatively contribute to cell type-specific promoter activity and subsequent gene expression [46].

Single cell Hi-C was first reported in 2013 to explore the cell-to-cell variability of chromatin structures using a single copy X-chromosome model in isolated mouse nuclei [47]. More recently, the use of nucleic acid barcodes to index single cell nuclei eliminated the need to isolate individual nuclei for Hi-C, thus providing a more streamlined approach [48]. As single cell technologies improve along with analytical methods, we anticipate rapid adoption of single cell 3D genome approaches for many experimental designs.

Protein-mediated genome-wide methodologies (Table 1) include additional steps to isolate regions of interacting DNA based on the architectural proteins that influence those interactions, such as loop boundary markers (CTCF, cohesin, etc.), epigenetic markers of enhancers (acetylation of histone H3 on lysine 27 (H3K27ac)), or transcription factors [15, 33, 49–51]. Targeting specific proteins involved in chromatin organization reduces the background signal and the required sequencing depth—number of sequencing reads—necessary to achieve meaningful semi-quantitative results. Furthermore, these improvements have significantly reduced the number of

cells required, making it possible to now study DNA looping in primary cells. Recently, Mumbach et al. [52] reported using between 0.5 and one million cells to identify H3K27ac (a histone modification of active enhancers) looping profiles on naïve T cells, T-helper, and Th17 cells isolated from a primary T-cell population using HiChIP technology. The study demonstrated unique and differentially active enhancer loop clusters that corresponded with altered gene expression in each cell type [52], thus supporting current models suggesting different cell types and cell states adopt modified regulatory networks with specific enhancer–promoter loops to drive unique gene expression profiles.

3D genome-wide exploration generates tremendous amounts of sequencing data that require advanced algorithms and pipelines for processing, visualizing, and interpreting the functional significance of these 3D features. Fortunately, several robust software packages are publicly available and more are in development. Each algorithm uses different alignment strategies and filtering criteria to generate heatmaps based on interaction frequencies [43, 53] or looping diagrams that map protein-mediated DNA looping events in the context of linear chromatin [54]. Improvements to capture technologies that select for specific chromatin characteristics, such as histone marks or protein factors, and sequencing technologies that allow for sample barcoding and deeper sequencing continue to improve throughput and reduce background. Simultaneous improvements to the analysis pipelines that define the 3D genome continue to improve the base-pair resolution and quantitative capabilities of 3D technologies, allowing investigations of how disease-associated SNPs alter gene expression through modified 3D genome structures.

Application of 3C technologies to uncover new insights from GWAS in autoimmune disease

Autoimmune diseases, like most complex genetic diseases, result from the collective influence of multiple genetic variants on gene expression and responses to potentially damaging environmental conditions [2]. Investigating the functional significance of GWAS variants in the context of the 3D genome is essential for mechanistic understanding of how these variants, most of which are enriched in largely uncharacterized enhancer regions, influence disease pathology by reducing or enhancing interactions between enhancers and promoters within the enhancer regulatory network (Fig. 4a, b). For example, GWAS and fine-mapping revealed several autoimmune disease risk variants in the chromosome 6q23 locus, including a tandem pair of systemic lupus erythematosus (SLE)-associated polymorphisms, rs148314165 (−T) and rs200820567 (T > A) (referred to as the TT > A

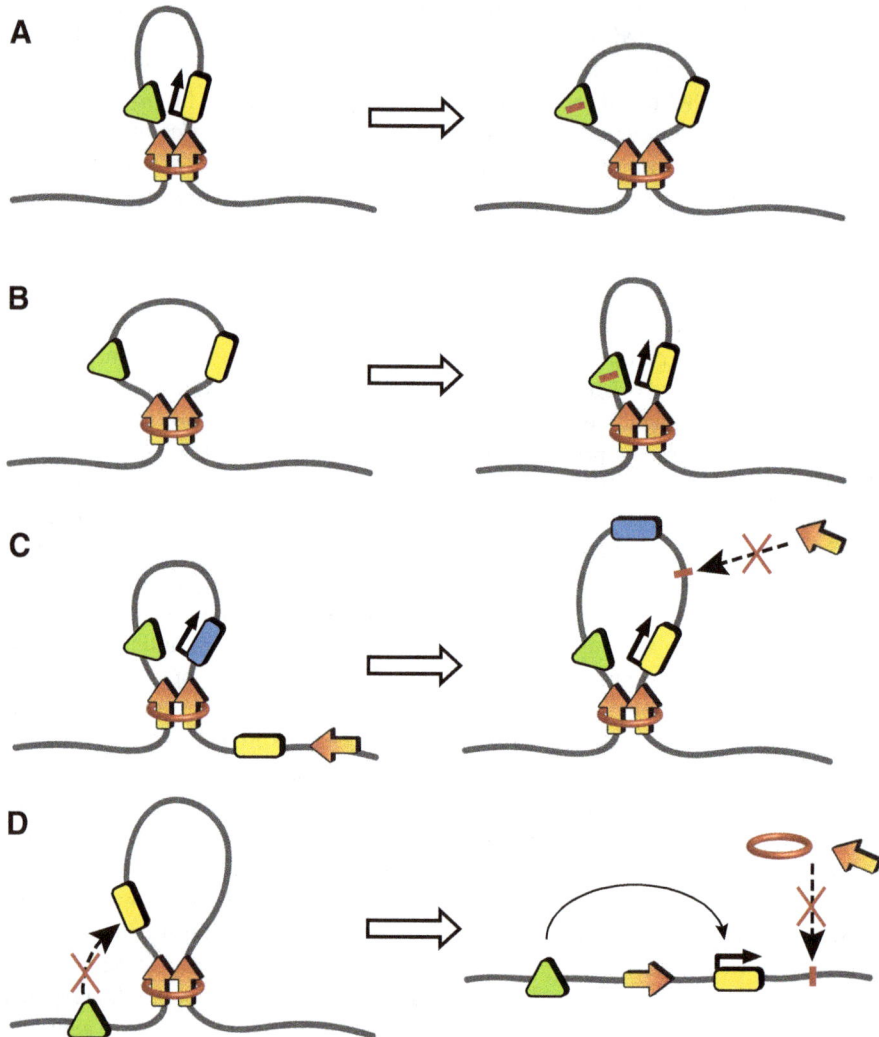

Fig. 4 Altering the 3D genome architecture disrupts gene expression regulation. **a**, **b** An enhancer (*green triangle*) can modulate gene expression by interacting with and delivering transcription factors to its target gene promoter (*yellow rectangle*) through long-range enhancer–promoter interactions. A causal mutation (*red bar*) in the enhancer can alter gene expression by modulating the frequency of this interaction. Impairing the frequency of the long-range interaction reduces delivery of transcription factors to the promoter, thus hindering gene expression (**a**). Enhancing interactions between the enhancer and promoter facilitates gene expression (**b**). **c**, **d** Insulated neighborhoods can regulate gene expression by restricting interactions between active enhancers (*green triangle*) and target gene promoters (*blue rectangle*) within an insulated loop boundary. Causal mutations (*red bar*) that disrupt CTCF anchor motifs can modify (**c**) or disrupt (**d**) existing loops, allowing the once-restricted enhancer (*green triangle*) to now interact with gene promoters (*yellow rectangle*) outside of the original insulated neighborhood

variants), located in an ENCODE-identified putative enhancer region located ~ 42 kb downstream of the tumor necrosis factor alpha-induced protein 3 (*TNFAIP3*) gene promoter [55, 56]. *TNFAIP3* is a critical negative regulator of pro-inflammatory nuclear factor kappa B (NF-κB) signaling implicated in many autoimmune diseases, and therefore a suspected target gene of the identified enhancer [55–57]. Functional studies using the quantitative-PCR-based 3C method determined that this enhancer facilitated *TNFAIP3* gene expression by bringing transcription factors, including NF-κB, to the *TNFAIP3* promoter region via

long-range enhancer–promoter interactions [55]. Importantly, the presence of the risk allele (−A/−A) in the enhancer was shown to significantly disrupt NF-κB binding and inhibit DNA looping of the enhancer to the *TNFAIP3* promoter, effectively suppressing *TNFAIP3* expression [57].

3D genome analysis is also a powerful method for identifying unsuspected candidate genes whose expression could be altered by risk variants in enhancers. For example, an enhancer harboring GWAS risk variants for rheumatoid arthritis was identified between oligodendrocyte transcription factor 3 (*OLIG3*) and *TNFAIP3*. In contrast to the well characterized role of *TNFAIP3* in regulating inflammatory signaling pathways, *OLIG3* is an important regulator of neuronal development and has no established role in the immune system [58], suggesting that *TNFAIP3* was the likely target of this enhancer. To test this hypothesis, Capture Hi-C studies in both B and T cells from patients with rheumatoid arthritis were performed. Interestingly, these studies revealed that chromatin loops formed not only between the enhancer and the downstream promoter of *TNFAIP3*, but also with the promoters of interleukin 20 receptor subunit alpha (*IL20RA*) and interferon gamma receptor 1 (*IFNGR1*) located 180 kb upstream [59]. Functional follow-up studies using 3C confirmed that the presence of the risk allele of SNP, rs6927172, in the enhancer resulted in increased looping to the promoter and a concomitant increase in *IL20RA* gene expression [59]. Importantly, no long-range interactions were observed between the enhancer and the *OLIG3* promoter, effectively eliminating this gene from further consideration. Together, these studies demonstrate the utility of targeted 3D genome applications to test and refine hypotheses regarding loop formation with enhancers harboring GWAS risk variants and their impact on gene expression.

Variants that disrupt anchor protein motifs, such as CTCF motifs that define TAD and insulated neighborhood boundaries, also have the potential to disrupt gene expression regulation by permitting aberrant boundary formation and allowing unrestricted enhancer activation of genes normally excluded from the neighborhood (Fig. 4c, d). An example of this occurs in T-cell acute lymphoblastic leukemia (T-ALL) where a mutation in a CTCF anchor motif disrupts the insulated neighborhood where the T-ALL-associated oncogene, TAL BHLH transcription factor 1 (*TAL1*), resides [60]. Importantly, this insulated neighborhood is devoid of a promoter, effectively inhibiting *TAL1* expression. Disrupting this CTCF boundary allows the promoter of a nearby gene, STIL centriolar assembly protein (*STIL*), to reposition near *TAL1* and activate expression [60]. This is one of many reported mutations in CTCF anchor motifs that have been shown to promote tumorigenesis by modifying looping activities around specific oncogenes [32, 61, 62].

3D genome technologies that typically require tens of millions of input cells have largely limited investigations into the potential implications of disrupting CTCF boundaries in primary immune cells involved in autoimmune disease pathogenesis. However, a recent report using 4C with NGS demonstrated that two asthma risk variants at the chromosome 17q21 locus, rs4065275 and rs12936231, individually altered CTCF binding motifs in CD4+ and CD8+ T cells [63]. In both cases, the 3D regulatory networks at this locus were significantly altered, resulting in increased expression of ORMDL sphingolipid biosynthesis regulator 3 (*ORMDL3*), a gene that facilitates cytokine production in the lung [63]. This study is one of the first to demonstrate that chromatin conformation methodologies can be used in primary cells to show that variants disrupting specific insulator boundaries can significantly alter the expression of genes implicated in disease pathogenesis. As more of these studies emerge in the future, we anticipate this to be a recurring theme, not only for cancer but complex diseases as well.

Conclusions

Analysis of 3D chromatin topology is an essential component for a complete mechanistic understanding of how genetic variants associated with complex human disease drive disease pathogenesis. As large-scale 3D chromatin technologies improve, we anticipate many of their current shortcomings will dissipate. In particular, we look forward to improvements in analytical methods that would facilitate truly quantitative comparisons of relative loop frequencies and enhancer–promoter interactions between different cell types and conditions. This, combined with reductions in chromatin input requirements such that small numbers of primary cells could be analyzed, would scale the potential of 3D chromatin studies in a manner that is now common for transcriptome studies.

The recently established 4D Nucleome Project supported by the NIH Common Fund [64] is charged with developing a "wiring diagram" for how the "parts list" discovered by the ENCODE and NIH-Roadmap consortiums is connected in 3D space and time to orchestrate proper gene transcription. Importantly, this consortium will work to innovate single-cell applications and establish quantitative analytical and innovative visualization platforms to bring 3D genome information into the mainstream of complex disease genetic analysis. As we have attempted to highlight in this review, this knowledge will be necessary for us to fully translate GWAS information into a more precise mechanistic understanding of how genetic variation influences disease risk. Ultimately, we hope that this will lead to improvements in our ability to predict, diagnose, and treat autoimmune diseases.

Abbreviations
3C: Chromatin conformation capture; 3D: Three-dimensional; CTCF: CCCTC-binding factors; ENCODE: Encyclopedia of DNA Elements; GWAS: Genome-wide association study(ies); H3K27ac: Acetylation of histone H3 on lysine 27; IDH: Isocitrate dehydrogenase; IFNGR1: Interferon gamma receptor 1; IGF2: Insulin-like growth factor 2; IHEC: International Human Epigenome Consortium; IL20RA: Interleukin 20 receptor subunit alpha; NF-κB: Nuclear factor kappa B; NGS: Next generation sequencing; NIH: National Institutes of Health; OLIG3: Oligodendrocyte transcription factor 3; ORMDL3: ORMDL Sphingolipid biosynthesis regulator 3; PCR: Polymerase chain reaction; PDGFRA: Platelet-derived growth factor receptor alpha; SLE: Systemic lupus

erythematosus; SNP: Single nucleotide polymorphism; TAD: Topologically associating domain; TAL1: TAL BHLH Transcription Factor 1; T-ALL: T-cell acute lymphoblastic leukemia; TNFAIP3: Tumor necrosis factor alpha-inducible protein 3

Funding

Research in the Gaffney lab is funded by the Presbyterian Health Foundation and NIH grants, P30 GM110766, R01 AR056360, U19 AI082714, and R01 AR063124.

Authors' contributions

YF, KLT, and PMG all contributed in writing the manuscript. YF and CL created the figures. All authors have read and approved the final manuscript.

Consent for publication

Not applicable.

Competing interests

The authors declare that they have no competing interests.

Author details

[1]Division of Genomics and Data Sciences, Arthritis and Clinical Immunology Research Program, Oklahoma Medical Research Foundation, 825 Northeast 13th Street, Oklahoma City, OK 73104, USA. [2]School of Electrical and Computer Engineering, University of Oklahoma, Devan Energy Hall 150, 110 West Boyd Street, Norman, OK 73019, USA.

References

1. Gutierrez-Arcelus M, Rich SS, Raychaudhuri S. Autoimmune diseases - connecting risk alleles with molecular traits of the immune system. Nat Rev Genet. 2016;17(3):160–74.
2. Ramos PS, Shedlock AM, Langefeld CD. Genetics of autoimmune diseases: insights from population genetics. J Hum Genet. 2015;60(11):657–64.
3. Visscher PM, Wray NR, Zhang Q, Sklar P, McCarthy MI, Brown MA, Yang J. 10 years of GWAS discovery: biology, function, and translation. Am J Hum Genet. 2017;101(1):5–22.
4. Manolio TA, Collins FS, Cox NJ, Goldstein DB, Hindorff LA, Hunter DJ, McCarthy MI, Ramos EM, Cardon LR, Chakravarti A, et al. Finding the missing heritability of complex diseases. Nature. 2009;461(7265):747–53.
5. Farh KK-H, Marson A, Zhu J, Kleinewietfeld M, Housley WJ, Beik S, Shoresh N, Whitton H, Ryan RJ, Shishkin AA. Genetic and epigenetic fine mapping of causal autoimmune disease variants. Nature. 2015;518(7539):337–43.
6. Consortium EP. An integrated encyclopedia of DNA elements in the human genome. Nature. 2012;489(7414):57–74.
7. Bernstein BE, Stamatoyannopoulos JA, Costello JF, Ren B, Milosavljevic A, Meissner A, Kellis M, Marra MA, Beaudet AL, Ecker JR, et al. The NIH Roadmap Epigenomics Mapping Consortium. Nat Biotechnol. 2010;28(10): 1045–8.
8. Bujold D, Morais DAL, Gauthier C, Cote C, Caron M, Kwan T, Chen KC, Laperle J, Markovits AN, Pastinen T, et al. The International Human Epigenome Consortium Data Portal. Cell Syst. 2016;3(5):496–9 e492.
9. Heinz S, Romanoski CE, Benner C, Glass CK. The selection and function of cell type-specific enhancers. Nat Rev Mol Cell Biol. 2015;16(3):144–54.
10. Heintzman ND, Stuart RK, Hon G, Fu Y, Ching CW, Hawkins RD, Barrera LO, Van Calcar S, Qu C, Ching KA. Distinct and predictive chromatin signatures of transcriptional promoters and enhancers in the human genome. Nat Genet. 2007;39(3):311–8.
11. Bonev B, Cavalli G. Organization and function of the 3D genome. Nat Rev Genet. 2016;17(11):661–78.
12. Gómez-Díaz E, Corces VG. Architectural proteins: regulators of 3D genome organization in cell fate. Trends Cell Biol. 2014;24(11):703–11.
13. Nichols MH, Corces VG. A CTCF code for 3D genome architecture. Cell. 2015;162(4):703–5.
14. Krijger PHL, De Laat W. Regulation of disease-associated gene expression in the 3D genome. Nat Rev Mol Cell Biol. 2016;17(12):771–82
15. Yu M, Ren B. The three-dimensional organization of mammalian genomes. Annu Rev Cell Dev Biol. 2017;33:265–89.
16. Schaffner W. Enhancers, enhancers–from their discovery to today's universe of transcription enhancers. Biol Chem. 2015;396(4):311–27.
17. Martin P, McGovern A, Orozco G, Duffus K, Yarwood A, Schoenfelder S, Cooper NJ, Barton A, Wallace C, Fraser P, Worthington J, Eyre S. Capture Hi-C reveals novel candidate genes and complex long-range interactions with related autoimmune risk loci. Nat Commun. 2015;6:10069.
18. Dixon JR, Selvaraj S, Yue F, Kim A, Li Y, Shen Y, Hu M, Liu JS, Ren B. Topological domains in mammalian genomes identified by analysis of chromatin interactions. Nature. 2012;485(7398):376–80.
19. Cremer T, Kurz A, Zirbel R, Dietzel S, Rinke B, Schröck E, Speicher MR, Mathieu U, Jauch A, Emmerich P. Role of chromosome territories in the functional compartmentalization of the cell nucleus. Cold Spring Harb Symp Quant Biol. 1993;58:777–92.
20. Bouwman BA, de Laat W. Getting the genome in shape: the formation of loops, domains and compartments. Genome Biol. 2015;16:154.
21. Lieberman-Aiden E, Van Berkum NL, Williams L, Imakaev M, Ragoczy T, Telling A, Amit I, Lajoie BR, Sabo PJ, Dorschner MO. Comprehensive mapping of long-range interactions reveals folding principles of the human genome. Science. 2009;326(5950):289–93.
22. Fortin JP, Hansen KD. Reconstructing A/B compartments as revealed by Hi-C using long-range correlations in epigenetic data. Genome Biol. 2015;16:180.
23. Wang SY, Su JH, Beliveau BJ, Bintu B, Moffitt JR, Wu CT, Zhuang XW. Spatial organization of chromatin domains and compartments in single chromosomes. Science. 2016;353(6299):598–602.
24. Nora EP, Lajoie BR, Schulz EG, Giorgetti L, Okamoto I, Servant N, Piolot T, van Berkum NL, Meisig J, Sedat J. Spatial partitioning of the regulatory landscape of the X-inactivation centre. Nature. 2012;485(7398):381–5.
25. Sanborn AL, Rao SS, Huang S-C, Durand NC, Huntley MH, Jewett AI, Bochkov ID, Chinnappan D, Cutkosky A, Li J. Chromatin extrusion explains key features of loop and domain formation in wild-type and engineered genomes. Proc Natl Acad Sci U S A. 2015;112(47):E6456–65.
26. Hansen AS, Pustova I, Cattoglio C, Tjian R, Darzacq X. CTCF and cohesin regulate chromatin loop stability with distinct dynamics. eLife. 2017;6:e25776.
27. Fudenberg G, Pollard K. Chromatin features constrain structural variation across evolutionary timescales. bioRxiv. 2018:285205.
28. Schmitt AD, Hu M, Jung I, Xu Z, Qiu YJ, Tan CL, Li Y, Lin S, Lin YI, Barr CL, et al. A compendium of chromatin contact maps reveals spatially active regions in the human genome. Cell Rep. 2016;17(8):2042–59.
29. Hnisz D, Day DS, Young RA. Insulated neighborhoods: structural and functional units of mammalian gene control. Cell. 2016;167(5):1188–200.
30. Dowen JM, Fan ZP, Hnisz D, Ren G, Abraham BJ, Zhang LN, Weintraub AS, Schuijers J, Lee TI, Zhao K. Control of cell identity genes occurs in insulated neighborhoods in mammalian chromosomes. Cell. 2014;159(2):374–87.
31. Shen Y, Yue F, McCleary DF, Ye Z, Edsall L, Kuan S, Wagner U, Dixon J, Lee L, Lobanenkov VV. A map of the cis-regulatory sequences in the mouse genome. Nature. 2012;488(7409):116–20.
32. Katainen R, Dave K, Pitkänen E, Palin K, Kivioja T, Välimäki N, Gylfe AE, Ristolainen H, Hänninen UA, Cajuso T. CTCF/cohesin-binding sites are frequently mutated in cancer. Nat Genet. 2015;47(7):818–21.
33. Schmitt AD, Hu M, Ren B. Genome-wide mapping and analysis of chromosome architecture. Nat Rev Mol Cell Biol. 2016;17(12):743–55.
34. Dekker J, Rippe K, Dekker M, Kleckner N. Capturing chromosome conformation. Science. 2002;295(5558):1306–11.
35. Hagege H, Klous P, Braem C, Splinter E, Dekker J, Cathala G, De Laat W, Forné T. Quantitative analysis of chromosome conformation capture assays (3C-qPCR). Nat Protoc. 2007;2(7):1722.
36. Nakagawa H, Chadwick RB, Peltomäki P, Plass C, Nakamura Y, de la Chapelle A. Loss of imprinting of the insulin-like growth factor II gene occurs by biallelic methylation in a core region of H19-associated CTCF-binding sites in colorectal cancer. Proc Natl Acad Sci U S A. 2001;98(2):591–6.

37. Kurukuti S, Tiwari VK, Tavoosidana G, Pugacheva E, Murrell A, Zhao Z, Lobanenkov V, Reik W, Ohlsson R. CTCF binding at the H19 imprinting control region mediates maternally inherited higher-order chromatin conformation to restrict enhancer access to Igf2. Proc Natl Acad Sci U S A. 2006;103(28):10684–9.

38. Nativio R, Sparago A, Ito Y, Weksberg R, Riccio A, Murrell A. Disruption of genomic neighbourhood at the imprinted IGF2-H19 locus in Beckwith–Wiedemann syndrome and Silver–Russell syndrome. Hum Mol Genet. 2011; 20(7):1363–74.

39. Flavahan WA, Drier Y, Liau BB, Gillespie SM, Venteicher AS, Stemmer-Rachamimov AO, Suvà ML, Bernstein BE. Insulator dysfunction and oncogene activation in IDH mutant gliomas. Nature. 2016;529(7584):110–4.

40. Zhao Z, Tavoosidana G, Sjölinder M, Göndör A, Mariano P, Wang S, Kanduri C, Lezcano M, Sandhu KS, Singh U. Circular chromosome conformation capture (4C) uncovers extensive networks of epigenetically regulated intra- and interchromosomal interactions. Nat Genet. 2006;38(11):1341–7.

41. Dostie J, Richmond TA, Arnaout RA, Selzer RR, Lee WL, Honan TA, Rubio ED, Krumm A, Lamb J, Nusbaum C. Chromosome Conformation Capture Carbon Copy (5C): a massively parallel solution for mapping interactions between genomic elements. Genome Res. 2006;16(10):1299–309.

42. Hughes JR, Roberts N, McGowan S, Hay D, Giannoulatou E, Lynch M, De Gobbi M, Taylor S, Gibbons R, Higgs DR. Analysis of hundreds of cis-regulatory landscapes at high resolution in a single, high-throughput experiment. Nat Genet. 2014;46(2):205.

43. Durand NC, Robinson JT, Shamim MS, Machol I, Mesirov JP, Lander ES, Aiden EL. Juicebox provides a visualization system for Hi-C contact maps with unlimited zoom. Cell Syst. 2016;3(1):99–101.

44. Jin F, Li Y, Dixon JR, Selvaraj S, Ye Z, Lee AY, Yen C-A, Schmitt AD, Espinoza CA, Ren B. A high-resolution map of the three-dimensional chromatin interactome in human cells. Nature. 2013;503(7475):290.

45. Belaghzal H, Dekker J, Gibcus JH. Hi-C 2.0: An optimized Hi-C procedure for high-resolution genome-wide mapping of chromosome conformation. Methods. 2017;123:56–65.

46. Javierre BM, Burren OS, Wilder SP, Kreuzhuber R, Hill SM, Sewitz S, Cairns J, Wingett SW, Varnai C, Thiecke MJ, et al. Lineage-specific genome architecture links enhancers and non-coding disease variants to target gene promoters. Cell. 2016;167(5):1369–1384.e19.

47. Nagano T, Lubling Y, Stevens TJ, Schoenfelder S, Yaffe E, Dean W, Laue ED, Tanay A, Fraser P. Single-cell Hi-C reveals cell-to-cell variability in chromosome structure. Nature. 2013;502(7469):59–64.

48. Ramani V, Deng X, Qiu R, Gunderson KL, Steemers FJ, Disteche CM, Noble WS, Duan Z, Shendure J. Massively multiplex single-cell Hi-C. Nat Methods. 2017;14(3):263–6.

49. Fullwood MJ, Liu MH, Pan YF, Liu J, Xu H, Mohamed YB, Orlov YL, Velkov S, Ho A, Mei PH. An oestrogen-receptor-α-bound human chromatin interactome. Nature. 2009;462(7269):58–64.

50. Mumbach MR, Rubin AJ, Flynn RA, Dai C, Khavari PA, Greenleaf WJ, Chang HY. HiChIP: efficient and sensitive analysis of protein-directed genome architecture. Nat Methods. 2016;13(11):919–22.

51. Fang R, Yu M, Li G, Chee S, Liu T, Schmitt AD, Ren B. Mapping of long-range chromatin interactions by proximity ligation-assisted ChIP-seq. Cell Res. 2016;26(12):1345–48.

52. Mumbach MR, Satpathy AT, Boyle EA, Dai C, Gowen BG, Cho SW, Nguyen ML, Rubin AJ, Granja JM, Kazane KR. Enhancer connectome in primary human cells identifies target genes of disease-associated DNA elements. Nat Genet. 2017;49(11):1602–12.

53. Kerpedjiev P, Abdennur N, Lekschas F, McCallum C, Dinkla K, Strobelt H, Luber JM, Ouellette SB, Ahzir A, Kumar N, Hwang J, Lee S, Alver BH, Pfister H, Mirny LA, Park PJ, Gehlenberg N. HiGlass: Web-based visual exploration and analysis of genome interaction maps. Genome Biology. 2018;19:125.

54. Lareau CA, Aryee MJ. Hichipper: a preprocessing pipeline for calling DNA loops from HiChIP data. Nat Methods. 2018;15(3):155.

55. Wang S, Wen F, Wiley GB, Kinter MT, Gaffney PM. An enhancer element harboring variants associated with systemic lupus erythematosus engages the TNFAIP3 promoter to influence A20 expression. PLoS Genet. 2013;9(9):e1003750.

56. Graham RR, Cotsapas C, Davies L, Hackett R, Lessard CJ, Leon JM, Burtt NP, Guiducci C, Parkin M, Gates C. Genetic variants near TNFAIP3 on 6q23 are associated with systemic lupus erythematosus. Nat Genet. 2008;40(9):1059–61.

57. Wang S, Wen F, Tessneer KL, Gaffney PM. TALEN-mediated enhancer knockout influences TNFAIP3 gene expression and mimics a molecular

phenotype associated with systemic lupus erythematosus. Genes Immun. 2016;17(3):165–70.

58. Hernandez-Miranda LR, Ruffault P-L, Bouvier JC, Murray AJ, Morin-Surun M-P, Zampieri N, Cholewa-Waclaw JB, Ey E, Brunet J-F, Champagnat J. Genetic identification of a hindbrain nucleus essential for innate vocalization. Proc Natl Acad Sci U S A. 2017;114(30):8095–100.

59. McGovern A, Schoenfelder S, Martin P, Massey J, Duffus K, Plant D, Yarwood A, Pratt AG, Anderson AE, Isaacs JD. Capture Hi-C identifies a novel causal gene, IL20RA, in the pan-autoimmune genetic susceptibility region 6q23. Genome Biol. 2016;17(1):212.

60. Hnisz D, Weintraub AS, Day DS, Valton A-L, Bak RO, Li CH, Goldmann J, Lajoie BR, Fan ZP, Sigova AA. Activation of proto-oncogenes by disruption of chromosome neighborhoods. Science. 2016;351(6280):1454–58.

61. Witcher M, Emerson BM. Epigenetic silencing of the p16INK4a tumor suppressor is associated with loss of CTCF binding and a chromatin boundary. Mol Cell. 2009;34(3):271–84.

62. Xiang J-F, Yin Q-F, Chen T, Zhang Y, Zhang X-O, Wu Z, Zhang S, Wang H-B, Ge J, Lu X. Human colorectal cancer-specific CCAT1-L lncRNA regulates long-range chromatin interactions at the MYC locus. Cell Res. 2014;24(5):513–31.

63. Schmiedel BJ, Seumois G, Samaniego-Castruita D, Cayford J, Schulten V, Chavez L, Ay F, Sette A, Peters B, Vijayanand P. 17q21 asthma-risk variants switch CTCF binding and regulate IL-2 production by T cells. Nat Commun. 2016;7:13426.

64. Dekker J, Belmont AS, Guttman M, Leshyk VO, Lis JT, Lomvardas S, Mirny LA, O'shea CC, Park PJ, Ren B. The 4D nucleome project. Nature. 2017;549(7671):219.

23

VZV-specific T-cell levels in patients with rheumatic diseases are reduced and differentially influenced by antirheumatic drugs

David Schub[1], Gunter Assmann[2], Urban Sester[3], Martina Sester[1] and Tina Schmidt[1]* ⓘ

Abstract

Background: Varicella zoster virus (VZV)-specific cellular immunity is essential for viral control, and the incidence of VZV reactivation is increased in patients with rheumatic diseases. Because knowledge of the influence of antirheumatic drugs on specific cellular immunity is limited, we analyzed VZV-specific T cells in patients with rheumatoid arthritis (RA) and seronegative spondylarthritis (SpA), and we assessed how their levels and functionality were impacted by disease-modifying antirheumatic drugs (DMARDs). A polyclonal stimulation was carried out to analyze effects on general effector T cells.

Methods: CD4 T cells in 98 blood samples of patients with RA ($n = 78$) or SpA ($n = 20$) were quantified by flow cytometry after stimulation with VZV antigen and the polyclonal stimulus *Staphylococcus aureus* enterotoxin B (SEB), and they were characterized for expression of cytokines (interferon-γ, tumor necrosis factor [TNF]-α, interleukin [IL]-2) and markers for activation (CD69), differentiation (CD127), or functional anergy programmed death 1 molecule [PD-1], cytotoxic T-lymphocyte antigen 4 [CTLA-4]. Results of patients with RA were stratified into subgroups receiving different antirheumatic drugs and compared with samples of 39 healthy control subjects. Moreover, direct effects of biological DMARDs on cytokine expression and proliferation of specific T cells were analyzed in vitro.

Results: Unlike patients with SpA, patients with RA showed significantly lower percentages of VZV-specific CD4 T cells (median 0.03%, IQR 0.05%) than control subjects (median 0.09%, IQR 0.16%; $p < 0.001$). Likewise, SEB-reactive CD4 T-cell levels were lower in patients (median 2.35%, IQR 2.85%) than in control subjects (median 3.96%, IQR 4.38%; $p < 0.05$); however, expression of cytokines and cell surface markers of VZV-specific T cells did not differ in patients and control subjects, whereas SEB-reactive effector T cells of patients showed signs of functional impairment. Among antirheumatic drugs, biological DMARDs had the most pronounced impact on cellular immunity. Specifically, VZV-specific CD4 T-cell levels were significantly reduced in patients receiving TNF-α antagonists or IL-6 receptor-blocking therapy ($p < 0.05$ and $p < 0.01$, respectively), whereas SEB-reactive T-cell levels were reduced in patients receiving B-cell-depleting or IL-6 receptor-blocking drugs (both $p < 0.05$).

Conclusions: Despite absence of clinical symptoms, patients with RA showed signs of impaired cellular immunity that affected both VZV-specific and general effector T cells. Strongest effects on cellular immunity were observed in patients treated with biological DMARDs. These findings may contribute to the increased susceptibility of patients with RA to VZV reactivation.

Keywords: T cells, Varicella zoster virus, bDMARDs, Antirheumatic medication, Rheumatic patients

* Correspondence: tina.schmidt@uks.eu
[1]Department of Transplant and Infection Immunology, Saarland University, 66421 Homburg, Germany
Full list of author information is available at the end of the article

Background

The varicella zoster virus (VZV) establishes lifelong persistence, thereby requiring permanent control by the host immune system. As a consequence, viral reactivation, mainly presenting as herpes zoster with a median incidence of 4–4.5 per 1000 person-years in the general population [1], preferentially occurs in individuals with impaired immune function. Large observational studies demonstrated a higher rate of herpes zoster in patients with rheumatic disease [2–4]; comparison between different autoimmune diseases revealed the highest age-standardized incidence of herpes zoster in patients with systemic lupus erythematosus (SLE), followed by inflammatory bowel disease and rheumatoid arthritis (RA) [4].

During the last several years, cellular immunity was identified as a main contributor to efficient control of VZV in both immunocompetent and immunocompromised persons [5–8]. This also holds true for patients with autoimmune diseases, where VZV-specific CD4 T cells seem crucial to preventing reactivation [8, 9]. We have previously found in immunocompetent individuals and various groups of immunocompromised patients with and without herpes zoster that VZV-specific CD4 T cells show distinct changes in phenotype and functionality in association with herpes zoster [10]. Interestingly, when compared with control subjects, first evidence suggests that patients with rheumatic diseases showed lower levels of VZV-specific CD4 T cells and an increased expression of the inhibitory molecule cytotoxic T-lymphocyte antigen 4 (CTLA-4) on polyclonally stimulated effector T cells, even in the absence of acute VZV reactivation [10]. This indicates a general impairment of cellular immunity that may be a consequence of the autoimmune disease itself or be caused at least in part by treatment with immunomodulatory antirheumatic drugs such as conventional and biological disease-modifying antirheumatic drugs (cDMARDs and bDMARDs, respectively). Although these immunological alterations may predispose for an increased zoster incidence in patients with rheumatic diseases, evidence on the association of different treatment modalities and the risk for herpes zoster is conflicting (reviewed in [11, 12]). In addition, studies on the influence of antirheumatic medication on VZV-specific cellular immunity are limited. Therefore, the aim of the present study was to analyze the impact of disease entity and antirheumatic medication on VZV-specific and general effector T-cell immunity in patients with RA and seronegative spondylarthritis (SpA). Furthermore, the effect of different antirheumatic drugs on effector T cells was analyzed in vitro.

Methods

Recruitment of the study population

Patients with rheumatic diseases, including RA and different types of seronegative spondylarthritis (SpA, including psoriatic arthritis [PsA] and ankylosing spondylitis [AS]), were recruited. Seven patients with RA had more than one blood sample analyzed because their antirheumatic medication was changed at least once during the period of patient enrollment. Because VZV-specific T-cell levels and phenotype are altered in patients with herpes zoster and were shown to normalize within 3 months after resolution [10], patients who had experienced active herpes zoster within the last 3 months before sample acquisition were excluded from major analyses. Likewise, VZV-immunoglobulin G (IgG)-seronegative individuals were excluded. Healthy immunocompetent individuals were recruited as control subjects. Patients had received treatment with cDMARDs or bDMARDs for at least 12 weeks to ensure sufficient exposure to the antirheumatic agent. Patients who did not receive any antirheumatic therapy (except steroids) for at least 12 weeks before blood sampling were termed "therapy-naïve." If steroids were given, the dosage ranged from 1.5 mg to 40 mg prednisolone equivalent daily (mean 6.4 ± 7.4 mg/d). Additional information regarding history of previous episodes of herpes zoster was collected from the study participants and the treating physician.

Quantification and characterization of VZV-specific and SEB-reactive T cells

T cells from heparinized whole blood were stimulated in vitro and incubated for 6 h exactly as described before [10]. In brief, blood samples were stimulated with a lysate of VZV-infected fibroblasts, uninfected control lysate (negative control; Virion/Serion, Würzburg, Germany), and 2.5 µg/ml *Staphylococcus aureus* enterotoxin B (SEB) (positive control; Sigma-Aldrich, St. Louis, MO, USA), respectively. All stimulations were performed in the presence of 1 µg/ml anti-CD28 and anti-CD49d (BD Biosciences, San Jose, CA, USA). The last 4 h of stimulation was carried out in the presence of 10 mg/ml brefeldin A. Thereafter, cells were fixed and immunostained with antibodies toward CD4, CD69, interferon (IFN)-γ, interleukin (IL)-2, tumor necrosis factor (TNF)-α, CTLA-4, the programmed death 1 molecule (PD-1) (all from BD Biosciences), and CD127 (eBioscience, San Diego, CA, USA). Flow cytometric analyses were performed on a FACSCanto II using FACSDiva version 6.1.3 software (BD Biosciences). Percentages of VZV-specific CD4 T cells were calculated by subtracting the results obtained after VZV-specific stimulation by those of the negative control. The experimental approach including the detection limit of 0.02% VZV-specific CD4 T cells was established before [10]. Based on serology as a gold standard, this assay has a sensitivity of 92% and a specificity of 74% [10], and the stimuli are able to detect VZV-specific T cells in both infected individuals [10] and after varicella vaccination (Additional file 1: Figure S1).

For analysis of late cytokine expression and proliferation, blood samples were processed as described above, but incubation time was prolonged to 36 h. Proliferation was assessed as described before [13] by incorporation of 500 mM bromodeoxyuridine (BrdU) (Sigma-Aldrich) that was added after 28 h. After fixation, cells were stained with antibodies toward CD4, CD8, CD69, IFN-γ, and BrdU (all from BD Biosciences).

Preincubation of immune cells with antirheumatic and other immunosuppressive agents

Whole blood (300 µl) was preincubated at 37 °C, 5% CO_2, for 4 h with estimated maximum plasma levels of different antirheumatic and other immunosuppressive agents as well as with fivefold lower and fivefold higher concentrations (tenfold for methylprednisolone [MP]), respectively. Estimated maximum plasma levels were 150 µg/ml for abatacept, 100 µg/ml for adalimumab, 2.5 µg/ml for etanercept, 300 µg/ml for rituximab and tocilizumab, 1 µg/ml for MP, 0.8 µg/ml for cyclosporine A (CyA), 0.4 µg/ml for methotrexate, and 50 ng/ml for tofacitinib. CyA was chosen as a positive control drug with a known dose-dependent inhibitory effect on T-cell effector function and proliferation [13, 14]. After preincubation, samples were processed for cytokine secretion and proliferation analyses as described above. Because abatacept acts as a T-cell costimulation inhibitor by blocking the CD28-CD80/86 interaction, analyses of its effect on T-cell stimulation were performed in both the presence and absence of anti-CD28 antibody, which was routinely added together with CD49d to all stimulatory reactions (*see above*).

Quantification of VZV-specific antibodies

VZV-specific antibodies were quantified using a commercial anti-IgG enzyme-linked immunosorbent assay (Euroimmun AG, Lübeck, Germany). IgG levels < 80 IU/L were scored negative, levels 80–110 IU/L were scored intermediate, and levels > 110 IU/L were scored positive according to the manufacturer's instructions.

Statistical analysis

Statistical data analysis was carried out using Prism version 5.03 software (GraphPad Software, La Jolla, CA, USA). Analyses of continuous variables (leukocyte count, percentage of lymphocytes, C-reactive protein [CRP],

erythrocyte sedimentation rate [ESR], VZV- and SEB-reactive CD4 T-cell frequencies) were performed using the Mann-Whitney U test for two groups and the Kruskal-Wallis test (with Dunn's posttest) for more than two groups. Differences in age, time since disease onset, Disease Activity Score 28-joint count (DAS28), and T-cell cytokine expression were analyzed using an unpaired t test for comparison between two groups and one-way analysis of variance (with Bonferroni posttest) for comparison of more than two groups. Comparison of categorical variables (erosive course, gender, history of herpes zoster) was performed using Fisher's exact test and the χ^2 test for two or more groups, respectively. Correlations were analyzed according to Spearman (rank-sum).

Results
Study population

VZV-specific immunity was analyzed in 98 samples of 90 patients with rheumatic diseases, including 70 patients (78 samples) with RA and 20 patients with different types of seronegative spondylarthritis (SpA, including 17 patients with PsA and 3 patients with AS). Samples from 39 age-matched immunocompetent individuals served as controls. Four patients (three RA, one SpA) showed VZV-specific IgG below the detection limit and were excluded from all subsequent analyses. Moreover, one sample of a patient who had an episode of zoster 1 month prior to sampling was excluded from major analyses. Their patient characteristics were not different from the remaining study participants, which are shown in Table 1. The three groups did not show any significant differences in gender, leukocyte counts, and percentages of lymphocytes. Likewise, time since onset of disease, DAS28, ESR, and the percentage of patients with an erosive course did not differ between patients with RA and patients with SpA, whereas CRP was significantly higher in patients with SpA ($p = 0.03$). In contrast to healthy control subjects, 12 of the 85 VZV-seropositive patients (11 RA, 1 SpA) reported a history of herpes zoster 8.2 ± 9.2 years ago ($p = 0.03$).

Lower percentages of VZV-specific and SEB-reactive CD4 T cells in patients with rheumatoid arthritis

To compare VZV-specific T-cell immunity in patients with RA, with SpA, and in healthy control subjects, whole-blood samples ($n = 74$, 19, and 39, respectively) were stimulated with VZV lysate and subsequently analyzed using flow cytometry. Stimulation with uninfected control lysate served as a negative control, and stimulation with SEB was performed for general assessment of polyclonally activated effector T cells. Reactive CD4 T cells were identified by coexpression of the activation marker CD69 and the cytokine IFN-γ after stimulation.

Table 1 Characteristics of the study population[a]

	Healthy control subjects	Patients with RA	Patients with seronegative SpA	p Value
Total number of tested samples	39	74	19[b]	–
Age, years, mean ± SD	58.6 ± 16.2	60.6 ± 13.0	51.4 ± 11.9	0.04[c,d]
Female sex, n (%)	22 (56.4)	56 (75.7)	11 (57.9)	0.07[e]
Leukocyte count median (IQR), cells/μl	7320 (3072) (n = 36)	7800 (4240) (n = 73)	7400 (4200) (n = 19)	0.42[f]
Lymphocytes median (IQR), %	26.0 (11.1) (n = 28)	23.0 (13.6) (n = 73)	26.0 (10.0) (n = 19)	0.12[f]
Time since disease onset, years, mean ± SD	–	8.0 ± 6.4 (n = 67)	7.9 ± 8.8 (n = 19)	0.93[g]
DAS28, mean ± SD	–	3.76 ± 1.27 (n = 50)	3.72 ± 1.48 (n = 3)	0.96[g]
CRP median (IQR), mg/L	–	1.9 (3.7) (n = 64)	4.3 (14.1) (n = 16)	0.03[h]
ESR median (IQR), mm/h	–	13.0 (18.5) (n = 52)	14.0 (18.0) (n = 15)	0.57[h]
Erosive course, %	–	40.0 (n = 60)	46.7 (n = 15)	0.77[i]
History of herpes zoster > 3 months ago, n (%)	0	11 (14.9)	1 (5.3)	0.03[e]

Abbreviations: CRP C-reactive protein, DAS28 Disease Activity Score 28-joint count, ESR Erythrocyte sedimentation rate, RA Rheumatoid arthritis, SpA Seronegative spondylarthritis
The numbers in parentheses (n) refer to the samples for which the respective information was available
[a]VZV-IgG negative individuals (3 female RA patients (50, 58, and 77 years of age) and 1 male SpA patient (37 years of age), and one sample of an 80 years old female RA patient with an episode of herpes zoster 1 month before sampling were excluded (their leukocyte counts and clinical characteristics were not different from the remaining patients)
[b]Sixteen patients with psoriatic arthritis, three patients with ankylosing spondylitis
[c]In posttest, $p < 0.05$ only between RA and SpA
[d]One-way analysis of variance
[e]χ^2 test
[f]Kruskal-Wallis test
[g]Unpaired t test
[h]Mann-Whitney U test
[i]Fisher's exact test

Representative examples of flow cytometric dotplots are shown in Fig. 1a. CD4 T-cell frequencies in patients with RA and patients with SpA were lower than in control subjects, which held true for both VZV-specific ($p < 0.0001$) (Fig. 1b, left panel) and SEB-reactive CD4 T cells ($p = 0.013$) (Fig. 1b, right panel). In contrast, no differences were observed in VZV-specific IgG levels (Fig. 1c). As described before [10], there was an inverse correlation of VZV-specific T-cell levels with age ($r = -0.306$, $p = 0.008$), which was not observed for SEB-reactive T cells ($r = -0.030$, $p = $ n.s.) (Additional file 1: Table S1). However, the lower percentage of reactive CD4 T cells in patients with RA was associated with neither disease activity (DAS28) (Fig. 1d) nor other clinical parameters (Additional file 1: Table S1). Likewise, no differences were found in VZV-specific and SEB-reactive CD4 T-cell frequencies between patients with and without a history of previous herpes zoster (gray and white symbols in Fig. 1). Interestingly, however, the patient who was excluded from the analyses owing to an episode of herpes zoster 1 month before sampling had a markedly higher percentage of VZV-specific CD4 T cells (0.396%) than in the time before zoster (0.010%; data not shown).

To characterize functional and phenotypical properties of VZV- and SEB-reactive T cells, the expression profiles of the cytokines IFN-γ, IL-2, and TNF-α were analyzed, where a total of seven subpopulations expressing either one, two, or all three cytokines were considered. In addition, surface markers associated with functional anergy (CTLA-4, PD-1) and differentiation (CD127) were analyzed. Representative examples of the flow cytometric dotplots are depicted in Additional file 1: Figure S2. As shown in Fig. 2, VZV-specific CD4 T cells in patients did not exhibit any signs of functional impairment. In contrast, when compared with those of control subjects, SEB-reactive CD4 T cells of patients with RA showed lower percentages of cells expressing all three cytokines ($p = 0.0004$) or IFN-γ alone ($p = 0.005$) or in combination with IL-2 ($p = 0.006$) (Fig. 2a, lower panel). Likewise, SEB-reactive T cells from patients with RA and patients with SpA had higher expression levels of the anergy marker CTLA-4 ($p < 0.05$) (Fig. 2b, upper panel), whereas PD-1 expression was significantly higher in patients with SpA only ($p < 0.05$) (Fig. 2b, middle panel). In contrast, expression of the differentiation marker CD127 did not differ in any of the groups (Fig. 2b, lower panel).

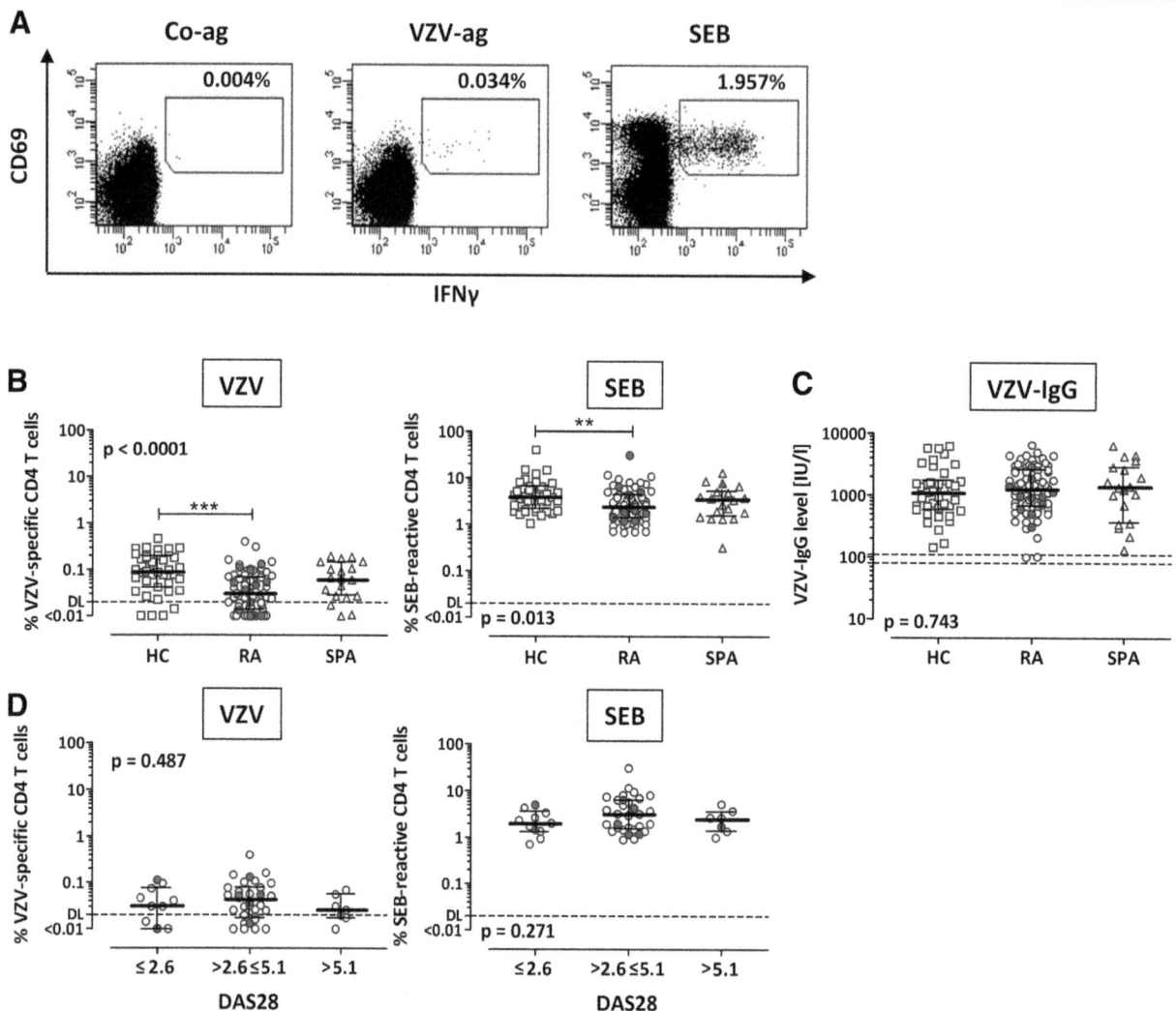

Fig. 1 Varicella zoster virus (VZV)-specific and *Staphylococcus aureus* enterotoxin B (SEB)-reactive CD4 T cells show reduced frequencies in patients with rheumatoid arthritis (RA). Whole blood was stimulated with control antigen (Co-ag, negative control), VZV antigen (VZV-ag), and the polyclonal stimulus SEB, respectively, and reactive CD4 T cells (CD69$^+$IFN-γ$^+$) were analyzed using flow cytometry. **a** Typical dotplots of a 39-year-old patient with RA are shown. Numbers indicate the percentages of reactive CD4 T cells. **b** Frequencies of VZV-specific CD4 T cells corrected for the negative control (*left*) and of SEB-reactive CD4 T cells (*right*), comparing samples of healthy control subjects (HC, $n = 39$), patients with RA ($n = 74$) and seronegative spondylarthritis (SpA, $n = 19$). **c** Levels of VZV-specific antibodies (immunoglobulin G [IgG]) in HC, RA, and SpA determined by IgG enzyme-linked immunosorbent assay of plasma samples. **d** Stratification of VZV-specific (*left panel*) and SEB-reactive CD4 T-cell frequencies (*right panel*) of patients with RA according to disease activity (three DAS28 categories; ≤ 2.6, full remission, low disease activity, $n = 11$; > 2.6 to ≤ 5.1, moderate disease activity, $n = 32$; and > 5.1, high disease activity, $n = 7$). *Bars* indicate median values and IQRs; *dotted lines* depict the respective detection limits (DLs) as determined before (VZV 0.02%, SEB 0.05% [10]) or as indicated by the manufacturer (IgG). Gray symbols represent patients with known history of herpes zoster. Statistical analysis was performed using the Kruskal-Wallis test and Dunn's posttest. Significant differences in posttest are marked by asterisks (*$p < 0.05$; ***$p < 0.001$)

Together, the results show significantly lower percentages of reactive CD4 T cells in patients with RA, but not in patients with SpA, when compared with control subjects (median threefold lower VZV-specific and median 1.7-fold lower SEB-reactive T cells). Functionality of VZV-specific CD4 T cells does not seem to be impaired, whereas polyclonally activated effector T cells showed minor but significant alterations in functionality in patients with RA and in patients with SpA.

Influence of antirheumatic therapy on VZV-specific and SEB-reactive CD4 T cells in patients with RA

Because the immunological alterations in patients with rheumatic diseases were most pronounced in patients with RA, further analyses were restricted to this patient group. To evaluate potential effects of antirheumatic drugs on antigen-specific cellular immunity, patients were subdivided according to their specific antirheumatic medication (Fig. 3a), with or without corticosteroids,

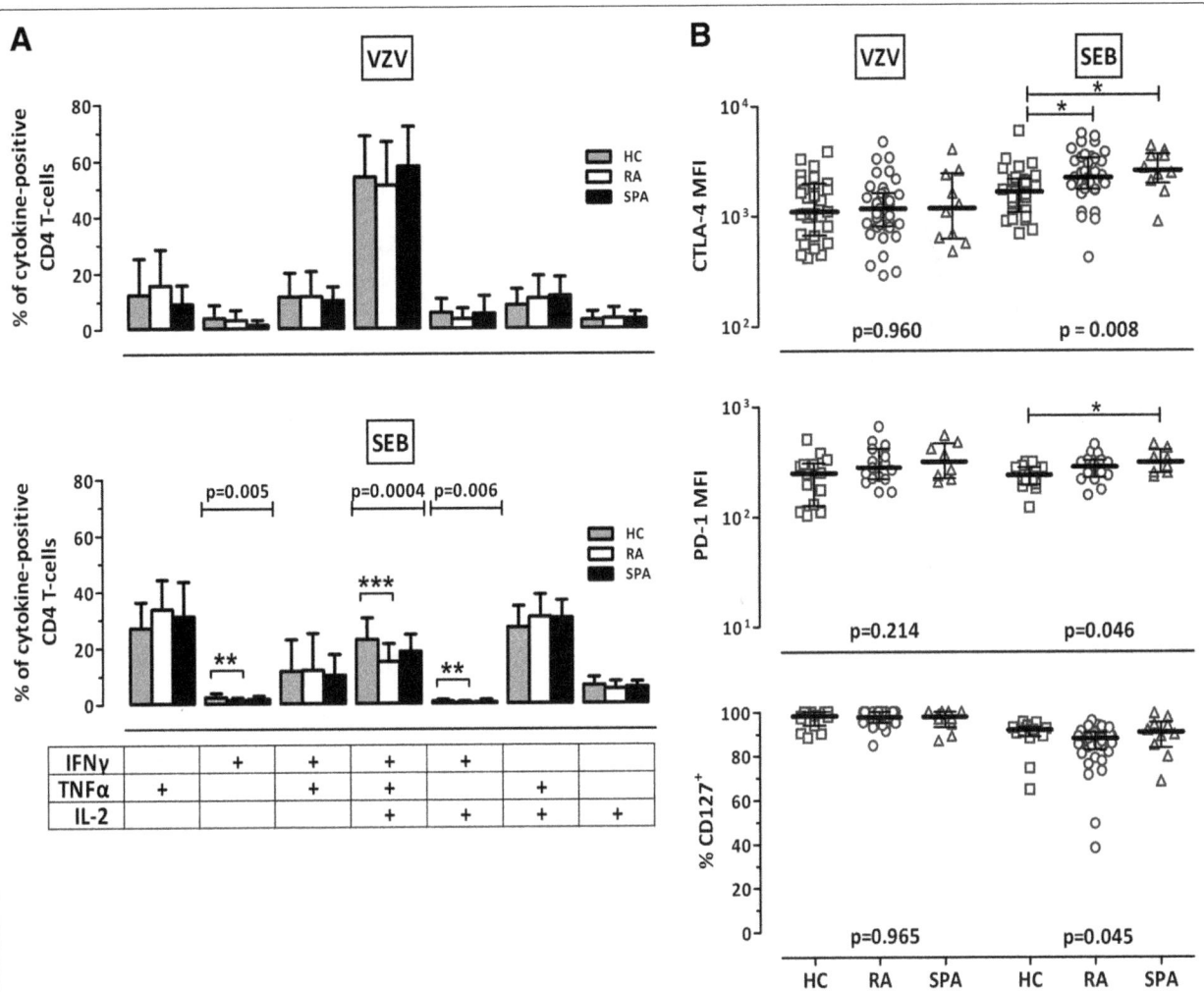

Fig. 2 Moderate functional differences in polyclonally stimulated CD4 T cells of control subjects (HC) and patients with rheumatoid arthritis (RA). **a** Cytokine-expressing CD4 T cells of HC (*gray*), patients with RA (*white*), and patients with seronegative spondylarthritis (SpA; *black*) are divided according to their expression of interferon (IFN)-γ, interleukin (IL)-2, and tumor necrosis factor (TNF)-α after stimulation with varicella zoster virus antigen (VZV, *upper panel*) or *Staphylococcus aureus* enterotoxin B (SEB, *lower panel*). To ensure robust statistics, this analysis was restricted to all VZV-positive samples where at least 30 cytokine-producing CD4 T cells were detectable (29 samples for HC, 27 for RA, and 10 for SpA, respectively). Bars represent subpopulations of single-, double-, or triple-cytokine-producing cells among all VZV- or SEB-reactive CD4 T cells, including means and SDs. **b** Expression of the cytotoxic T-lymphocyte antigen 4 (CTLA-4), the programmed death 1 molecule (PD-1), and CD127 was analyzed on reactive (CD69+/IFN-γ+) CD4 T cells of HC, RA, and SpA. Only samples with at least 20 VZV-specific CD4 T cells were analyzed (n = 29 HC, 37 RA, and 10 SpA for CTLA-4; n = 14 HC, 17 RA, and 8 SpA for PD-1; and n = 15 HC, 37 RA, and 10 SpA for CD127). Statistical significance was assessed using one-way analysis of variance with Bonferroni posttest (**a**) or the Kruskal-Wallis test with Dunn's posttest (**b**). Significant differences in posttests are marked by asterisks (*p < 0.05; **p < 0.01; ***p < 0.001)

bDMARDs, cDMARDs, or combined cDMARDs/bDMARDs. Interestingly, VZV-specific T-cell levels were low in patients both with and without steroids, but they did not differ between the two groups (p < 0.001 when compared with control subjects, respectively) (Fig. 3b, upper panel). In contrast, the decrease in SEB-reactive T-cell levels was more pronounced for patients receiving steroids, indicating a potential role of this drug (Fig. 3b, lower panel). However, direct comparisons of VZV- and SEB-reactive cells between patients with and without steroids revealed no significant differences between the

groups (p = 0.492 and p = 0.250, respectively). After stratifying the patients according to bDMARDs and nonbiological medications, significantly lower VZV-specific T-cell levels than in control subjects were found in both patients with and without bDMARDs, with lowest median frequencies in patients with bDMARDs (Fig. 3c, upper panel) (p < 0.001 and p < 0.01, respectively). Of note, the more pronounced impact of bDMARDs on VZV-specific T-cell frequencies was additionally evident by the fact that T-cell levels were low not only in patients who received bDMARDs alone but also in those who received them in

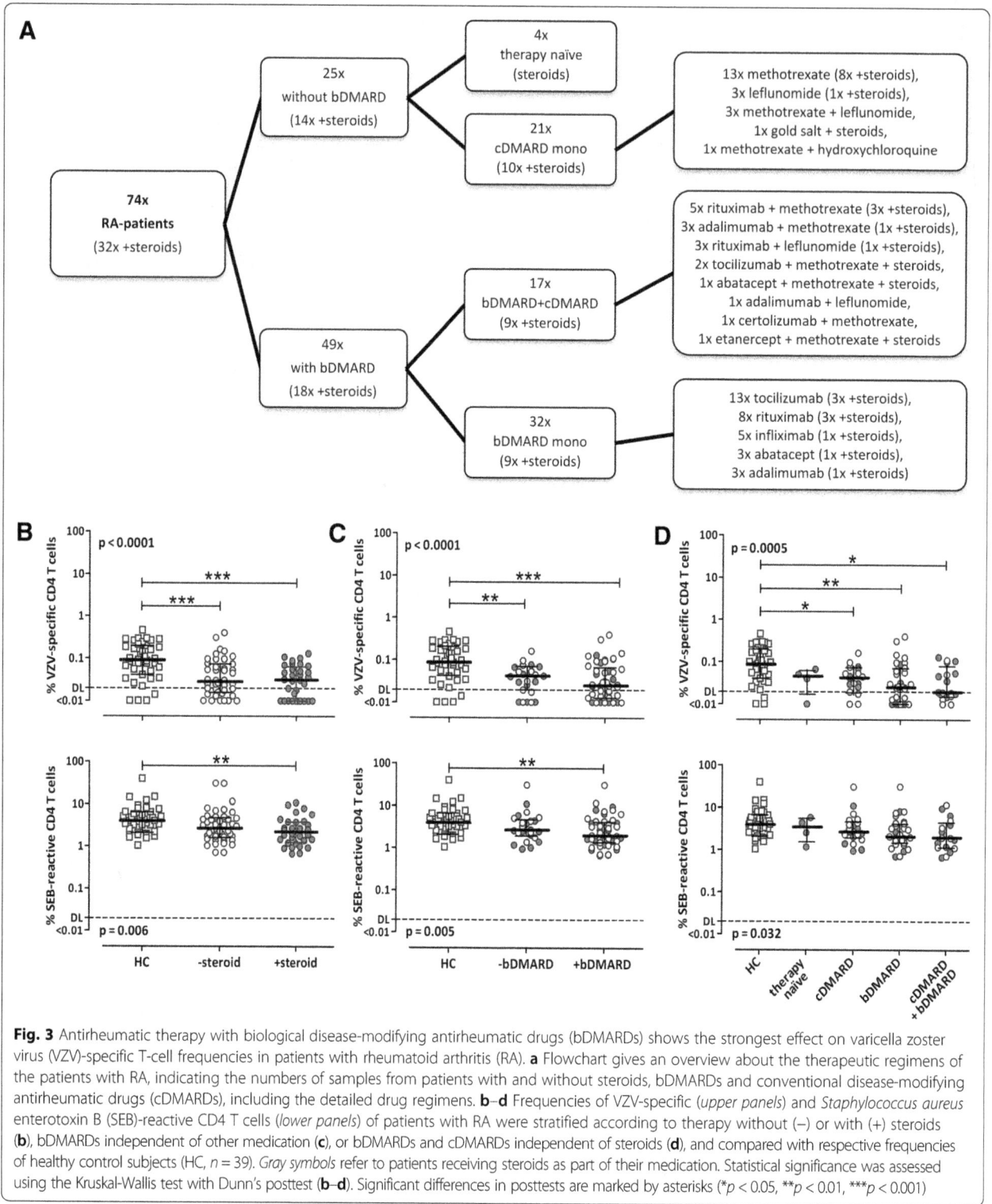

Fig. 3 Antirheumatic therapy with biological disease-modifying antirheumatic drugs (bDMARDs) shows the strongest effect on varicella zoster virus (VZV)-specific T-cell frequencies in patients with rheumatoid arthritis (RA). **a** Flowchart gives an overview about the therapeutic regimens of the patients with RA, indicating the numbers of samples from patients with and without steroids, bDMARDs and conventional disease-modifying antirheumatic drugs (cDMARDs), including the detailed drug regimens. **b–d** Frequencies of VZV-specific (*upper panels*) and *Staphylococcus aureus* enterotoxin B (SEB)-reactive CD4 T cells (*lower panels*) of patients with RA were stratified according to therapy without (−) or with (+) steroids (**b**), bDMARDs independent of other medication (**c**), or bDMARDs and cDMARDs independent of steroids (**d**), and compared with respective frequencies of healthy control subjects (HC, $n = 39$). *Gray symbols* refer to patients receiving steroids as part of their medication. Statistical significance was assessed using the Kruskal-Wallis test with Dunn's posttest (**b–d**). Significant differences in posttests are marked by asterisks (*$p < 0.05$, **$p < 0.01$, ***$p < 0.001$)

combination with cDMARDs ($p < 0.01$ and $p < 0.05$, respectively) (Fig. 3d, upper panel). Likewise, SEB-reactive CD4 T-cell levels were lowest in patients with bDMARDs ($p < 0.01$) (Fig. 3c, lower panel), whereas no specific differences were found when stratified into treatment subgroups

(Fig. 3d, lower panel). As highlighted by gray symbols, steroids did not have any influence on specific T-cell levels among the different treatment subgroups (Fig. 3c and d). Interestingly, there was also no correlation between the dosage of steroids and VZV-reactive ($r = 0.098$, $p = $ n.s.) or

SEB-reactive T-cell levels ($r = -0.191$, p = n.s.) (Additional file 1: Table S1). Among cDMARDs, most patients received methotrexate ($n = 30$). Although cDMARDs decreased VZV-specific T-cell levels to some extent (Fig. 3d), T-cell levels did not differ between patients with and without methotrexate (Additional file 1: Figure S3). Taken together, among antirheumatic medications, bDMARDs had the most pronounced decreasing effect on VZV-specific T-cell frequencies, whereas SEB-reactive effector T cells seemed to be negatively influenced by glucocorticoids and/or bDMARDs.

Differential impact of bDMARDs on T-cell immunity depending on their mechanism of action

Because bDMARDs, which have the strongest influence on cellular immunity in patients with RA, differ in their mechanisms of action, we further analyzed their impact on VZV-specific and SEB-reactive T cells. Therefore, patients were divided into four groups receiving (1) the T-cell costimulation blocking agent abatacept; (2) TNF blocker adalimumab, etanercept, infliximab, or certolizumab; (3) the B-cell-depleting drug rituximab; or (4) the IL-6-receptor blocker tocilizumab. Comparison of the CD4 T-cell frequencies with those of healthy control subjects revealed a significant reduction, especially in patients receiving the IL-6 receptor blocker, both after VZV-specific ($p < 0.01$) (Fig. 4a) and after polyclonal stimulation ($p < 0.05$) (Fig. 4b). Three of four patients on abatacept had low levels of VZV-specific T cells, although statistical analysis of this effect is limited by the low number of patients available for recruitment. In addition, significant differences were detected for VZV-specific T cells of patients on TNF-blocking therapy ($p < 0.05$) and for SEB-reactive cells of patients receiving rituximab ($p < 0.05$) compared with healthy control subjects. Again, treatment with steroids did not have any influence on specific T-cell levels among subgroups of bDMARDs (gray symbols in Fig. 4).

To further evaluate the net effect of antirheumatic drugs independent of the disease background, whole-blood samples of three healthy control persons were supplemented in vitro with increasing concentrations of the different drugs and subsequently stimulated with VZV lysate or SEB as described before. Blood of nonimmunocompromised healthy control subjects was chosen to study direct effects of the drugs at defined dosages added in vitro without being confounded by effects of drugs that patients had received as part of their medication. The baseline VZV-specific T-cell levels of these individuals (0.061%, 0.086%, and 0.124%) were in the range of what is found for healthy control subjects (*see* Fig. 1b). Although CyA is not used in patients with RA, this drug served as an internal control for a known dose-dependent immunosuppressive effect on CD4 T-cell effector function in this in vitro system [13]. After 6 h of stimulation, coexpression of the activation marker CD69 with cytokine IFN-γ, IL-2, or TNF-α was determined by flow cytometry (Additional file 1: Figure S4A). Although the number of replicates was low (three VZV and three SEB stimulations),

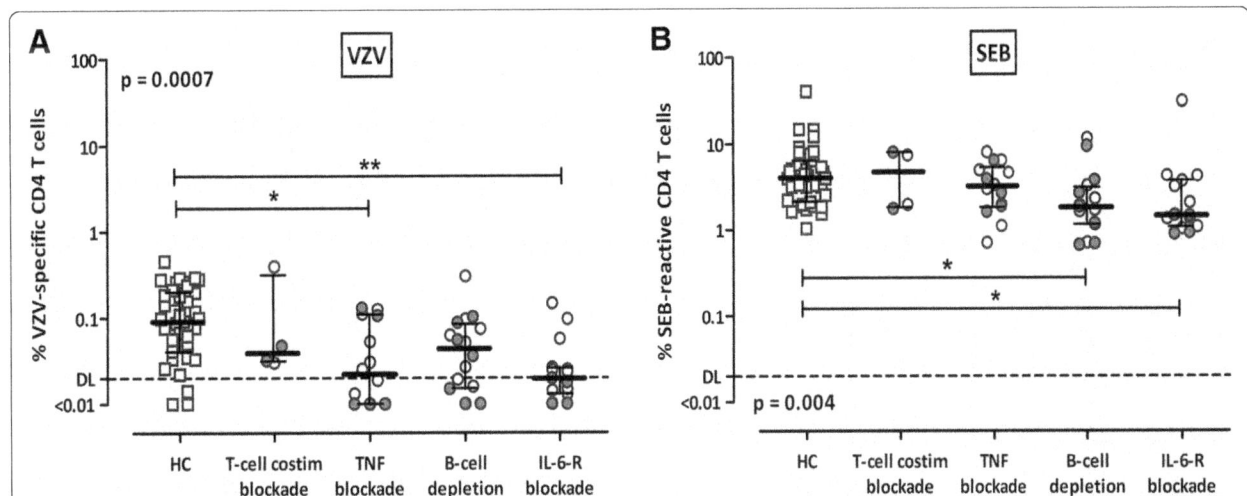

Fig. 4 Specific biological disease-modifying antirheumatic drugs (bDMARDs) show differences in their effect on reactive CD4 T cells of patients with rheumatoid arthritis (RA). Scatterplots depict frequencies of varicella zoster virus (VZV)-specific (a) and *Staphylococcus aureus* enterotoxin B (SEB)-reactive (b) CD4 T cells of healthy control subjects (HC, $n = 39$) as well as patients with RA receiving biological disease-modifying bDMARDs, stratified according to the mechanism of action of the respective bDMARD (abatacept, T-cell costimulation blockade, $n = 4$; adalimumab, etanercept, infliximab, certolizumab, TNF blockade, $n = 14$; rituximab, B-cell depletion, $n = 16$; tocilizumab, interleukin [IL]-6R blockade, $n = 15$). Bars indicate median values and IQRs, *dotted lines* are detection limits for VZV-specific and SEB-reactive CD4 T cells as determined before (VZV 0.02%, SEB 0.05% [10]), respectively. *Gray symbols* refer to patients receiving steroids as part of their medication. Statistical differences were assessed using the Kruskal-Wallis test with Dunn's posttest. Significant differences in posttests are marked by asterisks (*$p < 0.05$; **$p < 0.01$)

a pronounced dose-dependent decrease in cytokine-expressing T-cell frequencies was observed after incubation with the positive control drug CyA. To a lesser extent, this effect was also observed with MP. Interestingly, the only bDMARD that led to a similar dose-dependent decrease in VZV-specific and SEB-reactive T-cell frequencies was the TNF blocker adalimumab, but this inhibitory effect was restricted to the expression of TNF-α (Additional file 1: Figure S4A, lower panel), whereas there was no detectable effect on IFN-γ or IL-2 expression (Additional file 1: Figure S4A, upper or middle panel, respectively). All other tested drugs did not have any pronounced decreasing effect on cytokine induction in vitro. This also held true for methotrexate and the Janus kinase (JAK) inhibitor tofacitinib, which were tested in an independent series of five healthy individuals (Additional file 1: Figure S5A). When analyzing late cytokine expression (Additional file 1: Figure S4B and S5B) and proliferation (Additional file 1: Figure S4C and S5C) after 36 h of stimulation with SEB, CyA and MP had a clear dose-dependent inhibitory effect on both CD4 and CD8 T cells, whereas all other drugs had either no or no pronounced effect.

Discussion

Patients with rheumatic diseases are at increased susceptibility for VZV reactivations. In line with this observation, the present study shows lower levels of VZV-specific T cells in patients with RA than in healthy control subjects. While this effect was not associated with disease severity, treatment regimens had a decreasing influence on cellular immunity, with regimens including bDMARDs showing the most pronounced effects.

Because VZV-specific CD4 T cells were shown to be essential for effective VZV control [8], the significantly lower frequencies of VZV-specific CD4 T cells in patients with RA may be the main explanation for their increased susceptibility to VZV reactivations. The pronounced role of the cellular arm of adaptive immunity is supported by the fact that VZV IgG levels were not concomitantly impaired. This is consistent with observations in patients with SLE who showed a significant reduction in VZV-specific T-cell frequencies, even in the presence of increased VZV IgG levels [9]. This lends support to the assumption that a poor VZV-specific cellular but not humoral immunity may be the main contributor to increased zoster incidence in patients with RA. In our study, the median percentage of VZV-specific T cells in patients with SpA was also lower than in control subjects, but this effect was less pronounced than that in patients with RA, which may indicate that the extent of immune impairment may depend on the

entity of rheumatic disease. Indeed, the incidence of herpes zoster in different groups of patients with autoimmune and inflammatory diseases ranges from 6.8 per 1000 person-years in patients with gout to 19.9 per 1000 person-years in patients with SLE [4]. Interestingly, consistent with effects on VZV-specific CD4 T cells in our study, the incidence rate in patients with RA was higher than that of patients with PsA and AS [4].

We have previously shown that patients with herpes zoster [10] and VZV-associated meningitis [15] show increased levels of VZV-specific T cells with limited ability to produce cytokines and with increased expression levels of markers of functional anergy such as CTLA-4 or PD-1. These parameters were typical characteristics of VZV-specific T cells not only in immunocompetent symptomatic patients but also in patients with immunodeficiency, including RA, which normalized after resolution of zoster within approximately 3 months to levels comparable to those of individuals without history of zoster [10]. Although patients with a history of zoster were included in the present study, their zoster episode was several years ago, and none of the patients showed any evidence of herpes zoster or other clinical signs of VZV reactivation at the time of analysis. As with our findings in immunocompetent control subjects [10], VZV-specific T-cell levels in patients with a history of herpes zoster did not differ from those of patients who never experienced a VZV reactivation. Despite absence of clinical symptoms, quantitative differences in VZV-specific T-cell levels were observed between patients and control subjects, whereas functionality and cell surface expression of anergy markers were largely unaffected. When analyzing SEB-reactive T cells as a surrogate for T cells with other specificities, those also showed decreased levels. Moreover, there was also evidence for a reduced percentage of multifunctional T cells and increased expression of CTLA-4 and PD-1, which were similar to those in asymptomatic transplant recipients receiving immunosuppressive therapy [10, 16–18]. Notably, however, the detected changes were less pronounced than those found in patients with active infection. These data are consistent with recent findings that bulk CD4 T cells from patients with RA and SpA were shown to have slightly elevated expression levels of CTLA-4 or PD-1 [19]. Together, this may reflect increased susceptibility for infections and/or may be the result of a history of more frequent infections of patients with rheumatic diseases than in immunologically healthy persons.

The decrease in T-cell levels may be a direct effect of immunosuppressive and immunomodulatory drugs and further influenced by the underlying disease. Because patients typically received immunosuppressive drug combinations at the time of recruitment, the net influence of individual drugs is difficult to assess. In line with a clear dose-dependent association between the use of corticosteroids and zoster risk [20–23], our in vitro experiments in which MP was supplemented in concentrations equivalent to 4 and 400 mg/d indicate an involvement of steroids in reducing effector T-cell frequencies. The observation that differences in patients with RA with and without steroids were only significant for polyclonally stimulated T cells may be due to the fact that steroid dosage in our patients varied from as little as 1.5 to up to 40 mg/d with only four patients receiving ≥ 10 mg/d, and most patients received additional immunomodulatory drugs such as bDMARDs, which may have unmasked the effect of an individual drug. Thus, differences may result from the fact that the in vitro experiments analyzed potential direct effects of each individual immunosuppressive drug on T-cell effector function, whereas T-cell analyses in patients in vivo are influenced by the combined action of several immunosuppressive drugs that most patients received simultaneously.

Up to now, several studies have reported an increased incidence and severity of VZV reactivations in patients with rheumatic disease receiving therapy with bDMARDs [20, 24–26]. In line with that, we observed significantly reduced cellular immune responses in patients receiving therapy with different bDMARDs. Among those, the IL-6 receptor blocker and TNF antagonists had the most pronounced effect on VZV-specific CD4 T-cell frequencies in patients with RA. TNF antagonists may have both direct and indirect effects on VZV replication. Given the role of TNF-α as an effective inhibitor of VZV replication [27], a causative role of TNF antagonist therapy for an increased incidence of VZV reactivations is conceivable. Moreover, stimulation of blood samples from healthy control subjects in the presence of the TNF blocker adalimumab dose-dependently impaired TNF-α induction in CD4 T cells while not affecting IFN-γ or IL-2, which indicates an immediate drug effect on effector T-cell function independent of the underlying disease. In patients on TNF antagonist therapy, a decrease in TNF-α signaling may negatively affect nuclear factor (NF)-κB activation, which may have a direct inhibitory effect on immune cells. TNF antagonists may also negatively affect VZV-infected cells in addition to the gene product of VZV-ORF61, which is capable of inhibiting NF-κB activation owing to its E3 ubiquitin ligase activity [28]. Together, both processes may synergistically favor VZV reactivation events. As with effects of TNF antagonists on the VZV-specific immune response, patients receiving the IL-6 receptor blocker tocilizumab showed significantly lower VZV-specific CD4 T-cell frequencies than

control subjects. However, because frequencies of SEB-reactive T cells were also reduced, the inhibitory effect may be less specific. In patients with SLE, treatment with tocilizumab led to a decrease in the percentage of HLA-DR$^+$ activated T cells [29]. Given that IL-6 inhibits regulatory T-cell (Treg) development by inducing a shift towards T-helper type 17 cell development, blocking of IL-6 signal transduction by tocilizumab induces higher amounts of Tregs, which might result in suppression of cytokine expression in effector T cells [30, 31]. We finally also found that polyclonal T-cell responses were significantly reduced in patients receiving rituximab, whereas its effect on VZV-specific CD4 T cells was less pronounced. Although this drug primarily targets B cells via binding to CD20, adverse effects on T cells are also known [32]. Apart from reduced T-cell responses by missing antigen presentation of B cells, rituximab may directly influence cytokine expression of T cells by binding to CD20-positive T cells [33]. If so, it is tempting to speculate whether VZV-specific T cells are largely CD20-negative and thus less susceptible to rituximab treatment. More recently, treatment regimens including JAK inhibitors such as tofacitinib and baricitinib were also shown to be associated with a high rate of herpes zoster [34, 35]. Although we did not find any pronounced effect of tofacitinib on T-cell effector function in vitro, studying the effect of these novel drugs on VZV-specific cellular immunity in vivo may be an interesting area of future research to better understand increased susceptibility for VZV reactivations.

Our study may be limited by sample size and lack of follow-up data to study quantitative levels of specific T-cell immunity in relation to clinical reactivation events. Therefore, future longitudinal studies in larger cohorts of patients with RA should address whether a progressive decrease in specific immunity and functional impairment may be used as a predictor for VZV reactivations. This type of study with a larger sample size will also allow simultaneous characterization of VZV-specific immunity in association with the frequency of VZV infections on therapy with different bDMARDs.

Conclusions

Patients with RA show a decreased level of antigen-specific CD4 T cells, with VZV-specific T cells being particularly influenced by bDMARDs such as TNF antagonists and IL-6 receptor blockers, which may account for an increased incidence of VZV reactivations. Our findings are relevant for clinical practice because they emphasize the importance of preventive measures such as zoster vaccinations. Moreover, together with our findings on phenotypical and functional changes of specific immunity in patients with active VZV infection [10, 15], this knowledge may be useful for cellular diagnostics to assess individual immunocompetence toward this clinically relevant pathogen. Finally, this study may be extended to study VZV-specific immunocompetence in patients with novel synthetic disease-modifying antirheumatic drugs known to be associated with increased risk of herpes zoster.

Additional file

Additional file 1: Table S1. Correlation between VZV-specific or SEB-reactive CD4 T-cell levels and demographic and clinical parameters in patients with RA. **Figure S1.** VZV-specific CD4 T cells are detectable after varicella vaccination. **Figure S2.** Representative examples of flow cytometric analyses. **Figure S3.** Analysis of the influence of methotrexate on VZV-specific and SEB-reactive CD4 T cells. **Figure S4.** In vitro effect of antirheumatic drugs on cytokine expression and proliferation of reactive T cells. **Figure S5.** In vitro effect of tofacitinib and methotrexate on cytokine expression and proliferation of reactive T cells. (DOC 2282 kb)

Abbreviations

AS: Ankylosing spondylitis; BrdU: Bromodeoxyuridine; cDMARD/bDMARD: Conventional/biologic disease-modifying antirheumatic drug; CRP: C-reactive protein; CTLA-4: Cytotoxic T-lymphocyte antigen 4; CyA: Cyclosporine A; DMARD: Disease-modifying antirheumatic drug; ESR: Erythrocyte sedimentation rate; IFN-γ: Interferon-γ; IgG: Immunoglobulin G; IL: Interleukin; JAK: Janus kinase; MP: Methylprednisolone; NF-κB: Nuclear factor-κB; PD-1: Programmed death 1 molecule; PsA: Psoriatic arthritis; RA: Rheumatoid arthritis; SEB: *Staphylococcus aureus* enterotoxin B; SLE: Systemic lupus erythematosus; SpA: Seronegative spondylarthritis; TNF-α: Tumor necrosis factor–α; Treg: Regulatory T cell; VZV: Varicella zoster virus

Acknowledgements

The authors thank Candida Guckelmus and Lisa Lieblang for excellent technical assistance and the clinical collaborators for indispensable help in sample acquisition.

Funding

This work was supported in part by grants from HOMFORexzellent (to TS) and from Chugai Pharma Marketing Ltd. (to GA). The funding bodies did not have any role in the design of the study; in the collection, analysis, and interpretation of data; or in writing the manuscript.

Authors' contributions

DS performed the experiments, analyzed the data, and was a contributor to the writing of the manuscript. GA was involved in the study design, was the main contributor in patient recruitment and sample acquisition, and contributed to writing the manuscript. US contributed to the study design and data interpretation. MS contributed to the study design and data analysis and interpretation and was a contributor to the writing of the manuscript. TS contributed to study design and data analysis and interpretation and was the main contributor in writing the manuscript. All authors read and approved the final manuscript.

Consent for publication

Not applicable.

Competing interests

The authors declare that they have no competing interests.

Author details

[1]Department of Transplant and Infection Immunology, Saarland University, 66421 Homburg, Germany. [2]Department of Internal Medicine I, Saarland University, Homburg, Germany. [3]Department of Internal Medicine IV, Saarland University, Homburg, Germany.

References

1. Yawn BP, Gilden D. The global epidemiology of herpes zoster. Neurology. 2013;81(10):928–30.
2. Chakravarty EF, Michaud K, Katz R, Wolfe F. Increased incidence of herpes zoster among patients with systemic lupus erythematosus. Lupus. 2013; 22(3):238–44.
3. McDonald JR, Zeringue AL, Caplan L, Ranganathan P, Xian H, Burroughs TE, et al. Herpes zoster risk factors in a national cohort of veterans with rheumatoid arthritis. Clin Infect Dis. 2009;48(10):1364–71.
4. Yun H, Yang S, Chen L, Xie F, Winthrop K, Baddley JW, et al. Risk of herpes zoster in autoimmune and inflammatory diseases: implications for vaccination. Arthritis Rheum. 2016;68(9):2328–37.
5. Malavige GN, Jones L, Black AP, Ogg GS. Rapid effector function of varicella-zoster virus glycoprotein I-specific CD4+ T cells many decades after primary infection. J Infect Dis. 2007;195(5):660–4.
6. Sadaoka K, Okamoto S, Gomi Y, Tanimoto T, Ishikawa T, Yoshikawa T, et al. Measurement of varicella-zoster virus (VZV)-specific cell-mediated immunity: comparison between VZV skin test and interferon-γ enzyme-linked immunospot assay. J Infect Dis. 2008;198(9):1327–33.
7. Vossen MT, Gent MR, Weel JF, de Jong MD, van Lier RA, Kuijpers TW. Development of virus-specific CD4+ T cells on reexposure to varicella-zoster virus. J Infect Dis. 2004;190(1):72–82.
8. Park HB, Kim KC, Park JH, Kang TY, Lee HS, Kim TH, et al. Association of reduced CD4 T cell responses specific to varicella zoster virus with high incidence of herpes zoster in patients with systemic lupus erythematosus. J Rheumatol. 2004;31(11):2151–5.
9. Rondaan C, de Haan A, Horst G, Hempel JC, van Leer C, Bos NA, et al. Altered cellular and humoral immunity to varicella-zoster virus in patients with autoimmune diseases. Arthritis Rheum. 2014;66(11):3122–8.
10. Schub D, Janssen E, Leyking S, Sester U, Assmann G, Hennes P, et al. Altered phenotype and functionality of varicella zoster virus-specific cellular immunity in individuals with active infection. J Infect Dis. 2015;211(4):600–12.
11. Humphreys J, Hyrich K, Symmons D. What is the impact of biologic therapies on common co-morbidities in patients with rheumatoid arthritis? Arthritis Res Ther. 2016;18:282.
12. Ramiro S, Sepriano A, Chatzidionysiou K, Nam JL, Smolen JS, van der Heijde D, et al. Safety of synthetic and biological DMARDs: a systematic literature review informing the 2016 update of the EULAR recommendations for management of rheumatoid arthritis. Ann Rheum Dis. 2017;76(6):1101–36.
13. Leyking S, Wolf M, Mihm J, Schaefer M, Bohle RM, Fliser D, et al. Alloreactive T cells to identify risk HLA alleles for retransplantation after acute accelerated steroid-resistant rejection. Transplant Proc. 2015;47(8):2425–32.
14. Leyking S, Budich K, van Bentum K, Thijssen S, Abdul-Khaliq H, Fliser D, et al. Calcineurin inhibitors differentially alter the circadian rhythm of T-cell functionality in transplant recipients. J Transl Med. 2015;13:51.
15. Schub D, Fousse M, Fassbender K, Gartner BC, Sester U, Sester M, et al. CTLA-4-expression on VZV-specific T cells in CSF and blood is specifically increased in patients with VZV related central nervous system infections. Eur J Immunol. 2018;48(1):151–60.
16. Schmidt T, Adam C, Hirsch HH, Janssen MW, Wolf M, Dirks J, et al. BK polyomavirus-specific cellular immune responses are age-dependent and strongly correlate with phases of virus replication. Am J Transplant. 2014; 14(6):1334–45.

17. Sester U, Presser D, Dirks J, Gartner BC, Kohler H, Sester M. PD-1 expression and IL-2 loss of cytomegalovirus-specific T cells correlates with viremia and reversible functional anergy. Am J Transplant. 2008;8(7):1486–97.

18. Sester U, Fousse M, Dirks J, Mack U, Prasse A, Singh M, et al. Whole-blood flow-cytometric analysis of antigen-specific CD4 T-cell cytokine profiles distinguishes active tuberculosis from non-active states. PLoS One. 2011;6(3):e17813.

19. Frenz T, Grabski E, Buschjager D, Vaas LA, Burgdorf N, Schmidt RE, et al. CD4+ T cells in patients with chronic inflammatory rheumatic disorders show distinct levels of exhaustion. J Allergy Clin Immunol. 2016;138(2):586–9 e10.

20. Liao TL, Chen YM, Liu HJ, Chen DY. Risk and severity of herpes zoster in patients with rheumatoid arthritis receiving different immunosuppressive medications: a case-control study in Asia. BMJ Open. 2017;7(1):e014032.

21. Pappas DA, Hooper MM, Kremer JM, Reed G, Shan Y, Wenkert D, et al. Herpes zoster reactivation in patients with rheumatoid arthritis: analysis of disease characteristics and disease-modifying antirheumatic drugs. Arthritis Care Res. 2015;67(12):1671–8.

22. Winthrop KL, Baddley JW, Chen L, Liu L, Grijalva CG, Delzell E, et al. Association between the initiation of anti-tumor necrosis factor therapy and the risk of herpes zoster. JAMA. 2013;309(9):887–95.

23. Yun H, Xie F, Delzell E, Chen L, Levitan EB, Lewis JD, et al. Risks of herpes zoster in patients with rheumatoid arthritis according to biologic disease-modifying therapy. Arthritis Care Res. 2015;67(5):731–6.

24. Segan J, Staples MP, March L, Lassere M, Chakravarty EF, Buchbinder R. Risk factors for herpes zoster in rheumatoid arthritis patients: the role of tumour necrosis factor-α inhibitors. Intern Med J. 2015;45(3):310–8.

25. Singh JA, Cameron C, Noorbaloochi S, Cullis T, Tucker M, Christensen R, et al. Risk of serious infection in biological treatment of patients with rheumatoid arthritis: a systematic review and meta-analysis. Lancet. 2015; 386(9990):258–65.

26. Strangfeld A, Listing J, Herzer P, Liebhaber A, Rockwitz K, Richter C, et al. Risk of herpes zoster in patients with rheumatoid arthritis treated with anti-TNF-α agents. JAMA. 2009;301(7):737–44.

27. Ito M, Nakano T, Kamiya T, Kitamura K, Ihara T, Kamiya H, et al. Effects of tumor necrosis factor α on replication of varicella-zoster virus. Antivir Res. 1991;15(3):183–92.

28. Whitmer T, Malouli D, Uebelhoer LS, DeFilippis VR, Fruh K, Verweij MC. The ORF61 protein encoded by simian varicella virus and varicella-zoster virus inhibits NF-κB signaling by interfering with IκBα degradation. J Virol. 2015; 89(17):8687–700.

29. Shirota Y, Yarboro C, Fischer R, Pham TH, Lipsky P, Illei GG. Impact of anti-interleukin-6 receptor blockade on circulating T and B cell subsets in patients with systemic lupus erythematosus. Ann Rheum Dis. 2013;72(1):118–28.

30. Dienz O, Rincon M. The effects of IL-6 on CD4 T cell responses. Clin Immunol. 2009;130(1):27–33.

31. Kikuchi J, Hashizume M, Kaneko Y, Yoshimoto K, Nishina N, Takeuchi T. Peripheral blood CD4+CD25+CD127low regulatory T cells are significantly increased by tocilizumab treatment in patients with rheumatoid arthritis: increase in regulatory T cells correlates with clinical response. Arthritis Res Ther. 2015;17:10.

32. Melet J, Mulleman D, Goupille P, Ribourtout B, Watier H, Thibault G. Rituximab-induced T cell depletion in patients with rheumatoid arthritis: association with clinical response. Arthritis Rheum. 2013;65(11):2783–90.

33. Stroopinsky D, Katz T, Rowe JM, Melamed D, Avivi I. Rituximab-induced direct inhibition of T-cell activation. Cancer Immunol Immunother. 2012; 61(8):1233–41.

34. Genovese MC, Kremer J, Zamani O, Ludivico C, Krogulec M, Xie L, et al. Baricitinib in patients with refractory rheumatoid arthritis. N Engl J Med. 2016;374(13):1243–52.

35. Winthrop KL, Curtis JR, Lindsey S, Tanaka Y, Yamaoka K, Valdez H, et al. Herpes zoster and tofacitinib: clinical outcomes and the risk of concomitant therapy. Arthritis Rheumatol. 2017;69(10):1960–8.

Permissions

All chapters in this book were first published in AR&T, by BioMed Central; hereby published with permission under the Creative Commons Attribution License or equivalent. Every chapter published in this book has been scrutinized by our experts. Their significance has been extensively debated. The topics covered herein carry significant findings which will fuel the growth of the discipline. They may even be implemented as practical applications or may be referred to as a beginning point for another development.

The contributors of this book come from diverse backgrounds, making this book a truly international effort. This book will bring forth new frontiers with its revolutionizing research information and detailed analysis of the nascent developments around the world.

We would like to thank all the contributing authors for lending their expertise to make the book truly unique. They have played a crucial role in the development of this book. Without their invaluable contributions this book wouldn't have been possible. They have made vital efforts to compile up to date information on the varied aspects of this subject to make this book a valuable addition to the collection of many professionals and students.

This book was conceptualized with the vision of imparting up-to-date information and advanced data in this field. To ensure the same, a matchless editorial board was set up. Every individual on the board went through rigorous rounds of assessment to prove their worth. After which they invested a large part of their time researching and compiling the most relevant data for our readers.

The editorial board has been involved in producing this book since its inception. They have spent rigorous hours researching and exploring the diverse topics which have resulted in the successful publishing of this book. They have passed on their knowledge of decades through this book. To expedite this challenging task, the publisher supported the team at every step. A small team of assistant editors was also appointed to further simplify the editing procedure and attain best results for the readers.

Apart from the editorial board, the designing team has also invested a significant amount of their time in understanding the subject and creating the most relevant covers. They scrutinized every image to scout for the most suitable representation of the subject and create an appropriate cover for the book.

The publishing team has been an ardent support to the editorial, designing and production team. Their endless efforts to recruit the best for this project, has resulted in the accomplishment of this book. They are a veteran in the field of academics and their pool of knowledge is as vast as their experience in printing. Their expertise and guidance has proved useful at every step. Their uncompromising quality standards have made this book an exceptional effort. Their encouragement from time to time has been an inspiration for everyone.

The publisher and the editorial board hope that this book will prove to be a valuable piece of knowledge for researchers, students, practitioners and scholars across the globe.

Contributors

Anna Neumann, Arnd Kleyer, Louis Schuster, Matthias Englbrecht, Andreas Berlin, David Simon, Jürgen Rech and Georg Schett
Department of Internal Medicine 3, Friedrich Alexander University Erlangen-Nurnberg and Universitätsklinikum Erlangen, Ulmenweg 18, 91054 Erlangen, Germany

Judith Haschka
Department of Internal Medicine 3, Friedrich Alexander University Erlangen-Nurnberg and Universitätsklinikum Erlangen, Ulmenweg 18, 91054 Erlangen, Germany
St. Vincent Hospital, VINFORCE Study Group, Medical University of Vienna, Vienna, Austria.

Camille P. Figueiredo
Department of Internal Medicine 3, Friedrich Alexander University Erlangen-Nurnberg and Universitätsklinikum Erlangen, Ulmenweg 18, 91054 Erlangen, Germany
Division of Rheumatology, Faculdade de Medicina da Universidade de São Paulo, São Paulo, Brazil

Christian Muschitz, Roland Kocijan and Heinrich Resch
St. Vincent Hospital, VINFORCE Study Group, Medical University of Vienna, Vienna, Austria

Jiannan Li, Jin-wei Wang, Min Chen and Zhao Cui
Renal Division, Department of Medicine, Peking University First Hospital, Peking University Institute of Nephrology, Key Laboratory of Renal Disease, Ministry of Health of China, Key Laboratory of CKD Prevention and Treatment, Ministry of Education of China, Beijing, China

Luxia Zhang
Renal Division, Department of Medicine, Peking University First Hospital, Peking University Institute of Nephrology, Key Laboratory of Renal Disease, Ministry of Health of China, Key Laboratory of CKD Prevention and Treatment, Ministry of Education of China, Beijing, China
Peking University, Center for Data Science in Health and Medicine, Beijing, China

Ming-hui Zhao
Renal Division, Department of Medicine, Peking University First Hospital, Peking University Institute of Nephrology, Key Laboratory of Renal Disease, Ministry of Health of China, Key Laboratory of CKD Prevention and Treatment, Ministry of Education of China, Beijing, China
Peking-Tsinghua Center for Life Sciences, Beijing, People's Republic of China

Jian-yan Long
Clinical Trial Unit, First Affiliated Hospital of Sun Yat-Sen University, Guangzhou, China

Haibo Wang
Clinical Trial Unit, First Affiliated Hospital of Sun Yat-Sen University, Guangzhou, China
China Standard Medical Information Research Center, Shenzhen, Guangdong, China

Wei Huang
Department of Occupational and Enviromental Health, Peking University School of Public Health, Beijing, China

Ji-Yih Chen, Yeong-Jian Jan Wu and Jing-Chi Lin
Department of Medicine, Division of Allergy, Immunology and Rheumatology, Chang Gung Memorial Hospital, Chang Gung University College of Medicine, No. 5, Fu-Shin St. Kwei-Shan, Tao-Yuan, Taiwan

Chin-Man Wang
Department of Rehabilitation, Chang Gung Memorial Hospital, Chang Gung University College of Medicine, No. 5, Fu-Shin St. Kwei-Shan, Tao-Yuan, Taiwan

Tai-Di Chen
Department of Anatomic Pathology, Chang Gung Memorial Hospital, Chang Gung University College of Medicine, Tao-Yuan, Taiwan

Ling Ying Lu
Department of Medicine, Division of Allergy Immunology and Rheumatology, Kaohsiung Veterans General Hospital, No. 386, Dazhong 1st Rd, Zuoying District, Kaohsiung City 81362, Taiwan

Jianming Wu
Department of Veterinary and Biomedical Sciences, Department of Medicine, University of Minnesota, 235B Animal Science/Vet. Med. Bldg, 1988 Fitch Avenue, St. Paul, MN 55108, USA

Xiuhong Weng and Bo Cheng
Department of Stomatology, Zhongnan Hospital of Wuhan University, 169 Donghu Road, Wuhan 430071, Hubei Province, China

Yi Liu
Department of Stomatology, Union Hospital, Tongji Medical College, Huazhong University of Science and Technology, 1277 Jiefang Ave, Jianhan District, Wuhan 430022, Hubei Province, China

Shun Cui
Department of Rheumatology, Union Hospital, Tongji Medical College, Huazhong University of Science and Technology, 1277 Jiefang Ave, Jianghan District, Wuhan 430022, Hubei Province, China

Ashika Chhana, Bregina Pool, Karen E. Callon, Mei Lin Tay, David Musson, Dorit Naot and Jillian Cornish
Department of Medicine, Bone and Joint Research Group, University of Auckland, Auckland, New Zealand

Nicola Dalbeth
Department of Medicine, Bone and Joint Research Group, University of Auckland, Auckland, New Zealand.

Department of Medicine, Faculty of Medical and Health Sciences, University of Auckland, 85 Park Rd, Grafton, Auckland, New Zealand

Geraldine McCarthy
Department of Rheumatology, Mater Misericordiae University Hospital, Dublin, Ireland

Susan McGlashan
Department of Anatomy and Medical Imaging, University of Auckland, Auckland, New Zealand

Anna Deminger, Eva Klingberg, Hans Carlsten and Lennart T. Jacobsson
Department of Rheumatology and Inflammation Research, Sahlgrenska Academy at University of Gothenburg, Box 480, 405 30 Gothenburg, Sweden

Helena Forsblad-d'Elia
Department of Rheumatology and Inflammation Research, Sahlgrenska Academy at University of Gothenburg, Box 480, 405 30 Gothenburg, Sweden
Department of Public Health and Clinical Medicine, Rheumatology, 901 87 Umeå University, Umeå, Sweden

Mats Geijer
Department of Radiology, Skåne University Hospital, 221 85 Lund, Sweden
Faculty of Medicine, Lund University, Box 117, 221 00 Lund, Sweden

Jan Göthlin
Department of Radiology, Sahlgrenska University Hospital, Mölndal, 431 80 Mölndal, Sweden

Martin Hedberg
Section of Rheumatology, Södra Älvsborg Hospital, 501 82 Borås, Sweden

Eva Rehnberg
Section of Rheumatology, Alingsås Hospital, 441 33 Alingsås, Sweden

Hui Deng, Nan Hu, Chen Wang, Min Chen and Ming-Hui Zhao
Renal Division, Department of Medicine, Peking University First Hospital, Peking University Institute of Nephrology, Beijing 100034, China
Key Laboratory of Renal Disease, Ministry of Health of China, Beijing 100034, China
Key Laboratory of Chronic Kidney Disease Prevention and Treatment, Ministry of Education, Peking University, Beijing 100034, China
Peking-Tsinghua Center for Life Sciences, Beijing 100034, China

Charles McWherter and Yun-Jung Choi
CymaBay Therapeutics, Inc., Newark, California, USA

Ramon L. Serrano, Sushil K. Mahata, Robert Terkeltaub and Ru Liu-Bryan
VA San Diego Healthcare System, 111K, 3350 La Jolla Village Drive, San Diego, CA 92161, USA.
University of California San Diego, La Jolla, California, USA

Rosaline van den Berg
Department of Rheumatology, Erasmus Medical Center, Rotterdam, The Netherlands

Annette H. M. van der Helm-van Mil
Department of Rheumatology, Erasmus Medical Center, Rotterdam, The Netherlands
Department of Rheumatology, Leiden University Medical Center, Leiden, The Netherlands

Marion C. Kortekaas
Department of Rheumatology, Leiden University Medical Center, Leiden, The Netherlands

Sarah Ohrndorf
Department of Rheumatology, Leiden University Medical Center, Leiden, The Netherlands
Department of Rheumatology and Clinical Immunology, Charité – Universitätsmedizin Berlin, Berlin, Germany

Miranda Houtman, Louise Ekholm, Espen Hesselberg, Karine Chemin, Vivianne Malmström, Ingrid E. Lundberg and Leonid Padyukov
Division of Rheumatology, Department of Medicine, Karolinska Institutet, Karolinska University Hospital, Stockholm, Sweden

Ann M. Reed
Department of Pediatrics, Duke Children's Hospital, Duke University Medical Center, Durham, USA

Emilie H. Regner, Mark E. Gerich and Blair P. Fennimore
Division of Gastroenterology, Department of Medicine, University of Colorado School of Medicine, Aurora, CO, USA
Mucosal Inflammation Program, University of Colorado School of Medicine, Aurora, CO, USA

Andrew Stahly
Division of Rheumatology, Department of Medicine, University of Colorado School of Medicine, Aurora, CO, USA

Neha Ohri, Widian K. Jubair and Kristine A. Kuhn
Division of Rheumatology, Department of Medicine, University of Colorado School of Medicine, Aurora, CO, USA
Mucosal Inflammation Program, University of Colorado School of Medicine, Aurora, CO, USA

Liron Caplan
Division of Rheumatology, Department of Medicine, University of Colorado School of Medicine, Aurora, CO, USA
Denver Veterans Affairs Medical Center (Denver VAMC), Denver, CO, USA

Diana Ir, Charles E. Robertson and Daniel N. Frank
Division of Infectious Disease, Department of Medicine, University of Colorado School of Medicine, Aurora, CO, USA

Carsten Görg and Janet Siebert
Computational Bioscience Program, University of Colorado School of Medicine, Aurora, CO, USA

Gwen Sascha Fernandes
Academic Rheumatology, Division of Rheumatology, Orthopedics and Dermatology, Nottingham City Hospital, University of Nottingham, Clinical Sciences Building, Nottingham NG5 1PB, UK
Arthritis Research UK Centre for Sports, Exercise and Osteoarthritis, Queen's Medical Centre, Derby Road, Nottingham NG7 2UH, UK
Arthritis Research UK Pain Centre, University of Nottingham, Nottingham NG5 1PB, UK

Ana Marie Valdes, David Andrew Walsh, Weiya Zhang and Michael Doherty
Academic Rheumatology, Division of Rheumatology, Orthopedics and Dermatology, Nottingham City Hospital, University of Nottingham, Clinical Sciences Building, Nottingham NG5 1PB, UK
Arthritis Research UK Centre for Sports, Exercise and Osteoarthritis, Queen's Medical Centre, Derby Road, Nottingham NG7 2UH, UK

Arthritis Research UK Pain Centre, University of Nottingham, Nottingham NG5 1PB, UK
NIHR Nottingham Biomedical Research Centre, University of Nottingham, Nottingham NG5 1PB, UK

Marwa Qadri and Khaled A. Elsaid
Department of Biomedical and Pharmaceutical Sciences, Chapman University School of Pharmacy, Rinker Health Sciences Campus, 9401 Jeronimo Road, Irvine, CA 92618, USA

Ling X. Zhang and Wendy Wong
Department of Emergency Medicine, Rhode Island Hospital, Providence, RI, USA

Gregory D. Jay
Department of Emergency Medicine, Rhode Island Hospital, Providence, RI, USA
Department of Biomedical Engineering, Brown University, Providence, RI, USA

Anthony M. Reginato and Changqi Sun
Division of Rheumatology and Department of Dermatology, Rhode Island Hospital, Providence, RI, USA

Tannin A. Schmidt
Biomedical Engineering Department, School of Dental Medicine, University of Connecticut Health Center, Farmington, CT, USA

Ericka N. Merriwether
Department of Physical Therapy, Steinhardt School of Culture, Education, and Human Development, New York University, New York, NY, USA

Dana L. Dailey, Carol G. T. Vance, Katherine M. Geasland and Ruth Chimenti
Department of Physical Therapy and Rehabilitation Science, University of Iowa, Iowa City, IA, USA

Laura A. Frey-Law
Department of Physical Therapy and Rehabilitation Science, University of Iowa, Iowa City, IA, USA
College of Nursing, University of Iowa, Iowa City, IA,USA

Kathleen A. Sluka
Department of Physical Therapy and Rehabilitation Science, University of Iowa, Iowa City, IA, USA
College of Nursing, University of Iowa, Iowa City, IA,USA
Department of Physical Therapy and Rehabilitation Science, 1-242 MEB, University of Iowa Carver College of Medicine, Iowa City, IA 52422-1089, USA

Barbara A. Rakel
College of Nursing, University of Iowa, Iowa City, IA,USA

Miriam B. Zimmerman
College of Public Health, University of Iowa, Iowa City, IA, USA

Meenakshi Golchha and Leslie J. Crofford
Department of Medicine/Rheumatology and Immunology, Vanderbilt University, Nashville, TN, USA

Johanna M. W. Hazes
Department of Rheumatology, Erasmus MC, Rotterdam, the Netherlands

Wendy Dankers, Claudia González-Leal, Nadine Davelaar, Patrick S. Asmawidjaja and Adriana M. C. Mus
Department of Rheumatology, Erasmus MC, Rotterdam, the Netherlands
Department of Immunology, Erasmus MC, Rotterdam, the Netherlands

Erik Lubberts
Department of Rheumatology, Erasmus MC, Rotterdam, the Netherlands
Department of Immunology, Erasmus MC, Rotterdam, the Netherlands
Erasmus MC University Medical Center, Wytemaweg 80, 3015CN Rotterdam, The Netherlands

Edgar M. Colin
Department of Internal Medicine, Erasmus MC, Rotterdam, the Netherlands

Roy M. Fleischmann
Southwestern Medical Center, Metroplex Clinical Research Center, University of Texas, 8144 Walnut Hill Lane, Suite 810, Dallas, TX 75231, USA

Rieke Alten
Schlosspark-Klinik, University Medicine Berlin, Heubnerweg 2, Berlin 14059,Germany

Margarita Pileckyte
Department of Rheumatology, Hospital of Lithuanian University of Health Sciences, Eiveniu str.2, Kaunas, LT 50161, Lithuania

Kasia Lobello, Carol Cronenberger and Daniel Alvarez
Pfizer Inc., 500 Arcola Road Collegeville, Collegeville, PA 19426, USA

Steven Y. Hua
Pfizer Inc., 10777 Science Center Drive, CB1/2103, San Diego, CA 92121, USA

Amy E. Bock and K. Lea Sewell
Pfizer Inc., 300 Technology Square, Cambridge, MA 02139, USA

Marco Lanzillotta, Emanuel Della-Torre, Emanuele Bozzalla-Cassione, Lucrezia Rovati and Lorenzo Dagna
Università Vita-Salute San Raffaele, IRCCS-San Raffaele Scientific Institute, Milan, Italy
Unit of Immunology, Rheumatology, Allergy and Rare Diseases (UnIRAR), IRCCS-San Raffaele Scientific Institute, via Olgettina 60, 20132 Milan, Italy

Fabio Ciceri
Università Vita-Salute San Raffaele, IRCCS-San Raffaele Scientific Institute, Milan, Italy
Hematology and Bone Marrow Transplantation Unit, IRCCS-San Raffaele Scientific Institute, Milan, Italy

Enrica Bozzolo
Unit of Immunology, Rheumatology, Allergy and Rare Diseases (UnIRAR), IRCCS-San Raffaele Scientific Institute, via Olgettina 60, 20132 Milan, Italy

Raffaella Milani
Unit of Immunohematology and Transfusion Medicine, IRCCS-San Raffaele Scientific Institute, Milan, Italy

Paolo Giorgio Arcidiacono
Pancreato-Biliary Endoscopy and Endosonography Division, IRCCS-San Raffaele Scientific Institute, Milan, Italy

Stefano Partelli and Massimo Falconi
Division of Pancreatic Surgery, Pancreas Translational and Clinical Research Center, IRCCS-San Raffaele Scientific Institute, Milan, Italy

Shasha Hu, Yong Hou, Qian Wang, Mengtao Li, Dong Xu and Xiaofeng Zeng
Department of Rheumatology and Clinical Immunology, Peking Union Medical College Hospital, Chinese Academy of Medical Sciences and Peking Union Medical College, Beijing 100730, China

Akihiko Hiyama, Kosuke Morita, Daisuke Sakai and Masahiko Watanabe
Department of Orthopaedic Surgery, Surgical Science, Tokai University School of Medicine, 143 Shimokasuya, Isehara, Kanagawa 259-1193, Japan
Research Center for Regenerative Medicine, Tokai University School of Medicine, 143 Shimokasuya, Isehara, Kanagawa 259-1193, Japan

Benjamin Rauwel
Centre de Physiopathologie Toulouse Purpan, INSERM-CNRS-UPS, UMR 1043, CHU Purpan, 1 Place Baylac, 31024 Toulouse Cedex, France

Jean-Luc Davignon and Jean-Fredéric Boyer
Centre de Physiopathologie Toulouse Purpan, INSERM-CNRS-UPS, UMR 1043, CHU Purpan, 1 Place Baylac, 31024 Toulouse Cedex, France
Centre de Rhumatologie, CHU de Toulouse, 31059 Toulouse, France

Yannick Degboé, Arnaud Constantin and Alain Cantagrel
Centre de Physiopathologie Toulouse Purpan, INSERM-CNRS-UPS, UMR 1043, CHU Purpan, 1 Place Baylac, 31024 Toulouse Cedex, France
Centre de Rhumatologie, CHU de Toulouse, 31059 Toulouse, France
Faculté de Médecine, Université Paul Sabatier Toulouse III, 31062 Toulouse, France

Andrey Kruglov
Lomonosov Moscow State University, 119991 Moscow, Russia
German Rheumatism Research Center (DRFZ), 10117 Berlin, Germany

Amber T Collins, Micaela L Kulvaranon, Gangadhar M Utturkar and Wyatt A R Smith
Department of Orthopaedic Surgery, Duke University, Box 3093, Duke University Medical Center, Durham, NC 27710, USA

Hattie C Cutcliffe
Department of Orthopaedic Surgery, Duke University, Box 3093, Duke University Medical Center, Durham, NC 27710, USA
Department of Biomedical Engineering, Duke University, Campus Box 90281, 101 Science Drive, Durham 27708, NC, USA

Louis E DeFrate
Department of Orthopaedic Surgery, Duke University, Box 3093, Duke University Medical Center, Durham, NC 27710, USA
Department of Biomedical Engineering, Duke University, Campus Box 90281, 101 Science Drive, Durham 27708, NC, USA

Department of Mechanical Engineering and Materials Science, Duke University, Campus Box 90300, Hudson Hall, Durham 27708, NC, USA

Charles E Spritzer
Department of Radiology, Duke University, Box 3808, Duke University Medical Center, Durham 27710, NC, USA

Farshid Guilak
Department of Orthopaedic Surgery, Washington University and Shriners Hospitals for Children, Campus Box 8233, Couch Research Building, Room 3121, St. Louis 63110, MO, USA

Yao Fu, Kandice L Tessneer and Patrick M Gaffney
Division of Genomics and Data Sciences, Arthritis and Clinical Immunology Research Program, Oklahoma Medical Research Foundation, 825 Northeast 13th Street, Oklahoma City, OK 73104, USA

Chuang Li
School of Electrical and Computer Engineering, University of Oklahoma, Devan Energy Hall 150, 110 West Boyd Street, Norman, OK 73019, USA

David Schub, Martina Sester and Tina Schmidt
Department of Transplant and Infection Immunology, Saarland University, 66421 Homburg, Germany

Gunter Assmann
Department of Internal Medicine I, Saarland University, Homburg, Germany

Urban Sester
Department of Internal Medicine IV, Saarland University, Homburg, Germany

Index